9.7.08

Essential Endodontology

Essential Endodontology

Prevention and Treatment of Apical Periodontitis

Second edition

Edited by

Dag Ørstavik
cand. odont. & dr. odont.
Professor and Head
Department of Endodontics
Institute of Clinical Dentistry
University of Oslo
Oslo, Norway

Thomas Pitt Ford
BDS, PhD, FD, RCPS
Professor of Endodontology
Dental Institute
King's College London
London, UK

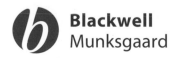

Blackwell
Munksgaard

© 2008 by Blackwell Munksgaard Ltd
© 1998 by Blackwell Science Ltd

Blackwell Munksgaard, a Blackwell Publishing Company,
Blackwell Publishing Ltd, 9600 Garsington Road, Oxford OX4 2DQ, UK
    Tel: +44 (0)1865 776868
Blackwell Publishing Professional, 2121 State Avenue, Ames, Iowa 50014-8300, USA
    Tel: +1 515 292 0140
Blackwell Publishing Asia Pty Ltd, 550 Swanston Street, Carlton, Victoria 3053, Australia
    Tel: +61 (0)3 8359 1011

First published 1998 by Blackwell Science Ltd
Second edition published 2008 by Blackwell Munksgaard Ltd

ISBN: 978-14051-4976-1

Library of Congress Cataloging-in-Publication Data
Essential endodontology : prevention and treatment of apical periodontitis / edited by Dag Ørstavik, Thomas Pitt Ford.
-- 2nd ed.
     p. ; cm.
   Includes bibliographical references and index.
   ISBN-13: 978-1-4051-4976-1 (hardback : alk. paper)
   ISBN-10: 1-4051-4976-0 (hardback : alk. paper) 1.
Periodontis--Prevention. 2.   Periodontis--Treatment. 3.   Endodontics.   I. Ørstavik, Dag. II. Pitt Ford, T.
   [DNLM: 1. Periodontitis--prevention & control. 2. Endodontics. 3. Periodontitis--therapy. WU 242 E78 2008]
   RK450.P4E85 2008
   617.6′32--dc22

                                                                                                    2007029630

A catalogue record for this title is available from the British Library

Set in Times
by Gray Publishing, Tunbridge Wells, Kent, UK
Printed and bound in Singapore
by Markono Print Media Pte Ltd

For further information on Blackwell Munksgaard, visit our website:
www.dentistry.blackwellmunksgaard.com

Contents

Contributors

Gilberto Debelian
Institute of Clinical Dentistry
Faculty of Dentistry
University of Oslo
0455 Oslo, Norway

Harald M. Eriksen
Institute of Clinical Dentistry
Faculty of Medicine
University of Tromsø
9037 Tromsø, Norway

Shimon Friedman
Discipline of Endodontics
Faculty of Dentistry
University of Toronto
124 Edward Street
Toronto, Ontario
Canada M5G 1G6

Gunnar Hasselgren
College of Dental Medicine
Columbia University Medical
  Center
630 West 168th
New York, NY 10032-3702, USA

Karin Heyeraas
Department of Biomedicine
Faculty of Medicine
University of Bergen
Jonas Lies vei 91
N-5009 Bergen, Norway

Nobuyuki Kawashima
Department of Restorative
  Sciences
Graduate School
Tokyo Medical and Dental
  University
1-5-45 Yushima
Bunkyo-Ku, Japan 113-8549

Tore A. Larheim
Institute of Clinical Dentistry
Faculty of Dentistry
University of Oslo
0455 Oslo, Norway

Ivar A. Mjör
University of Florida College of
  Dentistry
Department of Operative
  Dentistry
P.O. Box 100415
Gainesville, FL 32610-0415, USA

P.N.R. Nair
Institute for Oral Biology
Section of Oral Structures and
  Development
Center of Dental and Oral
  Medicine
University of Zurich
CH-8028 Zurich, Switzerland

Dag Ørstavik
Institute of Clinical Dentistry
Faculty of Dentistry
University of Oslo
0455 Oslo, Norway

Heather Pitt Ford
Department of Paediatric
  Dentistry
Guy's Hospital
Guy's and St. Thomas' NHS
  Foundation Trust
London SE1 9RT, UK

Thomas Pitt Ford
Dental Institute
King's College London
Guy's Hospital
London SE1 9RT, UK

Asgeir Sigurdsson
Hávallagata 15
Reykjavik 101, Iceland

José F. Siqueira Jr
Department of Endodontics
School of Dentistry
Estácio de Sá University
Rio de Janeiro, RJ, Brazil

Larz S.W. Spångberg
Department of Oral Health and
  Diagnostic Sciences
University of Connecticut Health
  Center
263 Farmington Avenue
Farmington, CT 06030, USA

Hideaki Suda
Pulp Biology and Endodontics
Department of Restorative
  Sciences
Graduate School
Tokyo Medical and Dental
  University
I-5-45 Yushima
Bunkyo-Ku, Japan 113-8549

Martin Trope
Department of Endodontics
School of Dentistry
University of North Carolina
  at Chapel Hill
Chapel Hill, NC 27599-7450, USA

Preface to the Second Edition

Our aim for the first edition of *Essential Endodontology* was to develop a text on apical periodontitis as a specific disease entity. In the years that have passed it has become apparent that the concept of apical periodontitis as the disease of reference in endodontics is a very productive one. Within research, teaching, and clinical practice, greater emphasis is now being placed on disease diagnosis, prevention, and treatment. Endodontology, which has traditionally been a technical field with its focus on treatment methods and materials rather than on clinical and biological science, is coming of age and one can document increasing research activity on pulpal and periapical disease that forms a solid foundation for rational diagnosis and treatment.

Along with this augmented activity in basic and clinical research, it has also become evident that the original text needed updating and supplementation. The present edition is an attempt to consolidate the information from the first edition that has stood the test of time, and to complement this with relevant emerging new research findings. As editors we are again proud to have had the cooperation of so many outstanding clinicians and scientists in the production of this book.

While this text is aimed at graduate students of endodontology, specialists or the interested general practitioners, we have been pleased to learn that it is also used in undergraduate programs. We believe that this testifies to the need for scientifically founded texts for this segment and reflects the consolidation of endodontology as a science-based dental discipline.

We therefore hope the book will be useful to readers of all categories and that you will find its substance and style helpful in the striving for quality and excellence in our profession.

Dag Ørstuvik and Thomas Pitt Ford
Editors

Chapter 1
Apical Periodontitis: Microbial Infection and Host Responses

Dag Ørstavik and Thomas Pitt Ford

1.1 Introduction

Traditionally, endodontology includes pulp and periapical biology and pathology. Clinically, however, endodontics is perceived as treatment of the root canal with files and the placement of a root filling, or treatment by surgical endodontics. The vital pulp and the treatment measures to preserve its vitality are usually considered a part of conservative dentistry, and include specific techniques in dental traumatology. In both principle and practice, the situation changes when pulp extirpation or root canal treatment is considered necessary. While the initial diagnoses and the difficulties associated with treatment may be related to the state of the pulp, the purpose of treatment is no longer the preservation of the pulp, but the prevention and elimination of infection in the root canal system. The ultimate biological aim of this treatment is *either to prevent or cure apical periodontitis* (Fig. 1.1). Of the endodontic diseases, apical periodontitis is therefore prominent as it is a primary indication for root canal treatment and because it is by far the most common sequel when treatment is inadequate or fails.

Research in recent decades has documented particularly the importance of microbial factors in the initiation, development and persistence of apical periodontitis [3,12,13,20,21,26,27,30,35] (Fig. 1.2). Emphasis must therefore be on the infectious etiology of apical

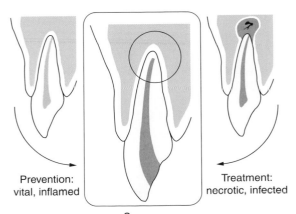

Prevention:
vital, inflamed

Treatment:
necrotic, infected

Success =
absence of apical periodontitis:
clinically, radiographically, histologically

Fig. 1.1 Prevention or treatment of apical periodontitis.

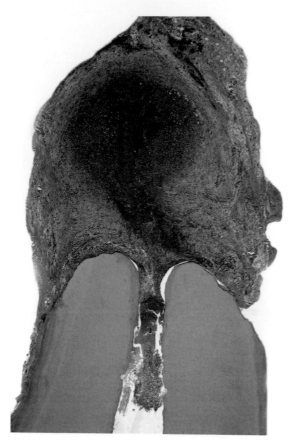

Fig. 1.2 A longitudinal section of a root with apical periodontitis. The root canal contains bacteria. (Courtesy of Dr D. Ricucci.)

periodontitis and on the importance of aseptic and antiseptic principles during treatment. Similarly, research findings have an immediate and extensive impact on aspects of diagnosis, treatment, prognosis and evaluation of outcome in endodontics. It is important to use the acquired knowledge to build treatment principles logically, and to show how these principles may and should be applied in clinical practice.

1.2 Terminology

Both pulp and pulp–periodontal diseases have been subject to almost innumerable diagnostic schemes, classification systems, and terminology. Periodontitis caused by infection of the pulp canal system has been termed apical periodontitis, apical granuloma/

cyst, periapical osteitis, periradicular periodontitis, among other terms. Sub-classifications have been acute/chronic/exacerbating/Phoenix abscess, and symptomatic/asymptomatic [39]. There are arguments in favor of each of these schemes. The present text makes use of the more conservative terms, i.e., acute/chronic/exacerbating apical periodontitis as principal terminology (Table 1.1). The following is a brief argument for the retention of these terms.

Symptomatic/asymptomatic apical periodontitis has been suggested as the primary diagnostic term instead of acute/chronic apical periodontitis. This is based on the assumption that the diagnosis of chronic or acute stages of the disease is difficult or impossible when a histological definition of acute/chronic forms the reference. It is also attractive to use a terminology that may seem (relatively) unambiguous. However, as the terms chronic and acute in fact belong principally to the temporal and clinical aspects of disease, there is no basic conflict between these two schemes of classification. Furthermore, acute and chronic are generally perceived as diagnostic terms, whereas symptomatic and asymptomatic traditionally are descriptions used during history taking and examination of the patient.

Periradicular periodontitis is an alternative term that has gained increasing support [1]. Periradicular periodontitis literally means "inflammation around the tooth around the root", and could be conceived as tautologically excessive. It includes lateral and furcal locations of inflammation, but it does not distinguish etymologically pulp-induced periodontitis from marginally derived periodontitis. "Apical" distinguishes the disease from marginally derived periodontitis, and while it does not purport to include lateral and furcal locations, these are by comparison scarce and are easily perceived as variants of their more frequent disease of reference.

Apical periodontitis includes dental abscess, granuloma and cyst as manifestations of the same basic disease; these latter terms are not in conflict with other classification schemes. The historical emphasis on the differential diagnosis of a cyst versus a granuloma may have been overstated, particularly as radiographs are poor discriminators [29]. Cysts and granulomas have the same etiology [23] (Chapters 3 and 5) and basic disease processes (Chapter 4); their treatment and prognosis are also similar (Chapters 11 and 12). However, there are studies indicating that true cysts may show impaired healing [24,26].

Table 1.1 Main terminology used in the present text

Primary term	Alternative term
Apical periodontitis	Periradicular periodontitis
Granuloma	Periapical osteitis
Cyst	
Furcal apical periodontitis	Interradicular apical periodontitis
Lateral apical periodontitis	
Acute apical periodontitis	Symptomatic apical periodontitis
	Acute apical abscess
Exacerbating apical periodontitis	Phoenix abscess
	Symptomatic apical periodontitis
Chronic apical periodontitis	Asymptomatic apical periodontitis
Apical periodontitis with sinus tract	Suppurative apical periodontitis
	Apical periodontitis with fistula
Condensing apical periodontitis	Condensing osteitis
	Periapical osteosclerosis
Transient apical periodontitis	Transient apical breakdown

The use of the term "periapical osteitis" has been limited and the connotation that bone is inflamed seems incorrect. Rather, the inflammation of the apical periodontium causes resorption of the bone and prevents it from becoming infected.

In summary, "apical periodontitis" takes preference by etymology and usage; "acute" and "chronic" are preferred and used as clinical supplementary terms of disease. On the other hand, terminology should not be used as a straightjacket for authors. Therefore, variants of the terms and references to other diagnostic schemes, in this book and other texts, are inevitable, even desirable.

1.3 Oral and dental infection

The oral cavity is an extension of the skin/mucosal barrier to the external environment. In the digestive tract, it may be viewed as the first battleground for the body's efforts to maintain homeostasis and keep infection away from the vulnerable interior parts of the body [5]. Infection occurs when pathogenic or opportunistic microorganisms infiltrate or penetrate the body surface. In the oral/dental sphere, the body surface is either the mucosa or the enamel/dentine coverage of underlying soft tissue (Fig. 1.3).

Teeth, cheek cells, tongue crypts, tonsillar irregularities, gingival sulci and other anatomical structures are safe havens for microbial populations of the mouth. From these areas, microbes of varying virulence may emigrate and cause infections such as tonsillitis, gingivitis, pericoronitis, marginal periodontitis, dental caries, pulpitis and apical periodontitis. Whereas physiological and mechanical cleansing activities tend to reduce the level of microorganisms in the mouth, environmental factors sometimes favor infection rather than its prevention. Current research on oral microbial communities emphasizes the concept of biofilm formation and development, with particular physiological, genetic and pathogenic properties of the organisms expressed as a consequence of the conditions within the biofilm (Chapters 4 and 5).

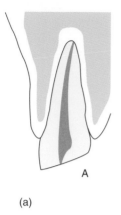
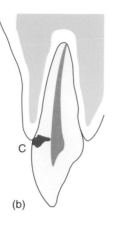
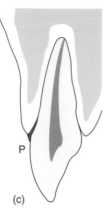

(a)   (b)   (c)

Fig. 1.3   Breaks in the mucocutaneous barrier associated with teeth. (a) Attrition (A), abrasion or trauma exposes the pulp. (b) Dental caries (C) reaches the pulp with subsequent infection of the pulp and periapical tissues. (c) Dental plaque (P) penetrates the gingival cuff and bacteria invade the gingival and periodontal tissues.

1.3.1 Marginal periodontitis

The gingival sulcus is potentially a weak link in the surface cover, combining a thin epithelial coverage with a topographic structure that favors the accumulation of bacteria on the adjoining tooth. With time, the microbial challenge in this area frequently overwhelms the body defenses and causes gingivitis and subsequent marginal periodontitis. Untreated, the ensuing inflammation is often followed by loosening of the tooth, its loss and, finally, reestablishment of the mucosal barrier. Biologically, the inflammation has a surface localization with easy drainage of pus, and deeper infection of tissues is not often seen. Moreover, tooth loss from marginal periodontitis usually happens late in the lifecycle of the individual, with limited consequences for the survivability of the individual, group or species.

1.3.2 Dental caries

Clinical dentistry and dental science have emerged in response largely to the other major, visible infection of the oral cavity: dental caries. The disease has primarily, but not exclusively, affected children and young adults; and the pain, impaired appearance, and tooth loss at an early age associated with dental caries have made it a major challenge to societies where it has become widespread. However, the epidemic of dental caries may have had a relatively short history in the lifespan of man. Although the history of dental caries goes back to the Iron Age and earlier, archaeological material and historical sources do not indicate that dental caries was widespread until a few centuries ago. Greater use of preventive measures in developed countries has caused a downturn in disease, although

it still constitutes a significant health concern for some population groups and individuals.

1.3.3 Pulp infection and periapical inflammation

Infection and inflammation of the pulp and periapical tissues have long been regarded as an extension of the dental caries process. This has been a reasonable interpretation in view of the dominance of caries as a source of infection of dentin during the last few cen-

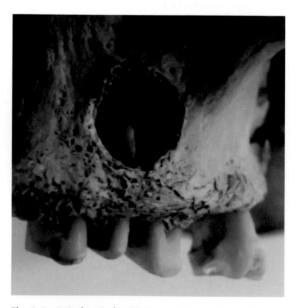

Fig. 1.4   Apical periodontitis in an upper premolar of a woman's skull found in Iceland and dating to the twelfth century. Trauma or wear caused exposure of the pulp with infection and lesion development.

turies. However, infection of the pulp and periapical tissues and the tissue responses are probably an older and more general biological occurrence than dental caries (Fig. 1.4). Despite the common origin of infecting organisms, the microbial floras of dental caries and endodontic infections differ in many respects. The evolutionary biological development of the permanent dentition, which has nonreplaceable teeth, must also have included the development of effective responses to trauma and subsequent infection of the deeper tissues.

Apical periodontitis may thus be viewed as a tissue response to pulp infection from trauma such as blows to or fracture of the teeth, attrition from mastication, and abrasion from the use of teeth as tools for survival. Essentially, apical periodontitis may be seen as the body's means of coping with the threat of infection following breaches in the mucosal/tooth barrier from trauma to, or attrition of, the teeth. An exposed pulp potentially leaves the body open to infection; the processes of apical periodontitis then usually work to create a second barrier within the body to prevent further spread of potentially threatening microbes [14,23] (Figs 1.5 and 1.6).

Treatment of apical periodontitis must be seen in the context of preventing microbial access to the jawbone and the body beyond, and needs to be achieved by effective disinfection and obturation. A complete seal from the coronal to the apical end of the treated root reestablishes the mucocutaneo-odonto barrier, whereas voids or leaks may present an opportunity for bacteria to establish a foothold close to the body's

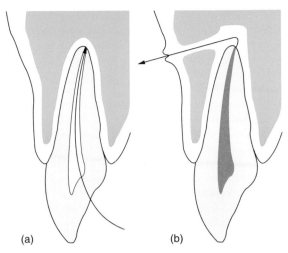

Fig. 1.6 Infection of the pulp (a) is externalized by development of a sinus tract from apical periodontitis (b).

interior. The recent emphasis on coronal leakage of bacteria and bacterial products as opposed to apical leakage is a reflection of this more scientifically based line of reasoning [18,40].

1.4 Biological and clinical significance of apical periodontitis

1.4.1 Infection theory

In the pre-antibiotic era, infections of the pulp and periapical tissues were considered potentially serious and in need of close monitoring. In the early days of antibiotics, it was found that most of these infections were readily susceptible to penicillin, and therefore the spread of infection to regional spaces was believed to be easily controllable by antibiotics. Today, it is recognized that pulp infection may be caused by organisms of different virulence [36] (Chapter 5), and that control of the infection is not always easily obtained, particularly when endodontic treatment is ineffective.

The flora of the mouth is fortunately composed of few species of pathogenic organisms, which usually have low virulence (Chapter 5). Most may be considered opportunistic, causing disease only in mixed infections or in hosts compromised by other diseases. Teleologically, it is usually not to the advantage of microbial species living on other organisms to cause disease; the basis for their presence is rather the preservation of the host.

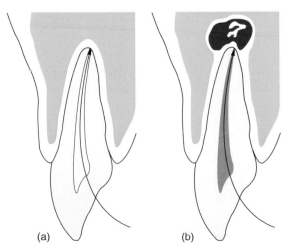

Fig. 1.5 Infection of the pulp (a) is contained by development of an apical granuloma/cyst (b).

Organisms that are not normally pathogenic in the oral cavity may exhibit features of virulence if allowed access to the pulp or periapical tissues. Studies of the infected pulp have shown the presence of oral bacteria that normally inhabit the mouth in the absence of disease. The apical periodontitis response to pulp infection may be viewed as a way of taming and coping with expressions of virulence by the infecting organisms. Thus, the pain frequently encountered in the early stages of disease development usually subsides in response to the tissue reactions. Furthermore, the initial expansion of the lesion of apical periodontitis is soon followed by periods of quiescence [34], possibly even regression or at least consolidation of the lesion. This dynamic process is accompanied in time by changes in the composition of the flora recoverable from the root canal [13].

Research has also documented that some forms of apical periodontitis may be associated with particular species dominating in the pulp canal flora (Chapter 5). Evidence from molecular analysis implies that endodontic infections may be more opportunistic than specific, and may include more species than previously thought [22] (Chapter 5). There is a need for more research into microbiological causes and interactions in apical periodontitis to improve diagnosis and treatment. Specifically, this would apply to the so-called "therapy-resistant" cases of apical periodontitis [2,7,25,42], in which infection persists despite apparently adequate root canal treatment, and to retreatment cases in which *Enterococcus faecalis* has been implicated [11].

1.4.2 Endodontic infection and general health

The focal infection theory has been a source of both frustration and inspiration in dental practice and research [6]. There has been frustration, first because irrelevant and sometimes incorrect arguments and concepts were used to dictate an unnecessary wave of tooth extractions in healthy individuals for decades; and secondly because unsubstantiated opinions on the subject for too long a time afterwards restricted clinical developments in the field of endodontics. The controversy, however, sparked important new discoveries, and it is, even today, an important part of the frame of reference that is applied to endodontic microbiology and host defense mechanisms.

Focal infection originally implied dissemination of pathogens from the focus to remote part of the body, where secondary disease arose [6]. With time,

the concept was expanded to include immune products "homing" to other organs and causing disease or symptoms there. Fortunately, most, if not all, concerns of the proponents of the focal infection theory have been proven unsubstantiated. There remains, however, a recognition that apical periodontitis is a response to microbial infection that needs to be contained, cured and eliminated for optimum general health.

In view of the many patients with compromised general health who now retain their teeth into old age, it is reassuring that current research demonstrates that while bacteremias during endodontic treatment occur, the incidence or magnitude is not alarming, and indeed is comparable to, or less than, that of most routine dental procedures [9]. However, the nature of the infecting organism may possibly be a source of concern [10]. The risks of antibiotic prophylaxis need to be weighed against the consequences of bacteremia.

1.4.3 Infection control

The outcome of endodontic treatment is dependent on using an aseptic technique and antiseptic measures to eliminate infection. However, the critical role of infection control may not always be given the prominence that it deserves. The transmission of hepatitis viruses has been an issue for a long time, but there has been more recent concern about prion transmission via contaminated instruments [32]. There has been debate about reuse of root canal files from the biological perspective [17] as distinct from the mechanical perspective; protocols for instrument decontamination have been developed in the face of increasing governmental regulation.

1.4.4 Microbial specificity and host defense

The host responses to root canal infection have been the subject of much research in recent years. There is great similarity between the pathogenic processes in marginal and apical periodontitis, and many of the findings in periodontal research have direct relevance to apical periodontitis. A clearer concept of the immunological processes involved in the development of apical periodontitis is emerging [14,34] (Chapter 3). Microbiological variability and virulence factors in infected root canals have been demonstrated, and data are emerging which indicate that the bacterial flora varies systematically with the clinical condition of the tooth involved (persistent infection, therapy-resistant infection) (Chapters 5 and 11). Thus, different strategies of antimicrobial measures may have to be applied depending on the microbiological diagnosis in a given case.

1.4.5 The compromised host

A characteristic feature of dentistry as it is practiced today is the shift of care from young to elderly people. The success of preventive dentistry in controlling and containing dental caries has resulted in a larger part of the population retaining their natural teeth longer and aspiring to keep them into old age. The improvement in dental health as regards dental caries has therefore not resulted in a decrease in demand for endodontic treatment; rather, more people in the older age groups are seeking to preserve their teeth by endodontic intervention. The net result is a stable, or increasing, demand for endodontic treatment (Chapter 8) rather than a decline. With the increased demand for endodontic care among the elderly, there is also concern for the consequences of apical periodontitis and its treatment sequels in relation to other medical conditions. Fortunately, many of the concerns which previously were held as restrictions to endodontic treatment of the elderly have not been substantiated: both the prevention and cure of apical periodontitis by endodontics seem to be as successful in the old as in the young. Moreover, initial concerns about treatment outcome in HIV-positive patients seem unfounded [28].

There are a number of medical conditions that may influence the indications for, and choice of, endodontic treatment and that occur more frequently among elderly patients. Generally, any disease for which bacteremia poses an additional hazard is of concern when endodontic treatment is being considered. Particularly, a history of infective endocarditis, congenital heart disease, rheumatic heart fever or the presence of an artificial heart valve or other susceptible implants may necessitate the implementation of an antibiotic regimen in conjunction with the endodontic procedures. The progression, possibly also prognosis and healing pattern in diabetic patients may differ from that in people not affected by the disease [16,31]. Special consideration must be given to patients who are being treated with immunosuppressants, or otherwise have compromised immune systems [37,44]. A number of the blood dyscrasias, notably leukemias, are associated with

potentially serious sequels to apical periodontitis: infection spreads easily and may require extensive antimicrobial therapy [41]. A special case is presented by the irradiated patient: the high incidence of osteoradionecrosis after oral surgical procedures places high demands on effective, conservative treatment of endodontic conditions. Smoking has been shown to have an adverse effect on marginal periodontitis and wound healing; the effect of smoking on apical periodontitis has largely been overlooked, and the limited evidence is conflicting [4,19].

1.4.6 Tooth loss and replacement

Untreated apical periodontitis represents a chronic infection of the oral tissues at locations closer to more vital organs than many other oral infections. While these infections may remain quiescent for decades, they may also develop and spread with serious consequences for the individual [8,33]. In the face of the risks of such chronic infection from involved teeth, their extraction and replacement by implants has been put forward and discussed as a viable alternative to endodontic treatment [43]. The variable success rates (by strict criteria) of treatment procedures for the cure of apical periodontitis [15] (Chapter 14) are sometimes put forth as arguments for the implant "treatment" concept. However, what little evidence there is does not indicate a lower survival rate of endodontically treated teeth [38], and the superiority of tooth preservation compared to its replacement should be evident as a biological principle of preference. On the other hand, the challenge from other treatment concepts to endodontics as a discipline should act as a driving force to produce more and scientifically solid evidence for the modalities of cure and prevention applied to our disease of interest, apical periodontitis.

1.5 Conclusion

Pulp and periapical inflammation, the associated pain and the consequences of root canal infection remain significant aspects of dentistry today. New knowledge and insights provide better treatment opportunities and stimulate further research activities. The prevention and control of apical periodontitis has a solid scientific base, but the many variations in the clinical manifestations of the disease still leave technical and biological problems that need to be solved. Despite

recent technological advances in treatment, evidence
of improved outcome is still lacking. Alternative
treatment involving implants is promoted as being
better, but the criteria of evaluation of the outcome
of the two forms of treatment are dissimilar; there is
no true evidence-based comparison.

1.6 References

1. American Association of Endodontists (2003) *Glossary of endodontic terms*, 7th edn. Chicago, IL: American Association of Endodontists.
2. Barnard D, Davies J, Figdor D (1996) Susceptibility of *Actinomyces israelii* to antibiotics, sodium hypochlorite and calcium hydroxide. *International Endodontic Journal* **29**, 320–6.
3. Bergenholtz G (1974) Micro-organisms from necrotic pulp of traumatized teeth. *Odontologisk Revy* **25**, 347–58.
4. Bergström J, Babcan J, Eliasson S (2004) Tobacco smoking and dental periapical condition. *European Journal of Oral Science* **112**, 115–20.
5. Bernard C (1927) *An introduction to the study of experimental medicine, 1865*. English translation by Henry Copley Greene, Macmillan & Co., 1927.
6. Billings F (1913) Chronic focal infection as a causative factor in chronic arthritis. *Journal of the American Medical Association* **61**, 819–23.
7. Byström A, Claeson R, Sundqvist G (1985) The antibacterial effect of camphorated paramonochlorophenol, camphorated phenol and calcium hydroxide in the treatment of infected root canals. *Endodontics and Dental Traumatology* **1**, 170–5.
8. Caruso PA, Watkins LM, Suwansaard P, Yamamoto M, Durand ML, Romo LV, Rincon SP, Curtin HD (2006) Odontogenic orbital inflammation: clinical and CT findings – initial observations. *Radiology* **239**, 187–94.
9. Debelian GJ, Olsen I, Tronstad L (1994) Systemic diseases caused by oral microorganisms. *Endodontics and Dental Traumatology* **10**, 57–65.
10. Debelian GJ, Olsen I, Tronstad L (1995) Bacteremia in conjunction with endodontic therapy. *Endodontics and Dental Traumatology* **11**, 142–9.
11. Evans M, Davies JK, Sundqvist G, Figdor D (2002) Mechanisms involved in the resistance of *Enterococcus faecalis* to calcium hydroxide. *International Endodontic Journal* **35**, 221–8.
12. Fabricius L, Dahlén G, Holm SE, Möller ÅJR (1982) Influence of combinations of oral bacteria on periapical tissues of monkeys. *Scandinavian Journal of Dental Research* **90**, 200–6.
13. Fabricius L, Dahlén G, Öhman AE, Möller ÅJR (1982) Predominant indigenous oral bacteria isolated from infected root canals after varied time of closure. *Scandinavian Journal of Dental Research* **90**, 134–44.
14. Kawashima N, Okiji T, Kosaka T, Suda H (1996) Kinetics of macrophages and lymphoid cells during the development of experimentally induced periapical lesions in rat molars: a quantitative immunohistochemical study. *Journal of Endodontics* **22**, 311–16.
15. Kirkevang LL, Vaeth M, Hörsted-Bindslev P, Wenzel A (2006) Longitudinal study of periapical and endodontic status in a Danish population. *International Endodontic Journal* **39**, 100–7.
16. Kohsaka T, Kumazawa M, Yamasaki M, Nakamura H (1996) Periapical lesions in rats with streptozotocin-induced diabetes. *Journal of Endodontics* **22**, 418–21.
17. Linsuwanont P, Parashos P, Messer HH (2004) Cleaning of rotary nickel-titanium endodontic instruments. *International Endodontic Journal* **37**, 19–28.
18. Madison S, Wilcox LR (1988) An evaluation of coronal microleakage in endodontically treated teeth. III. In vivo study. *Journal of Endodontics* **14**, 455–8.
19. Marending M, Peters OA, Zehnder M (2005). Factors affecting the outcome of orthograde root canal therapy in a general dentistry hospital practice. *Oral Surgery, Oral Medicine, Oral Pathology, Oral Radiology, and Endodontics* **99**, 119–24.
20. Möller ÅJR, Fabricius L, Dahlén G, Öhman AE, Heyden G (1981) Influence on periapical tissues of indigenous oral bacteria and necrotic pulp tissue in monkeys. *Scandinavian Journal of Dental Research* **89**, 475–84.
21. Molven O, Olsen I, Kerekes K (1991) Scanning electron microscopy of bacteria in the apical part of root canals in permanent teeth with periapical lesions. *Endodontics and Dental Traumatology* **7**, 226–9.
22. Munson MA, Pitt Ford T, Chong B, Weightman A, Wade WG (2002) Molecular and cultural analysis of the microflora associated with endodontic infections. *Journal of Dental Research* **81**, 761–6.
23. Nair PN (2004) Pathogenesis of apical periodontitis and the causes of endodontic failures. *Critical Reviews in Oral Biology and Medicine* **15**, 348–81.
24. Nair PNR, Pajarola G, Schroeder HE (1996) Types and incidence of human periapical lesions obtained with extracted teeth. *Oral Surgery, Oral Medicine, Oral Pathology* **81**, 93–102.
25. Nair PNR, Sjögren U, Kahnberg KE, Sundqvist G (1990) Intraradicular bacteria and fungi in root-filled asymptomatic human teeth with therapy-resistant periapical lesions: a long-term light and electron microscopic follow-up study. *Journal of Endodontics* **16**, 580–88.
26. Nair PNR, Sjögren U, Schumacher E, Sundqvist G (1993) Radicular cyst affecting a root-filled human tooth: a long-term post-treatment follow-up. *International Endodontic Journal* **26**, 225–33.
27. Nair R (1987) Light and electron microscopic studies of root canal flora and periapical lesions. *Journal of Endodontics* **13**, 29–39.
28. Quesnell BT, Alves M, Hawkinson RW Jr, Johnson BR, Wenckus CS, BeGole EA (2005) The effect of human immunodeficiency virus on endodontic treatment outcome. *Journal of Endodontics* **31**, 633–6.
29. Ricucci D, Mannocci F, Pitt Ford TR (2006) A study of periapical lesions correlating the presence of a radiopaque lamina with histological findings. *Oral Surgery, Oral Medicine, Oral Pathology, Oral Radiology, and Endodontics* **101**, 389–94.
30. Ricucci D, Pascon EA, Pitt Ford TR, Langeland K (2006) Epithelium and bacteria in periapical lesions.

Oral Surgery, Oral Medicine, Oral Pathology, Oral Radiology, and Endodontics **101**, 239–49.

31. Segura-Egea JJ, Jimenez-Pinzon A, Rios-Santos JV, Velasco-Ortega E, Cisneros-Cabello R, Poyato-Ferrera M (2005) High prevalence of apical periodontitis amongst type 2 diabetic patients. *International Endodontic Journal* **38**, 564–9.

32. Smith AJ, Bagg J, Ironside JW, Will RG, Scully C (2003) Prions and the oral cavity. *Journal of Dental Research* **82**, 769–75.

33. Stalfors J, Adielsson A, Ebenfelt A, Nethander G, Westin T (2004) Deep neck space infections remain a surgical challenge. A study of 72 patients. *Acta Otolaryngol* **124**, 1191–6.

34. Stashenko P, Wang CY, Tani-Ishii N, Yu SM (1994) Pathogenesis of induced rat periapical lesions. *Oral Surgery, Oral Medicine, Oral Pathology* **78**, 494–502.

35. Sundqvist G (1976) Bacteriological studies of necrotic dental pulps. Umeå, Sweden: Umeå University Odontological Dissertations.

36. Sundqvist G (1994) Taxonomy, ecology, and pathogenicity of the root canal flora. *Oral Surgery, Oral Medicine, Oral Pathology* **78**, 522–30.

37. Teixeira FB, Gomes BP, Ferraz CC, Souza-Filho FJ, Zaia AA (2000) Radiographic analysis of the development of periapical lesions in normal rats, sialoadenectomized rats and sialoadenectomized-immunosuppressed rats. *Endodontics and Dental Traumatology* **16**, 154–7.

38. Torabinejad M, Goodacre CJ (2006) Endodontic or dental implant therapy: The factors affecting treatment planning. *Journal of the American Dental Association* **137**, 973–7.

39. Tronstad L (2003) *Clinical endodontics*, 2nd edn. Stuttgart: Thieme.

40. Trope M, Chow E, Nissan R (1995) In vitro endotoxin penetration of coronally unscaled endodontically treated teeth. *Endodontics and Dental Traumatology* **11**, 90–4.

41. Walsh LJ (1997) Serious complications of endodontic infections: Some cautionary tales. *Australian Dental Journal* **42**, 156–9.

42. Weiger R, Manncke B, Werner H, Löst C (1995) Microbial flora of sinus tracts and root canals of non-vital teeth. *Endodontics and Dental Traumatology* **11**, 15–19.

43. Wolcott J, Meyers J (2006) Endodontic re-treatment or implants: a contemporary conundrum. *The Compendium of Continuing Education in Dentistry* **27**, 104–10.

44. Zyrianov GV, Apollonova LA, Bogomazov MIa, Frolova TM (1991) The characteristics of the development of experimental apical periodontitis in irradiation-induced immunodeficiency. [In Russian.] *Stomatologiia (Mosk)* Nov–Dec;(6), 13–15.

Chapter 2
Pulp–Dentin and Periodontal Anatomy and Physiology

Ivar A. Mjör and Karin Heyeraas

2.1 Introduction

Pulp and dentin develop from the dental papilla during the bell stage of the enamel organ (Fig. 2.1). Odontoblasts differentiate from ectomesenchymal cells at the periphery of the dental papilla through interaction with the cells of the inner enamel epithelium. They form predentin which subsequently mineralizes. Although the dentin and pulp are basically different in that dentin is a mineralized tissue and the pulp is a soft tissue, they remain anatomically and functionally closely integrated throughout the life of the tooth. Thus, the two tissues are often referred to as the pulp–dentin organ or the pulp–dentin complex.

The soft tissue of the dental pulp communicates directly with the periodontal ligament (PDL) through the apical foramen or foramina. Sometimes the apical area consists of a delta of accessory canals with several communications between the pulp and the PDL. The rest of the PDL is separated from the pulp–dentin organ by the cementum (Fig. 2.2). Fibers from the periodontal ligament are embedded in the cementum and alveolar bone as Sharpey's fibers, and in this manner they attach the teeth to the alveolar bone.

The PDL and the cementum develop from the dental sac which is the mesodermal tissue found between the enamel organ and the developing alveolar processes of the mandible and maxilla. Proliferation of the Hertwig's root epithelium, which comprises the inner and outer enamel epithelium, maps out the shape of the root. As it breaks down, cytodifferentiation leading to cementogenesis occurs adjacent to the already formed root dentin. The rest of the dental sac then forms the PDL.

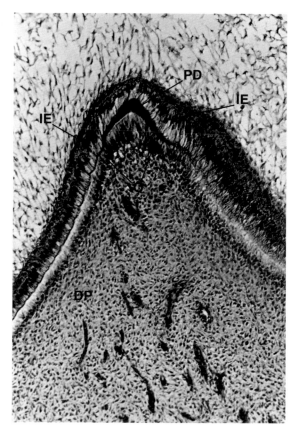

Fig. 2.1 Initiation of dentinogenesis at the bell stage of tooth development (DP, dental papilla; O, odontoblasts; PD, pre-dentin; IE, inner dental epithelium).

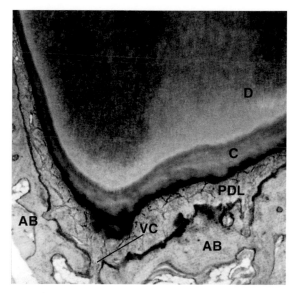

Fig. 2.2 The apical portion of a tooth showing alveolar bone (AB), periodontal ligament (PDL), cementum (C), dentin (D), Volkmann's canal (VC).

tial to act on the cells in the dental papilla to induce odontoblast differentiation. If the cells do not possess the power to induce odontoblast differentiation after breakdown of the root sheath, the cell rests will remain as Malassez's epithelial rests, either in the periodontal ligament (Fig. 2.3) or in the pulp (Fig. 2.4).

The formation of lateral root canals and an apical delta of accessory canals rather than a single apical foramen may be a normal variant or it may be due to disturbances of Hertwig's root epithelium. Such disturbances may be induced by external factors such as orthodontic tooth movement [87] or other local influences [31]. If cells of the inner dental epithelium of Hertwig's root epithelium do not fully differentiate to induce odontoblast formation in a small area, then no dentin will be found in that location. When Hertwig's sheath then breaks down, a canal of connective tissue through the dentin will connect the pulp and the periodontal ligament.

Fragmentation of Hertwig's root sheath may also occur on the pulpal side [87]. True pulp stones will form if this breakdown occurs while the cells in the inner dental epithelium still maintain their poten-

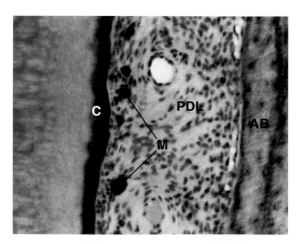

Fig. 2.3 Section through the periodontal ligament (PDL) showing Malassez's epithelial rests (M) adjacent to cementum (C) (AB, alveolar bone).

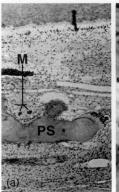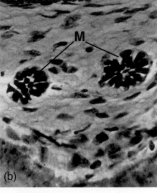

Fig. 2.4 (a) An irregularly shaped pulp stone (PS) and two Malassez's epithelial rests (M) in the pulp. (b) Higher magnification of two epithelial cell rests.

2.2 The pulp–dentin organ

The odontoblasts lining the predentin represent the link between dentin and pulp. This layer of cells (Fig. 2.5) sometimes gives the appearance of being pseudostratified in fully formed teeth, due to a crowding of the odontoblasts as they move from the dentinoenamel junction (DEJ) or the cemento-enamel junction (CEJ) towards the center of the dental papilla during dentinogenesis.

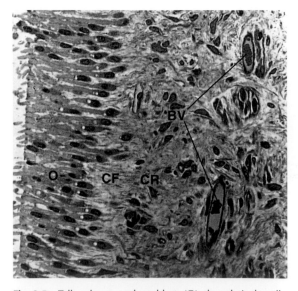

Fig. 2.5 Tall, columnar odontoblasts (O), the relatively cell free zone (CF) and the relatively cell-rich zone (CR) in the dental pulp. (BV, blood vessels.)

2.2.1 The odontoblast

The odontoblasts are matrix-producing cells and show all the characteristic features associated with protein synthesis (Fig. 2.6). They belong to the unique group of specialized cells, like nerve cells, that normally lasts the entire life of the tooth. If destroyed by trauma, inflammation or other means, replacement odontoblasts may be differentiated from undifferentiated cells in the dental pulp under favorable conditions.

The fully differentiated odontoblasts are tall columnar cells (Fig. 2.5). They are attached to each other through intercellular junctions that are local specializations of the cell membranes (Fig. 2.7). The nucleus is polarized and located at the distal end of the cell. The cytoplasm comprises accumulations of rough-surfaced endoplasmic reticulum (RER) (Fig. 2.6) located mainly peripherally in the odontoblast. It surrounds the Golgi apparatus and a number of secretory granules, vesicles and microtubules. Mitochondria are found everywhere in the cell body.

The odontoblast process, also referred to as Tomes' process, is housed within the dentinal tubule, and extends from the body of the odontoblast along the entire length of the tubules [46]. The histologic detection of a process is not synonymous with the presence of cytoplasm in the process; it may merely demonstrate the presence of a sheet-like structure of the odontoblast process within the tubules. A structure referred to as lamina limitans lines the dentinal tubules [89]. It has a high content of glycosaminoglycans and may be important in the regulation of peritubular dentin formation.

The odontoblast process is normally devoid of the typical organelles associated with protein synthesis. Its ultrastructure demonstrates microtubules, microfilaments, granules and vesicles (Fig. 2.6). The full extent of the cytoplasmic components of the odontoblast process has not been verified, but it is clearly present in the pulpal 200 μm of the dentin. It is also known that tissue changes occur in dentin, e.g., growth of the peritubular dentin leading to obturation of the tubules. Such physiological processes indicate the existence of cytoplasm in the full length of the tubules, at least in newly erupted teeth.

2.3 The pulp tissue

The cells in the dental pulp, in common with all other cells in the body, are dependent on the extra-

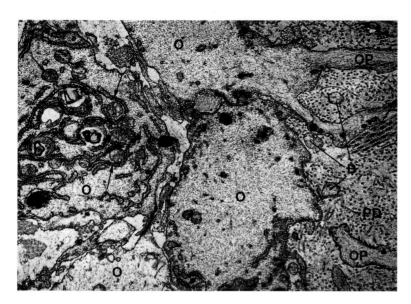

Fig. 2.6 Electron micrograph showing odontoblasts (O) and longitudinal and cross-sectioned odontoblast processes (OP) in the predentin (PD) from the root of the tooth. Note abundance of major organelles (arrows) associated with protein production in parts of the odontoblast some distance from the pre-dentin. The odontoblast process and the adjacent cytoplasm of the odontoblasts are almost devoid of the major organelles, but contain microtubules, microfilaments and secretory granules (B, branches of the odontoblast process). (Reproduced from [22] with permission from *Scandinavian Journal of Dental Research*.)

cellular fluids, i.e., blood and interstitial fluid, to remain vital and have normal functions. Every cell must have nutrition and the means to rid itself of waste products, and these metabolic requirements are taken care of by the extracellular fluids. All cells, including the pulpal cells, are surrounded by interstitial fluid (Fig. 2.8), which is similar in composition to plasma except for less plasma proteins. Accordingly, the interstitial fluid acts as the intermediary link between cells and blood or as an extension of the plasma.

The dental pulp in newly erupted teeth is composed of loose connective tissue of an immature nature. It is characterized by a large number of cells and few fibers. In teeth of older individuals fewer cells are present and the fibrous components predominate. The connective tissue fibers present in young teeth are limited to locations around the nerves and blood vessels (Fig. 2.13). Collagen type I and III has been shown to be present.

2.3.1 Cells of the dental pulp

The pulp cells are embedded in a gelatinous ground substance, the composition and physiological significance of which has not been studied in detail. However, chondroitin sulfates, hyaluronates and proteoglycans are present and constitute the main

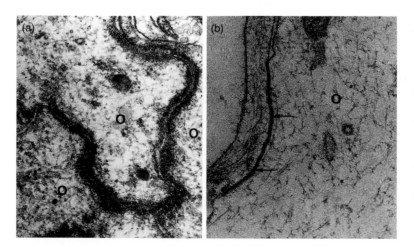

Fig. 2.7 Electron micrograph showing electron dense junctional complexes between (a) odontoblasts (O) from root dentin and (b) between an odontoblast (O) and a cytoplasmic process (arrows) similar to complexes found between odontoblasts and nerves. (a) Reproduced from [27] with permission from *Scandinavian Journal of Dental Research* and (b) reproduced from [18] with permission from *Acta Odontologica Scandinavica*.

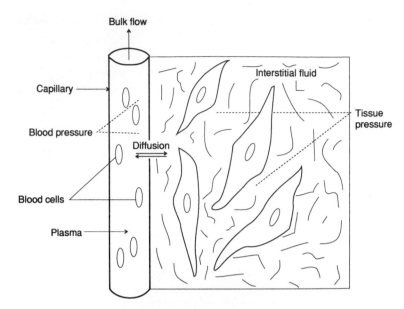

Fig. 2.8   Schematic diagram illustrating capillary, cells and interstitial fluid. Blood is brought to the capillaries by bulk flow, and diffusion links plasma and interstitial fluid. The cells are surrounded by interstitial fluid acting as an extension of the plasma.

part of the ground substance. The gelatinous consistency of the pulp comprises the extracellular, clear interstitial fluid. Due to its low content of plasma proteins, the interstitial fluid has a lower colloidal osmotic pressure than blood plasma, favoring capillary absorption. The function of the peripheral

lymphatic vessels is to remove proteins and other macromolecules from the tissue, thus maintaining and restoring this difference in colloidal osmotic pressures between interstitial fluid and plasma. If no difference in colloidal osmotic pressure between blood plasma and interstitial fluid prevailed, the fil-

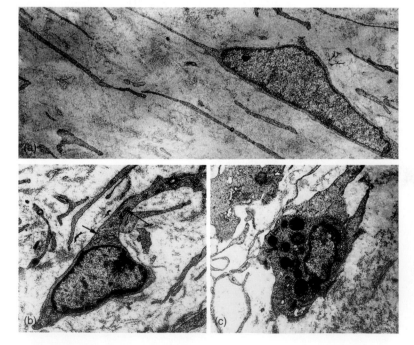

Fig. 2.9   Electron micrographs of cells in the human dental pulp from a recently erupted tooth. (a) An undifferentiated mesenchymal cell or an inactive fibroblast. The nucleus occupies the main part of the cell body. Note long, slender cytoplasmic processes with no major organelles and lack of collagen fibers. (b) Stellate-shaped fibroblast with a few organelles (arrows) in the cytoplasm. (c) A macrophage with characteristic intracytoplasmic granules. (Reproduced from [68] with permission from Munksgaard.)

tration force would be active, and the tissue pressure would rise to the same level as the blood pressure causing ischemia and necrosis. The hydrostatic pressure in the interstitial fluid of the pulp, so-called tissue pressure, is normally about 5–20 mmHg.

The cells of the pulp in newly erupted teeth are mainly undifferentiated cells and fibroblasts (Fig. 2.9). Occasionally, macrophages (Fig. 2.9) and white blood cells may be found. Dendritic, presumably immunocompetent cells are also normally present in the pulp [40]. Fat cells are not present. Mast cells are rarely present in normal healthy pulp, but they are commonly found in inflamed pulps.

The undifferentiated cells and the fibroblasts are difficult to differentiate from each other. Both have a relatively large nucleus with little cytoplasm and few of the organelles associated with protein synthesis. They both have long, slender cellular extensions which make them stellate shaped. These cellular extensions may be in desmosomal contact. The undifferentiated cells can develop into fibroblasts and replacement odontoblasts under special circumstances.

A special arrangement of cells is characteristic for the human coronal pulp (Fig. 2.5). On the pulpal side of the odontoblasts, a layer with few or no cells is present, sometimes referred to as the basal layer of Weil. Pulpally to this relatively cell free layer, a cell rich zone is present. The rest of the pulp tissue is fairly uniform in structure.

Nerves and blood vessels enter the pulp through the apical foramen or foramina (Fig. 2.10). They run close together until the main branching takes place in the coronal pulp. Both the nerves and the blood vessels (Fig. 2.11) branch profusely in the odontoblast/sub-odontoblast region.

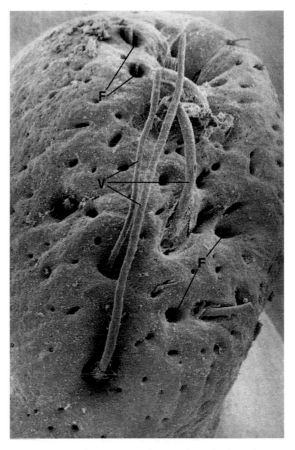

Fig. 2.10 Vessels (V) entering/leaving the pulp through numerous apical foramina (F) in a dog tooth. The number of foramina is not representative for human teeth. (Reproduced from [88] with permission from *Journal of Endodontics*.)

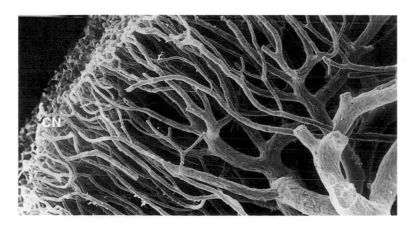

Fig. 2.11 Blood vessels in the pulp. Note terminal capillary network (CN) subjacent to the predentin. (Reproduced from [88] with permission from *Journal of Endodontics*.)

2.3.2 Nerves in the dental pulp

The distribution and types of nerves in the dental pulp have received renewed interest during the last few decades owing to their importance in the inflammatory response. Release of neuropeptides from pulpal nerve endings may in fact be the earliest reaction in the sequence of events leading to pulp inflammation.

Myelinated and unmyelinated nerves are present in the pulp [17] (Fig. 2.12). The majority of nerves are sensory, whereas sympathetic nerves have been reported to make up no more than 10% in fully developed teeth [25]. Both the sympathetic and sensory nerves can affect the pulpal circulation by release of vasoactive neuropeptides. The sympathetic neuro-peptide Y (NPY) and noradrenaline (NA) cause vasoconstriction, and the sensory neuropeptides such as CGRP, SP and NKA induce vasodilatation. Myelinated A-fibers and nonmyelinated C-fibers are somatic afferent nerves which carry sensory pain impulses. Most of the nerves terminate in the coronal pulp, and less than 10% of the nerve endings are found in the root pulp. An abundant plexus of nerves is found in the subodontoblastic region and between the odontoblasts (Fig. 2.13). Naked nerve endings, including gap junctions [55], are found on odontoblasts and in the walls of blood vessels. Nerves also extend into the periodontoblastic space of the predentin (Fig. 2.14) and the mineralized dentin (Fig. 2.14) in close proximity to the odontoblast process.

2.3.3 Blood vessels in the dental pulp

Arterioles and venules enter and leave the dental pulp through the apical foramen, but some also pass through lateral root canals which may be located anywhere in the root. Sometimes several apical foramina exist forming an apical delta (Fig. 2.10). Some arterioles pass directly to the coronal pulp through the central part of the pulp. Others supply the root pulp.

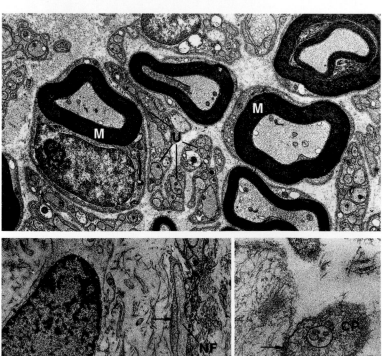

Fig. 2.12 Electron micrograph illustrating details of a nerve from the central part of a pulp with myelinated (M) and unmyelineated (U) nerve fibers. All fibers are invested by Schwann cell cytoplasm (pointers). Reproduced from [18] with permission from *Acta Odontologica Scandinavica*.

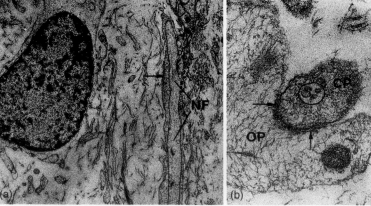

Fig. 2.13 (a) Nerve fiber (NF) enfolded by Schwann cell cytoplasm (arrows) in the odontoblast layer and (b) cytoplasmic process (CP) with a membrane-limited structure (arrow) similar to that of a nerve fiber in tight junction with the adjacent odontoblast (OP). Reproduced from [18] with permission from *Acta Odontologica Scandinavica*.

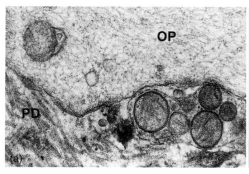
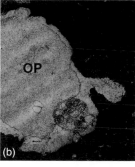

Fig. 2.14 Nerve fibers in the periodontoblastic space (a) in the predentin (PD) and (b) in dentin and close contact with the odontoblast processes (OP). (Reproduced from [18] with permission from *Acta Odontologica Scandinavica*.)

They branch and end up in a dense capillary network which is particularly predominant in the odontoblast and subodontoblastic region (Fig. 2.11). Some arterioles make U-turn loops. Venules largely follow the same course as the arterioles and a triad of arteriole, venule and nerve is often found centrally in the connective tissue of the pulp (Fig. 2.15).

Pulp vessels are thin-walled relative to the size of the lumen and also in absolute dimensions. The vessel walls may be discontinuous and pulp capillaries may be fenestrated (Figs 2.16 and 2.17). The

pulp is richly vascularized, but all capillaries in the subodontoblastic layer are normally not functional at the same time [17]. If required, the nonfunctional capillaries and arterioles (Fig. 2.18) may be filled quickly and an almost instantaneous local or general hyperemia may be established in the odontoblast/subodontoblastic region. Blood is brought to the vessels by bulk flow due to the blood pressure created by the heart contractions and substances are transported between the blood and interstitial fluid by diffusion. The smallest blood vessels, the capillaries, are

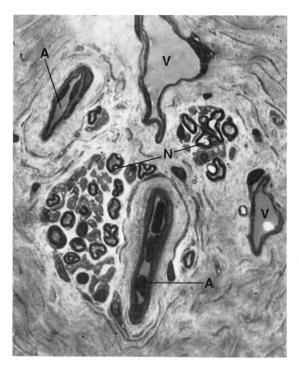

Fig. 2.15 Area from the central part of the pulp showing the triad arteriole (A), venule (V) and nerve (N).

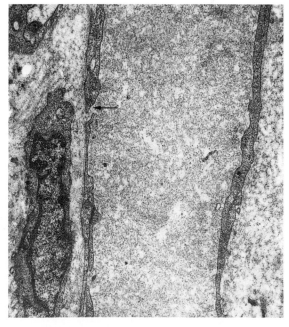

Fig. 2.16 A vessel in the pulp with discontinued epithelium (arrow) and lack of a basement membrane, possibly a lymph vessel. (Reproduced from [17] with permission from *Acta Odontologica Scandinavica*.)

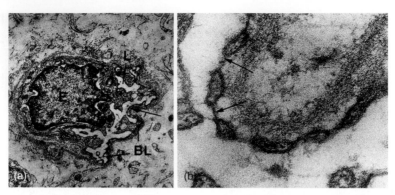

Fig. 2.17 (a) A capillary with a collapsed lumen (L) and typical fenestrations (arrows) in the vessel wall. (b) The fenestrations shown in higher magnification (E, endothelial cell, BL, Basement Lamina). (Reproduced from [17] with permission from *Acta Odontologica Scandinavica*.)

so well distributed that no cells are further away from a vessel than 50–100 μm. Due to the short distances between the capillaries and the cells, the thin and sometimes discontinuous vessel walls and capillary fenestrations, the exchange of substances between blood and interstitial fluid may take place rapidly by diffusion (Fig. 2.8). Lymph vessels are also present

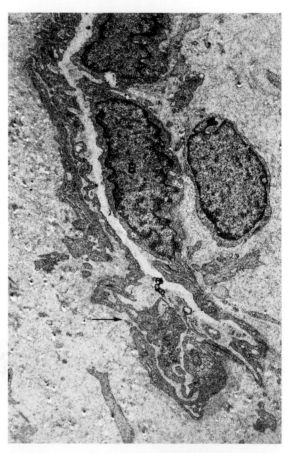

Fig. 2.19 A possible lymphatic vessel with irregular lumen, lack of basement membrane and irregular endothelial cells (E) with a possible discontinuation of the endothelial lining (arrow). (Reproduced from [17] with permission from *Acta Odontologica Scandinavica*.)

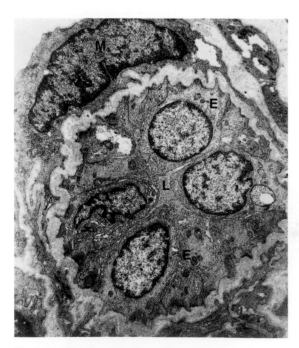

Fig. 2.18 Blood vessel with a collapsed lumen (L) (E, endothelial cell; M, myoendothelial cell). (Reproduced from [17] with permission from *Acta Odontologica Scandinavica*.)

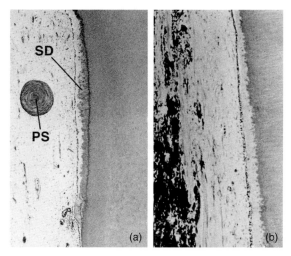

Fig. 2.20 Mineralized structures within the pulp. (a) A free pulp stone (PS), dentin, irregular secondary dentin (SD), and (b) irregular hematoxyphilic, dark staining areas of diffuse mineralizations in the pulp from a 67-year-old individual.

in the pulp [5] (Fig. 2.19). Their main function is to remove excess filtered fluid and plasma proteins.

2.3.4 Pulp stones

Pulp stones or denticles are mincralized structures within the pulp tissue. Different types of denticles have been described. They have been classified according to their location, as free (Fig. 2.20), attached or embedded (Fig. 2.21). On the basis of their structure, true pulp stone exhibits typical dentin structure while false pulp stones do not (Fig. 2.21). Diffuse minerali-

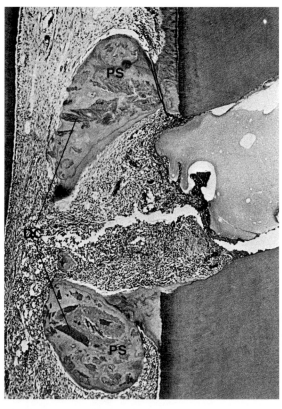

Fig. 2.22 Attached pulp stones (PS) which have formed around dentin chips (DC) which have entered the pulp as a result of pulp exposure.

zations are irregular in shape and do not have dentin structure (Fig. 2.20).

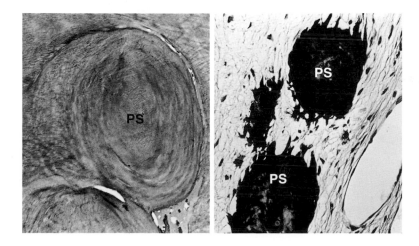

Fig. 2.21 Different types of pulp stones (PS). (a) Embedded pulp stones surrounded by dentin. (b) Free pulp stones without dentin structure.

Pulp stones may form under a number of different conditions. True pulp stones with dentin structure probably develop from fragmented portions of Hertwig's epithelium on the pulpal side. Odontoblasts may also be differentiated from immature cells in the dental pulp and initiate histogenesis of denticles. In addition, dentin fragments introduced into the pulp following pulp exposure may act as foci for pulp stone formation (Fig. 2.22). Diffuse mineralizations and false pulp stones may start forming in the wall of blood vessels.

2.4 The dentin

The odontoblast is the cellular component of dentin. It is located at the predentin/pulp border (Figs 2.5 and 2.6). The odontoblast processes are located within the dentinal tubules which extend from the pulp to the enamel and cementum.

Two mineralized structural entities can be identified in dentin [64]. The peritubular dentin lines the periphery of the tubules (Fig. 2.23) and its branches (Fig. 2.24). In teeth from older individuals, the peritubular dentin may completely obturate the tubules (Figs 2.23 and 2.25). It is highly mineralized (Fig. 2.25) and contains little organic material. The other mineralized component, intertubular dentin, is distinctly less mineralized than the peritubular dentin. It has a dense collagen matrix which constitutes about 93% of the organic matrix by weight or 17% of the dentin. Other components of the dentin comprise fractions of lipids, glycosaminoglycans, protein components other than collagen and citric acid, all in amounts less than 1% of the organic material by weight.

The predentin is the unmineralized dentin matrix that lines the entire pulpal side of the tissue. Sites of mineralization grow into spheres in the predentin and fuse resulting in a fairly uniform degree of mineralization. The globular calcospherites are recognized at the dentin–predentin border throughout the life of the tooth (Fig. 2.26). If the calcospherites do not fuse completely, unmineralized interglobular areas

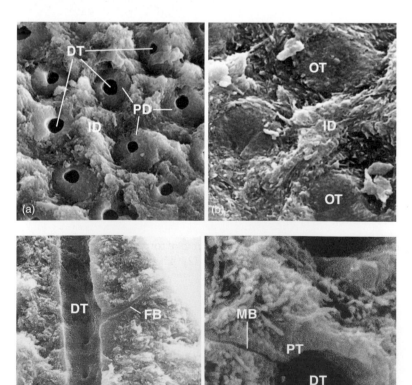

Fig. 2.23 Fractured dentin showing intertubular dentin (ID), peritubular dentin (PD) and dentinal tubules (DT): (a) newly erupted tooth; (b) obturated dentinal tubules (OT) in a tooth from an old individual.

Fig. 2.24 (a) Dentinal tubule (DT) from the root portion of a fractured section of a newly erupted tooth. Note many openings of branches from the tubule and one longitudinally fractured fine branch (FB) lined by peritubular dentin forking off at about a 45° angle from the main tubule. (b) Dentinal tubule also from a fractured section of a newly erupted tooth. Note microbranch (MB) with peritubular dentin (PT) leaving the main tubule at a 90° angle.

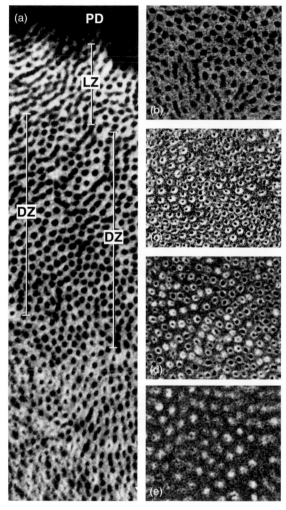

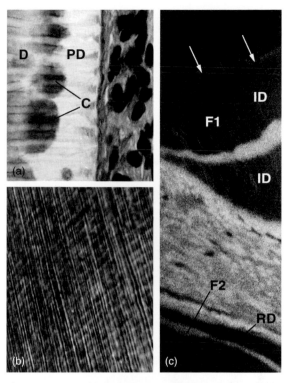

Fig. 2.26 Mineralization patterns of dentin. (a) Calcospherites (C) at the dentin (D)/predentin (PD) border. (b) Microradiograph showing incremental lines running obliquely across the field. (c) Fluorescent line (F1) is seen in the irregular secondary dentin (ID) and in the regularly secondary dentin (RD) at the floor of the pulp chamber (F2) in a tooth from a monkey which had received Procion Brilliant Red dye. Note also vague labeling (arrows) at the dentin/irregular secondary dentin interface.

Fig. 2.25 Microradiographs of undemineralized sections of dentin. Note that highly mineralized peritubular dentin is not found adjacent to the predentin (PD) in newly erupted teeth (a, b), but is found in the main bulk of the circumpulpal dentin (a, c). In teeth from older individuals, partly (d) and completely (e) obturated tubules are found. Note that a slightly darker (less mineralized) band of dentin can be discerned in (a), and (b) is from this dark zone (DZ) (LZ, lighter zone of higher mineral content). (Reproduced from [65] with permission from *Archives of Oral Biology*.)

will persist in the dentin (Fig. 2.27). Superimposed on the globular type of mineralization, an incremental pattern is found (Fig. 2.26). Such a linear pattern of mineralization is also found in secondary dentin formation (Fig. 2.26).

2.4.1 Primary and secondary dentin

Primary dentin is the term used to refer to the bulk of tissue formed during dentinogenesis until the tooth has erupted. The rate of formation is about 4 μm/day in monkey teeth [2]. The formation of dentin will also continue at a slow rate (0.8 μm/day) after the tooth has become functional. This secondary dentin is also called *physiologic* or *regular secondary dentin*. It is part of the continuous dentinogenesis that takes place during the life of the tooth. More regular secondary dentin forms on the ceiling and floor of the pulp chamber than in other locations which results in an uneven reduction in the size of the pulp chamber (Fig. 2.28 left). It should be noted that primary

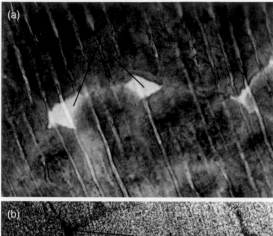

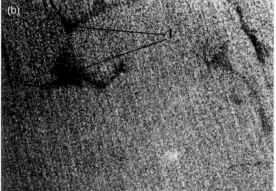

Fig. 2.27 Interglobular dentin (I) seen (a) in a hematoxylin and eosin stained section, and (b) in a microradiograph. Note that dentinal tubules pass through the interglobular areas (a).

dentin and physiological secondary dentin form a continuum without any distinct characteristics, or border, differentiating the two.

2.4.2 Tertiary dentin

Tertiary dentin is formed locally in response to irritations such as caries, attrition, operative procedures, and restorative materials (Figs 2.28 right and 2.29). Two types of tertiary dentin are recognized. A type formed by primary odontoblasts following a mild stimulus is referred to as *reactionary dentin*. Tertiary dentin formed by newly differentiated or secondary odontoblasts is termed *reparative dentin*. Other names used to describe tertiary dentin include irregular and irritation dentin.

Tertiary dentin may be looked on as a mineralized form of scar tissue. This dentin forms at a rate of 3 µm/day in monkey teeth [96]. Stanley [85] indicated its rate of formation in human teeth to average 1.5 µm/day. It makes the pulp chamber irregular in shape, but the term "irregular dentin" primarily reflects the irregular course of the dentinal tubules (Fig. 2.30).

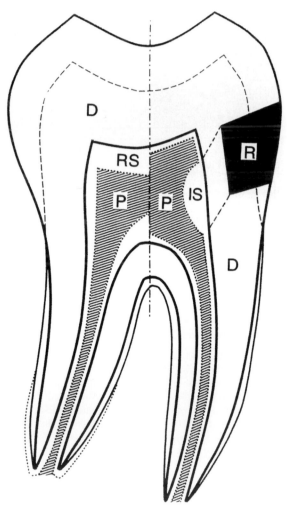

Fig. 2.28 Left half of diagram illustrates regular or physiological secondary dentin formation. Note that more regular secondary (RS) dentin forms on a ceiling and floor of the pulp chamber than on the walls. Right half of diagram illustrates tertiary dentin (IS) subjacent to a restoration (R) (P, pulp; D, primary dentin).

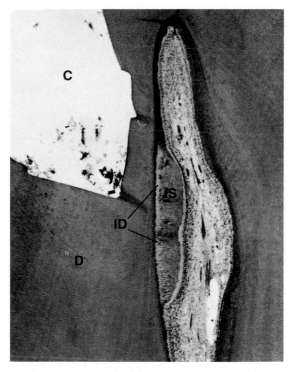

Fig. 2.29 Tertiary dentin (IS) subjacent to a cavity (C). Note interface dentin (ID) between the primary dentin (D) and the tertiary dentin. The extent of the tertiary dentin indicates the extent of cavity tubules.

Interface dentin

The first formed tertiary dentin of the reparative type is often particularly atypical in structure. It may have cellular inclusions and be atubular (Figs 2.29 and 2.31). This dentin has been referred to as *interface dentin* [56] and it has a marked physiological effect because it locally reduces the permeability of the dentin. A "barrier effect" is established in the affected area because the interface dentin prevents or markedly reduces direct communication between physiologic, primary or secondary, and tertiary dentin.

The irregular structure of the interface dentin is a result of destruction of the primary odontoblasts and the differentiation of secondary or replacement odontoblasts. The interface dentin is, therefore, the first dentin formed by the secondary odontoblasts. In many ways, it is similar to the first dentin formed by the original odontoblasts, i.e., the mantle dentin, which is relatively poorly mineralized but has a high content of organic material and much intertubular dentin with many terminal branches of the tubules present. Since the tubules

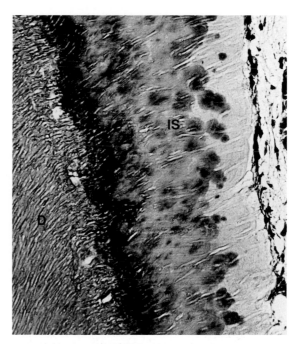

Fig. 2.30 Irregular secondary dentin (IS) showing aberrant course of the dentinal tubules. Note the irregular staining and structure of the first formed tertiary dentin, the interface dentin, adjacent to the regular, secondary dentin (D).

of the primary and irregular secondary dentin are not formed by the same odontoblasts, no direct communication exists between the two which also contributes to the "barrier effect". If the primary odontoblasts are not destroyed, but are stimulated to form more dentin in a localized area, the structure remains much the same as that of physiological secondary dentin.

2.4.3 Mineralization fronts in dentin

During dentinogenesis the intertubular and peritubular dentin mineralize at the same time, i.e., one mineralization front exists at the dentin/predentin border. Both the intertubular and the peritubular dentin mineralize as primary structures, and the peritubular dentin forms as a highly mineralized entity. At the time of eruption after the crown is fully formed, for some unknown reason dentinogenesis results in mineralization of the intertubular dentin only. Two mineralization fronts are then present in newly erupted teeth [65], one at the dentin–predentin border and one about 150 μm from this border. The mineralization at the dentin–predentin border at

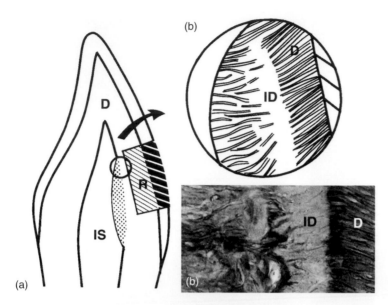

(a)

(b)

Fig. 2.31   (a) Diagram of a tooth with a restoration (R) and subjacent tertiary (IS) dentin. (b) Enlarged part of encircled area in (a). Note that the tubules in the dentin (D) are separated from the tertary dentin by the interface dentin (ID) and that the tubules in the dentin do not communicate with the tubules in the tertiary dentin. (c) Part of a section showing the dentin/tertiary dentin interface (D, dentin; ID, interface dentin which is part of the tertiary dentin).

this stage deals with the intertubular dentin only (Fig. 2.25). The degree of mineralization of the intertubular matrix is relatively low during a period of dentin formation (dark zone, Fig. 2.25), but soon reaches the normal degree of mineralization (light zone, Fig. 2.25). The peritubular dentin formation lags behind. Thus, the highly mineralized peritubular dentin in the most pulpal part of the dentin is a secondarily formed structure.

As development and aging continue, the intratubular mineralization continues and the peritubular dentin will eventually catch up with the slowly progressing regular secondary dentin formation. The two mineralization fronts will be adjacent to each other (Fig. 2.32). It is only after tooth eruption the two mineralization fronts merge.

It may be noted that the description of the two mineralization fronts at the time of completed crown formation and eruption of the teeth corresponds to the time when primary dentinogenesis is replaced by physiological secondary dentin formation. Thus, there may be a structural basis for differentiating between primary and secondary dentin. It should also be noted that this particular relationship is limited to crown dentin, and it is generally agreed that root dentin has only one mineralization front, although this aspect of dentinogenesis has not been studied in detail.

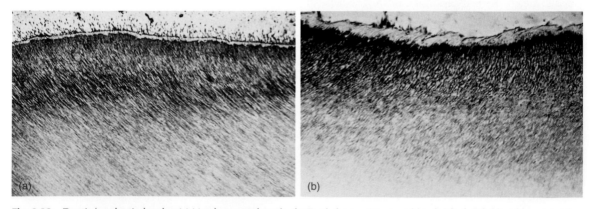

(a)

(b)

Fig. 2.32   Dentin/predentin border. (a) Newly erupted tooth. (b) Tooth from a 71-year-old individual. Toluidine blue stained sections. Note the difference in the staining of the dentin.

Continued intratubular mineralization of dentin occurs as an age change and may result in complete obturation of the tubules (Figs 2.23 and 2.25). This process may be accelerated by external stimuli of various types, including certain restorative materials. Another type of intratubular mineralization includes precipitation of mineral salts within the tubules, for example, as found in the "transparent zone" of dentin subjacent to a slowly progressing caries lesion. Both types of intratubular remineralizations are collectively referred to as *sclerotic dentin*.

2.4.4 The dentinal tubules

The tubules in the dentin are up to 2 μm in diameter and house the odontoblast process during dentinogenesis. The extent of the odontoblast process in erupted teeth has been a controversial topic for a long time [36], and it cannot be regarded as finally settled.

The density of the tubules varies depending on the location in the tooth. The most extreme values range from about 5000 to 90,000 tubules per mm², but a more common range is 8000 to 57,000 [70]. In general, the number of tubules is low peripherally and increases towards the pulp. The lowest number of tubules per mm² is found in the peripheral dentin subjacent to the occlusal fissure and the highest number is found in the innermost coronal dentin. The number of dentinal tubules in root dentin does not vary as markedly from the periphery towards the pulp

as in coronal dentin, the range being approximately 10,000–45,000 tubules at the level of the cemento-enamel junction. In the apical region, the dentin structure is irregular and the number of tubules per mm² ranges from about 3000 peripherally to about 15,000 pulpally. The range pulpally, which is of prime interest to endodontics, extends from 5000 to 30,000 per mm² and the branching of the tubules is quite pronounced. Some areas are devoid of tubules [71]). The structure of apical dentin does not favor adhesive techniques based on penetration of resin into dentinal tubules. The difficulty in controlling the wetness of a hybrid layer in this location represents another problem in using adhesive techniques for sealing off the apical part of the root canal.

Different types of branches of dentinal tubules can be identified on the basis of size, direction and location. The types and number of branches are affected by the density of the tubules. Mjör and Nordahl [70] have described three types of branches: (1) major branches, 0.5–1.0 μm in diameter found peripherally in the crown and the root, (2) fine branches, 300–700 nm in diameter, particularly numerous in areas where the densities of tubules are low, like in the root and under the occlusal fissure, and (3) microbranches, 25–200 nm in diameter, found anywhere in dentin. The major branches are typical peripheral delta branches (Fig. 2.33), fine branches leave the main tubules at a 45° angle (Figs 2.24 and 2.34) and the microbranches fork off at a 90° angle from the tubules (Fig. 2.24). The presence of branches is

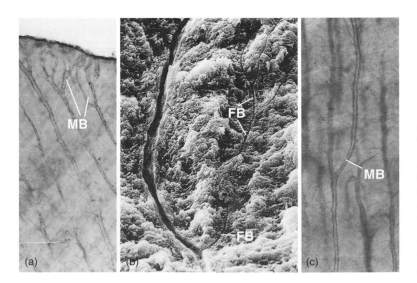

Fig. 2.33 Major branching (MB) of dentinal tubules in stained, demineralized sections (a,c) and ramifications of a fine branch (FB) in a fractured undermineralized section of dentin (b). Major branches fork off at an acute angle from the tubules. Major branches are 0.5–1.0 μm in diameter and are typically found in peripheral dentin (a, b), but may be found anywhere (c). (Reproduced from [70] with permission from *Archives of Oral Biology*.)

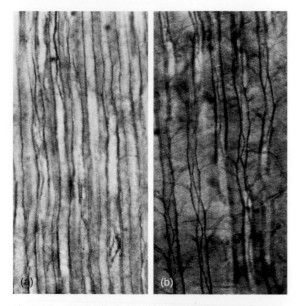

Fig. 2.34 Longitudinal view of dentinal tubules: (a) in the crown; (b) in the root. Note that the tubules are further apart in the root than in the crown and that numerous fine branches are found in the root. Hematoxylin and eosin stained sections.

related to the density of tubules, e.g., in the crown where the density of tubules is high, fine branches are rarely seen, but in the main bulk of root dentin, they are abundant (Fig. 2.34).

The branches of the tubules make up a profuse canalicular anastomosing system within the intertubular dentin (Fig. 2.35). Unusual branching of individual tubules may also be found (Fig. 2.36). The development of the different types of branches has not been studied, but it is well known that differentiating odontoblasts show multiple, peripheral cytoplasmic extensions during the initial phase of dentinogenesis.

These extensions explain the presence of the typical delta branches. Numerous branches of the odontoblast process during root formation (Fig. 2.35) also substantiate the presence of fine branches in the root (Fig. 2.35).

All types of branches will undoubtedly have effects on the permeability of the dentin and possibly on its sensitivity. Detailed characterization of dentin substrates for testing of adhesive materials is imperative in order to obtain meaningful results. Permeability studies of dentin must also take into account the number of tubules and the type of branching of tubules in dentin samples investigated. The branches may also play a role in the infection of the dentin.

Unusually large dentinal tubules, "giant tubules", have been described. They are present in cuspal and incisal areas and may represent vestigial remnants of the pulp chamber in these locations due to the crowding of the odontoblasts during dentinogenesis [67]. These areas are clinically important because they may represent easy accessible pathways to the pulp, e.g., after fracture of an incisal edge.

2.5 Pulpal blood flow

The volume of blood flowing through vessels per unit time is called blood flow. It is mainly the blood flow that determines the speed of the diffusion between blood and interstitial fluid: the higher the blood flow the faster the diffusion. Thus, the regulation of an adequate blood flow is a crucial point for survival and normal function in any tissue.

The dominating mechanism for regulation of pulpal blood flow is the nerve component. The pulp has a considerably denser nerve supply than the PDL and alveolar bone [44]. It is supplied by both autonomic

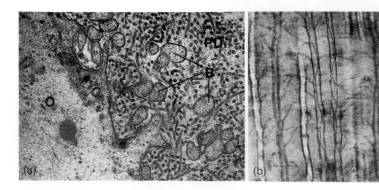

Fig. 2.35 (a) Electron micrograph showing numerous branches (B) from an odontoblast (O) in the predentin (PD) from the root of a young tooth. (Reproduced from [28] with permission from *Scandinavian Journal of Dental Research.*) (b) Numerous fine branches in root dentin in a stained demineralized section.

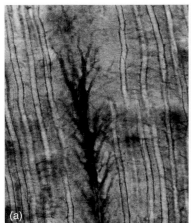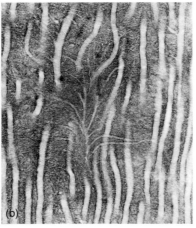

(a)   (b)

Fig. 2.36 Irregular branching of two dentinal tubules in stained demineralized sections: (a) from the cervical area near the cementoenamel junction in a newly erupted premolar; (b) from an incisor from a 64 year-old individual. (Reproduced from [70] with permission from *Archives of Oral Biology*.)

efferent adrenergic nerves of sympathetic origin and afferent sensory nerve fibers from the trigeminal ganglion [11,44]. The main innervation is sensory, whereas the sympathetic part has a smaller contribution. Activation of the sympathetic fibers causes pulpal vasoconstriction and a *decrease* in blood flow due to activation of α-receptors [21,45,53]. These receptors are also activated through the carotid baroreceptor reflex [39]. Neuropeptide Y (NPY), a 36-amino-acid peptide which is stored and coreleased together with noradrenalin (NA) in the sympathetic fibers, also cause a nonadrenergic fall in pulpal blood flow [20]. However, the sensory nerve fibers, which are responsible for tooth sensation, have a profound impact on pulpal circulation. The sensory pulpal nerves contain vasoactive peptides such as neurokinin A (NKA), calcitonin gene-related peptide (CGRP) and substance P (SP). The nerves release these neuropeptides from their pulpal nerve endings in response to afferent activation (Fig. 2.37) [30,38,75]. Thus, infusion of these neuropeptides [30], or tooth stimulation [38], causes a relatively long-lasting *increase* in pulpal blood flow.

Most of the pulpal nerves have been shown to contain CGRP. Approximately three times more fibers are labeled with CGRP than SP [44]. In the central pulp most of the nerves containing CGRP, SP and NPY are localized as a network in the walls of blood vessels (Fig. 2.38), clearly indicating their participation in blood flow regulation. In general, activation of sensory nerve fibers causes release of neuropeptides such as NKA, CGRP and SP from their nerve endings. The released neuropeptides act in a complex manner to cause vascular smooth muscle relaxation

and thus increase blood flow (Fig. 2.37). A direct receptor-mediated mechanism [32,64] and also an indirect mechanism via release of vasoactive substances from endothelial cells (endothelium-derived relaxing factor or EDRF) have been proposed in some tissues [10,38,64], and may be operating in the pulp.

Evidence that sensory neuropeptides, in particular SP, will initiate release of inflammatory agents such as histamine, bradykinin and prostaglandins has been reported by several investigators [8,26,47,83]. In the dental pulp, it has been found that vasodilation induced by sensory nerve stimulation can be inhibited by mepyramin [29] and by indomethacin [90]. Noxious stimuli to the pulp are found to increase the release of bradykinin and also the pulpal content of opioid enkephaline-like peptides [48], whereas sensory denervation causes a reduced blood flow during increased bradykinin infusion [74]. Hence, there is substantial evidence that the pulpal sensory nerves, when stimulated, play a significant role in regulating the release of vasoactive inflammatory agents in the pulp (Fig. 2.37).

2.5.1 Tissue fluid pressure

The hydrostatic pressure in the interstitial fluid surrounding the pulpal cells (Fig. 2.8) is called the pulpal tissue fluid pressure. Compared to most other tissues, the pulpal tissue pressure seems high, 5–20 mmHg above atmospheric pressure [42,87,94]. As the pulp is enclosed between rigid dentin walls, i.e., with low compliance, even modest changes in pulpal fluid volume will be reflected in the tissue pressure. Thus, any increase in fluid volume will increase pulpal tis-

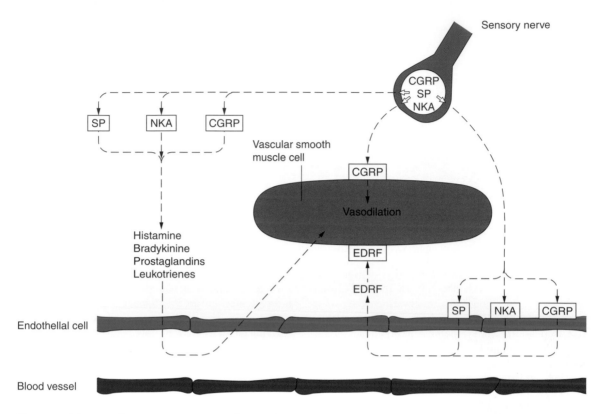

Fig. 2.37   Schematic drawing summarizing mechanisms for neuropeptide modulation of vascular tension. Release of the neuropeptides CGRP, SP and NKA from sensory nerve endings may cause vasodilation through a direct receptor-mediated mechanism, or indirectly via release of vasoactive substances from endothelial cells (EDRF), from the blood or from the tissue. (Reproduced from [43] with permission from *Proceedings of the Finnish Dental Society.*)

sue pressure and a decrease will act conversely. The significance of a relatively high pulpal tissue pressure in a low compliance environment has long been discussed and may be linked to a neurogenic defense mechanism that helps protect the pulp against entry of harmful agents via exposed dentinal tubules (Fig. 2.39) [63,94]. Most nerve fibers entering the dentinal tubules in rat [13,54,82] and cat [44] teeth contain the sensory vasodilating neuropeptide CGRP. Mechanical stimulation of dentin causes pulpal vasodilation [75,94] and therefore increased tissue pressure. Thus, an axon reflex, triggering reduced masticatory activity and thus protecting the teeth and pulp mechanism that helps protect the pulp, might be established when dentin tubules are exposed [63]: as outlined in Fig. 2.39, the sensory nerve fibers in the odontoblast/dentin area, when excited by the hydrodynamic mechanism [9], may release neuropeptides that cause

pulpal vasodilation with resultant increased tissue pressure. The increased tissue pressure will promote augmented outward flow of fluid through the exposed dentinal tubules. Increased outward flow of fluid in the dentinal tubules will protect the pulp against entry of harmful substances. It seems, therefore, beneficial for the pulp to have a high physiological tissue pressure, which promptly increases when blood flow increases due to its low compliance.

2.6 Inflammatory reactions

In general, inflammation is the protective response of tissues to injury. It is a fundamental process that enables the tissues to survive an insult and prepares the tissues for the reparative process. When injured, the loose connective tissue of the pulp will respond with

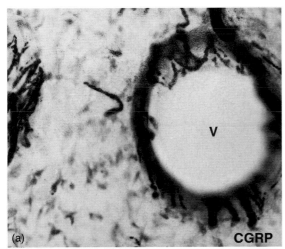

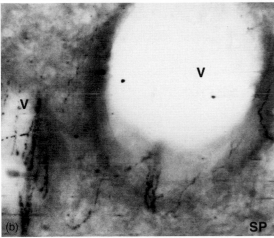

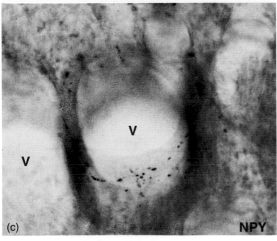

an inflammatory reaction like other connective tissue. However, in contrast to inflammation elsewhere in connective tissue, these reactions take place under special conditions, in a rigid dentin chamber, which to some extent makes the pulp vulnerable. As the pulp space cannot expand, any gain in blood volume or interstitial fluid volume will increase the pulpal tissue pressure. If the tissue pressure rises to the level of blood pressure, it might compress the vessels, thus counteracting any beneficial effect of increased blood flow during pulpitis [41]. As the initial reactions during any inflammation are vasodilation and increased vascular permeability, which increases both the volume of blood and interstitial fluid, the pulp will, necessarily, respond with an increased tissue pressure when inflamed (Fig. 2.40). However, it has also been shown that the tissue pressure increase during pulpal inflammation may be a local phenomenon [42,86,92], like the histopathology of pulp abscesses (Fig. 2.41). It is also possible that the pressure may only be transitorily increased [38].

Depending on the degree, severity and state of inflammation, the absolute magnitude and duration of the increased tissue pressure in the inflamed pulp will vary, because it simply reflects the increased pulpal fluid volume. It may exceed 60 mmHg in localized inflamed areas [86]. However, as long as the pulp is not severely damaged and the local feedback mechanisms counteracting the volume and thus the pressure increase are functioning (Fig. 2.40), the spread and increase in tissue pressure will be limited. The main feedback mechanisms counteracting a build-up and spread in tissue pressure are: (1) net absorption in capillaries in adjacent uninflamed tissue and (2) increased lymph flow (Figs 2.37 and 2.42). Both factors will transport fluid volume out of the affected area and then out of the tooth [43] and consequently lower the pressure. Accordingly, in spite of increased blood flow and vascular permeability due to inflammation, the effective removal of plasma and lymph ensures that the tissue pressure does not rise to the level of vessel compression and resulting necrosis. Thus, local coronal pulpitis may persist without spreading to the root pulp. Therefore, the pulp may heal provided the injurious agents are permanently

Fig. 2.38 Serial cross-sections of vessels (V) from cat canine pulp. Network of sensory nerve fibers containing the neuropeptides CGRP (a), substance P (b), and neuropeptide Y (c) in the vessel walls. (Reproduced from [44] with permission from *Acta Odontologica Scandinavica*.)

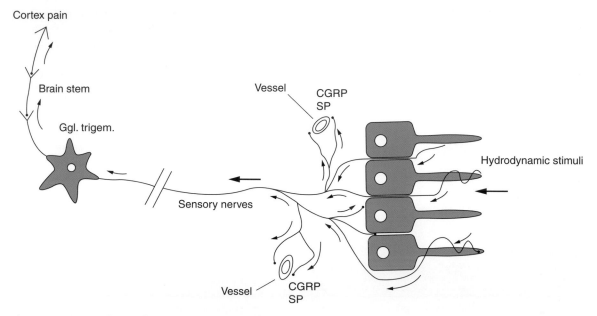

Fig. 2.39 Diagram showing how hydrodynamic stimuli will excite nerves in dentin odontoblast area causing pain and release of sensory neuropeptides (CGRP, SP) from nerve endings in the pulp. The neuropeptides induce vasodilation, which in turn promptly increases the tissue pressure locally in the low-compliant pulp. The increased tissue pressure will raise the outward flow of fluid in the exposed dentinal tubules, thus protecting the pulp against inward diffusion of harmful substances.

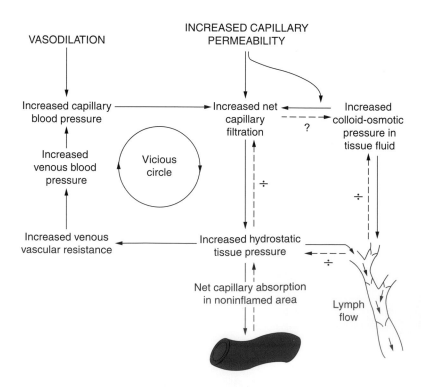

Fig. 2.40 Schematic build-up of a so-called vicious circle during local pulpal inflammation. The edema-preventing mechanisms that serve to keep the pulpal fluid volume relatively constant, and thus oppose a rise in tissue pressure and break the vicious circle, are indicated with dotted arrows. This vicious circle was the basis for the former theory of self-strangulation by pulp inflammation. (Reproduced from [40] with permission from *Acta Odontologica Scandinavica*.)

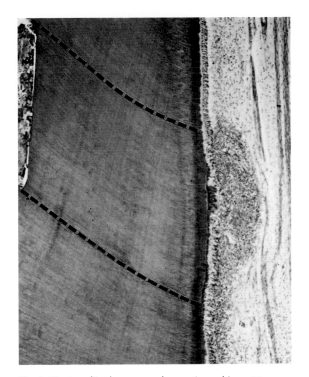

Fig. 2.41 Localized, severe pulp reaction subjacent to a cavity subjected to an experimental procedure intended to cause pulp reactions. Dotted lines outline the extent of cavity tubules.

removed or sealed off by reactions in dentine. In the case of severe persistent irritants, however, the increased tissue pressure may spread in an apical direction and cause total pulp necrosis.

Studies have indicated that both the sensory and sympathetic nerves play an important role in the pulpal inflammatory reactions [33,43,74]. As for the sensory nerves, an axon reflex similar to that involved in the triple response in skin inflammation [59] seems most likely and might be activated by local insults to dentin or pulp. It is well known that stimulation of pulpal sensory nerves causes vasodilation and increased vascular permeability [37,53,74], often referred to as neurogenic inflammation. In addition, studies have indicated that neuropeptides released from peripheral sensory nerve endings may act directly on the target tissue by stimulating leukocyte chemotaxis, regulating release of inflammatory mediators from macrophages and lymphocytes, and also by enhancing the proliferation of fibroblasts [7,49,62,73,78,79]. Furthermore, long lasting tooth stimulation [37] causes enhanced emigration of white cells out of blood vessels and into the tissue (Fig. 2.44). This reaction was abolished by inferior alveolar nerve axotomy (Fig. 2.44), indicating that neuropeptides released from peripheral nerve endings have an impact on the inflammatory white cell emigration.

Recent findings clearly show that the sympathetic nervous system (SNS) also has a profound impact on inflammation and immune responses (for references see [22]). Postganglionic sympathetic nerve terminals

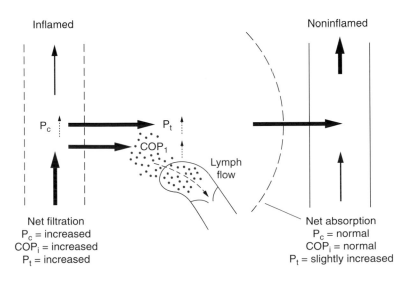

Inflamed

P_c P_t COP$_i$

Lymph flow

Net filtration
P_c = increased
COP_i = increased
P_t = increased

Noninflamed

Net absorption
P_c = normal
COP_i = normal
P_t = slightly increased

Fig. 2.42 Fluid and plasma protein (dots) removal from inflamed (left) and noninflamed tissue (right). Black arrows indicate relative magnitude and direction of fluid transport (P_c, capillary blood pressure; P_t, tissue pressure; COP_i, colloidal osmotic pressure in interstitial fluid). (Reproduced from [43] with permission from *Proceedings of the Finnish Dental Society*.)

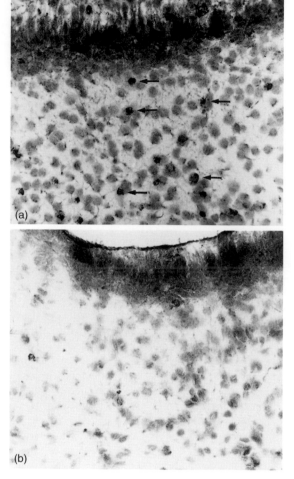

(a)

(b)

Fig. 2.43 Immunohistochemical micrographs from rat first molar pulps after long-term intermittent electrical stimulation of the crown. (a) Increased number of immunocompetent cells (arrows) in innervated pulp. (b) Absence of such cells in denervated pulp. Sections were incubated with W3/13 antibody, specific for leukocytes, plasma cells and granulocytes. (Courtesy of Dr I. Fristad.)

contain vesicles with noradrenaline (NA) and NPY which are released on stimulation (Fig. 2.44). Locally released NA and NPY are shown to affect circulation, lymphocyte traffic and proliferation as well as cytokine production [24]. Convincing evidence has been obtained that sympathetic neurotransmitters inhibit production of proinflammatory and increase antiinflammatory cytokines [93].

The SNS in the dental pulp is important for recruitment of inflammatory cells such as CD43+ granulo-

cytes as demonstrated by electrical tooth stimulation [16]. Sympathetic nerves appear to have an inhibitory effect on osteoclasts, odontoclasts, and on IL-1α production [6,36]. The SNS stimulates reparative dentin production, as reparative dentin formation was reduced after sympathectomy, and sprouting of sympathetic nerve fibers occurs in chronically inflamed dental pulp [35]. Furthermore, the sympathetic nerves exert a tonic regulatory effect over lymphocyte proliferation and migration, and neural imbalance caused by unilateral sympathectomy recruits immunoglobulin-producing cells to the noninflamed dental pulp [35]. Thus, the sensory and sympathetic nerves seem not only to take part in the vascular reactions during inflammation, but also to have an impact on emigration of white cells, immunological processes and proliferation, thereby promoting healing and repair after pulpal injury.

2.7 The periodontium

The periodontium includes the gingiva, the periodontal ligament (PDL), the alveolar bone and the dental cementum (Fig. 2.45). Its main function is to provide an attachment for the teeth to the alveolar bone by a fibrous joint of the gomphosis type. The joint allows minor adjustments in the position of the teeth. Thus, it provides a resilient suspensory apparatus that will provide optimal conditions for masticatory functions. The apical periodontium, including the PDL, cementum and the alveolar bone, is of prime importance for endodontology and these parts of the periodontium will be described in some detail.

2.8 The periodontal ligament

The PDL is a dense connective tissue with islands of interstitial loose connective tissue interspersed between the dense bundles of collagen fibers (Figs 2.3 and 2.45). The principal fibers of the PDL extend from the cementum to the alveolar bone. However, each fiber does not reach the entire distance between cementum and bone, and collectively they constitute an intricate branching and reuniting pattern of fibers. They are deeply embedded in the two mineralized tissues as Sharpey's fibres (Figs 2.45 and 2.46). The fibers inserting into cementum are smaller and more numerous than those entering into alveolar bone.

Four groups of principle fibers are recognized in the PDL. The *alveolar crest fibers* pass downward from the cementum in the cervical region of the tooth to the alveolar crest; the *horizontal fibers* comprise the cervical third of the PDL; the *oblique fibers* run from the alveolar bone somewhat apically to the cementum; and the *apical fibres* radiate from the cementum towards the alveolar bone in all directions.

The principal fibers of the PDL have a functional arrangement in that groups of fibers act against different types of forces, including resistance to rotation of the teeth. Although collagen is inelastic, slight movement of the teeth is possible due to the wavy course of the fibers allowing them to stretch during stress. Changes in the blood flow and blood pressure of the PDL will induce minor movement of the teeth [1,19]. The blood and tissue fluid also act as a hydrodynamic system which absorbs occlusal forces.

2.8.1 Cells of the PDL

Fibroblasts are the prevailing cell of the PDL. Those that are located between the principle fibers are long, slender cells, but those in the interstitial tissue are irregular or stellate-shaped. The function of the fibroblasts is to maintain the collagen fibers and the glycosaminoglycans and glycoproteins which constitute the ground substance during the normal turnover processes and during repair. Macrophages and mast cells, including associated cytokines, are

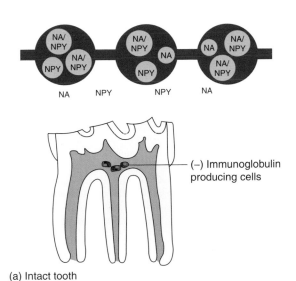

(a) Intact tooth

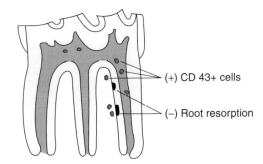

(b) Effect of electrical stimulation or OTM

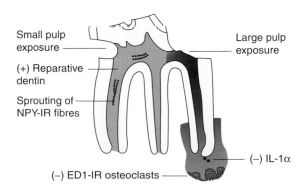

(c) Effect of pulp exposure

Fig. 2.44   Schematic illustrations summarizing potential effects of sympathetic nerves on dental tissues. Stimulating effects of sympathetic nerves are indicated with +, and inhibitory effects by –. Top panel illustrates a peripheral postganglionic sympathetic nerve terminal containing vesicles with noradrenalin (NA) or neuropeptide Y (NPY) which are released upon stimulation. Illustrations below show rat molar teeth in three different conditions. (a) Normal uninflamed pulp with sympathetic imbalance caused by unilateral sympathectomy recruits immunoglobulin producing cells. (b) Electrical stimulation of sympathetic nerves causes recruitment of CD43+ granulocytes in dental pulp. During orthodontic tooth movement (OTM), sympathetic nerves have an inhibitory effect on hard tissue resorption and a stimulating effect on CD43+ cell recruitment in the dental pulp and PDL. (c) The locally inflamed pulp shows increased reparative dentin formation and sprouting of sympathetic nerve fibers while the periapical lesion shows decreased IL-1α production and number of osteoclasts when compared to a denervated sympathectomized tooth. (Modified from [36].)

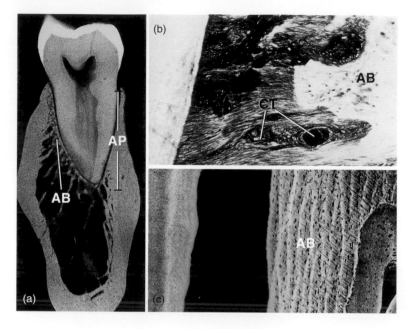

Fig. 2.45 Radiograph (a) and microradiographs (b, c) of alveolar bone (AB) in undermineralized (a, c) and demineralized sections (b). Note islands of blood vessels and loose connective tissue (CT) among the fibers of the periodontal ligament and radiolucent Sharpey's fibers that attach to alveolar bone (AP, alveolar process of the mandible).

also found in the normal PDL and they increase markedly during inflammation. On the cementum side of the PDL, cementoblasts are found and on the alveolar bone side osteoblasts are present. Osteoclasts and odontoclasts allow bone and tooth resorption. They play important roles in the turnover of the PDL, during periodontal, including apical, disease and during orthodontic movement of teeth. They also play an essential role in the development of apical periodontitis associated with pulp infection. Odontoclasts and osteoclasts also play a central role in shedding of primary teeth and during eruption of the permanent teeth.

Sympathectomy increases osteoclast-mediated bone resorption [57,81] and root dentin resorption [36], indicating that sympathetic nerves have an inhibitory effect on osteoclasts as well as odontoclasts (Fig. 2.44).

Sympathetic nerves in the PDL are also important for the recruitment of granulocytes as demonstrated by experimental tooth movement [36]. In experimentally induced periapical lesions, sympathetic nerves have an inhibitory effect on the size of the lesion, number of osteoclasts lining the lesion and amount of IL-1α within the lesion [35].

2.8.2 Epithelial cell remnants

Both the developing and mature tooth are surrounded by a continuous, netlike pattern of epithelial cells originating from the Hertwig's root sheath. These so-called Malassez's epithelial rests (Fig. 2.3) are locat-

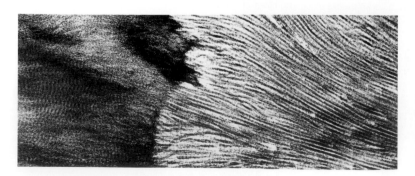

Fig. 2.46 Electron micrograph showing fine collagen fibers inserting into a cellular cementum as Sharpey's fibers. (Reproduced from [27] with permission from *Acta Odontologica Scandinavica*.)

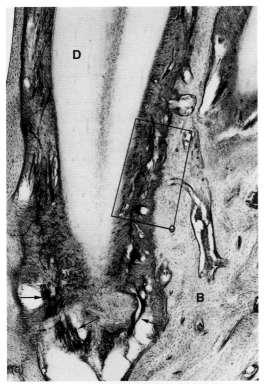

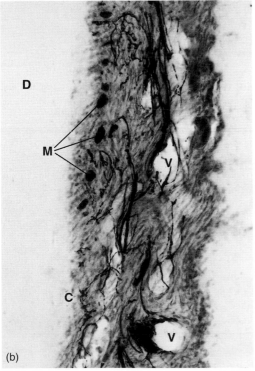

ed close to the root cementum in its entire length, and are shown to persist within the periodontal membrane throughout the life of the tooth [84,97]. The reason why the epithelial rests of Malassez persist in the PDL is unknown, but it has been proposed that these cells are important to prevent ankylosis and hinder bone ingrowth [61]. Stimulation of these epithelial cells may induce cell proliferation [31], which may form cyst linings at the periphery of lesions. Recent studies have hypothesized that the Malassez's cells may function as targets for developing periodontal nerves. Ruffini-like receptors and free nerve endings are closely related to these cells (Fig. 2.47) [44,60]. Furthermore, immunohistochemical studies have shown that Malassez's cells contain neuropeptides such as CGRP and SP and may therefore be classified as endocrine cells [44]. Thus, Malassez's cells in the PDL may have functional endocrine roles. Malassez's epithelial rests may also play a role in the formation of cementicles by undergoing mineralization. They may be attached or free and may contain cell rests much like pulp stones which may be found in the apical area of the teeth (Fig. 2.48).

2.8.3 Turnover

It is important to note that bone is a more dynamic tissue than cementum. The normal turnover of bone also affects the alveolar processes. Cementum is usually covered by a thin, unmineralized precementum, and slow cementogenesis compensates for wear of the teeth. Bone, on the other hand, is only covered by osteoid during bone formation. Unmineralized matrix tends to resist odontoclastic activity [87]. Thus, osteoclastic activity seems to predominate over odontoclastic or cementoclastic activity in the PDL and Howship's lacunae in bone defects develop more commonly than in teeth. Both resorptive processes may take place simultaneously. Reparative cementum formation by cellular cementum may fill in resorption defects.

Fig. 2.47 (a) Apical periodontal ligament of cat incisor richly supplied with protein gene product (PGP) immunoreactive nerves (arrows) from apical bone (B). (b) Enlargement of framed area showing nerve fibers supplying the blood vessels (V) and extensive branching of nerves towards the root cementum (C) and Malassez's epithelial cells (M) (D, dentin). (Reproduced from [44] with permission from *Acta Odontologica Scandinavica*.)

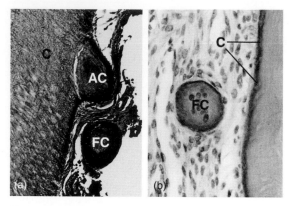

Fig. 2.48   (a) Attached (AC) and (b) free cementicles (FC) in the periodontal ligament (C, cementum).

The difference in resorptive activity between bone and cementum in the PDL is the basis for orthodontic tooth movement. Moderate forces applied to a tooth will result in bone resorption on the pressure side and bone formation on the tension side without resorption of the cementum. Thus, the tooth will move in the direction of the force applied. The use of excessive force may also result in resorption of the cementum and may reach clinically significant proportions.

2.8.4 Circulation in the PDL

The blood supply to the PDL is complex. It receives its blood via vessels from the alveolar bone, periosteum, gingiva and pulp. The main vessel supply originates from the intra-osseous arteries. As the arterial supply arises from different sources and the venules and veins drain both into the bone marrow and gingiva, the vascular bed of the PDL should not be regarded as an isolated functional unit. This implies that inflammatory and pathological changes in blood flow, tissue fluid pressure or blood pressure in the surrounding adjacent tissues, will also influence the periodontal circulation. Inflammatory vasodilation in parallel-coupled vessels in the alveolar bone or gingiva may cause reduced blood flow in the PDL due to a fall in pressure in the arterioles feeding the PDL.

Although tendinous, the PDL is highly vascularized. The total vascular volume has been calculated to be approximately 20% of the tissue, compared to only 3–4% in most other tissues.

The main vessels of the ligament run parallel to the long axis of the tooth in compartments of loose connective tissue between the fibers. The arterioles branch to form capillaries arranged in a flat, basket-like network that surrounds the root surface. The capillary network is located closer to the alveolar bone than to the cementum, and the vessels perforating the alveolar walls are most abundant in the apical third.

Blood flow in the PDL seems mainly to be controlled by sympathetic fibers causing vasoconstriction and by sensory fibers for vasodilation [19, 51]. However, due to the lack of suitable methods to measure blood flow in a tissue with such a tiny volume and a position secluded between bone and tooth as the PDL, quantitative measurements of blood flow in the PDL are almost lacking.

Qualitative measurements of PDL blood have shown that sympathetic vasoconstrictor fibers take part in regulation of PDL blood flow. Both α_1 and α_2 postjunctional adrenoreceptors are involved in the sympathetic vasoconstriction [19]. The constrictor effect is greatly reduced by α-adrenoceptor antagonists, but never abolished, indicating that some of the sympathetic fibers innervating the PDL contain NPY, which has been confirmed by immunohistochemical studies [44,76] (Fig. 2.49). Sympathetic induced vasodilations, due to activation of β-receptors that are most probably located in postcapillary resistance vessels, have also been found in the PDL [1].

Changes in PDL blood flow have been shown to affect the tooth position, and external forces applied to the tooth crown may greatly influence PDL blood flow [19,77]. Such changes in the normal conditions may possibly be related to changes in PDL tissue fluid pressure [19,56]. In common with the pulp, the PDL is also enclosed in a rigid, low compliance environment between alveolar bone and tooth. Changes in blood volume induced by venous stasis or cardiac arrest are thus within seconds transmitted to the PDL tissue fluid pressure [56]. This pressure has been recorded as relatively high compared to most other tissues [56,77,95]. It is claimed to affect tooth position, blood flow, the eruptive force of teeth, and probably pain sensation.

Unlike the pulp, where the main sensation is pain, the PDL has receptors for touch, pressure, movements and position of teeth, and pain. A variety of Ruffini-like mechanoreceptor structures are found in the PDL [14]. Some of the fully encapsulated mechanoreceptor structures are located in the interstitial loose connective tissue next to blood vessels. Thus, increased PDL blood flow causing increased tissue pressure would most probably cause excitation of mechanoreceptors. An increased blood volume in the PDL has been shown to raise the tissue pressure and cause tooth extrusion, whereas decreased blood volume causes tooth intrusion and reduces the tissue pressure [1,19,56]. Another aspect of the low compliance in the PDL is that changes in tissue pressure most likely will affect pain sensation, i.e., increased tissue fluid pressure causes increased activity in sensory A-δ and C-fibers, much the same way as in the pulp.

2.8.5 Innervation of PDL

Although less innervated than the dental pulp, the PDL is richly supplied with nerves entering both from the apical and lateral alveolar bone (Figs 2.40 and 2.52). The apical part of the ligament is most heavily innervated and the major part seems to be of sensory origin, whereas sympathetic, NPY-carrying fibers are rarely found. However, some larger vessels in the mandibular canal are densely innervated by NPY fibres in their walls [44]. Sprouting of sympathetic NPY-containing nerves may be observed in the inflamed PDL 20 days after pulp exposure [35]. The significance of this sprouting is not clearly understood, but it may affect blood flow and immunomodulation. Since it is known that peripheral endogenous sympathetic neurotransmitters are important regulators of vascular growth factors [3,98], it might suggest that sympathetic nerves play a role in revascularization during repair and healing processes in the inflamed PDL.

The periodontal ligament contains myelinated and unmyelinated nerve fibers. CGRP-IR fibres appear more frequently than SP-IR fibers at all levels in the PDL [44,80]. Most nerves in the PDL are localized in the apical third, closely associated with blood vessels. Periapical inflammation and orthodontic tooth movement have been found to induce a transient periapical sprouting of sensory CGRP-IR axons [15,80]. Similarly, increased occurrences of SP-IR periodontal fibres after application of orthodontic forces have been reported in cat canines [72]. Larger axons often form specialized terminals, predominantly in the apical area, described as Ruffini-like endings. Thin axons usually terminate as free nerve endings [12,60]. Both electrophysiological and histological data suggest that the Ruffini-like terminals as well as free nerve endings may function as mechanoreceptors [12,60]. Cementum appears not to be innervated [12,44], but extensive branching of sensory nerves is

often found adjacent to the apical cellular cementum, where few blood vessels are located (Fig. 2.47). As an osteogenic stimulating effect of CGRP on bone colonies *in vitro* has been observed [4], CGRP-containing fibers located adjacent to cementum might possess a stimulating effect on the apical cementum. These fibers may carry SP and CGRP. They are frequently observed on the exact border between PDL and cellular cementum where some form round, coiled, nerve-like endings. Others are closely associated with periodontal epithelial rests of Malassez's cells (Fig. 2.47) [44, 60]. In the apical part of cat PDL, immunoreactive cells forming a net-like pattern are regularly displayed in Malassez's epithelial rests surrounded by numerous nerve fibers. Some of the cells located in Malassez's rests are shown to contain CGRP and SP. Thus, in common with epithelium from other locations [23,91], it seems the Malassez's epithelium comprises cells that may be classified as endocrine cells due to their content of neuropeptides.

2.9 Cementum

Cementum is the avascular, mineralized connective tissue that covers the root of the tooth. Fine Sharpey's fibers representing the terminal fibers of the PDL, penetrate the cementum (Fig. 2.46). The coronal half of the cementum is typically acellular while the apical part has cementocytes embedded in its matrix.

The thickness of the cellular cementum increases with age. Compensatory cementum deposition occurs in the apical area to counterbalance occlusal attrition. Occasionally cementum formation may exceed this physiologic limit and result in hypercementosis, which may affect a single tooth or all the teeth. Local abnormal thickening of the cementum may be found in connection with chronic periapical inflammation. A more generalized hypercementosis may be associated with certain systemic disorders. Cementomas, cement-producing tumors, have also been described. If a root fractures, cementum may form between the root fragments and at the peripheral site of the fracture. If root resorption occurs, repair of the defects by cellular cementum formation may take place.

Cementicles may be found free in the PDL or as attached cementicles (Fig. 2.48). They may be formed by mineralization of degenerating epithelial rests or from thrombosed vessels. When present, cementicles are often found on most teeth.

2.9.1 Cementum structure

Two types of collagen fibers are found in cementum, matrix fibers and Sharpey's fibers. The matrix fibers are oriented parallel to the root surface and they are interwoven with the Sharpey's fibers which represent the termination of the principal fibers of the PDL. The matrix fibers are formed by the cementoblasts while Sharpey's fibers are formed by the fibroblasts in the PDL. When the position of the tooth is altered, e.g., during tooth eruption or as a result of orthodontic tooth movement, new attachment of periodontal fibers will take place and the fibers in the cementum will be oriented at different angles to the surface.

The cellular components of cementum include cementoblasts and cementocytes. The cementoblasts that line the root surface have all the ultrastructural characteristics of cells capable of synthesizing collagen and protein–polysaccharide complexes. The cementocytes are harbored in lacunae that are embedded in the matrix of the cellular cementum. They have relatively few organelles; this signifies a low functional activity.

The ground substance contains protoglycans and glycoproteins like other periodontal tissues.

The precementum is a thin unmineralized layer that covers the cementum. It prevents, up to a certain point, the root from resorption. If it mineralizes, root resorption may occur.

2.10 Alveolar bone

The alveolar bone is that part of the alveolar processes of the mandible and maxilla which line the alveoli for the teeth (Fig. 2.50). It has all the features of cortical bone and it is further characterized by harboring the Sharpey's fibers from the PDL. Alveolar bone has numerous channels for blood and lymph vessels (Volkmann's canals) from the cancellous bone to the PDL and it is, therefore, often referred to as the cribriform plate. Despite all the channels passing, it appears as a radiopaque line on clinical radiographs (Fig. 2.51a), which gives it the name lamina dura. It is an important diagnostic landmark. A breach in its continuity on radiographs may be a sign of resorption, often associated with pulp infection or periodontal disease. However, the degree of mineralization of the alveolar bone is no different from that of the rest of the cortical bone in the alveolar process (Fig. 2.51b). Apparently the tangential superimposition of the alveolar bone on radiographs gives the lamina dura its characteristic radiodensity.

The buccal and lingual laminae of the alveolar processes of the mandible and maxilla vary depending on the location within the jaw. The buccal (vestibular) lamina is usually thinner than the lingual (palatal) lamina, except in the molar region of the mandible where the lingual lamina is the thinner of the two. This relationship is important to keep in mind when teeth are extracted and for draining abscesses from periapical areas since they tend to follow the path of least resistance. The close relationship between the alveoli and the maxillary sinus (Fig. 2.52a) is also

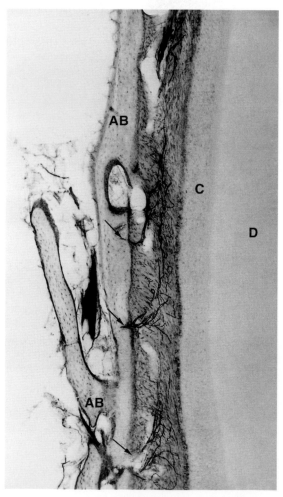

Fig. 2.49 Section through the periodontal ligament from apical third of cat canine showing numerous nerve fibers (arrows) approaching the ligament from alveolar bone (AB) (D, dentin; C, cementum). (Reproduced from [44] with permission from *Acta Odontologica Scandinavica*.)

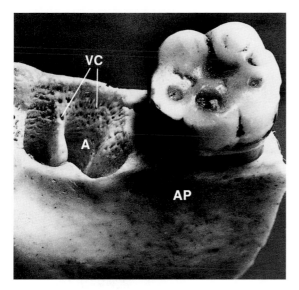

Fig. 2.50 Alveolus with Volkmann's canals (VC) perforating the alveolar bone (AP, alveolar process of the mandible). (Reproduced from [69] with permission from Munksgaard.)

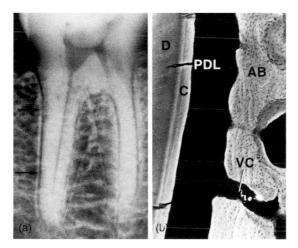

Fig. 2.51 (a) Radiograph of a molar tooth showing the radiodense alveolar bone (arrows) which gives it the name lamina dura. (b) Microradiograph of a ground section showing dentin (D), cementum (C), periodontal ligament space (PDL) and alveolar bone (AB) (VC, Volkmann's canal).

of importance during surgical extractions, implant placement and endodontic procedures. (Fig. 2.52b).

2.10.1 Alveolar bone structure

The alveolar bone has all the basic characteristics of bone tissue, including osteoblasts, osteocytes and

osteoclasts (Fig. 2.53). Its development is closely associated with the presence of teeth. If teeth are lost, the alveolar bone undergoes resorption. It should also be kept in mind that if teeth do not erupt, no alveolar bone will develop.

Osteoblasts are matrix-producing cells, with a well-developed Golgi apparatus, granular endoplasmic reticulum and mitochondria. Osteoblasts that become embedded in the bone matrix are referred to as osteocytes. They lose many of their organelles, but they maintain cytoplasmic contact with neighboring osteocytes. Collagen formation may take place in the periosteocytic space between the osteocytes and the wall of the lacunae. Mineralization of the lacunae

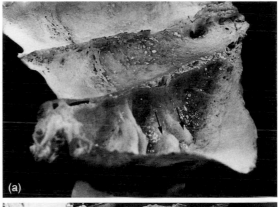

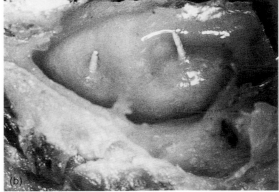

Fig. 2.52 (a) A split maxilla at the level of the hard palate showing apices of the roots of the first permanent molar (arrows) extending into the maxillary sinus. Reproduced from [69] with permission from Munksgaard. (b) A dissected specimen from a series of experimental endodontic procedures on monkeys showing perforation into the maxillary sinus by gutta-percha points. (Courtesy of Dr D. Ørstavik and Dr I.A. Mjör.)

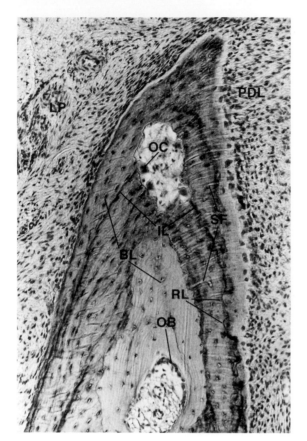

Fig. 2.53 Demineralized section showing human alveolar crest and adjacent tissues (PDL, periodontal ligament; OB, osteoblasts; SF, Sharpey's fibers; LP, lamina propria of attached gingiva; BL, bone lacunae with osteocytes, OC osteoclast; IL incremental lines; RL, reversal lines). (Courtesy of Dr K. Reitan.)

may occur, resulting in "plugged lacunae". Osteolysis may also occur in the lacunae and it represents a part of the mineral metabolism of bone tissue. However, the main part of the turnover associated with bone remodeling involves osteoclastic activity (Fig. 2.53) and new bone formation by osteoblasts.

The normal turnover rate results in bone tissue of different ages in the alveolar processes. Osteons with different degrees of mineralization are found (Fig. 2.51b). Bone lamella which are the incremental growth lines of bone tissue, are discernible. Osteoid is present anywhere bone formation takes place, but it does not cover fully formed bone. The unmineralized core of the relatively thick Sharpey's fibers inserting into the alveolar bone gives it a striated appearance in microradiographs (Fig. 2.45c).

2.11 References

1. Aars H (1982) The influence of vascular β-adreno-receptors on the position and mobility of the rabbit incisor tooth. *Acta Physiologica Scandinavica* **116**, 423–8.
2. Avery J (1981) Repair potential of the pulp. *Journal of Endodontics* **7**, 205–12.
3. Basu S, Sarkar C, Chakroborty D, Nagy J, Mitra RB, Dasgupta PS, Mukhopadhyay D (2004) Ablation of peripheral dopaminergic nerves stimulates malignant tumor growth by inducing vascular permeability factor/vascular endothelial growth factor-mediated angiogenesis. *Cancer Research* **64**, 5551–5.
4. Bernard GW, Shih C (1990) The osteogenic stimulating effect of neuroactive calcitonon gene-related peptide. *Peptides* **11**, 625–32.
5. Bishop M, Malhotra M (1990) An investigation of lymphatic vessels in the feline dental pulp. *American Journal of Anatomy* **187**, 247–53.
6. Bletsa A, Heyeraas KJ, Haug SR, Berggreen E (2004). IL-1 alpha and TNF-alpha expression in rat periapical lesions and dental pulp after unilateral sympathectomy. *Neuroimmunomodulation* **11**, 376–84.
7. Blottner D, Baumgarten HG (1994) Neurotrophy and regeneration in vivo. *Acta Anatomica* **150**, 235–45.
8. Brain SD, Williams TJ, Tippins JR, *et al.* (1985) Calcitonin gene-related peptide is a potent vasodilator. *Nature* **313**, 54–6.
9. Brännström MA (1963) A hydrodynamic mechanism in the transmission of pain-producing stimuli through the dentine. In: Anderson DJ, editor. *Sensory mechanisms in dentine.* Oxford: Pergamon Press, pp. 73–9.
10. Bråtveit M (1991) Regional differences in mechanisms for peptidergic vasodilation in the rat. Thesis. University of Bergen, Bergen.
11. Byers MR (1984) Dental sensory receptors. *International Review in Neurobiology* **25**, 39–94.
12. Byers MR (1985) Sensory innervation of periodontal ligament of rat molars consists of unencapsulated Ruffini-like mechanoreceptors and free nerve endings. *Journal of Comparative Neurology* **231**, 500–18.
13. Byers MR (1992) Effects of inflammation on dental sensory nerves and vice versa. *Proceedings of the Finnish Dental Society* **88**, Suppl I, 499–506.
14. Byers MR, Dong WK (1989) Comparison of trigeminal receptor location and structure in periodontal ligament of different types of teeth from rat, cat and monkey. *Journal of Comparative Neurology* **278**, 117–27.
15. Byers MR, Taylor PE, Khayat BG, Kimberly CL (1990) Effects of injury and inflammation on pulpal and periapical nerves. *Journal of Endodontics* **16**, 78–84.
16. Csillag M, Berggreen E, Fristad I, Haug SR, Bletsa A, Heyeraas KJ (2004). Effect of electrical tooth stimulation on blood flow and immunocompetent cells in rat dental pulp after sympathectomy. *Acta Odontologica Scandinavica* **62**, 305–12.
17. Dahl E, Mjör IA (1973) The fine structure of the vessels in the human dental pulp. *Acta Odontologica Scandinavica* **31**, 223–30.

18. Dahl E, Mjör IA (1973) The structure and distribution of nerves in the pulp-dentin organ. *Acta Odontologica Scandinavica* **31**, 349–56.

19. Edwall B (1987) Experimental studies on blood flow regulation in oral tissues. Thesis, Karolinska Institutet, Stockholm.

20. Edwall B, Gazelius B, Fazekas A, Theodorsson-Norheim E, Lundberg JM (1985) Neuropeptide Y (NPY) and sympathetic control of blood flow in oral mucosa and dental pulp in cat. *Acta Physiologica Scandinavica* **125**, 253–64.

21. Edwall L, Kindlova M (1971) The effect of sympathetic nerve stimulation on the rate of disappearance of tracers from various oral tissue. *Acta Odontologica Scandinavica* **29**, 387–400.

22. Elenkov IJ, Wilder RL, Chrousos GP, Vizi ES (2000). The sympathetic nerve – an integrative interface between two supersystems: the brain and the immune system. *Pharmacology Review* **52**, 595–638.

23. English KB, Wang ZZ, Stayner N, Stensaas LJ, Martin H, Tuckett R (1992) Serotonin-like immunoreactivity in Merkel cells and their afferent neurons in touch domes from hairy skin of rats. *Anatomical Record* **232**, 112–20.

24. Eskandari F, Sternberg EM (2002) Neural-immune interactions in health and disease. *Annals of New York Academy of Science* **966**, 20–7.

25. Feher E, Csanyi K, Vajda J (1979) Ultrastructure and degeneration analysis of the nerve fibers of the tooth pulp in the cat. *Archives of Oral Biology* **22**, 699–704.

26. Foreman JC, Jordan CC (1984) Neurogenic inflammation. *Trends in Pharmacological Science* **5**, 116–19.

27. Furseth R (1967) A microradiographic and electron microscopic study of the cementum of human deciduous teeth. *Acta Odontologica Scandinavica* **25**, 613–45.

28. Furseth R (1971) The fine structure of the odontoblast/predentin area in the root. *Scandinavian Journal of Dental Research* **79**, 141–50.

29. Gazelius B (1981) Studies on the release and effects of putative mediators of pain in the dental pulp. Thesis. Department of Pharmacology, Karolinska Institutet, Stockholm.

30. Gazelius B, Edwall B, Olgart L, Lundberg JM, Hökfelt T, Fischer JA (1987) Vasodilatory effects and coexistence of calcitonin gene-related peptide (CGRP) and substance P in sensory nerves in cat dental pulp. *Acta Physiologica Scandinavica* **130**, 33–40.

31. Gilhuus-Moe O, Kvam E (1972) Behavior of the epithelial rests of Malassez following experimental movement of rat molars. *Acta Odontologica Scandinavica* **30**, 139–49.

32. Hanko J, Hardebo JE, Kåhrström J, Owman C, Sundler F (1985) Calcitonin gene-related peptide is present in mammalian cerebrovascular nerve fibres and dilates pial and peripheral arteries. *Neuroscience Letters* **57**, 91–105.

33. Haug SR, Heyeraas KJ (2006) Modulation of dental inflammation by the sympathetic nervous system. *Journal of Dental Research* **85**, 488–95.

34. Haug SR, Heyeraas KJ (2005) Immunoglobulin producing cells in the rat dental pulp after unilateral sympathectomy. *Neuroscience* **136**, 571–7.

35. Haug SR, Heyeraas KJ (2003) Effects of sympathectomy on experimentally induced pulpal inflammation and periapical lesions in rats. *Neuroscience* **120**, 827–36.

36. Haug SR, Brudvik P, Fristad I, Heyeraas KJ (2003) Sympathectomy causes increased root resorption after orthodontic tooth movement in rats: immunohistochemical study. *Cell Tissue Research* **313**, 167–75.

37. Heyeraas KJ, Jacobsen EB, Fristad I, Raab WH-M (1996) Vascular and immunoreactive nerve fibre reactions in the pulp after stimulation and denervation. *Proceedings of the International Conference on Dentin/Pulp Complex*, pp. 162–8. Chicago, IL: Quintessence.

38. Heyeraas KJ, Kim S, Raab WH-M, Byers MR, Liu M (1994) Effect of electrical tooth stimulation on blood flow, interstitial fluid pressure and substance P and CGRP-immunoreactive nerve fibres in the low compliant cat dental pulp. *Microvascular Research* **47**, 329–43.

39. Heyeraas Tønder K (1975) The effect of variations in arterial blood pressure and baroreceptor reflexes on pulpal blood flow in dogs. *Archives of Oral Biology* **20**, 345–9.

40. Heyeraas Tønder K (1980) Blood flow and vascular pressure in the dental pulp. *Acta Odontologica Scandinavica* **38**, 135–44.

41. Heyeraas Tønder KJ (1989) Pulpal hemodynamics and interstitial fluid pressure: Balance of transmicrovascular fluid transport. *Journal of Endodontics* **15**, 468–72.

42. Heyeraas Tønder KJ, Kvinnsland L (1983) Micropuncture measurements of interstitial fluid pressure in normal and inflamed dental pulp in cats. *Journal of Endodontics* **9**, 105–9.

43. Heyeraas Tønder KJ, Kvinnsland I (1992) Tissue pressure and blood flow in pulpal inflammation. *Proceedings of the Finnish Dental Society* **88** Suppl I, 393–401.

44. Heyeraas Tønder KJ, Kvinnsland I, Byers MR, Jacobsen EB (1993) Nerve fibres immunoreactive to protein gene product 9.5, calcitonin gene-related peptide, substance P, and Neuropeptide Y in the dental pulp, periodontal ligament, and gingiva in cats. *Acta Odontologica Scandinavica* **51**, 207–21.

45. Heyeraas Tønder K, Næss G (1978) Nervous control of blood flow in the dental pulp in dogs. *Acta Physiologica Scandinavica* **104**, 13–23.

46. Holland GR (1985) The odontoblast process: Form and function. *Journal of Dental Research* **64** (Special Issue), 499–514.

47. Holzer P (1988) Local effector functions of capsaicin-sensitive sensory nerve endings: Involvement of tachykinins, calcitonin gene-related peptide and other neuropeptides. *Neuroscience* **24**, 739–68.

48. Inoki R, Kudo T (1986) Enkephalins and bradykinin in dental pulp. *Trends in Pharmacological Science* **7**, 275–7.

49. Ishida-Yamsmoto A, Tohyama M (1989) Calcitonin gene-related peptide in the nervous tissue. *Progress in Neurobiology* **33**, 335–86.

50. Jontell M, Gunraj M, Bergenholtz G (1987) Immunocompetent cells in the normal dental pulp. *Journal of Dental Research* **66**, 1149–53.

51. Karita K, Izumi H, Tabata T, Kuriwada S, Sasano T, Sanjo D (1989) The blood flow in the periodontal ligament regulated by the sympathetic and sensory nerves

in the cat. *Proceedings of the Finnish Dental Society* **85**, 289–94.

52. Kerezoudis NP (1993) The roles of afferent and efferent nerves in vascular reactions in oral tissues. An experimental study in the rat. Thesis, Departments of Physiology, Pharmacology and Endodontics, Karolinska Institutet, Stockholm.

53. Kim S (1981) Regulations of blood flow of the dental pulp: macrocirculation and microcirculations studies. Dissertation, Columbia University, New York.

54. Kimberly CL, Byers MR (1988) Inflammation of rat molar pulp and periodontium causes increased calcitonon gene-related peptide and axonal sprouting. *Anatomical Record* **222**, 289–300.

55. Köling A (1983) Membrane structures in the human pulp-dentin organ. An electron microscopic investigation of permanent teeth using freeze fracture technique. Thesis, Uppsala University, Uppsala.

56. Kristiansen AB, Heyeraas KJ (1989) Micropuncture measurements of interstitial fluid pressure in the rat periodontal ligament. *Proceedings of the Finnish Dental Society* **85**, 295–300.

57. Ladizesky MG, Cutrera RA, Boggio V, Mautalen C, Cardinali DP (2000) Effect of unilateral superior cervical ganglionectomy on bone mineral content and density of rat's mandible. *Journal Autonomic Nervous System* **78**, 113–16.

58. Lambrichts I, Creemers J, Van Steenberghe D (1993) Periodontal neural endings intimately related to epithelial rests of Malassez in humans. *Journal of Anatomy* **82**, 153–62.

59. Lewis T (1927) *The blood vessels of the human skin and their responses*. London: Shaw & Sons.

60. Linden RWA (1990) Periodontal mechanoreceptors and their functions. In Taylor A, editor. *Neurophysiology of the jaws and teeth*, pp. 52–95. London: Macmillan Press.

61. Lindskog S, Blomlöf L, Hammarström L (1988) Evidence for a role of odontogenic epithelium in maintaining the periodontal space. *Journal of Clinical Periodontology* **15**, 371–3.

62. Lotz M, Vaughan JH, Carson D (1988) Effect of neuropeptides on production of inflammatory cytokines by human monocytes. *Science* **241**, 1218–21.

63. Matthews B (1992) Sensory physiology: a reaction. *Proceedings of the Finnish Dental Society* **88** Suppl I, 529–32.

64. McEwans J, Legon S, Wimalwansa S, *et al.* (1989) Calcitonin gene-related peptide: A review of its biology and relevance to the cardiovascular system. In Laragh JH, Brenner BM, Kaplan NM, editors. *Endocrine mechanisms in hypertension*, pp. 287–306. New York: Raven Press.

65. Mjör IA (1966) Microradiography of human coronal dentine. *Archives of Oral Biology* **11**, 225–34.

66. Mjör IA (1966) Relationship between microradiography and stainability of human coronal dentine. *Archives of Oral Biology* **11**, 1317–23.

67. Mjör IA (1983) Effects of operative procedures on the dentin and the pulp-dentin interface. *Proceedings, University of Michigan Dental Research Institute Symposium*, pp. 35–49.

68. Mjör IA (1986a) Dentin and pulp. In: *Human oral embryology and histology*, pp. 90–130. Mjör IA, Fejerskov O, editors. Copenhagen: Munksgaard.

69. Mjör IA (1986) The maxillary sinus. In: *Human oral embryology and histology*, pp. 296–301. Mjör IA, Fejerskov O, editors. Copenhagen: Munksgaard.

70. Mjör IA, Nordahl I (1996) The density and branching of dentinal tubules in human teeth. *Archives of Oral Biology* **41**, 401–12.

71. Mjör IA, Smith MR, Ferrari M, Mannocci F (2001) The structure of dentine in the apical region of human teeth. *International Endodontic Journal* **34**, 346–53.

72. Nicolay OF, Davidovitch Z, Shanfield JL, Alley K (1990) Substance P immunoreactivity in periodontal tissues during orthodontic tooth movement. *Bone Mineralization* **11**, 19–29.

73. Nilsson J, von Euler AM, Dalsgaard CJ (1985) Stimulation of connective tissue cell growth by substance P and substance K. *Nature* **315**, 61–3.

74. Olgart L (1992) Involvement of sensory nerves in hemodynamic reactions. *Proceedings of the Finnish Dental Society* **88** Suppl I, 403–18.

75. Olgart L, Gazelius B, Brodin E, Nilsson G (1977) Release of substance P-like immunoreactivity from dental pulp. *Acta Physiologica Scandinavica* **101**, 510–12.

76. Oswald RJ, Byers MR (1993) The injury response of pulpal NPY-Ir sympathetic fibres differs from that of sensory fibres. *Neuroscience Letters* **164**, 190–4.

77. Palcanis KG (1973) Effect of occlusal trauma on interstitial pressure in the periodontal ligament. *Journal of Dental Research* **52**, 903–10.

78. Payan DG (1985) Receptor-mediated mitogenic effects of substance P on cultured smooth muscle cells. *Biochemical and Biophysical Research Communications* **130**, 104–9.

79. Payan DG, McGillis JP, Groetzl EJ (1986) Neuroimmunology. *Advances in Immunology* **39**, 299–318.

80. Saito I, Ishii K, Hanada K, Sato O, Maeda T (1991) Responses of calcitonin gene-related peptide-immunopositive nerve fibres in the periodontal ligament of rat molars to experimental tooth movement. *Archives of Oral Biology* **36**, 689–92.

81. Sandhu HS, Herskovits MS, Singh IJ (1987) Effect of surgical sympathectomy on bone remodeling at rat incisor and molar root sockets. *Anatomical Record* **219**, 32–8.

82. Silvermann JD, Kruger L (1987) An interpretation of dental innervation based upon the pattern of calcitonin gene-related peptide (CGRP)-immunoreactive thin sensory axons. *Somatosensory Research* **5**, 157–75.

83. Skofitsch G, Savitt JM, Jacobowitz DM (1985) Suggestive evidence for a functional unit between mast cells and substance P fibres in the rat diaphragm and mesentery. *Histochemistry* **82**, 5–6.

84. Spouge JD (1980) A new look at the rests of Malassez. A review of their embryological origin, anatomy, and possible role in periodontal health and disease. *Journal of Periodontology* **51**, 437–44.

85. Stanley HR (1981) *Human pulp response to restorative dental procedures*, p. 29. Gainesville, FL: Storter Printing Co.

86. Stenvik A, Iversen J, Mjör IA (1972) Tissue pressure and histology of normal and inflamed tooth pulps in Macaque monkeys. *Archives of Oral Biology* **17**, 1501–11.
87. Stenvik A, Mjör IA (1970) Epithelial remnants and denticle formation in the human dental pulp. *Acta Odontologica Scandinavica* **28**, 721–8.
88. Takahashi K, Kishi Y, Kim S (1982) An electronmicroscopic study of the blood vessels of dog pulps using corrosion casts. *Journal of Endodontics* **8**, 131–5.
89. Thomas HF (1985) The dentin–predentin complex: Anatomical overview. *Journal of Dental Research* **64**, 607–12.
90. Todoki K (1988) Effect of vasoactive substances and electric stimulation of the inferior alveolar nerve on blood flow in the dental pulp in dogs. *Nippon Yakurigaku Zasshi* **82**, 61–7.
91. Turner DF (1983) The morphology and distribution of Merkel cells in primate gingival mucosa. *Anatomical Record* **205**, 197–205.
92. van Hassel JH (1971) Physiology of the human dental pulp. *Oral Surgery, Oral Medicine, Oral Pathology* **32**, 126–34.
93. Vizi ES, Elenkov IJ (2002) Nonsynaptic noradrenaline release in neuro-immune responses. *Acta Biologica Hungarian* **53**, 229–44
94. Vongsavan N, Matthews B (1992) Changes in pulpal blood flow and fluid flow through dentin produced by autonomic and sensory nerve stimulation in the cat. *Proceedings of the Finnish Dental Society* **88** Suppl I, 491–7.
95. Walker TW, Ng GC, Burke PS (1978) Fluid pressure in the periodontal ligament of the mandibular canine tooth in dogs. *Archives of Oral Biology* **23**, 753–65.
96. Wennberg A, Mjör IA, Heide S (1982) Rate of formation of regular and irregular secondary dentin in monkey teeth. *Oral Surgery, Oral Medicine, Oral Pathology* **54**, 232–7.
97. Wesselink P, Beertsen W (1993) The prevalence and distribution of rests of Malassez in the mouse molar and their possible role in repair and maintenance of the periodontal ligament. *Archives of Oral Biology* **38**, 399–403.
98. Zukowska-Grojec Z, Karwatowska-Prokopczuk E, Fisher TA, Ji H (1998) Mechanisms of vascular growth-promoting effects of neuropeptide Y: role of its inducible receptors. *Regulation of Peptides* **75–76**, 231–8.

Chapter 3

Immunopathological Aspects of Pulpal and Periapical Inflammations

Nobuyuki Kawashima and Hideaki Suda

3.1 Introduction

Dental pulp is encased by hard tissues – enamel and dentin – that act as physical and mechanical barriers against antigenic challenges from the oral cavity [31]. Enamel and dentin are similar to the stratum corneum in the skin epidermis, which faces the outside of the body and protects the integrity of the inner components. The epidermis is equipped with an immunosurveillance system composed of Langerhans cells, dendritic cells (DCs) and T cells, so that it can catch and remove exogenous invaders [71]. Dental pulp possesses a similar immunosurveillance system consisting of DCs, macrophages and natural killer (NK) cells, and is prepared to fight against antigenic challenges via the dentinal tubules [123,124,134–7, 139,145,232,237,240,241,256,281,342,358]. When the pulpal surveillance system encounters excessive invasion of exogenous antigens, it evokes pulpal inflammation, which is characterized by inflammatory cell infiltration and the synthesis of various mediators [27, 70,87,149,153,177,180,205,222,223,284]. The initial reactions against such antigenic challenges are mediated by innate immune reactions. However, it is usually difficult for the innate immune system to cope with persistent and severe challenges, and therefore, adaptive immune reactions predominantly mediated by lymphocytes are quickly initiated. Although such defense mechanisms exist in the pulp, severe and long-lasting inflammatory reactions induce irreversible destruction of the dental pulp due to the limited circulation system and low-compliance environment [159]. Once inflammation has progressed in the pulp, the defense lines shift from the dental pulp to the periapical tissues. Specifically, immunocompetent cell infiltration around the apex and alveolar bone resorption are initiated, while the pulp vitality is still retained [150]. Similar to pulpal inflammation, periapical lesions represent inflammatory pathosis, which is characterized by immunocompetent cell infiltration and periapical bone destruction [5,6,10, 18,37,73,86,89,90,95,131–133,143,144,150,169, 181,183,193–195,197,203,239,264,288,294,310,311,317, 318,324,337,352,372]. Periapical lesion progression is also characterized and regulated by chemical mediators [20,23,27,34,60,101,119,151,184,196,204,276,277,312, 320,323,351,353,375], the syntheses and functions of which are controlled by one another. This situation is referred to as "a network of mediators" [154,293–295]. In this chapter, the properties and etiologies of pulpal and periapical inflammations are reviewed.

3.2 Overview of inflammation

3.2.1 Classification of inflammation

Inflammation represents self-defense reactions against infection or irritation. These reactions are mediated by the immune system and characterized by inflammatory cell infiltration and the synthesis of chemical mediators. The immune system is composed of *innate* and *adaptive* systems. In general, accumulation of neutrophils, macrophages and DCs, which are typical components of innate immunity, is observed at the beginning of inflammation. Cells infiltrating inflamed sites or tissues are generically called inflammatory cells, and the number of inflammatory cells and the area of infiltration are related to the volume and properties of the stimuli. Acute inflammation involves temporal host reactions, and is characterized by severe infiltration of such inflammatory cells, which actively synthesize copious chemical mediators. These acute phase proinflammatory chemical mediators induce vasodilation of blood vessels and upregulation of capillary permeability, resulting in loss of blood plasma into tissues, as well as the formation of edema and swelling, which are typical phenomena of acute inflammation. The four principal effects of acute inflammation, namely redness (*rubor*), heat (*calor*), swelling (*tumor*) and pain (*dolor*), were originally described nearly 2000 years ago by Celcus and can be attributed to vasodilation of small blood vessels, increased blood flow, accumulation of fluid in the extravascular space and the synthesis of some specific mediators, respectively. Loss of function (*functio laesa*), which is a well-known consequence of inflammation, was added as a fifth effect by Virchow (1821–1902).

Sustained exogenous stimuli that cannot be removed by phagocytes, such as neutrophils and macrophages,

cause a shift from acute to chronic inflammation. The major components of chronic inflammation are lymphocytes, which belong to adaptive immunity. However, chronic inflammation is sometimes the primary event with no apparent preceding period of acute inflammation. In practice, most acute imflammation in pulp and periapical tissues is a phase conversion of preceding chronic lesions, which may actually be primary lesions.

3.2.2 Innate immunity

Cellular components

The first stage of common pulpal inflammation involves innate immunity, which is characterized by infiltration of phagocytes, such as neutrophils, macrophages and DCs. These cells recognize exogenous antigens, including invading bacteria and their components or byproducts, with low-specific surface receptors, and subsequently engulf and ingest them. Various mediators are synthesized by the infiltrating phagocytes, and these molecules determine the characteristics of inflammation.

Neutrophils. In general, inflammation begins with infiltration of neutrophils, which are mainly adapted for short-term responses. These cells are abundantly observed in blood, but rare in normal tissues. Their lifespan is very short, and they die within a few hours after their production in the bone marrow. They exhibit high mobility and active phagocytosis, and engulf invading exogenous bacteria or their byproducts, which are digested into small peptides by lysosomal enzymes. Typical examples of these enzymes are myeloperoxidase and muramidase, and their release upregulates vascular permeability, thereby promoting further infiltration of neutrophils. C5a and lipopolysaccharide (LPS) are strong chemoattractants for neutrophils. Other chemokines responsible for neutrophil infiltration are related to the so-called CXC chemokines, and include interleukin (IL)-8, growth-regulated oncogene (GRO) alpha, beta and gamma, neutrophil-activating peptide-2, granulocyte chemotactic protein 2 and epithelial cell-derived neutrophil-activating peptide-78 [19]. Neutrophils recognize not only exogenous antigens coated with antibodies, but also bacterial cell walls. CD14 expressed on neutrophils is referred to as LPS-binding protein and is important for LPS recognition. Recently, killing of bacteria or fungi has been reported to be accomplished by movement of ions, which produces vacuolar conditions that lead to microbial killing [280].

Macrophages. Infiltration of macrophages into sites of inflammation is relatively slow compared to that of neutrophils, but they are capable of engulfing and digesting almost any foreign agent, and their infiltration lasts for a longer time. Macrophages develop from monocytes in the blood and move to local tissues. They are phagocytic, and digest exogenous antigens and bacteria in their lysosomes. Mannose receptors (CD206) expressed on their cell surface recognize glycoproteins on bacterial surfaces and contribute to their ability to phagocytose bacteria [3]. Scavenger receptors bind to components of both Gram-positive and -negative bacteria, including LPS and lipoteichoic acids, and further contribute to the ability of macrophages to phagocytose bacteria. Moreover, macrophages promote the clearance of apoptotic cells. Receptors for complement proteins are also expressed on the surface of macrophages, as well as three well-defined receptors for IgG that facilitate the uptake of immune complexes.

Macrophages also express several kinds of toll-like receptors (TLRs), which are members of a family of receptors involved in the recognition of a wide range of microbial molecules [42,128,319,329]. TLRs, which were first identified in *Drosophila* as being related to dorsal–ventral axis determination, are known to be important for the removal of infectious agents. Recently, human homologues have been determined and constitute a family comprised of TLR1 to TLR10. In particular, TLR4 is important for LPS recognition, and its signaling is mediated by myeloid differentiation primary response gene (Myd) 88-dependent or -independent pathways. The Myd88-dependent pathway, which is mediated by IL1 receptor-associated kinase (IRAK) and tumor necrosis factor (TNF) receptor-associated factor (TRAF) 6, finally leads to activation of nuclear factor kappa B (NFκB), which in turn induces further signaling molecules [319]. The Myd88-independent pathway is mainly mediated by c-Jun N-terminal kinase (JNK) and phosphoinositide 3-kinase (PI3K) [319]. TLR signaling eventually induces the productions of inflammatory cytokines, such as IL1, IL6 and TNFα, and chemokines, which represent an effective barrier against the expansion of infection. TLR signals are also important for the expression of costimulatory molecules on DCs [108,214], which are essential for the activation of T cells. A variety of TLRs exist for various kinds of exogenous pathogens,

and the costimulatory functions of DCs differ for each TLR signaling pathway.

Macrophages are a major source of chemical mediators, such as IL1, TNFα and interferon (IFN) γ, which play important roles in the activation or growth promotion of neighboring cells. Recently, macrophages have been classified into two subpopulations, designated M1 and M2, which are similar to Th1 and Th2, respectively [260].

DCs. Neutrophils and macrophages are typical phagocytes, whereas DCs are professional antigen-presenting cells (APCs) that are essential for the activation of T and B cells [21,146,176,211,299,332]. Among the known APCs, only DCs are able to activate naive T cells. DCs, which are derived from hematopoietic stem cells, were named after their dendritic appearance. They are composed of epidermal Langerhans cells, dermal DCs and connective tissue interdigitating cells in non-lymphoid tissues [299], and myeloid DCs (mDCs; CD11b$^+$B220$^-$CD11c$^+$), CD8+ resident DCs (CD8$^+$B220$^-$CD11c$^+$) and plasmacytoid DCs (pDCs; B220$^+$CD11c$^+$) in lymphoid tissues [15,285]. mDCs produce large amounts of IFNγ, and induce Th1 type immune reactions, whereas pDCs synthesize large amounts of type I IFNs.

Immature DCs (iDCs) express low levels of major histocompatibility complex (MHC) class II antigens and costimulatory molecules, such as CD80 and CD86, and possess phagocytic activity. Mature DCs show low phagocytic activity, but express high levels of MHC class II antigens and costimulatory molecules. iDCs that have captured exogenous antigens move to local lymphoid tissues, where they present the antigens conjugated with MHC class II antigens to T cells, thereby inducing their activation. Costimulatory factors are essential for mediating T cell and DC activations. Although the transcription factor T-bet is well known for its role in Th1 cell differentiation, its expression by DCs may also be required for proinflammatory cytokine production and T-cell priming [354]. Recently, DCs have been reported to induce antigen-specific unresponsiveness or tolerance in central lymphoid organs and the periphery [300].

Chemical mediators

Cytokines. Cytokines are soluble low-molecular weight proteins that are mainly produced by immune cells, and regulate systemic or local events in autocrine (active on secreting cell) or paracrine (active on neighboring cells) fashions. Cytokines have been broadly categorized into three groups, proinflammatory, Th1, and Th2 cytokines. *Proinflammatory cytokines* include IL1, IL6, and TNFα, which are mainly produced by macrophages and cause fever [1]. This increase in the body temperature limits the growth of bacteria and simultaneously promotes adaptive immunity. These cytokines are synthesized quite quickly during exogenous antigenic challenges and induce the production of acute phase proteins in the liver. A typical acute phase protein is C-reactive protein (CRP), which works as an opsonin. TNFα is also involved in the homing of lymphocytes to lymph nodes and induces the maturation of DCs, thereby leading to the switch from innate immunity to adaptive immunity. *Th1 cytokines* are defined as those produced by Th1 type helper cells, and major components of Th1 cytokines are IL2, IL12, and IFNγ. IL2 plays roles in the growth of not only T cells but also B and NK cells. IFNγ is especially important for macrophage and NK cell activation, and antiviral activity. It also downregulates Th2 type reactions. IL12, which is mainly produced by macrophages, induces the growth of NK cells and activates T cells. IL12 is an essential cytokine for the activation of Th2 type immunoreactions. *Th2 cytokines* are defined as those produced by Th2 type helper cells, and typical Th2 cytokines are IL4 and IL10. IL4 is essential for the activation, growth and differentiation of B cells. It is also important for the growth and induction of Th2 cells, and the inhibition of macrophage activation. IL10, which is produced by Th2 cells, B cells and macrophages, inhibits macrophage activation, IL12 production and the shift to Th1.

Chemokines. Chemokine is a synthetic word derived from the phrase chemotactic cytokine. The major functions of chemokines are to induce exudation and translocation of leukocytes from blood vessels to specific sites, following the gradient of the chemokine concentration [19]. Chemokines are secretory heparin-binding basic proteins of small molecular weight, that are classified into the following four groups depending on the cysteine motifs close to their N-termini: CXC(L), CC(L), C(L) and CXXXC(L). Each group is usually denoted with "L", representing "ligands", and their specific receptors are denoted with "R". Chemokines are important not only for cellular exudation from blood vessels, but also for the homing of mature naive T cells to lymphoid tissues. CXC chemokines include IL8 and GROs, which are essential for

neutrophil infiltration into tissues. The CC chemokine subfamily contains macrophage inflammatory protein (MIP) 1α, MIP1β, MIP3, regulated upon activation, normal T cell expressed and secreted (RANTES), and monocyte chemoattractant proteins (MCPs), which are important for infiltration of monocytes and T cells. Chemokine receptors appear to span the cell membrane seven times, and are linked to G proteins. Among the chemokine receptors, CCR7 has been the subject of major studies due to its importance in the homing of lymphocytes to lymphoid tissues [298].

Arachidonic acid metabolites. Arachidonic acid is a polyunsaturated fatty acid with twenty carbons and four *cis*-double bonds, and is present in cell membranes [40]. Arachidonic acid metabolites, also called eicosanoids, include prostaglandins (PGs), thromboxanes, prostacyclin and leukotrienes. These metabolites are formed by two major classes of enzymes, namely cyclooxygenases (cox) for prostaglandins and thromboxanes, and lipoxygenases for leukotrienes and lipoxins. They are involved in a variety of biological processes, including inflammation and homeostasis. The cox pathway is mediated by cox1 and cox2. Cox1 is constitutively expressed and has homeostatic functions, whereas cox2 is closely related to inflammatory reactions. The most important PGs in inflammation are PGE2, PGD2, PGF2α, PGI2 and TXA2. PGE2 mediates vasodilation, modulates sensitivity to pain and is related to osteoclast activation. The most common antiinflammatory drugs used in the clinic are nonsteroidal antiinflammatory drugs (NSAIDs), which are cox inhibitors.

Nitric oxide. NO, a short-lived endogenously produced gas, is highly soluble in lipids and therefore readily diffuses across the cell membrane to interact with many other molecules, including reactive oxygen species such as superoxide [121]. It acts in a paracrine or even autocrine fashion, but only affects cells near its point of synthesis [121]. Furthermore, it is a biological effector molecule or signaling molecule in various systems, and essential for these systems in the body [208]. NO is synthesized from arginine by a group of enzymes called nitric oxide synthases (NOSs), with the aid of molecular oxygen and the reduced form of nicotinamide adenine dinucleotide phosphate (NADPH). Three NOS isoforms have been characterized, namely neuronal NOS (nNOS), endothelial NOS (eNOS) and inducible NOS (iNOS) [191].

nNOS and eNOS are produced constitutively, while iNOS is induced in response to inflammatory stimuli, such as LPS and cytokines. Once iNOS is induced, it can produce copious quantities of NO for a prolonged period [208], further affecting the synthesis of chemical mediators, such as IL1 [112], IL6 [212], IL12 [265], TNFα [212] and PGs [257].

Neuropeptides. Neuropeptides, defined as any peptides produced in and by the neuronal system, function as neurotransmitters or ubiquitous chemical mediators [115]. Substance P (SP), which belongs to the tachykinin neuropeptide family, is related to mood disorders, anxiety, stress and pain in the central nervous system, as well as pain, vascular modulation and immunological reactions in local tissues. The biological effects of SP, neurokinin A (NKA; substance K) and neurokinin B (NKB; neurokinin K) are mediated by three distinct receptors, designated NK1, NK2 and NK3, which are probably associated with G proteins that activate phosphatidylinositol-calcium second messenger systems [39,72,116]. The presence of NK1 at sites of inflammation was reported to be important for the functions of SP [38]. In addition, some NK1 and calcitonin gene-related peptide (CGRP) 1 receptor molecules are located close to odontoblasts in dental pulp tissues [94]. NKA and NKB are also members of the tachykinin family and arise via cleavage of SP precursors. These peptides are widely distributed in both the central and peripheral nervous systems. The biological actions of NKA are similar to those of SP, including vasodilation and stimulation of smooth muscle contraction. NK2 and NK3 are the major receptors for NKA and NKB, respectively [188].

CGRP is a 37-amino acid residue peptide derived from alternative splicing of the calcitonin gene in a tissue-specific manner, and may exist in two forms, a and b, with similar biological functions [9]. This peptide is widely distributed in both the central and peripheral nervous systems [114,347]. There are two G protein-coupled CGRP receptors, namely CGRP1 and CGRP2, and their signal transduction is modified by receptor activity-modifying protein 1 (RAMP1) and receptor component protein (RCP) [47,84,201,360]. The major function of CGRP involves vascular modulation.

Neuropeptide Y (NPY) is the most abundant neuropeptide in the brain [8], and its biological functions are associated with feeding behavior, circadian rhythms and vascular resistance [82,279]. It also acts as a vaso-constrictor of local blood flow. Vasoactive intestinal peptide (VIP) is a 28-amino acid peptide structurally related to secretin [271,272,283], and exerts many biological effects through interactions with the serpentine class II G protein-coupled receptors VIPR1 and VIPR2 [122,289,321]. It was originally isolated from intestinal extracts, and found to be a potent vasodilator that causes smooth muscle relaxation. It is widely distributed in the central and peripheral nervous systems. Recently, VIP was reported to be produced by Th2 cells [76], and to function as an antiinflammatory modulator [258].

Kinins. Kinins are peptides of 9–11 amino acids. Bradykinin (BK) is a potent vasodilator [81] that upregulates vascular permeability [302]. It is also involved in pain sensation.

Defensin. Defensin is a basic peptide of around 30 amino acids, which contains six cysteine residues and intramolecular disulfide bonds [365]. Defensin creates holes in bacterial membranes, inducing bactericidal effects.

3.2.3 Adaptive immunity

The initial immune reactions are mediated by innate immunity, in which neutrophils and macrophages play leading roles. However, continuous or severe infections at levels beyond the capacity of innate immunity are mediated by adaptive immunity, which is much more specific toward exogenous antigens. Adaptive immunity is also called specific immunity, and possesses the ability to memorize and respond more vigorously to repeated exposures to the same antigen. The major components of adaptive immunity are T and B cells (lymphocytes).

T cells

T cells are classified into two categories according to their surface T cell receptors (TCRs), which are either the αβ or γδ type. Although the functions of TCRγδ-expressing cells are still uncertain, they are reportedly related to nonspecific defense systems against exogenous stimuli [57,107]. TCRαβ-expressing cells are generally classified into CD4-positive helper cells and CD8-positive effector cells. CD4-positive cells are further classified into Th1 and Th2 cells [182]. Th1 cells mainly produce IFNγ and IL2 and have roles in cellular immunity, while Th2 cells produce IL4, IL5 and IL10 and promote antibody synthesis from B cells, thereby playing roles in humoral immunity. The master molecule that induces Th1 cells is T-bet [313], while GATA binding protein 3 (GATA3) is essential for the induction of Th2 cells [374]. Recently, a third population of T cells regulating immune responses has been reported and designated CD4$^+$ regulatory T (Treg) cells. These naturally occurring cells, most of which constitutively produce CD25, actively suppress the activation and expansion of self-reactive T lymphocytes that have escaped thymic clonal deletion in the periphery [67,190,272]. Treg cells, which were named after their regulatory function on immunological reactions, are also a member of CD4$^+$ T cell lineages, and they are characterized by the expression of CD25 and a transcriptional factor, forkhead box P3 (Foxp3) [117]. Treg cells may be related to autoimmune diseases [261,274] and cancer immunity [228]. Recently, a new lineage of CD4$^+$ T cells, Th17 cells, has been reported [106]. Th17 cells are characterized by the expression of IL17 and also express IL6, TNF and GM-CSF but neither IFNγ nor IL4 [105,245]. Development of Th17 is promoted by IL6, IL23 and TGFβ, although IL23 may be involved in expanding and maintaining this population of cells rather than differentiation [326]. Th1 cytokine (IFNγ) and Th2 cytokine (IL4) down-regulate the development of Th17, but most prominent suppressor may be IL27, which repressed *de novo* Th17 cell differentiation driven by IL6 and TGFβ in a signal transducer and activator of transcription 1 (STAT-1)-dependent way [26,305]. Th17 cells influence inflammatory responses, including defense against extracellular bacteria, autoimmunity and cancer [326]. CD8-positive cells are known as cytotoxic T cells (CTLs). The initial binding of these cells to targets is mediated by adhesive molecules, and further processing is exclusively promoted by specific interactions between the antigens and their TCRs. When CTLs recognize target antigens, they induce cell death by means of granule- and FAS-mediated pathways. The granule-mediated pathways are induced by the pore-forming molecule perforin, which was initially thought to merely damage the target cell membrane, and mediated by the release of granzyme B that has a preference for the initiation of proteolytic cleavage [25]. CTLs also produce several cytokines, such as TNFα and IFNγ, that have cytotoxic effects when secreted in the vicinity of target cells.

B cells

B cells are generated in the bone marrow from pluripotent hematopoietic stem cells [202]. The principal events during the development and maturation of B cells are the expressions of various cell-surface markers or other molecules and the rearrangement of immunoglobulin genes. The first functional B cells are known as immature B cells, and are defined by the expression of immunoglobulin (Ig) M on their cell surface. Immature B cells exit the bone marrow and enter the spleen, where they further differentiate through several transitional stages and eventually become mature follicular or marginal-zone B cells. These cells can also undergo terminal differentiation to become plasma cells, which work as antibody-producing cells [199].

3.3 The defense system in dental pulp and periapical tissues

3.3.1 The defense system in dental pulp

Dental pulp is a unique connective tissue with a specific anatomical arrangement dictated by its position inside a rigid chamber and its role of forming a hard tissue on the wall of the chamber [31]. The rigid chamber of enamel and dentin is a physical and mechanical protector of the pulp tissues against invaders from outside of the body. Odontoblasts are responsible for dentin deposition, which is a mechanical defense system for dental pulp.

Cellular defense systems against exogenous invasion are present in dental pulp (Fig. 3.1). In normal pulp, the presence of an immunosurveillance system composed of various immunocompetent cells has been reported. Specifically, MHC class II antigen-expressing cells, including DCs and macrophages, were identified in normal pulp of both rodent [49,125, 134–137,139,232,237,240,342] and human [123,124, 234,241,273,281] teeth.

Numerous MHC class II antigen-expressing cells, which are mostly professional APCs and a mixed population of activated macrophages and DCs, are localized in the odontoblastic layer or para-odontoblastic layer. This corresponds to strategic areas where foreign antigens initially enter the pulp tissues. Penetration of their cytoplasmic processes into the dentinal tubules is sometimes observed, and is thought

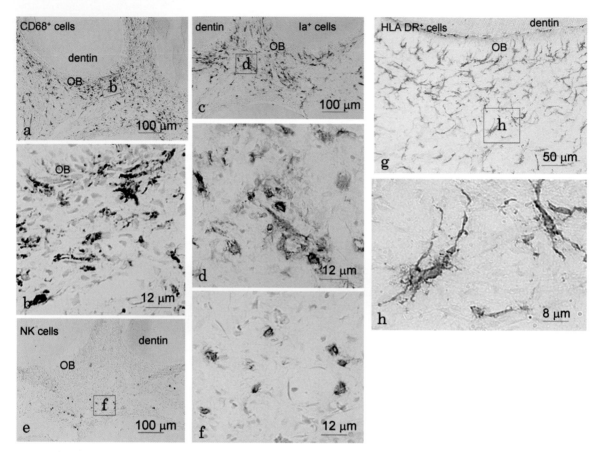

Fig. 3.1 Immunodefense system in normal pulp. Numerous CD68$^+$ cells (a, b) corresponding to macrophages/DCs and Ia$^+$ cells (c, d) are observed in rat normal pulp. These cells show various morphologies, such as oval, polygonal, spindle and dendritic. Numerous HLA-DR$^+$ cells are also observed in human normal pulp (g, h), and many of these extend dendritic cellular processes (photographs courtesy of Dr Sakurai). Many of the cells are located in the odontoblastic and sub-odontoblastic layers, suggesting that they are present in the pulp tissues to catch exogenous invaders via dentinal tubules. Although these cells may be able to remove a small number of antigenic challenges, specific immunological reactions by professional immune components, such as T cells, are induced when the challenge surpasses their capacity (Fig. 3.7) NK and NKT cells, members of the innate immune system, are predominantly located in the center of pulp tissues (e, f). OB: odontoblasts. (From Kawashima N *et al.* 2006 [154].)

to catch foreign antigens [233,234,266]. APCs activate Th cells, CTLs and B cells by presenting them with antigens derived from exogenous invaders. MHC class II antigen-expressing cells in rat dental pulp are capable of presenting antigens to Th cells [138]. Among the APCs, only DCs are specialized to direct naive T cells to lymphoid tissues [120]. Once DCs encounter foreign antigens in local tissues, such as dental pulp, they become activated and migrate into lymph nodes, where they activate naive T cells and initiate the immune response. Immature DCs possess phagocytic activity, digest foreign antigens and express them on their cell surfaces with not only MHC class II antigens but also costimulatory receptors, such as CD80 and CD86, during the course of maturation. The presence of these APCs has also been reported in deciduous tooth pulp [12,145].

NK cells and natural killer T (NKT) cells are also present in normal pulp [154]. NK cells can recognize foreign antigens nonspecifically, and attack these exogenous invaders using effector proteins, in a similar manner to CTLs [25]. Stimulation of NK cells through activated receptors can lead to the production of cytokines, such as IFNγ, TNFα and granulocyte-macrophage colony stimulating factor (GM-CSF) [14,160,242]. NK cells express three types of receptors, namely activating, inhibitory and costimulatory receptors [369]. Activating signals are mediated by adaptor molecules, such as DNAX-activating protein of 12-kDa (DAP12), while inhibitory signals are related to immunoreceptor tyrosine-based inhibitory motifs (ITIMs) and associated with intracellular phosphatases, such as SH2-domain-containing protein tyrosine phosphatase 1 (SHP1). NK-cell receptor protein 1 (Nkrp1; CD161) and Ly49 are the most common NK cell surface molecules, and are further classified into subgroups composed of activating and inhibitory signal mediators. Activation of NK cells is induced by IL12, TNFα and IFNs. NKT cells possess the phenotypes of both NK cells and T lymphocytes [173]. They express the NK receptors NK1.1 or NKR-P1A, and a semi-invariant T cell receptor a-chain (composed of Va14-Ja18 in mice and the homologous Va24-Ja18 in humans), that was recently shown to recognize CD1d-presented glyco-sphingolipids (isoglobotrihexosylceramide; iGb3) from Gram-negative bacteria lacking LPS [164,200]. Therefore, NKT cells are essential in innate immunity for the recognition and deletion of some specific microorganisms. Furthermore, NKT cells are also the major source of IL4 and IFNγ [172,325].

T and B cells are not common components of the defense system in normal pulp, and are sparsely observed [134,273]. Reparative dentin, which is produced by odontoblasts, represents a physical barrier against exogenous invaders. A close relationship between odontoblasts and MHC class II-positive cells in the para-odontoblastic layer has been reported [232]. The most abundant cellular components in dental pulp are pulpal cells (fibroblasts), and *in vitro* studies have revealed that these cells are capable of producing chemical mediators, such as IL1β, IL6, IL8 and MCP1 against bacteria or their components [24,63,118,180,185,198,216,248,308,333, 334,367].

3.3.2 The defense system in periapical tissues

Periapical tissues are dense fibrous connective tissues that occupy the apical periodontal space between the root apex of a tooth and the alveolus, where rich supplies of blood and nerve fibers are observed. The major immunocompetent cells of periapical tissues are macrophage-lineage cells [142,147], which are sparsely distributed. Other kinds of immunocompetent cells, such as lymphocytes, are rarely observed. Compared to pulp tissues, the defense system in periapical tissues appears to be immature, which may be attributed to the location: the periapical tissues are situated in an area of the body where they do not directly face antigenic challenges from the external environment.

3.4 Etiologies of pulpitis and apical periodontitis

3.4.1 Pulpitis

Bacterial infection

Most cases of pulpitis arise from bacterial infection through carious lesions. Even incipient carious lesions limited to the enamel can cause accumulation of MHC class II antigen-expressing cells in the superficial pulp through dentinal tubules corresponding to the carious lesions [123,124,273,370,371]. The accumulation of these immunocompetent cells is thought to be related to stimuli from the cariogenic biofilm, which are transmitted along the rod/inter-rod enamel and dentinal tubules [32,33]. Although bacteria cannot penetrate demineralized rod/inter-rod enamel, disruption of the enamel layer in carious lesions can allow bacterial invasion into the deep layer, further promoting the pulpal reaction via the dentinal tubules. If dental pulp is directly exposed to the oral environment by an accidental tooth fracture or mechanical pulp exposure, bacteria in the oral cavity rapidly invade the pulp tissues [104].

The importance of bacterial infection in the process of pulpal inflammation was established in the classical experiments with germ-free rats by Kakehashi *et al.* in 1965 [141]. Briefly, the pulp of the upper first molars was exposed and left open to the oral cavity in normal and germ-free rats. In the normal rats, pulpal inflammation occurred and progressed, before total necrosis was induced. In contrast, there were minimal inflammatory reactions in germ-free rats, and reparative dentin was formed.

Invasion by common oral bacteria induces pulpal inflammation [143,144,150,237,239,310]. Bacteria are also the source of carious and periodontal lesions, although the specific bacteria that trigger pulpal inflammation are still unknown. Significant positive associations between the detection of *Micromonas micros* and *Porphyromonas endodontalis* and inflammatory degeneration of pulpal tissues have been reported [192]. Furthermore, inoculation of four commonly isolated bacteria from pulpal inflammation, namely *Prevotella intermedia*, *Fusobacterium nucleatum*, *M. micros* and *Streptococcus intermedius*, into the oral cavity induced rapid progression of pulpal inflammation and pulpal necrosis in experimental mice [152,277,330]. Further studies are necessary to elucidate the specific bacteria responsible for pulpal inflammation.

Pulpal inflammation or necrosis has been implicated in anachoresis, which is defined as the transportation of microbes through blood or lymph to areas of inflammation [7,51,75,77,78,98,263,343]. However, evidence confirming penetration of blood-borne bacteria into the pulp via apical foramina with establishment of pulpal infection is still poor, and it is more likely that pulpal necrosis is caused by mechanisms other than anachoresis, such as microcracks or dentinal exposure, and that blood-borne bacteria may drift into the pulp chamber after total necrosis of the pulp.

Progression of periodontal diseases sometimes causes pulpal pathosis. Accessory canals are frequently found on the chamber floor of molars, in the bifurcation or trifurcation area, and a close anatomical relationship of pulp tissues with periodontal tissues via accessory canals has been reported [50,85,168, 186,227,348]. The deep periodontal pocket may expose the openings of accessory canals, allowing microorganisms or their components to access the pulp tissues [175]. If advanced periodontal diseases reach the apical foramina, which represent the major entrance to the circulation and nervous system of pulp tissues, degradation or inflammation of the pulp tissues would proceed from the apical portion. Such pulpal inflammation is called retrograde pulpitis. Progression of periapical lesions in neighboring teeth to the apex can also cause retrograde pulpitis.

Physical damage and chemical substances

Physical damage, such as cavity preparation [65], and chemical substances from dental materials [66] and disinfectants [35] are candidate factors for inducing inflammatory reactions in dental pulp.

Although heat generation during drilling or cutting of teeth using a dental engine or turbine was reported to be harmful to pulp tissues, exposure of dentinal tubules is probably a greater problem for the pulp tissue integrity. Some specific lasers, i.e., Nd:YAG and Er:YAG, that are clinically applied for cavity preparation, may generate heat by irradiation, which is thought to be a risk factor for pulp tissues [218].

Irritant effects of dental filling materials and disinfecting medicaments have been widely reported *in vivo* and *in vitro*. However, most pulpal reactions in teeth restored with dental filling materials are not related to the materials used, but rather to microleakage, which is defined as the passage of bacteria, fluids, molecules or ions between the cavity wall and the restorative material [247]. Microleakage has been reported to be associated with pulpal inflammation [2,44,45,213,247,275].

3.4.2 Apical periodontitis

Bacterial invasion

The popular etiology of periapical pathosis involves bacterial invasion via infected root canals, which results from progression of pulpal inflammation also caused by bacterial infection. Without pulpal tissues, there is no self-defense system. In other words, there is no effective clearance system to remove bacteria or exogenous components from the root canal, where various bacterial colonies are formed, and bacteria can exit the root canal into periapical tissues. Continuous bacterial invasion from infected root canals into periapical tissues is the trigger of periapical inflammatory reactions, including alveolar bone destruction, and chronic inflammation in periapical tissues is related to the establishment of periapical lesions.

The microflora of infected root canals are similar to those of deep periodontal pockets [157], and the most frequent genera in necrotic pulp are *Prevotella*,*Fusobacterium*,*Lactobacillus*,*Streptococcus*, *Clostridium*, and *Peptostreptococcus* for bacteria, and *Candida* and *Saccharomyces* for yeasts [174]. The presence of *Actinomyces* has also been reported [286,363]. To date, most research has focused on *Enterococcus faecalis*, which is thought to be implicated in persistent or recurrent apical periodontitis [102,156,209, 250,287,309]. Moreover, the presence of *E. faecalis* may be related to refractory endodontic cases [307].

The presence of fungi in root canals with primary periapical lesions [174,282] has also been reported, but their contribution to the progression or perpetuation of periapical lesions is still unclear.

Others

Several reports have mentioned the possible toxicity of root canal filling materials [56,97,243]. However, it is doubtful that exposure of endodontic materials to periapical tissues induces significant pathological reactions *in vivo*. Serum antibodies or delayed-type hypersensitivity reactions against various endodontic materials in experimental models have been reported [41], but have not been confirmed in patients following root canal treatments. Residual inflammation observed after such treatments probably reflects continued infection around the apex, which may be related to the complexity of the root canal anatomy [252,349], biofilm formation [179] or extraradicular infection. Infection of dentinal tubules [11,215,231] is also resistant to conventional root canal treatments [251]. Cementum possesses various irregular pores, some of which are located outside the immunosurveillance system, thereby providing settlement areas for endodontal or periodontal bacteria. Biofilms are resistant to conventional antibacterial treatments, such as the application of antibiotics, and the presence of biofilms around the apex has been reported [229]. Although root canal treatments effectively remove infection from the root canal, and the root canals are then hermetically obturated with guttapercha and endodontic sealers, recurrence or persistence of periapical lesions may result from poor sealing of the coronal portion that does not effectively block microleakage along the root filling, known as coronal leakage [4,262].

3.5 Classification of pulpitis and apical periodontitis

3.5.1 Pulpitis

Pulpitis is classified into reversible and irreversible types [62,210] (Fig. 3.2). Reversible pulpitis, including pulp hyperemia, does not show severe clinical symptoms and recovery to healthy pulp tissues is expected if adequate treatments are provided. Stimuli, such as thermal changes, can induce a momentary and painful response, which disappears as soon as the stimuli are removed, and no spontaneous pain is exhibited in reversible pulpitis. In other words, reversible pulpitis is reactive, and the responses, albeit exaggerated, are only produced following stimulation [62].

In general, irreversible pulpitis is accompanied by severe symptoms, such as spontaneous pain and prolonged induced pain, and diagnosed as acute pulpitis [13]. However, chronic pulpitis, which does not show any acute symptoms, but is suspected to involve total or partial inflammation, is also included in irreversible pulpitis. As the name suggests, irreversible pulpitis involves persistent inflammation of the pulp, and recovery is not expected by conservative pulpal treatments. Total pulp amputation, i.e., pulpectomy, is the only treatment modality for irreversible pulpitis. Histologically, inflammatory reactions in reversible pulpitis are limited, and most of the pulp tissues are intact. On the other hand, severe inflammatory reactions are usually observed in irreversible pulpitis. Chronic hyperplastic pulpitis (proliferative pulpitis or pulp polyp) is sometimes observed in young teeth, and characterized by the proliferation of pulpal fibroblasts in response to bacterial invasion, such as carious lesions [55,80]. Young teeth possess widely opened apical foramina that provide an abundant blood supply, thereby permitting effective self-defense reactions, including overgrowth of fibroblasts instead of pulpal necrosis, which is the common final stage in pulpal inflammation of mature teeth with narrow apical foramina. Internal resorption, the etiology of which is still unclear, is a nonsymptomatic lesion in the pulp, and globular resorption of dentin is typically observed [165,253,259]. Symptomatic irreversible pulpitis is characterized by spontaneous, intermittent or continuous paroxysms of pain, which are moderate to severe and can be sharp or dull, and localized or referred [62]. Most symptomatic irreversible pulpitis is histologically categorized into suppurative pulpitis, characterized by pulpal infiltration of inflammatory cells (neutrophils and macrophages), and the quantity and quality of chemical mediators in the lesion determine the occurrence of pain [226]. Chronic ulcerative pulpitis is used as a histological/clinical classification, and exhibits no severe symptoms other than long-lasting dull pain and discomfort in conjunction with pulpal exposure [230]. Various immunocompetent cells are observed, and the major components in both types of pulpitis are similar. Totally degenerated pulp tissues are diagnosed as pulp necrosis [210].

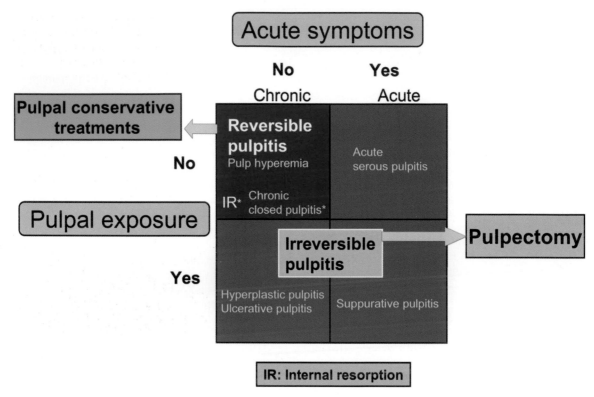

Fig. 3.2 Classification of pulpal inflammation (pulpitis). Conservative treatment of pulp with or without pulp capping is usually performed for reversible pulpitis (green), although total pulp removal (pulpectomy) is necessary for irreversible pulpitis (purple). The pathological classification of pulpal inflammation (pink letters), which used to be estimated from clinical symptoms, is determined by histological evaluation. However, this may not have potentially important clinical implications, since only pulpectomy is performed to treat irreversible pulpitis. *: Pulpectomy is also applied for internal resorption (IR) and chronic closed pulpitis, which are not generally accompanied with severe symptoms and pulp exposure.

3.5.2 Apical periodontitis

The clinical classifications of apical periodontitis include acute and chronic forms, which occur with and without severe clinical symptoms, respectively [62] (Fig. 3.3). Typical chronic apical periodontitis is accompanied by periapical bone destruction, which is radiographically observed as periapical radiolucency around the apex. Apical periodontitis is histologically classified into periapical granulomas and cysts [217]. Periapical granulomas are characterized by the accumulation of inflammatory cells, especially macrophages, although various kinds of inflammatory cells, such as neutrophils, T cells, B cells and plasma cells, are also observed. Periapical cysts are characterized by epithelium-lined cavities, which are open to or independent of the root canals, and sometimes called periapical pocket cysts and periapical true cysts, respectively [219]. The mechanisms of cyst cavity formation are hypothesized to involve nutrition deficiency or an abscess [220]. The possible involvement of nutrition deficiency is based on the assumption that epithelial strands block nutrition of cellular components in the lesions, which would undergo necrosis. Alternatively, degeneration of inner components of the cysts may be induced by destructive enzymes released from neutrophils in an abscess. The epithelium in the cysts is believed to be derived from the cell remnants of Malassez [331]. Periapical cysts often contain deposits of cholesterol crystals [17,341]. Periapical scars are closely related to the healing process. The

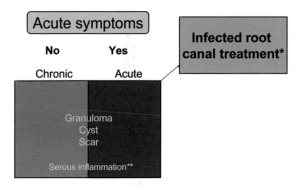

Fig. 3.3 Classification of periapical inflammation (apical periodontitis). The clinical classification of apical periodontitis is simple, and only involves acute or chronic periapical lesions. Treatment of infected root canals is usually performed for both types of periapical lesions, and the clinical goal is to thoroughly remove the infection, followed by complete sealing of the root canal space. Pathological classification is indicated by pink letters.
*: Periapical radiolucency is sometimes observed in vital teeth. In such situation, removal of carious and/or adjustment of occlusion and splint effectively promote healing of the lesions. **: Adjustment of occlusion is sometimes sufficient for some cases of serous periapical inflammation, which are induced by traumatic occlusion.

major components of scar lesions are fibroblasts and an inflammatory process is rarely observed [251].

3.6 Histological evaluation of the pathogenesis of pulpitis and apical periodontitis

Pulpal and periapical pathoses are characterized by inflammatory reactions, including inflammatory cell infiltration into the pulpal and periapical tissues and the synthesis of chemical mediators. The diversity of clinical samples is related to the variety of their histories, and experimental models are often used to analyze pulpal and periapical inflammatory processes.

3.6.1 Pulpal inflammation

Experimental models of pulpal inflammation

The maxillary incisors of rats or mice are popularly used to evaluate acute pulpal inflammation. Rat and mouse maxillary incisors are easy to access because of their anatomical location in the proximal portion of the oral cavity. Furthermore, the incisors are large compared to the overall body size. The availability of various kinds of antibodies against rodent antigens is attractive for immunohistochemical studies. Genetic modifications, such as transfer of transgenic genes or gene knockout, are commonly carried out in rodents. Application of LPS is the most frequently used method for inducing pulpitis in the incisors [29,149, 153,235,236,238]. However, there are several limitations to this experimental method. First, the incisors grow and erupt permanently, and second, the apex opens widely. Therefore, the pulpal inflammation model involving rodent incisors is only suitable for evaluating the initiation or acute phase of pulpal inflammation.

In contrast to incisors, molars of rats or mice are not permanently erupting teeth. They show apical root closure and are relatively small, rendering them somewhat difficult to handle. Pulpal exposure to the oral environment easily induces pulpal inflammation in molars [143,144,150,161,205,314,338]. However, their pulp tissues develop total pulp necrosis within 14–28 days, and chronic pulpal inflammation, which is commonly observed in humans, is hardly observed in rodent models. Cavity preparation in molars is a clever way to induce temporal acute pulpal inflammation, and has been widely used to analyze neural responses to localized pulpal inflammation [52,158,161,327,328]. Denervation studies are often performed in rodents to investigate the involvement of the neural system in pulpal inflammation [54,92,93,106].

Apart from rodents, cats [109,224,336], ferrets [30,43,59,126,267,268] and dogs [225,315,316,322] have been used for pulpal inflammation studies. From a clinical point of view, human or any species close to human, such as monkey and baboon, should be applied to reveal the properties of pulpal inflammation, and some experiments using human or monkey are reported [44,61,68,110,111,166,206,207,290,291, 301,335,346,356]. However, the number of reports using human or primate experimental models tends to be limited in these days because of ethical reasons.

Histology of pulpal inflammation

Cellular components. The initiation of experimentally induced pulpal inflammation, which represents an acute inflammation model, is characterized by infiltration of neutrophils [149] (Fig. 3.4). The peak of their accumulation is seen at 3 h after LPS application to pulp tissues, and rapidly decreases thereafter. Following the neutrophil infiltration, macrophages become the majority of the pulpal immunocompetent cells, and their number peaks at 9 h.

Chemical mediators and neuropeptides. Even normal pulp tissues express relatively low levels of several cytokines, such as IL1α and ILβ. However, inflamed pulp shows rapid increases in the expression levels of several proinflammatory cytokines, including IL1α, IL1β, IL6, IL12 and TNFα [153], which may contribute to further activation of macrophages

and other immunocompetent cells (Fig. 3.5). On the other hand, expression of IL10 is delayed compared to the proinflammatory cytokine expressions. IL10 is a typical antiinflammatory cytokine, and downregulates the synthesis of proinflammatory cytokines in experimentally induced mouse periapical lesions. Therefore, IL10 may be induced as a result of a negative feedback system in order to regulate proinflammatory cytokine synthesis during the progression of pulpal inflammation [153] (Fig. 3.6). NO also plays a role in the progression of pulpal inflammation (Fig. 3.4). Increased NADPH-diaforase and NOS immunoreactivities have been reported in inflamed rat pulp

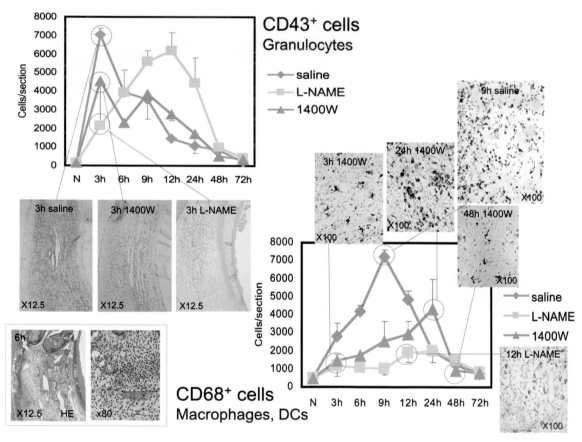

Fig. 3.4 Kinetics of CD43$^+$ neutrophils and CD68$^+$ macrophages/DCs in experimentally induced acute pulpal inflammation in rat incisors. LPS application to rat incisor pulp is a typical method for inducing acute pulpal inflammation. The peak infiltrations of CD43$^+$ neutrophils and CD68$^+$ macrophages/DCs into pulp tissues in response to LPS are observed at 3 and 9 h, respectively. N^G-nitro-L-arginine methyl ester (LNAME) and 1400W are typical NOS and specific iNOS inhibitors, respectively. Administration of 1400 W induces drastic decreases in the numbers of neutrophils and macrophages/DCs infiltrating the dental pulp. The anti-CD68 antibody used recognizes both macrophages and DCs. (From Kawanishi N *et al.* 2004 [149].)

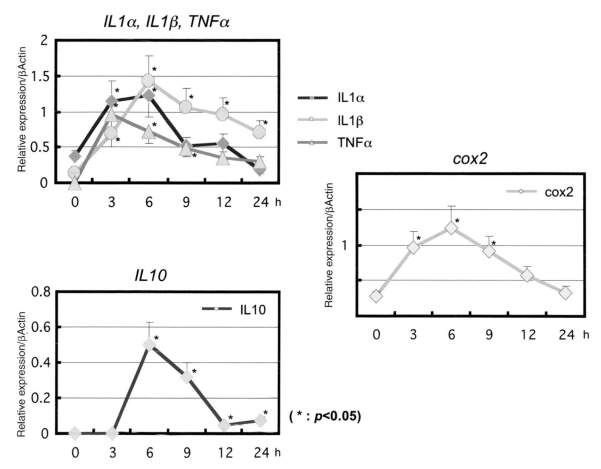

Fig. 3.5 Cytokine and cox2 mRNA expressions during experimentally induced rat pulpal inflammation. The expressions of proinflammatory cytokines (IL1α, IL1β, and TNFα) and cox2 peak at 6 h after LPS application. On the other hand, the expression of IL10, one of the antiinflammatory cytokines, is first observed at 6 h, indicating that its synthesis may be induced as a result of a feedback mechanism to downregulate the actions of the proinflammatory cytokines. (From Kawashima N et al. 1999 [152].)

[177]. NO is predicted to participate in the process of pulpal inflammation by accelerating the expressions of chemokines, which would further induce inflammatory cell infiltration and the expressions of proinflammatory cytokines and cox2 [149,153]. Upregulation of arachidonic-acid metabolites, such as PGE_2, has been reported in experimentally induced rat pulpal inflammation [235,236]. PGs may be related to the activation of an inflammatory response, as well as pain sensation in pulpal pathosis. Extensive sprouting of CGRP-immunoreactive nerve fibers has been detected in inflamed pulp tissues [52,158,161,327,328], and neuronal factors released from sensory or sympathetic nerves are thought to modulate the immunological

defense system in dental pulp, as evaluated by denervation studies [54,92,93,106].

Clinical pulpal inflammation

Human pulpal inflammation is characterized by the presence of a variety of immunocompetent cells, including those from both the innate and adaptive immune systems, suggesting a complicated history for pulpal pathosis (Figs 3.7 and 3.8). Carious lesions, which are the main cause of pulpal inflammation, are basically chronic infectious diseases, and the continuous invasion by bacteria via dentinal tubules induces not only innate, but also adaptive immuno-

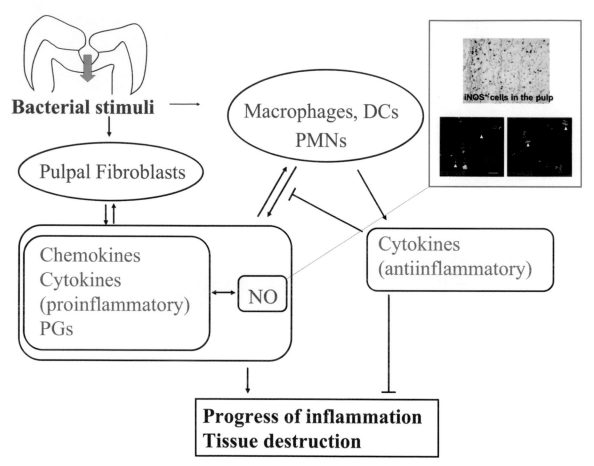

Fig. 3.6 Schematic diagram of the process of pulpal inflammation. Invasion by bacteria or bacterial components via dentinal tubules or directly from carious lesions into the pulp induces the productions of various chemical mediators by immunocompetent cells, such as neutrophils, macrophages, DCs and pulpal fibroblasts. These proinflammatory mediators include chemokines, proinflammatory cytokines, PGs and NO, which further promote the synthesis of proinflammatory mediators from immunocompetent cells and pulpal fibroblasts. Synergic effects are observed among the proinflammatory mediators. The production of the proinflammatory mediators is regulated by antiinflammatory mediators, and these mediator networks may determine the progress of pulpal inflammation.

logical reactions. Clinical pulpal inflammation gradually progresses through these immune reactions. The balance between innate and adaptive reactions depends on the volume and quality of the infection, as well as the conditions of the defense system in the body. Innate and adaptive reactions are characterized by the infiltration of neutrophils/macrophages and lymphocytes, respectively [123,124,273,371]. In inflamed human pulp tissues, upregulated levels of TNFα, IL6, IL8 and IL18 expression have been reported [100,254,373]. The production of NOS is also enhanced in human pulpal inflammation, and its expression is correlated with the progression of acute inflammation [80]. PGs produced by pulpal fibroblasts and infiltrating macrophages through cox2 expression are important modulators of pulpal inflammation [222]. Several neuropeptides released in inflamed pulp may be important regulators of pathophysiological conditions of pulp tissues [103].

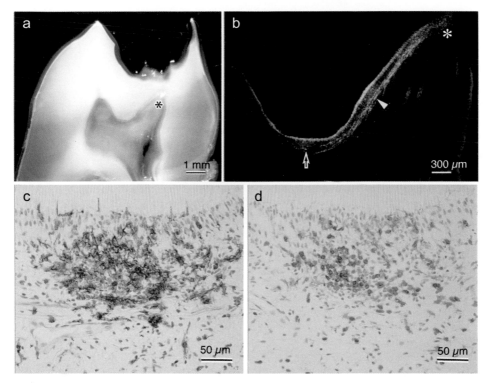

Fig. 3.7 Pulpal defense reactions against dental caries in humans. Pulpal immunological reactions were immunohistochemically determined in a moderately progressed carious human tooth (a) Accumulation of HLA-DR$^+$ cells is observed in the para-odontoblastic region under the carious lesion (b, c) Infiltration of T cells, some of which are surrounded by HLA-DR$^+$ cells, indicates that the lesion is chronic in nature. The arrow and arrowhead in (b) represent clusters of HLA-DR$^+$ cells. (From Yoshiba K *et al.* 2003 [370].)

3.6.2 Histology of apical periodontitis

Apical periodontitis is histologically characterized by the infiltration of various inflammatory cells [5,6,10, 18,37,73,86,89,90,95,131–133,143,144,150,169,181, 183,193–195,197,203,239,264,288,294,310,311,317, 318,324,337,352,372] and periapical bone destruction, which is clinically observed as periapical radiolucency on X-ray films. The most abundantly observed inflammatory cells in periapical lesions are macrophages, although DCs, T cells and B cells are also observed. Periapical bone destruction is sometimes initiated even when the root pulp tissues are still alive [150]. This phenomenon may occur when the level of exogenous invasion into the pulp overwhelms the capacity of the defense system, and the periapical tissues become the next defense front. These processes are clinically observed in vital teeth as periapical radiolucency on X-ray films.

Cellular components

Macrophages. Acute pulpal reaction is characterized by rapid accumulation of neutrophils, followed by infiltration of macrophages. However, the initiation of inflammatory reactions in periapical tissues while vital pulpal tissues still remain in the root canals is characterized by macrophage infiltration followed by periapical bone destruction in experimentally induced rat and mouse periapical lesions [143,150,239,312] (Fig. 3.9). Among established periapical lesions, macrophages represent the major population of inflammatory cells in human periapical granulomas [170,193,255,303] and rat periapical lesions [5,6, 143,144,150,183,203,310,340]. Macrophages are professional phagocytic cells, as well as the major source of various chemical mediators [203]. iNOS-producing macrophages were observed around abscess sites in experimentally induced rat periapical lesions, where

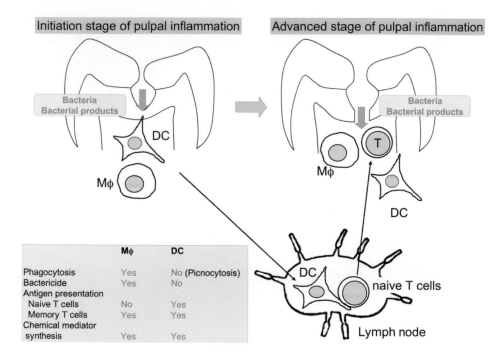

Initiation stage of pulpal inflammation

Advanced stage of pulpal inflammation

Bacteria
Bacterial products

Bacteria
Bacterial products

DC

Mφ

T

Mφ

DC

DC

naive T cells

Lymph node

	Mφ	**DC**
Phagocytosis	Yes	No (Picnocytosis)
Bactericide	Yes	No
Antigen presentation		
Naive T cells	No	Yes
Memory T cells	Yes	Yes
Chemical mediator synthesis	Yes	Yes

Fig. 3.8 Functional differences between macrophages and DCs. Macrophages are typical phagocytes that scavenge exogenous invaders by producing bactericidal molecules and chemical mediators. DCs are also an important source of chemical mediators. Both macrophages and DCs are typical APCs, but only DCs are able to educate naive T cells in specific lymphoid tissues.

the self-defense frontline is thought to be located [310]. NO is one of the most important bactericidal mediators produced by macrophages, and cox2 is also actively produced by macrophages in rat periapical lesions [184,185]. Macrophages are the major source of IL1 and TNFα, which are popular proinflammatory cytokines that contribute to the synthesis of osteoclasts, as well as the regulation of inflammatory processes [16,101,196,323].

DCs. In experimentally induced rat lesions, many MHC class II antigen-expressing cells are observed, which are morphologically identified as macrophages and DCs [143,144,194,239,310]. DC-like cells are located at the periphery of lesions, and increase in number at the late stage of lesion expansion [143]. Activated DCs expressing CD86 are also observed in experimentally induced periapical lesions [366], and their presence suggests that they have supportive effects on T and B cells.

T and B cells. The presence of T and B cells in human periapical lesions has been analyzed by immunohistochemical staining and FACS [18,22,28,69,255,264,288, 304,318,339,351]. Infiltration of CD4+ T helper (Th) cells and CD8+ CTLs, common subpopulations of T cells, into lesions has been reported. Several T cell

subpopulations, including CD4+ T cells and CD8+ T cells, are present, and their ratio is thought to be related to the lesion status [18,22,170,292,294,295]. However, the relationship between that ratio and the pathogenesis of periapical lesions is still unclear. Th cells are categorized into Th1 and Th2 subsets based on their cytokine productions. Th1 cytokine production is predominant at the early stage of lesion expansion, while Th2 cytokine production is induced at a relatively late stage [152]. Therefore, Th1 cells may contribute to the progression of apical lesions, while Th2 cells may be associated with lesion establishment. Th2 type cytokines induce humoral immunity, and the slow induction of Th2 cytokines during the course of lesion expansion may be related to the abundant infiltration of plasma cells into periapical lesions at the established stage [150,351].

Chemical mediators and neuropeptides

RANKL/RANK/OPG. Periapical lesions are characterized by periapical bone destruction, and this bone destruction is mediated by osteoclasts, which are multinuclear cells derived from macrophages [344,345]. Therefore, the synthesis of factors that are able to induce osteoclast differentiation and activation may be related to the expansion of periapical

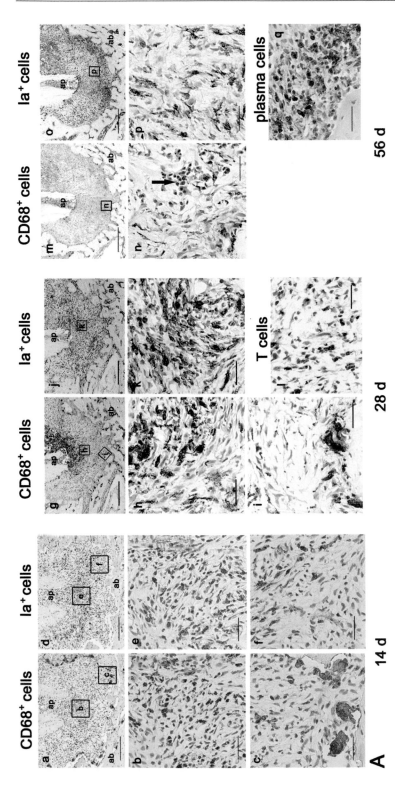

A   14 d   28 d   56 d

Fig. 3.9 Kinetics of immunocompetent cells in experimentally-induced rat periapical lesions. (A) Rat periapical lesions were induced by artificial pulpal exposure to the oral environment, and the localizations of CD68⁺ macrophages/DCs and Ia⁺ cells were determined immunohistochemically. Infiltration of immunocompetent cells into periapical tissues begins at 3 days after the pulpal exposure, and active lesion expansion with concomitant bone resorption is observed at 14 and 28 days (a, d, g, j). Various morphologies of CD68⁺ cells and Ia⁺ cells are observed in the lesions, although oval, irregular and polygonal cells are predominant in the center of the lesions (b, e, h, k). Spindle and dendritic cells are predominantly observed in the periphery of the lesions (c, f, i). The number of osteoclasts is increased at 14 days (a, c), and they are still observed at 28 days (g, i). Typical T cell infiltration begins at 28 days, and the cells are scattered throughout the lesions (l). Lesion expansion ceases at 56 days, although the periapical area is still filled with granular tissue. However, the surface of the alveolar bone is smooth (m, o). Many CD68⁺ cells and Ia⁺ cells show fibroblastic and dendritic morphologies (m, p). Accumulation of plasma cells is frequently observed close to the bone surface (m, o, q). The arrow represents a cluster of plasma cells (n) ap, apex; ab, alveolar bone. Bars: 150 mm (g, j, m, o); 120 mm (a, d); 30 mm (b, c, e, f, h, i, k, l, n, p, q).

[Part (B) is overleaf]

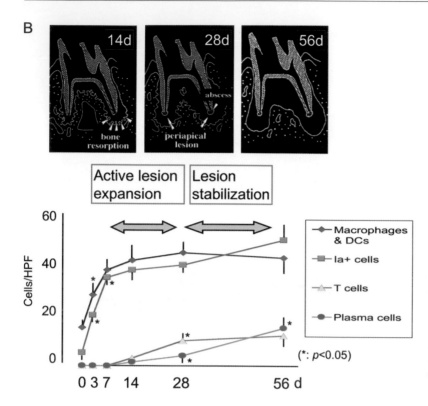

Fig. 3.9 (B) Changes in the densities of macrophages and lymphocytes were evaluated in the periapical tissue after pulp exposure. Increases in CD68[+] cells and Ia[+] cells are typically observed at the initiation stage of lesion expansion, and T cell and plasma cell infiltrations are predominantly observed in the late or stabilization stage of lesion expansion. (From Kawashima N *et al.* 1996 [150].)

lesions. Receptor activator of NFkB ligand (RANKL) was originally identified as TNF-related activation-induced cytokine receptor (TRANCE) and osteoclast differentiation factor (ODF), which were named according to their involvements in the activation and survival of DCs by T cells [361,362], and the differentiation and maturation of osteoclasts [306,368], respectively. RANKL is essential for osteoclastogenesis, and the presence of RANKL and M-CSF induces the differentiation of the precursor splenocytes into osteoclasts [368]. Vitamin D_3, parathyroid hormone (PTH), PGE2 and IL11 are popular inducers of bone resorption, and their functions in osteoclast induction are mediated by RANKL expression on stromal cells and osteoblasts. The receptor for RANKL is receptor activator of NFkB (RANK), which is expressed on osteoclast precursors. In order to regulate the osteoclastogenesis induced by RANKL, a natural decoy protein designated osteoprotegrin (OPG) is generated in the body. The presence of RANKL-positive cells is observed at the early stage of periapical lesion expansion [278,375], and the level of RANKL expression is thought to be correlated with periapical lesion expansion, which is followed by OPG expression [155]

(Fig. 3.10). RANKL mRNA expression has also been reported in human periapical lesions [269]. A close relationship between the kinetics of RANKL/RANK expression and the production of proinflammatory cytokines has also been observed [155].

Other mediators and neuropeptides. The syntheses of IL1 and TNFα, which are potent stimulators of bone resorption and formation, are first induced at the initiation stage of lesion expansion (Fig. 3.11). IL1 has been shown to enhance osteoclast differentiation by stimulating the fusion of pre-osteoclasts, and to act as a survival factor for mature osteoclasts [129,130,162,178]. Signals from IL-1-receptor and those from TNF-receptor could have a synergistic effect on RNAK-mediated TRAF6 activation [189]. Therefore, rapidly increasing expression levels of these cytokines at the initiation stage, and their dominant expressions at the lesion expansion stage would be correlated with the rapid induction and survival of osteoclasts, thereby inducing further periapical bone destruction [152]. Th1 cytokines, including IL12 and IFNγ, may participate in periapical bone destruction [152] by promoting proinflammatory cytokine pro-

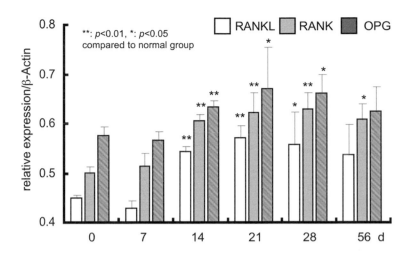

Fig. 3.10 RANKL expression in rat periapical lesions. Upregulation of RANKL expression was induced in the beginning of lesion expansion, and its expression tended to decrease in the end of lesion expansion. RANK and OPG expression followed the RANKL expression in the progress of periapical lesions. (From Kawashima *et al.* 2007 [155].)

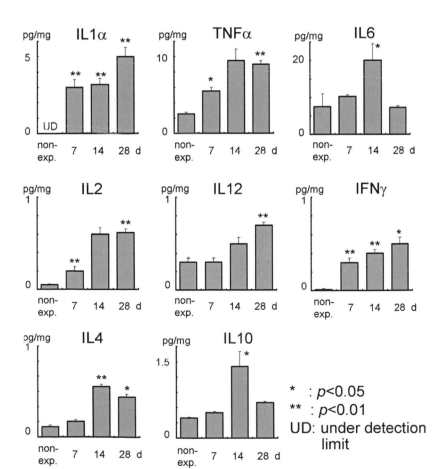

Fig. 3.11 Cytokine synthesis in mouse periapical lesions. Mouse periapical lesions were induced by infection of typical pathogens into exposed molar pulps. Active lesion expansion was observed at 7 days after pulp exposure, and the syntheses of various cytokines were measured by enzyme-linked immunosorbent assay. In particular, the syntheses of IL1α and TNFα, which are typical proinflammatory cytokines, and IL2, IL12 and IFNγ, which are Th1 cytokines, were promoted at this stage. Lesion expansion was stabilized at 28 days, and the syntheses of IL4 and IL10, which are important antiinflammatory cytokines, were initiated at 14 days. (From Kawashima N *et al.* 1999 [152].)

ductions by macrophages. Attenuation of periapical bone destruction was expected in the experimental periapical lesions of Th1-related cytokine deficient mice, however individual knockouts of the central Th1 mediator IFNγ, or the IFNγ-inducing cytokines IL-12 and IL-18, have no significant modification of bone destruction, suggestive of functional redundancy in proinflammatory pathways. On the other hand, IL-10/IL-12p40 double deficient mice exhibited significantly reduced proinflammatory IL-1 production in periapical lesions compared to IL-10 KO mice, suggesting that IL-12 keeps a potential to exaggerate periapical inflammation, though its function is generally regulated by IL-10 (private communication with Dr H Sasaki). On the other hand, syntheses of Th2 cytokines, including IL4 and IL10, follow those of proinflammatory and Th1 cytokines. The importance of IL10 for lesion stabilization was confirmed by a study involving IL10-deficient mice [276,278], in which enhanced expansion of experimentally induced periapical lesions was observed (Fig. 3.12). This lesion expansion induced by IL10 deficiency may be responsible for the upregulation of proinflammatory cytokine synthesis, which in turn is regulated by IL10 in periapical lesions. It is interesting that a regulatory function is observed for IL10, but not for IL4, among the Th2 cytokines. These findings suggest that periapical inflammation is a complicated process, which may be precisely regulated by a balance of proinflammatory and antiinflammatory cytokines in their network. IL6 deficiency was reported to increase inflammatory bone destruction, indicating that IL6 may function as a regulatory cytokine in periapical lesions [20].

Several studies have revealed that neuronal systems are involved in the development or stabilization of periapical lesions. Periapical tissues are innervated by both sensory and sympathetic [140,340,350] nerves, and sprouting of nerve fibers is induced during the

(a)

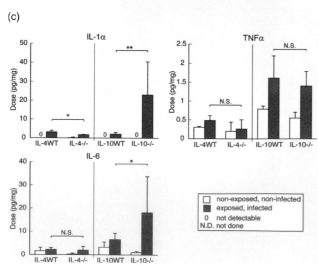

(b)

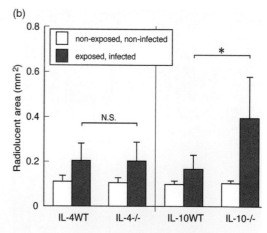

(c)

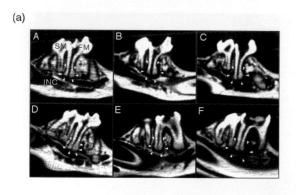

Fig. 3.12   IL-10 suppresses infection-stimulated bone resorption. The sizes of experimentally induced periapical lesions (A) in wild-type (a, d), IL4–/– (b, e) and IL10–/– (c, f) mice were observed radiographically. The progress of the lesion expansion is remarkable in IL10–/– mice (B), and the lesion expansion is correlated with increased expression of the typical proinflammatory cytokine IL1α (C), further suggesting the importance of a mediator network in the progress of periapical lesions. (From Sasaki H et al. 2000 [276].)

course of periapical inflammatory reactions [106,161]. The number of CGRP-containing nerve fibers is correlated with the size of experimentally induced rat periapical lesions [340], while SP-containing nerve fibers were observed in human periapical granuloma and associated with the accumulation of inflammatory cells [140]. Periapical inflammation induces sprouting of sympathetic nerve fibers, and sympathectomy upregulates the formation of osteoclasts, which further induces the expansion of periapical lesions [106]. These findings indicate that the neural system is tightly linked to the expansion or stabilization of periapical lesions, suggesting that neuroimmune interactions are important modulators for determining the progression of periapical lesions.

These mediators construct a network, in which the mediators or their syntheses are activated or suppressed by one another [152,278,293–295]. It should be noted that each mediator is simply a component of the network, and that the progression and stabilization of pulpal and periapical pathoses are determined by the status of the mediator network system (Fig. 3.13).

3.7 Modulators of pulpal and periapical inflammation

3.7.1 Neurogenic inflammation

Neurogenic inflammation [127] is defined as inflammation caused by the activation of peripheral neurons. It results in the release of neuropeptides that affect vasodilation and vascular permeability, and assists the initiation of proinflammatory and immune reactions at the site of injury. Unmyelinated C-fibers stimulated by injury release neuropeptides, such as SP and CGRP, which further induce histamine release from mast cells and BK liberation from kininogen via kallikrein, leading to upregulation of vascular permeability [64,359]. BK activates nerve fibers, and induces further neuropeptide release. Since the nerve fibers are branched and distributed over large areas, the release of neuropeptides is also caused in an axon reflex manner. It is believed that tooth hypersensitivity is related to this neurogenic inflammation [63]. Gingival redness corresponding to the portion of a root apex is sometimes clinically observed following pulpal inflammation, and this phenomenon may be related to neurogenic inflammation. Therefore, neuroimmune interactions may represent one of the

important modulators that determine the progression of pulpal and periapical inflammation.

3.7.2 Immunological disorders

Inflammatory reactions in the pulp or periapical tissues are modified by systemic immunological disorders. The modification of inflammation varies depending on the quantity and types of the immune system components involved.

Disorders of innate immunity

Since the innate immune system is the first defense front against exogenous antigenic challenges, disorders of innate immunity weaken the initial defense mechanism and induce further disturbances in the smooth shift from innate to adaptive immune reactions.

Emigration of white blood cells into inflammatory sites is believed to require at least three steps, namely rolling, adhesion and transendothelial migration. CD18, a member of the integrin-beta family, and CD11a (LFA1), CD11b (Mac1), CD11c or CD11d, which belong to the integrin-alpha family, form complexes that are present in cytoplasmic membranes and are important for binding of leukocytes to blood vessel walls. Mutations in CD18 are referred to as leukocyte adhesion deficiency type I (LAD I). P-selectin, which is stored in the alpha granules of platelets and Weibel–Palade bodies of endothelial cells [244], is quickly released in response to LTB4, C5a, TNFα and LPS, and induces further synthesis of E-selectin [376]. P/E selectins are responsible for rolling of leukocytes on endothelial cell walls, and P/E selectin-deficient mice mimic the clinical disease, leukocyte adhesion deficiency II (LAD II), which is a defect in fucose metabolism resulting in failure to express sialyl Lewis-X (CD15s), the ligand for P/E selectins [48,91]. A wide range of bacterial infections are observed in LAD I and II patients [83]. Experimentally induced periapical lesions in P/E selectin-deficient mice showed more severe bone destruction than those in wild-type mice [152] (Fig. 3.14). As the number of neutrophils in the lesions of the knockout mice was significantly smaller than that in the lesions of the wild-type mice, the initial defense system may not work adequately. This functional disturbance in the initiation of innate immunity may lead to ineffective removal of bacterial infection, thereby further inducing the

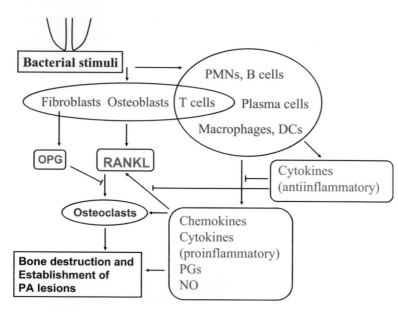

Fig. 3.13 Schematic process of periapical inflammation. Periapical lesions are characterized by periapical bone destruction by osteoclasts. One of the most important mediators in periapical lesions is RANKL, which promotes osteoclast synthesis. The natural antagonist of RANKL is OPG, and the balance between these two factors is critical for bone destruction. Various proinflammatory mediators, including IL1α and TNFα, also mediate osteoclast synthesis and activation directly or indirectly, and their syntheses are further modulated by antiinflammatory cytokines.

overproduction of proinflammatory cytokines, such as IL1, responsible for bone resorption.

Patients with neutropenia, who have very low numbers of blood neutrophils, face high risks of bacterial infection [36]. Furthermore, experimentally induced neutropenia exaggerates pulpal and periapical tissue destruction [148,221,357,364]. Chronic granulomatous disease, myeloperoxidase deficiency, glucose-6-phosphate dehydrogenase (G6PD) deficiency and Chediak Higashi syndrome are functional disorders of phagocytes, especially neutrophils, and expansion of inflammation is easily induced in these patients. The importance of innate immunity is thus demonstrated in these diseases. Acceleration of neutrophil functions by application of PGG glucan, a soluble highly purified yeast (1,3)-beta-glucan with broad antiinfective and immunomodulatory activities [296], may be effective to downregulate the progression of lesion expansion in these diseases.

Disorders of adaptive immunity

Severe combined immunodeficiency (SCID) is a primary immune deficiency [96]. Its characteristics are severe defects in T cell production and functions with defects in B-lymphocytes as primary or secondary problems, while defective NK cell production has also been reported in some genetic types. SCID patients usually show one or more serious infections. X-linked

SCID is the most common SCID, and is related to mutations of the IL2R gamma chain [355]. Autosomal SCID is caused by mutations of the following genes: Janus-associated kinase 3 (JAK3) [187], adenosine deaminase (ADA) [113], RAG1/RAG2 [46] or ZAP-70 [58]. Induction of periapical lesions by active bacterial infection through the exposed pulp chamber in RAG2-deficient mice was found to cause multiple abscess formation in the orofacial area [297,330]. It should be noted that disseminated bacterial infection may be caused not only by endodontic diseases but also by conventional (endodontic) treatments for patients.

Other immunodeficiency diseases are Wiskott–Aldrich syndrome, ataxia-telangiectasia and DiGeorge syndrome. Furthermore, defects in humoral immunity are observed in IgG deficiency, IgA deficiency, complement component deficiencies, C1 inhibitor deficiency, complement receptor deficiency, alternate complement pathway defects and hyper IgE syndrome.

Polymorphisms

Although bacterial infection is essential for initiating and perpetuating pulpal or periapical inflammatory diseases, environmental and genetic factors also contribute to individual variations in the pathogenesis and course of the diseases. Several reports have indi-

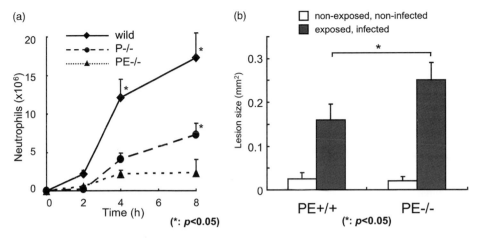

Fig. 3.14 Importance of neutrophils during lesion expansion. P/E selectin-deficient (PE–/–) mice lack rolling adhesion of leukocytes to the endothelium, and mimic the human syndrome LAD II. One of the typical findings of these mice is the presence of disturbed leukocyte behavior, especially of neutrophils infiltrating local lesions, such as periapical lesions (a) PE–/– mice exhibit significantly greater bone resorption than wild-type control mice (b), and this increase in bone resorption is correlated with decreased neutrophil infiltration into the periapical tissues of PE–/– mice. These findings suggest the importance of phagocytic leukocytes as a component of the defense system in periapical tissues/lesions. (From Kawashima N et al. 1999 [152].)

cated that polymorphisms in the IL-1β gene cluster may influence this variation and the severity of periodontal diseases [99,171,246]. Possible relationships between periodontal lesions and polymorphisms of the matrix metalloproteinase (MMP)-1 promoter [74], IgG Fc receptor [167], IL16 [88], IL10 and TNFα [163] have also been suggested.

3.8 Concluding remarks

In this chapter, we have described the pathogenesis of pulpal and periapical inflammations, and discussed the mechanisms of their development. Most instances of pulpitis result from pulpal infection as a consequence of carious lesions. Progression of pulpal inflammation may induce total pulp necrosis, allowing abundant bacterial penetration of the root canals, followed by periapical tissue destruction in response to the root canal infection, thereby inducing the establishment of periapical lesions. Pulpal and periapical inflammations are characterized by a variety of factors, among which chemical mediators play central roles. These chemical mediators, produced by inflammatory cells infiltrating the pulpal and periapical lesions, are sim-

ply classified into two categories of proinflammatory and antiinflammatory mediators, which are related to promotion and stabilization of the lesions, respectively. Proinflammatory mediators include IL1 and TNFα, which are "true" proinflammatory cytokines, and most of them are produced by macrophages. NO and PGs, which are mostly produced by iNOS and cox2 in macrophages, respectively, and IL12 and IFNγ, which are classified as Th1 cytokines, may be involved in the promotion of pulpal and periapical inflammations. Various chemokines produced by inflammatory cells induce further infiltration of inflammatory cells, which may upregulate the lesion expansion. Contrarily, the major antiinflammatory mediators are IL4, IL10 and IL13 produced by Th2 cells and classified as Th2 cytokines, which control and inhibit the continued expansion of pulpal and periapical inflammations. The typical phenomena of periapical lesions include periapical bone destruction, and RANKL plays an important role in lesion progression through osteoclastogenesis. The synthesis of this mediator is regulated positively or negatively by other regulating substances. This represents the essence of the mediator network, and the balance between proinflammatory and antiinflammatory mediators determines the progression or regression of pulpal and periapical lesions. Although self-defense systems are active in the pulp and periapical tissues, carious lesions or infected root canals are free from such self-defense mechanisms. The clinical conclusion is simply that the removal of infection and complete sealing of the root canal are essential for successful treatment of apical periodontitis and to prevent reinfection.

3.9 References

1. Abbas A, Lichtman A (2003) Cytokines. In *Cellular and molecular immunology*, pp. 243–74. Philadelphia, PA: Elsevier.
2. About I, Murray PE, Franquin JC, Remusat M, Smith AJ (2001) Pulpal inflammatory responses following non-carious class V restorations. *Operative Dentistry* **26**, 336–42.
3. Aderem A, Underhill DM (1999) Mechanisms of phagocytosis in macrophages. *Annual Review of Immunology* **17**, 593–623.
4. Adib V, Spratt D, Ng YL, Gulabivala K (2004) Cultivable microbial flora associated with persistent periapical disease and coronal leakage after root canal treatment: a preliminary study. *International Endodontic Journal* **37**, 542–51.
5. Akamine A, Anan H, Hamachi T, Maeda K (1994) A histochemical study of the behavior of macrophages during experimental apical periodontitis in rats. *Journal of Endodontics* **20**, 474–8.
6. Akamine A, Hashiguchi I, Toriya Y, Maeda K (1994) Immunohistochemical examination on the localization of macrophages and plasma cells in induced rat periapical lesions. *Endodontics and Dental Traumatology* **10**, 121–8.
7. Allard U, Nord CE, Sjöberg L, Strömberg T (1979) Experimental infections with *Staphylococcus aureus*, *Streptococcus sanguis*, *Pseudomonas aeruginosa*, and *Bacteroides fragilis* in the jaws of dogs. *Oral Surgery, Oral Medicine, Oral Pathology* **48**, 454–62.
8. Allen YS, Adrian TE, Allen JM, Tatemoto K, Crow TJ, Bloom SR, *et al.* (1983) Neuropeptide Y distribution in the rat brain. *Science* **221**, 877–9.
9. Amara SG, Jonas V, Rosenfeld MG, Ong ES, Evans RM (1982) Alternative RNA processing in calcitonin gene expression generates mRNAs encoding different polypeptide products. *Nature* **298**, 240–4.
10. Anan H, Akamine A, Maeda K (1993) An enzyme histochemical study of the behavior of rat bone cells during experimental apical periodontitis. *Journal of Endodontics* **19**, 83–6.
11. Ando N, Hoshino E (1990) Predominant obligate anaerobes invading the deep layers of root canal dentin. *International Endodontic Journal* **23**, 20–7.
12. Angelova A, Takagi Y, Okiji T, Kaneko T, Yamashita Y (2004) Immunocompetent cells in the pulp of human deciduous teeth. *Archives of Oral Biology* **49**, 29–36.
13. Antonelli JR (1990) Acute dental pain, Part II: Diagnosis and emergency treatment. *Compendium* **11**, 526, 528, 530–2.
14. Arase H, Arase N, Saito T (1996) Interferon gamma production by natural killer (NK) cells and NK1.1+ T cells upon NKR-P1 cross-linking. *Journal of Experimental Medicine* **183**, 2391–6.
15. Ardavin C (2003) Origin, precursors and differentiation of mouse dendritic cells. *Nature Reviews. Immunology* **3**, 582–90.
16. Artese L, Piattelli A, Quaranta M, Colasante A, Musani P (1991) Immunoreactivity for interleukin 1-beta and tumor necrosis factor-alpha and ultrastructural features of monocytes/macrophages in periapical granulomas. *Journal of Endodontics* **17**, 483–7.
17. Arwill T, Heyden G (1973) Histochemical studies on cholesterol formation in odontogenic cysts and granulomas. *Scandinavian Journal of Dental Research* **81**, 406–10.
18. Babal P, Brozman M, Jakubovsky J, Basset F, Jany Z (1989) Cellular composition of periapical granulomas and its function. Histological, immunohistochemical and electronmicroscopic study. *Czechoslovak Medicine* **12**, 193–215.
19. Baggiolini M, Dewald B, Moser B (1997) Human chemokines: an update. *Annual Review of Immunology* **15**, 675–705.
20. Balto K, Sasaki H, Stashenko P (2001) Interleukin-6 deficiency increases inflammatory bone destruction. *Infection and Immunity* **69**, 744–50.
21. Banchereau J, Steinman RM (1998) Dendritic cells and the control of immunity. *Nature* **392**, 245–52.
22. Barkhordar RA, Desouza YG (1988) Human T-lymphocyte subpopulations in periapical lesions. *Oral Surgery, Oral Medicine, Oral Pathology* **65**, 763–6.
23. Barkhordar RA, Hussain MZ, Hayashi C (1992) Detection of interleukin-1 beta in human periapical lesions. *Oral Surgery, Oral Medicine, Oral Pathology* **73**, 334–6.
24. Barkhordar RA, Ghani QP, Russell TR, Hussain MZ (2002) Interleukin-1beta activity and collagen synthesis in human dental pulp fibroblasts. *Journal of Endodontics* **28**, 157–9.
25. Barry M, Bleackley RC (2002) Cytotoxic T lymphocytes: all roads lead to death. *Nature Reviews. Immunology* **2**, 401–9.
26. Batten M, Li J, Yi S, Kljavin NM, Danilenko DM, Lucas S, *et al.* (2006) Interleukin 27 limits autoimmune encephalomyelitis by suppressing the development of interleukin 17-producing T cells. *Nature Immunology* **7**, 929–36.
27. Baumgardner KR, Law AS, Gebhart GF (1999) Localization and changes in superoxide dismutase immunoreactivity in rat pulp after tooth preparation. *Oral Surgery, Oral Medicine, Oral Pathology, Oral Radiology and Endodontics* **88**, 488–95.
28. Bergenholtz G, Lekholm U, Liljenberg B, Lindhe J (1983) Morphometric analysis of chronic inflammatory periapical lesions in root-filled teeth. *Oral Surgery, Oral Medicine, Oral Pathology* **55**, 295–301.

29. Bergenholtz G, Nagaoka S, Jontell M (1991) Class II antigen expressing cells in experimentally induced pulpitis. *International Endodontic Journal* **24**, 8–14.

30. Berggreen E, Heyeraas KJ (1999) The role of sensory neuropeptides and nitric oxide on pulpal blood flow and tissue pressure in the ferret. *Journal of Dental Research* **78**, 1535–43.

31. Berkovita BKB, Holland GR, Moxham BJ (2002) Dental pulp. In *Oral anatomy, histology and embryology*, pp. 149–67. Edinburgh: Mosby.

32. Bjorndal L, Darvann T, Thylstrup A (1998) A quantitative light microscopic study of the odontoblast and subodontoblastic reactions to active and arrested enamel caries without cavitation. *Caries Research* **32**, 59–69.

33. Bjorndal L, Darvann T (1999) A light microscopic study of odontoblastic and non-odontoblastic cells involved in tertiary dentinogenesis in well-defined cavitated carious lesions. *Caries Research* **33**, 50–60.

34. Bletsa A, Heyeraas KJ, Haug SR, Berggreen E (2004) IL-1 alpha and TNF-alpha expression in rat periapical lesions and dental pulp after unilateral sympathectomy. *Neuroimmunomodulation* **11**, 376–84.

35. Block RM, Lewis RD, Sheats JB, Burke SH (1981) Antibody formation to dog pulp tissue altered by camphor paramonochlorophenol via the root canal. *Oral Surgery, Oral Medicine, Oral Pathology* **51**, 637–42.

36. Bochud PY, Calandra T, Francioli P (1994) Bacteremia due to viridans streptococci in neutropenic patients: a review. *American Journal of Medicine* **97**, 256–64.

37. Bohne W (1990) Light and ultrastructural studies of human chronic periapical lesions. *Journal of Oral Pathology and Medicine* **19**, 215–20.

38. Bowden JJ, Garland AM, Baluk P, Lefevre P, Grady EF, Vigna SR, *et al.* (1994) Direct observation of substance P-induced internalization of neurokinin 1 (NK1) receptors at sites of inflammation. *Proceedings of the National Academy of Sciences of the United States of America* **91**, 8964–8.

39. Bozic CR, Lu B, Hopken UE, Gerard C, Gerard NP (1996) Neurogenic amplification of immune complex inflammation. *Science* **273**, 1722–5.

40. Brash AR (2001) Arachidonic acid as a bioactive molecule. *Journal of Clinical Investigation* **107**, 1339–45.

41. Bratel J, Jontell M, Dahlgren U, Bergenholtz G (1998) Effects of root canal sealers on immunocompetent cells in vitro and in vivo. *International Endodontic Journal* **31**, 178–88.

42. Brennan CA, Anderson KV (2004) Drosophila: the genetics of innate immune recognition and response. *Annual Review of Immunology* **22**, 457–83.

43. Browne RM, Plant CG, Tobias RS (1980) Quantification of the histological features of pulpal damage. *International Endodontic Journal* **13**, 104–11.

44. Browne RM, Tobias RS, Crombie IK, Plant CG (1983) Bacterial microleakage and pulpal inflammation in experimental cavities. *International Endodontic Journal* **16**, 147–55.

45. Browne RM, Tobias RS (1986) Microbial microleakage and pulpal inflammation: a review. *Endodontics and Dental Traumatology* **2**, 177–83.

46. Buckley RH (2004) Molecular defects in human severe combined immunodeficiency and approaches to immune reconstitution. *Annual Review of Immunology* **22**, 625–55.

47. Buhlmann N, Leuthauser K, Muff R, Fischer JA, Born W (1999) A receptor activity modifying protein (RAMP)2-dependent adrenomedullin receptor is a calcitonin gene-related peptide receptor when coexpressed with human RAMP1. *Endocrinology* **140**, 2883–90.

48. Bullard DC, Kunkel EJ, Kubo H, Hicks MJ, Lorenzo I, Doyle NA, *et al.* (1996) Infectious susceptibility and severe deficiency of leukocyte rolling and recruitment in E-selectin and P-selectin double mutant mice. *Journal of Experimental Medicine* **183**, 2329–36.

49. Bultzingslowen I, Jontell M (1999) Macrophages, dendritic cells and T lymphocytes in rat buccal mucosa and dental pulp following 5-fluorouracil treatment. *European Journal of Oral Sciences* **107**, 194–201.

50. Burch JG, Hulen S (1974) A study of the presence of accessory foramina and the topography of molar furcations. *Oral Surgery, Oral Medicine, Oral Pathology* **38**, 451–5.

51. Burke GW Jr, Knighton HT (1960) The localization of microorganisms in inflamed dental pulps of rats following bacteremia. *Journal of Dental Research* **39**, 205–14.

52. Byers MR, Taylor PE, Khayat BG, Kimberly CL (1990) Effects of injury and inflammation on pulpal and periapical nerves. *Journal of Endodontics* **16**, 78–84.

53. Byers MR, Swift ML, Wheeler EF (1992) Reactions of sensory nerves to dental restorative procedures. *Proceedings of the Finnish Dental Society* **88** Suppl 1, 73–82.

54. Byers MR, Taylor PE (1993) Effect of sensory denervation on the response of rat molar pulp to exposure injury. *Journal of Dental Research* **72**, 613–18.

55. Caliskan MK, Oztop F, Caliskan G (2003) Histological evaluation of teeth with hyperplastic pulpitis caused by trauma or caries: case reports. *International Endodontic Journal* **36**, 64–70.

56. Camps J, About I (2003) Cytotoxicity testing of endodontic sealers: a new method. *Journal of Endodontics* **29**, 583–6.

57. Carding SR, Egan PJ (2002) Gammadelta T cells: functional plasticity and heterogeneity. *Nature Reviews. Immunology* **2**, 336–45.

58. Chan AC, Kadlecek TA, Elder ME, Filipovich AH, Kuo WL, Iwashima M, *et al.* (1994) ZAP-70 deficiency in an autosomal recessive form of severe combined immunodeficiency. *Science* **264**, 1599–601.

59. Chattipakorn SC, Sigurdsson A, Light AR, Narhi M, Maixner W (2002) Trigeminal c-Fos expression and behavioral responses to pulpal inflammation in ferrets. *Pain* **99**, 61–9.

60. Chen CP, Hertzberg M, Jiang Y, Graves DT (1999) Interleukin-1 and tumor necrosis factor receptor signaling is not required for bacteria-induced osteoclastogenesis and bone loss but is essential for protecting the host from a mixed anaerobic infection. *American Journal of Pathology* **155**, 2145–52.

61. Cleaton-Jones P, Duggal M, Parak R, Williams S, Setzer S (2004) Pulpitis induction in baboon primary

teeth using carious dentine or *Streptococcus mutans*. *SADJ* **59**, 119–22.

62. Cohen S, Liewehr F (2002) Diagnostic procedures. In Cohen S, Burns R, editors. *Pathways of the pulp*, pp. 1–30. St Louis, MO: Mosby.

63. Coil J, Tam E, Waterfield JD (2004) Proinflammatory cytokine profiles in pulp fibroblasts stimulated with lipopolysaccharide and methyl mercaptan. *Journal of Endodontics* **30**, 88–91.

64. Costa SK, Moreno RA, Esquisatto LC, Juliano L, Brain SD, De Nucci G, *et al.* (2002) Role of kinins and sensory neurons in the rat pleural leukocyte migration induced by *Phoneutria nigriventer* spider venom. *Neuroscience Letters* **318**, 158–62.

65. Cotton WR (1967) Pulp response to an airstream directed into human cavity preparations. *Oral Surgery, Oral Medicine, Oral Pathology* **24**, 78–88.

66. Cotton WR (1979) Compatibility of various materials with oral tissues. II: Pulp responses to composite ingredients. Comments on Dr. Stanley's presentation. *Journal of Dental Research* **58**, 1518–21.

67. Coutinho A, Hori S, Carvalho T, Caramalho I, Demengeot J (2001) Regulatory T cells: the physiology of autoreactivity in dominant tolerance and "quality control" of immune responses. *Immunological Reviews* **182**, 89–98.

68. Cox CF, Bergenholtz G, Heys DR, Syed SA, Fitzgerald M, Heys RJ (1985) Pulp capping of dental pulp mechanically exposed to oral microflora: a 1–2 year observation of wound healing in the monkey. *Journal of Oral Pathology* **14**, 156–68.

69. Cymerman JJ, Cymerman DH, Walters J, Nevins AJ (1984) Human T lymphocyte subpopulations in chronic periapical lesions. *Journal of Endodontics* **10**, 9–11.

70. D'Souza R, Brown LR, Newland JR, Levy BM, Lachman LB (1989) Detection and characterization of interleukin-1 in human dental pulps. *Archives of Oral Biology* **34**, 307–13.

71. Daynes RA, Spangrude GJ, Roberts LK, Krueger GG (1985) Regulation by the skin of lymphoid cell recirculation and localization properties. *Journal of Investigative Dermatology* **85**, 14s–20s.

72. De Felipe C, Herrero JF, O'Brien JA, Palmer JA, Doyle CA, Smith AJ, *et al.* (1998) Altered nociception, analgesia and aggression in mice lacking the receptor for substance P. *Nature* **392**, 394–7.

73. de Oliveira Rodini C, Batista AC, Lara VS (2004) Comparative immunohistochemical study of the presence of mast cells in apical granulomas and periapical cysts: possible role of mast cells in the course of human periapical lesions. *Oral Surgery, Oral Medicine, Oral Pathology, Oral Radiology and Endodontics* **97**, 59–63.

74. de Souza AP, Trevilatto PC, Scarel-Caminaga RM, Brito RB, Line SR (2003) MMP-1 promoter polymorphism: association with chronic periodontitis severity in a Brazilian population. *Journal of Clinical Periodontology* **30**, 154–8.

75. Debelian GJ, Olsen I, Tronstad L (1994) Systemic diseases caused by oral microorganisms. *Endodontics and Dental Traumatology* **10**, 57–65.

76. Delgado M, Ganea D (2001) Cutting edge: is vasoactive intestinal peptide a type 2 cytokine? *Journal of Immunology* **166**, 2907–12.

77. Delivanis PD, Snowden RB, Doyle RJ (1981) Localization of blood-borne bacteria in instrumented unfilled root canals. *Oral Surgery, Oral Medicine, Oral Pathology* **52**, 430–2.

78. Delivanis PD, Fan VS (1984) The localization of blood-borne bacteria in instrumented unfilled and overinstrumented canals. *Journal of Endodontics* **10**, 521–4.

79. Di Nardo Di Maio F, Lohinai Z, D'Arcangelo C, De Fazio PE, Speranza L, *et al.* (2004) Nitric oxide synthase in healthy and inflamed human dental pulp. *Journal of Dental Research* **83**, 312–16.

80. Dixon AD, Peach R (1965) Fine structure of epithelial and connective tissue elements in human dental polyps. *Archives of Oral Biology* **10**, 71–81.

81. Dixon BS, Dennis MJ (1997) Regulation of mitogenesis by kinins in arterial smooth muscle cells. *American Journal of Physiology* **273**, C7–20.

82. Edwards CM, Abusnana S, Sunter D, Murphy KG, Ghatei MA, Bloom SR (1999) The effect of the orexins on food intake: comparison with neuropeptide Y, melanin-concentrating hormone and galanin. *Journal of Endocrinology* **160**, R7–12.

83. Etzioni A, Frydman M, Pollack S, Avidor I, Phillips ML, Paulson JC, *et al.* (1992) Brief report: recurrent severe infections caused by a novel leukocyte adhesion deficiency. *New England Journal of Medicine* **327**, 1789–92.

84. Evans BN, Rosenblatt MI, Mnayer LO, Oliver KR, Dickerson IM (2000) CGRP-RCP, a novel protein required for signal transduction at calcitonin gene-related peptide and adrenomedullin receptors. *Journal of Biological Chemistry* **275**, 31438–43.

85. Everett FG, Jump EB, Holder TD, Williams GC (1958) The intermediate bifurcational ridge: a study of the morphology of the bifurcation of the lower first molar. *Journal of Dental Research* **37**, 162–9.

86. Farber PA (1975) Scanning electron microscopy of cells from periapical lesions. *Journal of Endodontics* **1**, 291–4.

87. Felaco M, Di Maio FD, De Fazio P, D'Arcangelo C, De Lutiis MA, Varvara G, *et al.* (2000) Localization of the e-NOS enzyme in endothelial cells and odontoblasts of healthy human dental pulp. *Life Sciences* **68**, 297–306.

88. Folwaczny M, Glas J, Torok HP, Tonenchi L, Paschos E, Malachova O, *et al.* (2005) Prevalence of the –295 T-to-C promoter polymorphism of the interleukin (IL)-16 gene in periodontitis. *Clinical and Experimental Immunology* **142**, 188–92.

89. Fonzi L, Weber E, Kaitsas V, Rongione G (1988) Non specific acid esterase activity in human periapical inflammatory cells. *Journal of Submicroscopic Cytology and Pathology* **20**, 577–81.

90. Fouad AF, Walton RE, Rittman BR (1992) Induced periapical lesions in ferret canines: histologic and radiographic evaluation. *Endodontics and Dental Traumatology* **8**, 56–62.

91. Frenette PS, Mayadas TN, Rayburn H, Hynes RO, Wagner DD (1996) Susceptibility to infection and

altered hematopoiesis in mice deficient in both P- and E-selectins. *Cell* **84**, 563–74.

92. Fristad I, Heyeraas KJ, Jonsson R, Kvinnsland IH (1995) Effect of inferior alveolar nerve axotomy on immune cells and nerve fibres in young rat molars. *Archives of Oral Biology* **40**, 1053–62.

93. Fristad I, Heyeraas KJ, Kvinnsland IH, Jonsson R (1995) Recruitment of immunocompetent cells after dentinal injuries in innervated and denervated young rat molars: an immunohistochemical study. *Journal of Histochemistry and Cytochemistry* **43**, 871–9.

94. Fristad I, Vandevska-Radunovic V, Fjeld K, Wimalawansa SJ, Hals Kvinnsland I (2003) NK1, NK2, NK3 and CGRP1 receptors identified in rat oral soft tissues, and in bone and dental hard tissue cells. *Cell and Tissue Research* **311**, 383–91.

95. Gao Z, Mackenzie IC, Rittman BR, Korszun AK, Williams DM, Cruchley AT (1988) Immunocytochemical examination of immune cells in periapical granulomata and odontogenic cysts. *Journal of Oral Pathology* **17**, 84–90.

96. Gennery AR, Cant AJ (2001) Diagnosis of severe combined immunodeficiency. *Journal of Clinical Pathology* **54**, 191–5.

97. Gerosa R, Menegazzi G, Borin M, Cavalleri G (1995) Cytotoxicity evaluation of six root canal sealers. *Journal of Endodontics* **21**, 446–8.

98. Gier RE, Mitchell DF (1968) Anachoretic effect of pulpitis. *Journal of Dental Research* **47**, 564–70.

99. Gore EA, Sanders JJ, Pandey JP, Palesch Y, Galbraith GM (1998) Interleukin-1beta+3953 allele 2: association with disease status in adult periodontitis. *Journal of Clinical Periodontology* **25**, 781–5.

100. Guo X, Niu Z, Xiao M, Yue L, Lu H (2000) Detection of interleukin-8 in exudates from normal and inflamed human dental pulp tissues. *Chinese Journal of Dental Research* **3**, 63–6.

101. Hamachi T, Anan H, Akamine A, Fujise O, Maeda K (1995) Detection of interleukin-1 beta mRNA in rat periapical lesions. *Journal of Endodontics* **21**, 118–21.

102. Hancock HH, 3rd, Sigurdsson A, Trope M, Moiseiwitsch J (2001) Bacteria isolated after unsuccessful endodontic treatment in a North American population. *Oral Surgery, Oral Medicine, Oral Pathology, Oral Radiology and Endodontics* **91**, 579–86.

103. Hargreaves KM, Swift JQ, Roszkowski MT, Bowles W, Garry MG, Jackson DL (1994) Pharmacology of peripheral neuropeptide and inflammatory mediator release. *Oral Surgery, Oral Medicine, Oral Pathology* **78**, 503–10.

104. Harran-Ponce E, Holland R, Barreiro-Lois A, Lopez-Beceiro AM, Pereira-Espinel JL (2002) Consequences of crown fractures with pulpal exposure: histopathological evaluation in dogs. *Dental Traumatology* **18**, 196–205.

105. Harrington LE, Hatton RD, Mangan PR, Turner H, Murphy TL, Murphy KM, *et al.* (2005) Interleukin 17-producing CD4+ effector T cells develop via a lineage distinct from the T helper type 1 and 2 lineages. *Nature Immunology* **6**, 1123–32.

106. Haug SR, Heyeraas KJ (2003) Effects of sympathectomy on experimentally induced pulpal inflammation and periapical lesions in rats. *Neuroscience* **120**, 827–36.

107. Hayday A, Tigelaar R (2003) Immunoregulation in the tissues by gammadelta T cells. *Nature Reviews. Immunology* **3**, 233–42.

108. Hertz CJ, Kiertscher SM, Godowski PJ, Bouis DA, Norgard MV, Roth MD, *et al.* (2001) Microbial lipopeptides stimulate dendritic cell maturation via Toll-like receptor 2. *Journal of Immunology* **166**, 2444–50.

109. Heyeraas KJ, Kvinnsland I (1992) Tissue pressure and blood flow in pulpal inflammation. *Proceedings of the Finnish Dental Society* **88** Suppl 1, 393–401.

110. Heyeraas KJ, Berggreen E (1999) Interstitial fluid pressure in normal and inflamed pulp. *Critical Reviews in Oral Biology and Medicine* **10**, 328–36.

111. Heyeraas KJ, Sveen OB, Mjor IA (2001) Pulp–dentin biology in restorative dentistry. Part 3: Pulpal inflammation and its sequelae. *Quintessence International* **32**, 611–25.

112. Hill JR, Corbett JA, Kwon G, Marshall CA, McDaniel ML (1996) Nitric oxide regulates interleukin 1 bioactivity released from murine macrophages. *Journal of Biological Chemistry* **271**, 22672–8.

113. Hirschhorn R, Ellenbogen A, Tzall S (1992) Five missense mutations at the adenosine deaminase locus (ADA) detected by altered restriction fragments and their frequency in ADA – patients with severe combined immunodeficiency (ADA-SCID) *American Journal of Medical Genetics* **42**, 201–7.

114. Hokfelt T, Arvidsson U, Ceccatelli S, Cortes R, Cullheim S, Dagerlind A, *et al.* (1992) Calcitonin gene-related peptide in the brain, spinal cord, and some peripheral systems. *Annals of the New York Academy of Sciences* **657**, 119–34.

115. Hokfelt T, Broberger C, Xu ZQ, Sergeyev V, Ubink R, Diez M (2000) Neuropeptides – an overview. *Neuropharmacology* **39**, 1337–56.

116. Holst B, Hastrup H, Raffetseder U, Martini L, Schwartz TW (2001) Two active molecular phenotypes of the tachykinin NK1 receptor revealed by G-protein fusions and mutagenesis. *Journal of Biological Chemistry* **276**, 19793–9.

117. Hori S, Nomura T, Sakaguchi S (2003) Control of regulatory T cell development by the transcription factor Foxp3. *Science* **299**, 1057–61.

118. Hosoya S, Matsushima K (1997) Stimulation of interleukin-1 beta production of human dental pulp cells by Porphyromonas endodontalis lipopolysaccharide. *Journal of Endodontics* **23**, 39–42.

119. Huang GT, Do M, Wingard M, Park JS, Chugal N (2001) Effect of interleukin-6 deficiency on the formation of periapical lesions after pulp exposure in mice. *Oral Surgery, Oral Medicine, Oral Pathology, Oral Radiology and Endodontics* **92**, 83–8.

120. Hugues S, Fetler L, Bonifaz L, Helft J, Amblard F, Amigorena S (2004) Distinct T cell dynamics in lymph nodes during the induction of tolerance and immunity. *Nature Immunology* **5**, 1235–42.

121. Ignarro LJ, Buga GM, Wood KS, Byrns RE, Chaudhuri G (1987) Endothelium-derived relaxing factor produced and released from artery and vein is nitric

oxide. *Proceedings of the National Academy of Sciences of the United States of America* **84**, 9265–9.

122. Ishihara T, Shigemoto R, Mori K, Takahashi K, Nagata S (1992) Functional expression and tissue distribution of a novel receptor for vasoactive intestinal polypeptide. *Neuron* **8**, 811–19.

123. Izumi T, Kobayashi I, Okamura K, Sakai H (1995) Immunohistochemical study on the immunocompetent cells of the pulp in human non-carious and carious teeth. *Archives of Oral Biology* **40**, 609–14.

124. Izumi T, Kobayashi I, Okamura K, Matsuo K, Kiyoshima T, Ishibashi Y, *et al.* (1996) An immunohistochemical study of HLA-DR and alpha 1-antichymotrypsin-positive cells in the pulp of human non-carious and carious teeth. *Archives of Oral Biology* **41**, 627–30.

125. Izumi T, Inoue H, Matsuura H, Mukae F, Ishikawa H, Hirano H, *et al.* (2002) Age-related changes in the immunoreactivity of the monocyte/macrophage system in rat molar pulp after cavity preparation. *Oral Surgery, Oral Medicine, Oral Pathology, Oral Radiology and Endodontics* **94**, 103–10.

126. Jacobsen EB, Heyeraas KJ (1997) Pulp interstitial fluid pressure and blood flow after denervation and electrical tooth stimulation in the ferret. *Archives of Oral Biology* **42**, 407–15.

127. Jancso N, Jancso-Gabor A, Szolcsanyi J (1967) Direct evidence for neurogenic inflammation and its prevention by denervation and by pretreatment with capsaicin. *British Journal of Pharmacology and Chemotherapy* **31**, 138–51.

128. Janeway CA, Jr, Medzhitov R (2002) Innate immune recognition. *Annual Review of Immunology* **20**, 197–216.

129. Jimi E, Nakamura I, Amano H, Taguchi Y, Tsurukai T, Tamura M, *et al.* (1996) Osteoclast function is activated by osteoblastic cells through a mechanism involving cell-to-cell contact. *Endocrinology* **137**, 2187–90.

130. Jimi E, Akiyama S, Tsurukai T, Okahashi N, Kobayashi K, Udagawa N, *et al.* (1999) Osteoclast differentiation factor acts as a multifunctional regulator in murine osteoclast differentiation and function. *Journal of Immunology* **163**, 434–42.

131. Johannessen AC, Nilsen R, Skaug N (1983) Deposits of immunoglobulins and complement factor C3 in human dental periapical inflammatory lesions. *Scandinavian Journal of Dental Research* **91**, 191–9.

132. Johannessen AC, Nilsen R, Skaug N (1984) Enzyme histochemical characterization of mononuclear cells in human dental periapical chronic inflammatory lesions. *Scandinavian Journal of Dental Research* **92**, 325–33.

133. Johannessen AC (1986) Esterase-positive inflammatory cells in human periapical lesions. *Journal of Endodontics* **12**, 284–8.

134. Jontell M, Gunraj MN, Bergenholtz G (1987) Immunocompetent cells in the normal dental pulp. *Journal of Dental Research* **66**, 1149–53.

135. Jontell M, Bergenholtz G, Scheynius A, Ambrose W (1988) Dendritic cells and macrophages expressing class II antigens in the normal rat incisor pulp. *Journal of Dental Research* **67**, 1263–6.

136. Jontell M, Jiang WH, Bergenholtz G (1991) Ontogeny of class II antigen expressing cells in rat incisor pulp. *Scandinavian Journal of Dental Research* **99**, 384–9.

137. Jontell M, Bergenholtz G (1992) Accessory cells in the immune defense of the dental pulp. *Proceedings of the Finnish Dental Society* **88** Suppl 1, 344–55.

138. Jontell M, Eklof C, Dahlgren UI, Bergenholtz G (1994) Difference in capacity between macrophages and dendritic cells from rat incisor pulp to provide accessory signals to concanavalin-A-stimulated T-lymphocytes. *Journal of Dental Research* **73**, 1056–60.

139. Jontell M, Okiji T, Dahlgren U, Bergenholtz G (1998) Immune defense mechanisms of the dental pulp. *Critical Reviews in Oral Biology and Medicine* **9**, 179–200.

140. Kabashima H, Nagata K, Maeda K, Iijima T (2002) Involvement of substance P, mast cells, TNF-alpha and ICAM-1 in the infiltration of inflammatory cells in human periapical granulomas. *Journal of Oral Pathology and Medicine* **31**, 175–80.

141. Kakehashi S, Stanley HR, Fitzgerald RJ (1965) The effects of surgical exposures of dental pulps in germ-free and conventional laboratory rats. *Oral Surgery, Oral Medicine, Oral Pathology* **20**, 340–9.

142. Kan L, Okiji T, Kaneko T, Suda H (2001) Localization and density of myeloid leucocytes in the periodontal ligament of normal rat molars. *Archives of Oral Biology* **46**, 509–20.

143. Kaneko T, Okiji T, Kan L, Suda H, Takagi M (2001) An immunoelectron-microscopic study of class II major histocompatibility complex molecule-expressing macrophages and dendritic cells in experimental rat periapical lesions. *Archives of Oral Biology* **46**, 713–20.

144. Kaneko T, Okiji T, Kan L, Takagi M, Suda H (2001) Ultrastructural analysis of MHC class II molecule-expressing cells in experimentally induced periapical lesions in the rat. *Journal of Endodontics* **27**, 337–42.

145. Kannari N, Ohshima H, Maeda T, Noda T, Takano Y (1998) Class II MHC antigen-expressing cells in the pulp tissue of human deciduous teeth prior to shedding. *Archives of Histology and Cytology* **61**, 1–15.

146. Kapsenberg ML (2003) Dendritic-cell control of pathogen-driven T-cell polarization. *Nature Reviews. Immunology* **3**, 984–93.

147. Kawahara I, Takano Y, Sato O, Maeda T, Kannari K (1992) Histochemical and immunohistochemical demonstration of macrophages and dendritic cells in the lingual periodontal ligament of rat incisors. *Archives of Histology and Cytology* **55**, 211–17.

148. Kawahara T, Murakami S, Noiri Y, Ehara A, Takemura N, Furukawa S, *et al.* (2004) Effects of cyclosporin-A-induced immunosuppression on periapical lesions in rats. *Journal of Dental Research* **83**, 683–7.

149. Kawanishi HN, Kawashima N, Suzuki N, Suda H, Takagi M (2004) Effects of an inducible nitric oxide synthase inhibitor on experimentally induced rat pulpitis. *European Journal of Oral Sciences* **112**, 332–7.

150. Kawashima N, Okiji T, Kosaka T, Suda H (1996) Kinetics of macrophages and lymphoid cells during the development of experimentally induced periapical lesions in rat molars: a quantitative immunohistochemical study. *Journal of Endodontics* **22**, 311–16.

151. Kawashima N, Niederman R, Hynes RO, Ullmann-Cullere M, Stashenko P (1999) Infection-stimulated infraosseus inflammation and bone destruction is increased in P-/E-selectin knockout mice. *Immunology* **97**, 117–23.

152. Kawashima N, Stashenko P (1999) Expression of bone-resorptive and regulatory cytokines in murine periapical inflammation. *Archives of Oral Biology* **44**, 55–66.

153. Kawashima N, Nakano-Kawanishi H, Suzuki N, Takagi M, Suda H (2005) Effect of NOS inhibitor on cytokine and COX2 expression in rat pulpitis. *Journal of Dental Research* **84**, 762–7.

154. Kawashima N, Wongyaofa I, Suzuki N, Kawanishi HN, Suda H (2006) NK and NKT cells in the rat dental pulp tissues. *Oral Surgery, Oral Medicine, Oral Pathology, Oral Radiology and Endodontics* **102**, 558–63.

155. Kawashima N, Suzuki N, Yang G, Ohi C, Okuhara S, Nakano-Kawanishi H, *et al.* (2007). Kinetics of RANKL, RANK and OPG expressions in experimentally induced rat periapical lesions. *Oral Surgery, Oral Medicine, Oral Pathology, Oral Radiology and Endodontics* **103**, 707–11.

156. Kayaoglu G, Ørstavik D (2004) Virulence factors of *Enterococcus faecalis*: relationship to endodontic disease. *Critical Reviews in Oral Biology and Medicine* **15**, 308–20.

157. Kerekes K, Olsen I (1990) Similarities in the microfloras of root canals and deep periodontal pockets. *Endodontics and Dental Traumatology* **6**, 1–5.

158. Khayat BG, Byers MR, Taylor PE, Mecifi K, Kimberly CL (1988) Responses of nerve fibers to pulpal inflammation and periapical lesions in rat molars demonstrated by calcitonin gene-related peptide immunocytochemistry. *Journal of Endodontics* **14**, 577–87.

159. Kim S, Kim J (1990) Haemodynamic regulation of the dental pulp. In Inoki R, Kudo T, Olgart L, editors. *Dynamic aspects of dental pulp*, pp. 167–98. London: Chapman & Hall.

160. Kim S, Yokoyama WM (1998) NK cell granule exocytosis and cytokine production inhibited by Ly-49A engagement. *Cellular Immunology* **183**, 106–12.

161. Kimberly CL, Byers MR (1988) Inflammation of rat molar pulp and periodontium causes increased calcitonin gene-related peptide and axonal sprouting. *Anatomical Record* **222**, 289–300.

162. Kimble RB, Srivastava S, Ross FP, Matayoshi A, Pacifici R (1996) Estrogen deficiency increases the ability of stromal cells to support murine osteoclastogenesis via an interleukin-1 and tumor necrosis factor-mediated stimulation of macrophage colony-stimulating factor production. *Journal of Biological Chemistry* **271**, 28890–7.

163. Kinane DF, Hodge P, Eskdale J, Ellis R, Gallagher G (1999) Analysis of genetic polymorphisms at the interleukin-10 and tumour necrosis factor loci in early-onset periodontitis. *Journal of Periodontal Research* **34**, 379–86.

164. Kinjo Y, Wu D, Kim G, Xing GW, Poles MA, Ho DD, *et al.* (2005) Recognition of bacterial glycosphingolipids by natural killer T cells. *Nature* **434**, 520–5.

165. Kinomoto Y, Noro T, Ebisu S (2002) Internal root resorption associated with inadequate caries removal and orthodontic therapy. *Journal of Endodontics* **28**, 405–7.

166. Kitasako Y, Murray PE, Tagami J, Smith AJ (2002) Histomorphometric analysis of dentinal bridge formation and pulpal inflammation. *Quintessence International* **33**, 600–8.

167. Kobayashi T, Westerdaal NA, Miyazaki A, van der Pol WL, Suzuki T, Yoshie H, *et al.* (1997) Relevance of immunoglobulin G Fc receptor polymorphism to recurrence of adult periodontitis in Japanese patients. *Infection and Immunity* **65**, 3556–60.

168. Koenigs JF, Brilliant JD, Foreman DW (1974) Preliminary scanning electron microscope investigations of accessory foramina in the furcation areas of human molar teeth. *Oral Surgery, Oral Medicine, Oral Pathology* **38**, 773–82.

169. Kontiainen S, Ranta H, Lautenschlager I (1986) Cells infiltrating human apical inflammatory lesions. *Journal of Oral Pathology* **15**, 544–6.

170. Kopp W, Schwarting R (1989) Differentiation of T lymphocyte subpopulations, macrophages, and HLA-DR-restricted cells of apical granulation tissue. *Journal of Endodontics* **15**, 72–5.

171. Kornman KS, Crane A, Wang HY, di Giovine FS, Newman MG, Pirk FW, *et al.* (1997) The interleukin-1 genotype as a severity factor in adult periodontal disease. *Journal of Clinical Periodontology* **24**, 72–7.

172. Kronenberg M, Gapin L (2002) The unconventional lifestyle of NKT cells. *Nature Reviews. Immunology* **2**, 557–68.

173. Kronenberg M (2005) Toward an understanding of NKT cell biology: progress and paradoxes. *Annual Review of Immunology* **23**, 877–900.

174. Lana MA, Ribeiro-Sobrinho AP, Stehling R, Garcia GD, Silva BK, Hamdan JS, *et al.* (2001) Microorganisms isolated from root canals presenting necrotic pulp and their drug susceptibility in vitro. *Oral Microbiology and Immunology* **16**, 100–5.

175. Langeland K, Rodrigues H, Dowden W (1974) Periodontal disease, bacteria, and pulpal histopathology. *Oral Surgery, Oral Medicine, Oral Pathology* **37**, 257–70.

176. Lanzavecchia A, Sallusto F (2000) Dynamics of T lymphocyte responses: intermediates, effectors, and memory cells. *Science* **290**, 92–7.

177. Law AS, Baumgardner KR, Meller ST, Gebhart GF (1999) Localization and changes in NADPH-diaphorase reactivity and nitric oxide synthase immunoreactivity in rat pulp following tooth preparation. *Journal of Dental Research* **78**, 1585–95.

178. Lee SK, Gardner AE, Kalinowski JF, Jastrzebski SL, Lorenzo JA (2006) RANKL-stimulated osteoclast-like cell formation in vitro is partially dependent on endogenous interleukin-1 production. *Bone* **38**, 678–85

179. Leonardo MR, Rossi MA, Silva LA, Ito IY, Bonifacio KC (2002) EM evaluation of bacterial biofilm and microorganisms on the apical external root surface of human teeth. *Journal of Endodontics* **28**, 815–18.

180. Levin LG, Rudd A, Bletsa A, Reisner H (1999) Expression of IL-8 by cells of the odontoblast layer in vitro. *European Journal of Oral Sciences* **107**, 131–7.

181. Liapatas S, Nakou M, Rontogianni D (2003) Inflammatory infiltrate of chronic periradicular lesions: an immunohistochemical study. *International Endodontic Journal* **36**, 464–71.

182. Liew FY (2002) T(H)1 and T(H)2 cells: a historical perspective. *Nature Reviews. Immunology* **2**, 55–60.

183. Lin SK, Hong CY, Chang HH, Chiang CP, Chen CS, Jeng JH, *et al.* (2000) Immunolocalization of macrophages and transforming growth factor-beta 1 in induced rat periapical lesions. *Journal of Endodontics* **26**, 335–40.

184. Lin SK, Kok SH, Kuo MY, Wang TJ, Wang JT, Yeh FT, *et al.* (2002) Sequential expressions of MMP-1, TIMP-1, IL-6, and COX-2 genes in induced periapical lesions in rats. *European Journal of Oral Sciences* **110**, 246–53.

185. Lin SK, Kuo MY, Wang JS, Lee JJ, Wang CC, Huang S, *et al.* (2002) Differential regulation of interleukin-6 and inducible cyclooxygenase gene expression by cytokines through prostaglandin-dependent and -independent mechanisms in human dental pulp fibroblasts. *Journal of Endodontics* **28**, 197–201.

186. Lowman JV, Burke RS, Pelleu GB (1973) Patent accessory canals: incidence in molar furcation region. *Oral Surgery, Oral Medicine, Oral Pathology* **36**, 580–4.

187. Macchi P, Villa A, Giliani S, Sacco MG, Frattini A, Porta F, *et al.* (1995) Mutations of Jak-3 gene in patients with autosomal severe combined immune deficiency (SCID) *Nature* **377**, 65–8.

188. Maggi CA (1995) The mammalian tachykinin receptors. *General Pharmacology* **26**, 911–44.

189. Mak TW, Yeh WC (2002) Immunology: a block at the toll gate. *Nature* **418**, 835–6.

190. Maloy KJ, Powrie F (2001) Regulatory T cells in the control of immune pathology. *Nature Immunology* **2**, 816–22.

191. Marletta MA (1993) Nitric oxide synthase structure and mechanism. *Journal of Biological Chemistry* **268**, 12231–4.

192. Martin FE, Nadkarni MA, Jacques NA, Hunter N (2002) Quantitative microbiological study of human carious dentine by culture and real-time PCR: association of anaerobes with histopathological changes in chronic pulpitis. *Journal of Clinical Microbiology* **40**, 1698–704.

193. Marton IJ, Kiss C (1993) Characterization of inflammatory cell infiltrate in dental periapical lesions. *International Endodontic Journal* **26**, 131–6.

194. Marton IJ, Dezso B, Radics T, Kiss C (1998) Distribution of interleukin-2 receptor alpha-chain and cells expressing major histocompatibility complex class II antigen in chronic human periapical lesions. *Oral Microbiology and Immunology* **13**, 259–62.

195. Marton IJ, Kiss C (2000) Protective and destructive immune reactions in apical periodontitis. *Oral Microbiology and Immunology* **15**, 139–50.

196. Matsumoto A, Anan H, Maeda K (1998) An immunohistochemical study of the behavior of cells expressing interleukin-1 alpha and interleukin-1 beta within experimentally induced periapical lesions in rats. *Journal of Endodontics* **24**, 811–16.

197. Matsuo T, Ebisu S, Shimabukuro Y, Ohtake T, Okada H (1992) Quantitative analysis of immunocompetent cells in human periapical lesions: correlations with clinical findings of the involved teeth. *Journal of Endodontics* **18**, 497–500.

198. Matsushima K, Ohbayashi E, Takeuchi H, Hosoya S, Abiko Y, Yamazaki M (1998) Stimulation of interleukin-6 production in human dental pulp cells by peptidoglycans from *Lactobacillus casei*. *Journal of Endodontics* **24**, 252–5.

199. Matthias P, Rolink AG (2005) Transcriptional networks in developing and mature B cells. *Nature Reviews. Immunology* **5**, 497–508.

200. Mattner J, Debord KL, Ismail N, Goff RD, Cantu C, 3rd, Zhou D, *et al.* (2005) Exogenous and endogenous glycolipid antigens activate NKT cells during microbial infections. *Nature* **434**, 525–9.

201. McLatchie LM, Fraser NJ, Main MJ, Wise A, Brown J, Thompson N, *et al.* (1998) RAMPs regulate the transport and ligand specificity of the calcitonin-receptor-like receptor. *Nature* **393**, 333–9.

202. Medina KL, Garrett KP, Thompson LF, Rossi MI, Payne KJ, Kincade PW (2001) Identification of very early lymphoid precursors in bone marrow and their regulation by estrogen. *Nature Immunology* **2**, 718–24.

203. Metzger Z (2000) Macrophages in periapical lesions. *Endodontics and Dental Traumatology* **16**, 1–8.

204. Miyauchi M, Takata T, Ito H, Ogawa I, Kobayashi J, Nikai H, *et al.* (1996) Immunohistochemical detection of prostaglandins E2, F2 alpha, and 6-keto-prostaglandin F1 alpha in experimentally induced periapical inflammatory lesions in rats. *Journal of Endodontics* **22**, 635–7.

205. Miyauchi M, Takata T, Ito H, Ogawa I, Kobayashi J, Nikai H, *et al.* (1996) Immunohistochemical demonstration of prostaglandins E2, F2 alpha, and 6-keto-prostaglandin F1 alpha in rat dental pulp with experimentally induced inflammation. *Journal of Endodontics* **22**, 600–2.

206. Mjor IA, Tronstad L (1972) Experimentally induced pulpitis. *Oral Surgery, Oral Medicine, Oral Pathology* **34**, 102–8.

207. Mjor IA, Tronstad L (1974) The healing of experimentally induced pulpitis. *Oral Surgery, Oral Medicine, Oral Pathology* **38**, 115–21.

208. Moilanen E, Whittle B, Moncada S (1999) Nitric oxide as a factor in inflammation. In Gallin J, Snyderman R, editors. *Inflammation – basic principles and clinical correlates*, pp. 787–800. Philadelphia, PA: Lippincott Williams & Wilkins.

209. Molander A, Reit C, Dahlen G, Kvist T (1998) Microbiological status of root-filled teeth with apical periodontitis. *International Endodontic Journal* **31**, 1–7.

210. Morse DR, Seltzer S, Sinai I, Biron G (1977) Endodontic classification. *Journal of the American Dental Association* **94**, 685–9.

211. Moser M, Murphy KM (2000) Dendritic cell regulation of TH1–TH2 development. *Nature Immunology* **1**, 199–205.

212. Mossalayi MD, Paul-Eugene N, Ouaaz F, Arock M, Kolb JP, Kilchherr E, Debre P, Dugas B (1994) Involvement of Fc epsilon RII/CD23 and L-arginine-dependent

pathway in IgE-mediated stimulation of human mono-cyte functions. *International Immunology* **6**, 931–4.

213. Murray PE, Hafez AA, Smith AJ, Cox CF (2002) Bacterial microleakage and pulp inflammation associated with various restorative materials. *Dental Materials* **18**, 470–8.

214. Muzio M, Bosisio D, Polentarutti N, D'Amico G, Stoppacciaro A, Mancinelli R, *et al.* (2000) Differential expression and regulation of toll-like receptors (TLR) in human leukocytes: selective expression of TLR3 in dendritic cells. *Journal of Immunology* **164**, 5998–6004.

215. Nagaoka S, Miyazaki Y, Liu HJ, Iwamoto Y, Kitano M, Kawagoe M (1995) Bacterial invasion into dentinal tubules of human vital and nonvital teeth. *Journal of Endodontics* **21**, 70–3.

216. Nagaoka S, Tokuda M, Sakuta T, Taketoshi Y, Tamura M, Takada H, *et al.* (1996) Interleukin-8 gene expression by human dental pulp fibroblast in cultures stimulated with *Prevotella intermedia* lipopolysaccharide. *Journal of Endodontics* **22**, 9–12.

217. Nair PN (1998) Pathology of apical periodontitis. In Osrstavik D, Pit Ford TR, editors. *Essential endodontology*, pp. 68–105. Oxford: Blackwell.

218. Nair PN, Baltensperger MM, Luder HU, Eyrich GK (2003) Pulpal response to Er:YAG laser drilling of dentine in healthy human third molars. *Lasers in Surgery and Medicine* **32**, 203–9.

219. Ramachandran Nair PN, Pajarola G, Schroeder HE (1996) Types and incidence of human periapical lesions obtained with extracted teeth. *Oral Surgery, Oral Medicine, Oral Pathology, Oral Radiology and Endodontics* **81**, 93–102.

220. Ramachandran Nair PN (2002) Pathobiology of the periapex. In Cohen S, Burns RC, editors. *Pathways of the pulp*, pp. 457–500. St. Louis, MO: Mosby.

221. Nakamura K, Yamasaki M, Nishigaki N, Iwama A, Imaizumi I, Nakamura H, *et al.* (2002) Effect of metho-trexate-induced neutropenia on pulpal inflammation in rats. *Journal of Endodontics* **28**, 287–90.

222. Nakanishi T, Shimizu H, Hosokawa Y, Matsuo T (2001) An immunohistological study on cyclooxygenase-2 in human dental pulp. *Journal of Endodontics* **27**, 385–8.

223. Nakanishi T, Takahashi K, Hosokawa Y, Adachi T, Nakae H, Matsuo T (2005) Expression of macrophage inflammatory protein 3alpha in human inflamed dental pulp tissue. *Journal of Endodontics* **31**, 84–7.

224. Narhi M, Hirvonen T (1983) Functional changes in cat pulp nerve activity after thermal and mechanical injury of the pulp. *Proceedings of the Finnish Dental Society* **79**, 162–7.

225. Narhi MV, Hirvonen TJ, Hakumaki MO (1982) Responses of intradental nerve fibres to stimulation of dentine and pulp. *Acta Physiologica Scandinavica* **115**, 173–8.

226. Ngassapa D (1996) Correlation of clinical pain symptoms with histopathological changes of the dental pulp: a review. *East African Medical Journal* **73**, 779–81.

227. Niemann RW, Dickinson GL, Jackson CR, Wearden S, Skidmore AE (1993) Dye ingress in molars: furcation to chamber floor. *Journal of Endodontics* **19**, 293–6.

228. Nishikawa H, Kato T, Tanida K, Hiasa A, Tawara I, Ikeda H, *et al.* (2003) CD4+ CD25+ T cells responding to serologically defined autoantigens suppress anti-tumor immune responses. *Proceedings of the National Academy of Sciences of the United States of America* **100**, 10902–6.

229. Noiri Y, Ehara A, Kawahara T, Takemura N, Ebisu S (2002) Participation of bacterial biofilms in refractory and chronic periapical periodontitis. *Journal of Endodontics* **28**, 679–83.

230. Ogilvie A, Ingle J (1965) Pulpal pathosis. In *An atlas of pulpal and periapical biology*, pp. 295–348. Philadelphia, PA: Lea & Febiger.

231. Oguntebi BR (1994) Dentine tubule infection and end-odontic therapy implications. *International Endodontic Journal* **27**, 218–22.

232. Ohshima H, Kawahara I, Maeda T, Takano Y (1994) The relationship between odontoblasts and immuno-competent cells during dentinogenesis in rat incisors: an immunohistochemical study using OX6-monoclonal antibody. *Archives of Histology and Cytology* **57**, 435–47.

233. Ohshima H, Sato O, Kawahara I, Maeda T, Takano Y (1995) Responses of immunocompetent cells to cavity preparation in rat molars: an immunohistochemical study using OX6-monoclonal antibody. *Connective Tissue Research* **32**, 303–11.

234. Ohshima H, Maeda T, Takano Y (1999) The distribution and ultrastructure of class II MHC-positive cells in human dental pulp. *Cell and Tissue Research* **295**, 151–8.

235. Okiji T, Morita I, Kobayashi C, Sunada I, Murota S (1987) Arachidonic-acid metabolism in normal and experimentally-inflamed rat dental pulp. *Archives of Oral Biology* **32**, 723–7.

236. Okiji T, Morita I, Sunada I, Murota S (1989) Involvement of arachidonic acid metabolites in increases in vascular permeability in experimental dental pulpal inflammation in the rat. *Archives of Oral Biology* **34**, 523–8.

237. Okiji T, Kawashima N, Kosaka T, Matsumoto A, Kobayashi C, Suda H (1992) An immunohistochemical study of the distribution of immunocompetent cells, especially macrophages and Ia antigen-expressing cells of heterogeneous populations, in normal rat molar pulp. *Journal of Dental Research* **71**, 1196–202.

238. Okiji T, Morita I, Suda H, Murota S (1992) Pathophysiological roles of arachidonic acid metabolites in rat dental pulp. *Proceedings of the Finnish Dental Society* **88** Suppl 1, 433–8.

239. Okiji T, Kawashima N, Kosaka T, Kobayashi C, Suda H (1994) Distribution of Ia antigen-expressing nonlymphoid cells in various stages of induced periapical lesions in rat molars. *Journal of Endodontics* **20**, 27–31.

240. Okiji T, Kosaka T, Kamal AM, Kawashima N, Suda H (1996) Age-related changes in the immuno-reactivity of the monocyte/macrophage system in rat molar pulp. *Archives of Oral Biology* **41**, 453–60.

241. Okiji T, Jontell M, Belichenko P, Bergenholtz G, Dahlstrom A (1997) Perivascular dendritic cells of the human dental pulp. *Acta Physiologica Scandinavica* **159**, 163–9.

242. Ortaldo JR, Young HA (2003) Expression of IFN-gamma upon triggering of activating Ly49D NK receptors in vitro and in vivo: costimulation with IL-12 or IL-18

overrides inhibitory receptors. *Journal of Immunology* **170**, 1763–9.

243. Osorio RM, Hefti A, Vertucci FJ, Shawley AL (1998) Cytotoxicity of endodontic materials. *Journal of Endodontics* **24**, 91–6.

244. Papayianni A, Serhan CN, Brady HR (1996) Lipoxin A4 and B4 inhibit leukotriene-stimulated interactions of human neutrophils and endothelial cells. *Journal of Immunology* **156**, 2264–72.

245. Park H, Li Z, Yang XO, Chang SH, Nurieva R, Wang YH, *et al.* (2005) A distinct lineage of CD4 T cells regulates tissue inflammation by producing interleukin 17. *Nature Immunology* **6**, 1133–41.

246. Parkhill JM, Hennig BJ, Chapple IL, Heasman PA, Taylor JJ (2000) Association of interleukin-1 gene polymorphisms with early-onset periodontitis. *Journal of Clinical Periodontology* **27**, 682–9.

247. Pashley DH (1990) Clinical considerations of microleakage. *Journal of Endodontics* **16**, 70–7.

248. Patel T, Park SH, Lin LM, Chiappelli F, Huang GT (2003) Substance P induces interleukin-8 secretion from human dental pulp cells. *Oral Surgery, Oral Medicine, Oral Pathology, Oral Radiology and Endodontics* **96**, 478–85.

249. Patterson SS, Hillis PD (1972) Scar tissue associated with the apices of pulpless teeth prior to endodontic therapy. *Oral Surgery, Oral Medicine, Oral Pathology* **33**, 450–7.

250. Peciuliene V, Balciuniene I, Eriksen HM, Haapasalo M (2000) Isolation of Enterococcus faecalis in previously root-filled canals in a Lithuanian population. *Journal of Endodontics* **26**, 593–5.

251. Peters LB, Wesselink PR, Moorer WR (1995) The fate and the role of bacteria left in root dentinal tubules. *International Endodontic Journal* **28**, 95–9.

252. Peters OA, Laib A, Ruegsegger P, Barbakow F (2000) Three-dimensional analysis of root canal geometry by high-resolution computed tomography. *Journal of Dental Research* **79**, 1405–9.

253. Peterson DS, Taylor MH, Marley JF (1985) Calcific metamorphosis with internal resorption. *Oral Surgery, Oral Medicine, Oral Pathology* **60**, 231–3.

254. Pezelj-Ribaric S, Anic I, Brekalo I, Miletic I, Hasan M, Simunovic-Soskic M (2002) Detection of tumor necrosis factor alpha in normal and inflamed human dental pulps. *Archives of Medical Research* **33**, 482–4.

255. Piattelli A, Artese L, Rosini S, Quaranta M, Musiani P (1991) Immune cells in periapical granuloma: morphological and immunohistochemical characterization. *Journal of Endodontics* **17**, 26–9.

256. Pinzon RD, Kozlov M, Burch WP (1967) Histology of rat molar pulp at different ages. *Journal of Dental Research* **46**, 202–8.

257. Posadas I, Terencio MC, Guillen I, Ferrandiz ML, Coloma J, Paya M, *et al.* (2000) Co-regulation between cyclo-oxygenase-2 and inducible nitric oxide synthase expression in the time-course of murine inflammation. *Naunyn-Schmiedeberg's Archives of Pharmacology* **361**, 98–106.

258. Pozo D, Delgado M (2004) The many faces of VIP in neuroimmunology: a cytokine rather a neuropeptide? *FASEB Journal* **18**, 1325–34.

259. Rabinowitch BZ (1972) Internal resorption. *Oral Surgery, Oral Medicine, Oral Pathology* **33**, 263–82.

260. Rauh MJ, Ho V, Pereira C, Sham A, Sly LM, Lam V, *et al.* (2005) SHIP represses the generation of alternatively activated macrophages. *Immunity* **23**, 361–74.

261. Reddy J, Illes Z, Zhang X, Encinas J, Pyrdol J, Nicholson L, *et al.* (2004) Myelin proteolipid protein-specific CD4+CD25+ regulatory cells mediate genetic resistance to experimental autoimmune encephalomyelitis. *Proceedings of the National Academy of Sciences of the United States of America* **101**, 15434–9.

262. Ricucci D, Grondahl K, Bergenholtz G (2000) Periapical status of root-filled teeth exposed to the oral environment by loss of restoration or caries. *Oral Surgery, Oral Medicine, Oral Pathology, Oral Radiology and Endodontics* **90**, 354–9.

263. Robinson H, Boling L (1941) The anachoretic effect in pulpitis. I. Bacteriologic studies. *Journal of the American Dental Association* **28**, 268–82.

264. Rodini CO, Lara VS (2001) Study of the expression of CD68+ macrophages and CD8+ T cells in human granulomas and periapical cysts. *Oral Surgery, Oral Medicine, Oral Pathology, Oral Radiology and Endodontics* **92**, 221–7.

265. Rothe H, Hartmann B, Geerlings P, Kolb H (1996) Interleukin-12 gene-expression of macrophages is regulated by nitric oxide. *Biochemical and Biophysical Research Communications* **224**, 159–63.

266. Rungvechvuttivittaya S, Okiji T, Suda H (1998) Responses of macrophage-associated antigen-expressing cells in the dental pulp of rat molars to experimental tooth replantation. *Archives of Oral Biology* **43**, 701–10.

267. Rutherford RB, Gu K (2000) Treatment of inflamed ferret dental pulps with recombinant bone morphogenetic protein-7. *European Journal of Oral Sciences* **108**, 202–6.

268. Rutherford RB (2001) BMP-7 gene transfer to inflamed ferret dental pulps. *European Journal of Oral Sciences* **109**, 422–4.

269. Sabeti M, Simon J, Kermani V, Valles Y, Rostein I (2005) Detection of receptor activator of NF-kappa beta ligand in apical periodontitis. *Journal of Endodontics* **31**, 17–18.

270. Said SI, Mutt V (1970) Polypeptide with broad biological activity: isolation from small intestine. *Science* **169**, 1217–18.

271. Said SI, Mutt V (1972) Isolation from porcine-intestinal wall of a vasoactive octacosapeptide related to secretin and to glucagon. *European Journal of Biochemistry* **28**, 199–204.

272. Sakaguchi S (2000) Regulatory T cells: key controllers of immunologic self-tolerance. *Cell* **101**, 455–8.

273. Sakurai K, Okiji T, Suda H (1999) Co-increase of nerve fibers and HLA-DR- and/or factor-XIIIa-expressing dendritic cells in dentinal caries-affected regions of the human dental pulp: an immunohistochemical study. *Journal of Dental Research* **78**, 1596–608.

274. Salomon B, Lenschow DJ, Rhee L, Ashourian N, Singh B, Sharpe A, *et al.* (2000) B7/CD28 costimulation is essential for the homeostasis of the CD4+CD25+ immunoregulatory T cells that control autoimmune diabetes. *Immunity* **12**, 431–40.

275. Sasafuchi Y, Otsuki M, Inokoshi S, Tagami J (1999) The effects on pulp tissue of microleakage in resin composite restorations. *Journal of Medical and Dental Sciences* **46**, 155–64.

276. Sasaki H, Hou L, Belani A, Wang CY, Uchiyama T, Muller R, *et al.* (2000) IL-10, but not IL-4, suppresses infection-stimulated bone resorption in vivo. *Journal of Immunology* **165**, 3626–30.

277. Sasaki H, Balto K, Kawashima N, Eastcott J, Hoshino K, Akira S, *et al.* (2004) Gamma interferon (IFN-gamma) and IFN-gamma-inducing cytokines interleukin-12 (IL-12) and IL-18 do not augment infection-stimulated bone resorption in vivo. *Clinical and Diagnostic Laboratory Immunology* **11**, 106–10.

278. Sasaki H, Okamatsu Y, Kawai T, Kent R, Taubman M, Stashenko P (2004) The interleukin-10 knockout mouse is highly susceptible to Porphyromonas gingivalis-induced alveolar bone loss. *Journal of Periodontal Research* **39**, 432–41.

279. Schwartz MW, Woods SC, Porte D, Jr, Seeley RJ, Baskin DG (2000) Central nervous system control of food intake. *Nature* **404**, 661–71.

280. Segal AW (2005) How neutrophils kill microbes. *Annual Review of Immunology* **23**, 197–223.

281. Seltzer S, Rainey E, Gluskin AH (1977) Correlation of scanning electron microscope and light microscope findings in uninflamed and pathologically involved human pulps. *Oral Surgery, Oral Medicine, Oral Pathology* **43**, 910–28.

282. Sen BH, Piskin B, Demirci T (1995) Observation of bacteria and fungi in infected root canals and dentinal tubules by SEM. *Endodontics and Dental Traumatology* **11**, 6–9.

283. Sherwood NM, Krueckl SL, McRory JE (2000) The origin and function of the pituitary adenylate cyclase-activating polypeptide (PACAP)/glucagon superfamily. *Endocrine Reviews* **21**, 619–70.

284. Shiba H, Mouri Y, Komatsuzawa H, Ouhara K, Takeda K, Sugai M, *et al.* (2003) Macrophage inflammatory protein-3alpha and beta-defensin-2 stimulate dentin sialophosphoprotein gene expression in human pulp cells. *Biochemical and Biophysical Research Communications* **306**, 867–71.

285. Shortman K, Liu YJ (2002) Mouse and human dendritic cell subtypes, *Nature Reviews. Immunology* **2**, 151–61.

286. Siqueira JF, Jr, Rocas IN (2003) Polymerase chain reaction detection of Propionibacterium propionicus and Actinomyces radicidentis in primary and persistent endodontic infections. *Oral Surgery, Oral Medicine, Oral Pathology, Oral Radiology and Endodontics* **96**, 215–22.

287. Siqueira JF, Jr, Rocas IN (2004) Polymerase chain reaction-based analysis of microorganisms associated with failed endodontic treatment. *Oral Surgery, Oral Medicine, Oral Pathology, Oral Radiology and Endodontics* **97**, 85–94.

288. Sol MA, Tkaczuk J, Voigt JJ, Durand M, Sixou M, Maurette A, *et al.* (1998) Characterization of lymphocyte subpopulations in periapical lesions by flow cytometry. *Oral Microbiology and Immunology* **13**, 253–8.

289. Sreedharan SP, Patel DR, Huang JX, Goetzl EJ (1993) Cloning and functional expression of a human neuroendocrine vasoactive intestinal peptide receptor.

Biochemical and Biophysical Research Communications **193**, 546–53.

290. Stanley HR (1968) Design for a human pulp study. I. *Oral Surgery, Oral Medicine, Oral Pathology* **25**, 633–47.

291. Stanley HR (1968) Design for a human pulp study. II. *Oral Surgery, Oral Medicine, Oral Pathology* **25**, 756–64.

292. Stashenko P, Yu SM (1989) T helper and T suppressor cell reversal during the development of induced rat periapical lesions. *Journal of Dental Research* **68**, 830–4.

293. Stashenko P (1990) Role of immune cytokines in the pathogenesis of periapical lesions. *Endodontics and Dental Traumatology* **6**, 89–96.

294. Stashenko P, Yu SM, Wang CY (1992) Kinetics of immune cell and bone resorptive responses to endodontic infections. *Journal of Endodontics* **18**, 422–6.

295. Stashenko P, Wang CY, Tani-Ishii N, Yu SM (1994) Pathogenesis of induced rat periapical lesions. *Oral Surgery, Oral Medicine, Oral Pathology* **78**, 494–502.

296. Stashenko P, Wang CY, Riley E, Wu Y, Ostroff G, Niederman R (1995) Reduction of infection-stimulated periapical bone resorption by the biological response modifier PGG glucan. *Journal of Dental Research* **74**, 323–30.

297. Stashenko P, Teles R, D'Souza R (1998) Periapical inflammatory responses and their modulation. *Critical Reviews in Oral Biology and Medicine* **9**, 498–521.

298. Stein JV, Soriano SF, M'Rini C, Nombela-Arrieta C, de Buitrago GG, Rodriguez-Frade JM, *et al.* (2003) CCR7-mediated physiological lymphocyte homing involves activation of a tyrosine kinase pathway. *Blood* **101**, 38–44.

299. Steinman RM (1991) The dendritic cell system and its role in immunogenicity. *Annual Review of Immunology* **9**, 271–96.

300. Steinman RM, Hawiger D, Nussenzweig MC (2003) Tolerogenic dendritic cells. *Annual Review of Immunology* **21**, 685–711.

301. Stenvik A, Iversen J, Mjor IA (1972) Tissue pressure and histology of normal and inflamed tooth pulps in macaque monkeys. *Archives of Oral Biology* **17**, 1501–11.

302. Steranka LR, Farmer SG, Burch RM (1989) Antagonists of B2 bradykinin receptors. *FASEB Journal* **3**, 2019–25.

303. Stern MH, Dreizen S, Mackler BF, Selbst AG, Levy DM (1981) Quantitative analysis of cellular composition of human periapical granuloma. *Journal of Endodontics* **7**, 117–22.

304. Stern MH, Dreizen S, Mackler BF, Levy BM (1982) Isolation and characterization of inflammatory cells from the human periapical granuloma. *Journal of Dental Research* **61**, 1408–12.

305. Stumhofer JS, Laurence A, Wilson EH, Huang E, Tato CM, Johnson LM, *et al.* (2006) Interleukin 27 negatively regulates the development of interleukin 17-producing T helper cells during chronic inflammation of the central nervous system. *Nature Immunology* **7**, 937–45.

306. Suda T, Takahashi N, Martin TJ (1992) Modulation of osteoclast differentiation. *Endocrine Reviews* **13**, 66–80.

307. Sunde PT, Olsen I, Debelian GJ, Tronstad L (2002) Microbiota of periapical lesions refractory to endodontic therapy. *Journal of Endodontics* **28**, 304–10.

308. Sundqvist G, Lerner UH (1996) Bradykinin and thrombin synergistically potentiate interleukin 1 and tumour necrosis factor induced prostanoid biosynthesis in human dental pulp fibroblasts. *Cytokine* **8**, 168–77.

309. Sundqvist G, Figdor D, Persson S, Sjögren U (1998) Microbiologic analysis of teeth with failed endodontic treatment and the outcome of conservative re-treatment. *Oral Surgery, Oral Medicine, Oral Pathology, Oral Radiology and Endodontics* **85**, 86–93.

310. Suzuki N, Okiji T, Suda H (1999) Enhanced expression of activation-associated molecules on macrophages of heterogeneous populations in expanding periapical lesions in rat molars. *Archives of Oral Biology* **44**, 67–79.

311. Suzuki T, Kumamoto H, Ooya K, Motegi K (2001) Immunohistochemical analysis of CD1a-labeled Langerhans cells in human dental periapical inflammatory lesions – correlation with inflammatory cells and epithelial cells. *Oral Diseases* **7**, 336–43.

312. Suzuki T, Kumamoto H, Ooya K, Motegi K (2002) Expression of inducible nitric oxide synthase and heat shock proteins in periapical inflammatory lesions. *Journal of Oral Pathology and Medicine* **31**, 488–93.

313. Szabo SJ, Kim ST, Costa GL, Zhang X, Fathman CG, Glimcher LH (2000) A novel transcription factor, T-bet, directs Th1 lineage commitment. *Cell* **100**, 655–69.

314. Tagger M, Massler M (1975) Periapical tissue reactions after pulp exposure in rat molars. *Oral Surgery, Oral Medicine, Oral Pathology* **39**, 304–17.

315. Takahashi K (1990) Changes in the pulpal vasculature during inflammation. *Journal of Endodontics* **16**, 92–7.

316. Takahashi K (1992) Pulpal vascular changes in inflammation. *Proceedings of the Finnish Dental Society* **88** Suppl 1, 381–5.

317. Takahashi K (1998) Microbiological, pathological, inflammatory, immunological and molecular biological aspects of periradicular disease. *International Endodontic Journal* **31**, 311–25.

318. Takahashi K, MacDonald D, Murayama Y, Kinane D (1999) Cell synthesis, proliferation and apoptosis in human dental periapical lesions analysed by in situ hybridisation and immunohistochemistry. *Oral Diseases* **5**, 313–20.

319. Takeda K, Kaisho T, Akira S (2003) Toll-like receptors. *Annual Review of Immunology* **21**, 335–76.

320. Takeichi O, Saito I, Hayashi M, Tsurumachi T, Saito T (1998) Production of human-inducible nitric oxide synthase in radicular cysts. *Journal of Endodontics* **24**, 157–60.

321. Tan YV, Couvineau A, Van Rampelbergh J, Laburthe M (2003) Photoaffinity labeling demonstrates physical contact between vasoactive intestinal peptide and the N-terminal ectodomain of the human VPAC1 receptor. *Journal of Biological Chemistry* **278**, 36531–6.

322. Tang HM, Nordbo H, Bakland LK (2000) Pulpal response to prolonged dentinal exposure to sodium hypochlorite. *International Endodontic Journal* **33**, 505–8.

323. Tani-Ishii N, Wang CY, Stashenko P (1995) Immunolocalization of bone-resorptive cytokines in rat pulp and periapical lesions following surgical pulp exposure. *Oral Microbiology and Immunology* **10**, 213–19.

324. Tani N, Osada T, Watanabe Y, Umemoto T (1992) Comparative immunohistochemical identification and relative distribution of immunocompetent cells in sections of frozen or formalin-fixed tissue from human periapical inflammatory lesions. *Endodontics and Dental Traumatology* **8**, 163–9.

325. Taniguchi M, Harada M, Kojo S, Nakayama T, Wakao H (2003) The regulatory role of Valpha14 NKT cells in innate and acquired immune response. *Annual Review of Immunology* **21**, 483–513.

326. Tato CM, O'Shea JJ (2006) Immunology: what does it mean to be just 17? *Nature* **441**, 166–8.

327. Taylor PE, Byers MR, Redd PE (1988) Sprouting of CGRP nerve fibers in response to dentin injury in rat molars. *Brain Research* **461**, 371–6.

328. Taylor PE, Byers MR (1990) An immunocytochemical study of the morphological reaction of nerves containing calcitonin gene-related peptide to microabscess formation and healing in rat molars. *Archives of Oral Biology* **35**, 629–38.

329. Taylor PR, Martinez-Pomares L, Stacey M, Lin HH, Brown GD, Gordon S (2005) Macrophage receptors and immune recognition. *Annual Review of Immunology* **23**, 901–4.

330. Teles R, Wang CY, Stashenko P (1997) Increased susceptibility of RAG-2 SCID mice to dissemination of endodontic infections. *Infection and Immunity* **65**, 3781–7.

331. Ten Cate AR (1972) The epithelial cell rests of Malassez and the genesis of the dental cyst. *Oral Surgery, Oral Medicine, Oral Pathology* **34**, 956–64.

332. Thery C, Amigorena S (2001) The cell biology of antigen presentation in dendritic cells. *Current Opinion in Immunology* **13**, 45–51.

333. Tokuda M, Nagaoka S, Torii M (2002) Interleukin-10 inhibits expression of interleukin-6 and -8 mRNA in human dental pulp cell cultures via nuclear factor-kappaB deactivation. *Journal of Endodontics* **28**, 177–80.

334. Tokuda M, Miyamoto R, Sakuta T, Nagaoka S, Torii M (2005) Substance P activates p38 mitogen-activated protein kinase to promote IL-6 induction in human dental pulp fibroblasts. *Connective Tissue Research* **46**, 153–8.

335. Tonder KJ (1980) Blood flow and vascular pressure in the dental pulp. Summary. *Acta Odontologica Scandinavica* **38**, 135–44.

336. Tonder KJ, Kvinnsland I (1983) Micropuncture measurements of interstitial fluid pressure in normal and inflamed dental pulp in cats. *Journal of Endodontics* **9**, 105–9.

337. Torabinejad M, Bakland LK (1978) Immunopathogenesis of chronic periapical lesions. A review. *Oral Surgery, Oral Medicine, Oral Pathology* **46**, 685–99.

338. Torabinejad M, Bakland LK (1978) An animal model for the study of immunopathogenesis of periapical lesions. *Journal of Endodontics* **4**, 273–7.

339. Torabinejad M, Kettering JD (1985) Identification and relative concentration of B and T lymphocytes in human chronic periapical lesions. *Journal of Endodontics* **11**, 122–5.

340. Toriya Y, Hashiguchi I, Maeda K (1997) Immunohistochemical examination of the distribution of mac-

rophages and CGRP-immunoreactive nerve fibers in induced rat periapical lesions. *Endodontics and Dental Traumatology* **13**, 6–12.

341. Trott JR, Chebib F, Galindo Y (1973) Factors related to cholesterol formation in cysts and granulomas. *Journal/ Canadian Dental Association. Journal de l'Association Dentaire Canadienne* **39**, 550–5.

342. Tsuruga E, Sakakura Y, Yajima T, Shide N (1999) Appearance and distribution of dendritic cells and macrophages in dental pulp during early postnatal morphogenesis of mouse mandibular first molars. *Histochemistry and Cell Biology* **112**, 193–204.

343. Tziafas D (1989) Experimental bacterial anachoresis in dog dental pulps capped with calcium hydroxide. *Journal of Endodontics* **15**, 591–5.

344. Udagawa N, Takahashi N, Akatsu T, Tanaka H, Sasaki T, Nishihara T, *et al.* (1990) Origin of osteoclasts: mature monocytes and macrophages are capable of differentiating into osteoclasts under a suitable microenvironment prepared by bone marrow-derived stromal cells. *Proceedings of the National Academy of Sciences of the United States of America* **87**, 7260–4.

345. Udagawa N (2003) The mechanism of osteoclast differentiation from macrophages: possible roles of T lymphocytes in osteoclastogenesis. *Journal of Bone and Mineral Metabolism* **21**, 337–43.

346. Van Hassel HJ (1971) Physiology of the human dental pulp. *Oral Surgery, Oral Medicine, Oral Pathology* **32**, 126–34.

347. van Rossum D, Hanisch UK, Quirion R (1997) Neuroanatomical localization, pharmacological characterization and functions of CGRP, related peptides and their receptors. *Neuroscience and Biobehavioral Reviews* **21**, 649–78.

348. Vertucci FJ, Anthony RL (1986) A scanning electron microscopic investigation of accessory foramina in the furcation and pulp chamber floor of molar teeth. *Oral Surgery, Oral Medicine, Oral Pathology* **62**, 319–26.

349. Wada M, Takase T, Nakanuma K, Arisue K, Nagahama F, Yamazaki M (1998) Clinical study of refractory apical periodontitis treated by apicectomy. Part 1. Root canal morphology of resected apex. *International Endodontic Journal* **31**, 53–6.

350. Wakisaka S, Youn SH, Kato J, Takemura M, Kurisu K (1996) Neuropeptide Y-immunoreactive primary afferents in the dental pulp and periodontal ligament following nerve injury to the inferior alveolar nerve in the rat. *Brain Research* **712**, 11–18.

351. Walker KF, Lappin DF, Takahashi K, Hope J, Macdonald DG, Kinane DF (2000) Cytokine expression in periapical granulation tissue as assessed by immunohistochemistry. *European Journal of Oral Sciences* **108**, 195–201.

352. Walton RE, Garnick JJ (1986) The histology of periapical inflammatory lesions in permanent molars in monkeys. *Journal of Endodontics* **12**, 49–53.

353. Wang CY, Tani-Ishii N, Stashenko P (1997) Bone-resorptive cytokine gene expression in periapical lesions in the rat. *Oral Microbiology and Immunology* **12**, 65–71.

354. Wang J, Fathman JW, Lugo-Villarino G, Scimone L, von Andrian U, Dorfman DM, *et al.* (2006) Transcription factor T-bet regulates inflammatory arthritis through its function in dendritic cells. *Journal of Clinical Investigation* **116**, 414–21.

355. Wang X, Rickert M, Garcia KC (2005) Structure of the quaternary complex of interleukin-2 with its alpha, beta, and gammac receptors. *Science* **310**, 1159–63.

356. Warfvinge J (1986) Dental pulp inflammation; experimental studies in human and monkey teeth. *Swedish Dental Journal. Supplement* **39**, 1–36.

357. Waterman PA, Jr, Torabinejad M, McMillan PJ, Kettering JD (1998) Development of periradicular lesions in immunosuppressed rats. *Oral Surgery, Oral Medicine, Oral Pathology, Oral Radiology and Endodontics* **85**, 720–5.

358. Watts A, Paterson RC (1981) Cellular responses in the dental pulp: a review. *International Endodontic Journal* **14**, 10–19.

359. Weidner C, Klede M, Rukwied R, Lischetzki G, Neisius U, Skov PS, *et al.* (2000) Acute effects of substance P and calcitonin gene-related peptide in human skin – a microdialysis study. *Journal of Investigative Dermatology* **115**, 1015–1020.

360. Wimalawansa SJ (1996) Calcitonin gene-related peptide and its receptors: molecular genetics, physiology, pathophysiology, and therapeutic potentials. *Endocrine Reviews* **17**, 533–85.

361. Wong BR, Josien R, Lee SY, Sauter B, Li HL, Steinman RM, *et al.* (1997) TRANCE (tumor necrosis factor [TNF]-related activation-induced cytokine), a new TNF family member predominantly expressed in T cells, is a dendritic cell-specific survival factor. *Journal of Experimental Medicine* **186**, 2075–80.

362. Wong BR, Rho J, Arron J, Robinson E, Orlinick J, Chao M, *et al.* (1997) TRANCE is a novel ligand of the tumor necrosis factor receptor family that activates c-Jun N-terminal kinase in T cells. *Journal of Biological Chemistry* **272**, 25190–4.

363. Xia T, Baumgartner JC (2003) Occurrence of *Actinomyces* in infections of endodontic origin. *Journal of Endodontics* **29**, 549–52.

364. Yamasaki M, Kumazawa M, Kohsaka T, Nakamura H (1994) Effect of methotrexate-induced neutropenia on rat periapical lesion. *Oral Surgery, Oral Medicine, Oral Pathology* **77**, 655–61.

365. Yang D, Biragyn A, Kwak LW, Oppenheim JJ (2002) Mammalian defensins in immunity: more than just microbicidal. *Trends in Immunology* **23**, 291–6.

366. Yang G, Kawashima N, Kaneko T, Suzuki N, Okiji T, Suda H (2006) Kinetic study of immunohistochemical colocalization of antigen-presenting cells and nerve fibers in rat periapical lesions. *Journal of Endodontics* **33**, 132–6.

367. Yang LC, Huang FM, Lin CS, Liu CM, Lai CC, Chang YC (2003) Induction of interleukin-8 gene expression by black-pigmented Bacteroides in human pulp fibroblasts and osteoblasts. *International Endodontic Journal* **36**, 774–9.

368. Yasuda H, Shima N, Nakagawa N, Yamaguchi K, Kinosaki M, Mochizuki S, *et al.* (1998) Osteoclast differentiation factor is a ligand for osteoprotegerin/osteoclastogenesis-inhibitory factor and is identical to TRANCE/RANKL. *Proceedings of the National*

Academy of Sciences of the United States of America **95**, 3597–602.

369. Yokoyama WM, Plougastel BF (2003) Immune functions encoded by the natural killer gene complex. *Nature Reviews. Immunology* **3**, 304–16.

370. Yoshiba K, Yoshiba N, Iwaku M (2003) Class II antigen-presenting dendritic cell and nerve fiber responses to cavities, caries, or caries treatment in human teeth. *Journal of Dental Research* **82**, 422–7.

371. Yoshiba N, Yoshiba K, Iwaku M, Ozawa H (1998) Immunohistochemical localizations of class II antigens and nerve fibers in human carious teeth: HLA-DR immunoreactivity in Schwann cells. *Archives of Histology and Cytology* **61**, 343–52.

372. Yu SM, Stashenko P (1987) Identification of inflammatory cells in developing rat periapical lesions. *Journal of Endodontics* **13**, 535–40.

373. Zehnder M, Delaleu N, Du Y, Bickel M (2003) Cytokine gene expression – part of host defence in pulpitis. *Cytokine* **22**, 84–8.

374. Zhang DH, Cohn L, Ray P, Bottomly K, Ray A (1997) Transcription factor GATA-3 is differentially expressed in murine Th1 and Th2 cells and controls Th2-specific expression of the interleukin-5 gene. *Journal of Biological Chemistry* **272**, 21597–603.

375. Zhang X, Peng B (2005) Immunolocalization of receptor activator of NF kappa B ligand in rat periapical lesions. *Journal of Endodontics* **31**, 574–7.

376. Zimmerman BJ, Holt JW, Paulson JC, Anderson DC, Miyasaka M, Tamatani T, *et al.* (1994) Molecular determinants of lipid mediator-induced leukocyte adherence and emigration in rat mesenteric venules. *American Journal of Physiology* **266**, H847–53.

Chapter 4

Pathobiology of Apical Periodontitis

P.N.R. Nair

4.1 Introduction

Recent advances in microbiology have had a profound impact on the understanding of the etiology, pathogenesis and treatment of chronic diseases of persistent infections. It has become increasingly clear that unlike classical infectious diseases of single, specific etiological agents, there are several disease entities that are caused by a consortium of microbial species living together in an ecologically ordered communal form of living, now known as a biofilm [51]. Apical periodontitis belongs to this category of diseases. It is an inflammatory disorder of periradicular tissues caused by irritants of endodontic origin, mostly of persistent microbes living in the root canal system of the affected tooth [117,292]. The necrotic pulp offers a selective habitat for the endodontic microflora [71]. In the root canal the microbes grow in adhesive biofilms, aggregates,

coaggregates, and as planktonic cells suspended in the fluid phase of the canal [179]. A biofilm [51] is an extracellular matrix-embedded community of microorganisms that adhere to each other and/or to a moist surface in contrast with planktonic organisms, which are free-floating single microbial cells in an aqueous environment. Microorganisms are protected in biofilms where they have the remarkable ability to resist biocides several hundred times that of the same organisms in planktonic form [50,341]. Essentially apical periodontitis is the body's defense response to the destruction of tooth pulp and microbial settlement of the root canal system [132]. The microbes residing in the root canal can advance or their products can egress into the periapex. In response, the body mounts an array of defense consisting of several classes of cells, of intercellular messengers, of chemical weapons and of effector molecules. In spite of the formidable defense, the body cannot get rid of the microbes, mostly well entrenched as biofilms, in the sanctuary of the necrotic root canal. Therefore, apical periodontitis is not self-healing or self-limiting. The microbial factors and host defense clash, but strike an equilibrium that allows the persistence of pathogens in the root canal and limited host response, leading to the formation of various categories of lesion of apical periodontitis [180].

4.2 Classification and terminology

Apical periodontitis can be classified on several bases such as the etiology, symptoms and histopathological features. The World Health Organization [340] in the *Application of the International Classification of Diseases to Dentistry and Stomatology* classified apical periodontitis into various categories (Table 4.1). However, this clinically useful classification does not take into account the structural aspects of the lesions. As the architectural components of the lesion form the basis for an understanding of the disease process, a histopathological classification is followed in this chapter (Fig. 4.1). It is based on several criteria, which include the distribution of various cell populations within the lesion, the presence or absence of epithe-

lial cells, whether the lesion has been transformed into a cyst and the relationship of the cyst cavity to the root canal of the affected tooth [180,188].

4.2.1 Acute apical periodontitis

This is inflammation at the periapex. An *incipient* or *primary* acute apical periodontitis is inflammation of short duration and is initiated within a healthy periapex in response to irritants (Fig. 4.1a). When infection is involved this response may develop into a primary abscess. A *secondary acute* apical periodontitis (Fig. 4.1b) is an acute inflammatory response occurring in an already existing chronic apical periodontitis lesion. The latter form is also referred to as periapical flare-up, acute exacerbation, "Phoenix abscess" or secondary abscess. Depending on the presence or absence of epithelial cells the secondary acute apical periodontitis may be further subdivided into epithelialized or non-epithelialized lesions. The polymorphonuclear leucocyte (PMN) response may be restricted to a small area in the periapex forming a micro-abscess or may engulf the whole periapical area when it is referred to as dento-alveolar abscess which may "point" and open to the exterior by formation of a sinus tract.

Table 4.1   World Health Organization [340] classification of diseases of periapical tissues

Code No.	Category
K04.4	Acute apical periodontitis
K04.5	Chronic apical periodontitis (Apical granuloma)
K04.6	Periapical abscess with sinus (Dentoalveolar abscess with sinus, Periodontal abscess of pulpal origin)
K04.60	Periapical abscess with sinus to maxillary antrum
K04.61	Periapical abscess with sinus to nasal cavity
K04.62	Periapical abscess with sinus to oral cavity
K04.63	Periapical abscess with sinus to skin
K04.7	Periapical abscess without sinus (Dental abscess without sinus, Dentoalveolar abscess without sinus, Periodontal abscess of pulpal origin without sinus)
K04.8	Radicular cyst (Apical periodontal cyst, Periapical cyst)
K04.80	Apical and lateral cyst
K04.81	Residual cyst
K04.82	Inflammatory paradental cyst

Names in parentheses denote synonyms and conditions that are included in the category.

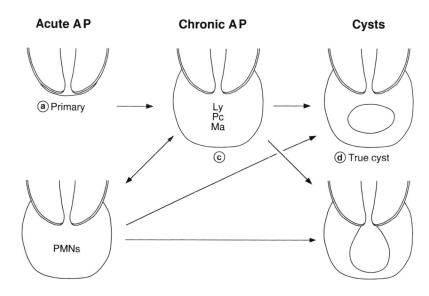

Fig. 4.1 Pathogenesis of apical periodontitis (AP) as acute (a, b), chronic (c) and cystic (d, e). The acute lesion may be primary (a) or secondary (b) and is characterized by the presence of a focus of neutrophils (PMNs). The major components of chronic lesions (c) are lymphocytes (Ly), plasma cells (Pc) and macrophage (Ma). Periapical cysts can be differentiated into true cysts (d) with completely enclosed lumina, and pocket cysts (e) with cavities open to the root canal. Arrows indicate the direction in which the lesions can change.

4.2.2 Chronic apical periodontitis

This is inflammation at the tooth apex of a long-standing nature and characterized by the presence of a granulomatous tissue predominantly infiltrated with lymphocytes, plasma cells and macrophages (Fig. 4.1c). These lesions may be epithelialized or non-epithelialized.

4.2.3 Periapical true cyst

This is an apical inflammatory cyst (Greek κυστις = bladder) with a distinct pathological cavity completely enclosed in an epithelial lining so that no communication to the root canal exists (Fig. 4.1d).

4.2.4 Periapical pocket cyst

This is an apical inflammatory cyst containing a sac-like, epithelium-lined cavity that is open to and continuous with the root canal (Fig. 4.1e).

4.3 Apical periodontitis

4.3.1 A disease of infection

More than a century ago, Miller [162] demonstrated the presence of several distinct types of bacteria in the necrotic dental pulp. Nevertheless, the etiological role of microorganisms in apical periodontitis remained

uncertain for several decades. Only bacteria found within intact solid lesions, particularly those found within phagocytic cells, were considered genuine [96] because of the problem of microbial contamination. As bacteria were detected only in a small fraction of the lesions, apical periodontitis was considered to be caused not necessarily by microbial infection alone, but by other primary and independent co-factors such as the necrotic pulp [136,280], stagnant tissue fluid [223] or root canal fillings. Several decades later Kakehashi *et al.* [117] reported that apical periodontitis did not develop in germ-free (gnotobiotic) rats when their molar pulps were exposed to the oral cavity, compared to control rats with a conventional oral microflora in which massive periapical radiolucencies occurred. Möller [166] showed the importance of asepsis in sampling of microorganisms from root canals of diseased teeth for culture studies and highlighted the great significance of obligate anaerobes in endodontic infections. Independent researchers confirmed the latter observations [22,118,344]. In the 1970s, advanced anaerobic techniques enabled the finding that the root canals of 18 out of 19 periapically affected teeth harbored a mixture of several species of bacteria that consisted predominantly of strict anaerobes [292]. A series of experimental studies [69] determined: (a) the conditions under which the endodontic flora develops and establishes itself, and (b) the biological properties and endodontic conditions which may favor the root canal flora to become pathogenic. Further clinical [64,125,303] and animal experimental [167,323] studies conclusively showed that *stagnant tissue fluid and sterile necrotic pulp tissue did not cause sustaining inflammation at the periapex*. The application of the precise technique of correlative light and transmission electron microscopy enabled the ultrastructural documentation of microorganisms within teeth, their strategic location in the apical root canal system and organization of the flora into biofilms [179]. Taken together, these studies provide a chain of evidence on the essential role of microorganisms in the development of apical periodontitis.

4.3.2 Portals of pulpal infection

There are several routes through which microorganisms can reach the dental pulp. Breaches in the hard tissue wall, resulting from caries, clinical procedures or trauma-induced fractures and cracks are the most frequent portals of pulpal infection. But microbes have also been isolated from teeth with necrotic pulps and apparently intact crowns [19,21,32,44,67,151,166, 292,344]. Endodontic infections of such teeth are preceded by pulp necrosis. It has been suggested that bacteria from the gingival sulci or periodontal pock-

ets might reach the root canals of these teeth through severed blood vessels of the periodontium [90]. However, it is very unlikely that microorganisms would survive the immunological defenses between the marginal gingiva and the apical foramen. An alternative possibility is that the teeth may clinically appear intact, but reveal microcracks in their hard tissues. The latter may provide portals of entry for bacteria. Pulpal infection can also occur through exposed dentinal tubules at the cervical root surface due to gaps in the cemental coating. It has been proposed that bacteria remaining in infected dentinal tubules (Fig. 4.2) can be a potential reservoir for endodontic reinfection [8,149,176,179,211,217,260,329]. Microbial infection has also been claimed to reach and seed in the necrotic pulp via the general blood circulation (anachoresis) [6,37,86,225]. However, bacteria could not be recovered from the root canal systems when the blood stream was experimentally infected unless the root canals were overinstrumented during the period of bacteremia [6,37,63,86,225]. Evidence that further discredits anachoresis as a potential source of necrotic pulpal infection comes from the study of Möller and others [167] in which all experimentally devitalised pulps ($n = 26$) in monkeys remained ster-

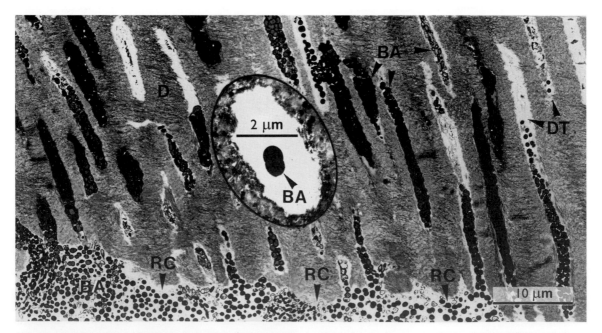

Fig. 4.2 Bacteria (BA) in dentinal tubules (DT) in the apical part of human root dentin (D). The bacteria invade the tubules from the infected root canal (RC). The presence of dividing forms (inset) is a clear sign of vitality of the microorganisms at the time of fixation (original magnifications: ×2480; inset ×9600).

ile for more than 6 months. Therefore, pulpal exposure to the oral cavity is the gateway of endodontic infection.

4.3.3 Endodontic flora

Following infection and pulp necrosis the root canal system provides a selective environment for the flora [71]. Morphologically, the endodontic flora consists of a mixed microbial population of cocci, rods, spirochetes and long filamentous organisms. Numerous dividing forms of cocci, rods and yeast cells are generally identifiable by transmission electron microscopy [179,186] which is a sign of vitality of the organisms at the time of fixation. These organisms are not uniformly distributed throughout the canal. The microbes can exist as aggregates of one microbial type (Fig. 4.3a–c), co-aggregates (Fig. 4.4) of several forms [48,179] and also as planktonic cells, suspended in the fluid phase of the infected and necrotic root canal. However, the undisturbed intracanal flora of an infected tooth with apical periodontitis is mostly organized as a matrix-embedded collection of multispecies organisms in ecosystems that may be immobile on the dentinal wall (Figs 4.3–4.5) [49–51,179,186]. This means that apical periodontitis is caused by an intraradicular growth of certain microorganisms that are ecologically organized into protected sessile biofilms [50,51] composed of cells embedded in a hydrated exopolysaccharide complex that cannot be eradicated by host defenses.

Cultivable microbes

The taxonomy of infected root canal flora is based on the application of advanced microbial culture techniques. This database is being reexamined and widened with the advent of molecular techniques in endodontic microbiology [175,228]. The results of early endodontic microbial culture studies have become irrelevant due to the difficulty of avoiding bacterial contamination from the oral surroundings [25,166,342] and to the absence of appropriate anaerobic methods for root canal sampling and cultivation of fastidious organisms. In order to recover such microorganisms from the necrotic pulp, stringent anaerobic sampling and cultivation techniques are necessary. These methods have been optimized only during the past three decades [107]. The two most significant advances in anaerobic technology have been (i) the innovative use of an anaerobic glovebox

[229,274] in which bacteria are protected from oxygen during isolation and cultivation, and (ii) the development of pre-reduced, anaerobically sterilized culture media for transport and growth [111,171]. Obligate anaerobes were believed to be killed by brief exposure to atmospheric O_2, but they can survive for several hours in media supplemented with hemolysed blood [42]. The enzyme, catalase, present in hemolysed blood, breaks down the toxic H_2O_2 in the medium to nontoxic O_2 and H_2O. These advances in anaerobic techniques have not only enabled the isolation and characterization of obligate anaerobes from the root canal systems of periapically affected teeth, but have also facilitated the study of their pathogenic properties [58,59,69–71,118,166,167,292,302,344].

A characteristic feature of the endodontic microflora is the small number of species that are usually isolated from such root canals. Application of advanced anaerobic techniques helped to establish that the root canal flora of teeth with clinically intact crowns but having necrotic pulps and diseased periapices is dominated (>90%) by obligate anaerobes [40,91,292,300] usually belonging to the genera *Fusobacterium*, *Porphyromonas* (formerly *Bacteroides* [254]), *Prevotella* (formerly *Bacteroides* [255]), *Eubacterium* and *Peptostreptococcus*. On the other hand, the microbial composition, even in the apical third of the root canal of periapically affected teeth with pulp canals exposed to the oral cavity by caries is not only different but also less dominated (<70%) by strict anaerobes [17]. Spirochetes have been found in necrotic root canals using microbial culture techniques [55,92,118], dark-field, [32,54,311] transmission electron microscopy [179] and molecular techniques [18,226,263]. Spirochetes are motile invasive pathogens (Fig. 4.6) that are associated with specific marginal periodontitis [145] and suspected etiological agents of acute necrotizing ulcerative gingivitis (ANUG) [146]. However, their role in apical periodontitis remains to be clarified. Culture studies, application of correlative light and transmission electron microscopy [186] (Figs 4.4 and 4.5) and scanning electron microscopy [253] revealed the presence of *fungi* in canals of teeth with primary apical periodontitis [334]. The presence of intraradicular *viruses* has so far been shown only in noninflamed dental pulps of patients infected with immunodeficiency virus [87]. As viruses cannot survive in a necrotic root canal without living cells to host them, they may not play an etiological role in primary apical periodontitis.

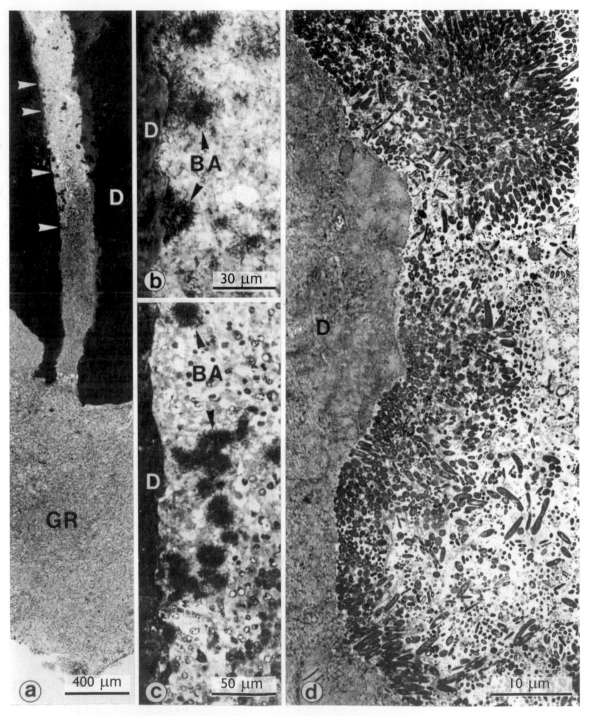

Fig. 4.3 Axial view of endodontic microbial biofilm in a human tooth with apical periodontitis (GR) and previously untreated root canal in axial view. The areas within the axial section of the tooth (a) in between the upper two and the lower two arrowheads are magnified in (b, c), respectively. Note the biofilm as dense bacterial aggregates (BA) sticking (b) to the dentinal (D) wall and also remaining suspended among neutrophilic granulocytes in the fluid phase of the root canal (c). A transmission electron microscopic view (d) of the pulp–dentin interface shows bacterial condensation on the surface of the dentinal wall forming a sessile biofilm (original magnifications: a ×46; b ×600; c ×370; d ×2350). (From Nair [180].)

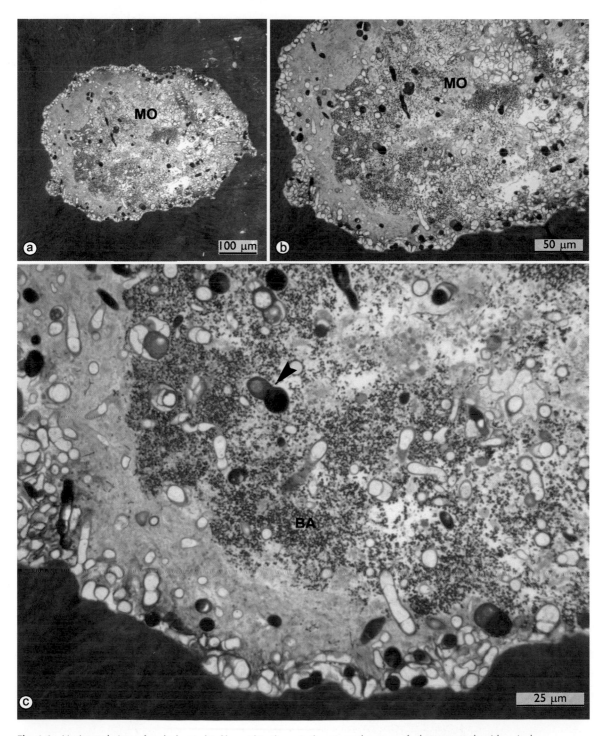

Fig. 4.4 Horizontal view of endodontic biofilm within the apical root canal system of a human tooth with apical periodontitis and previously untreated root canal. Stage-wise magnifications of a ramified segment of the canal system (a–c). Note the section of the canal system is filled with microorganisms (MO) of varying morphological forms; the small dot-like forms are bacteria (BA in c), and the large pleomorphic organisms showing filamentous and dividing forms (arrowhead) seem to be the yeast stage of fungi (original magnifications: a ×100, b ×280, c ×800). (From Nair *et al.* [186].)

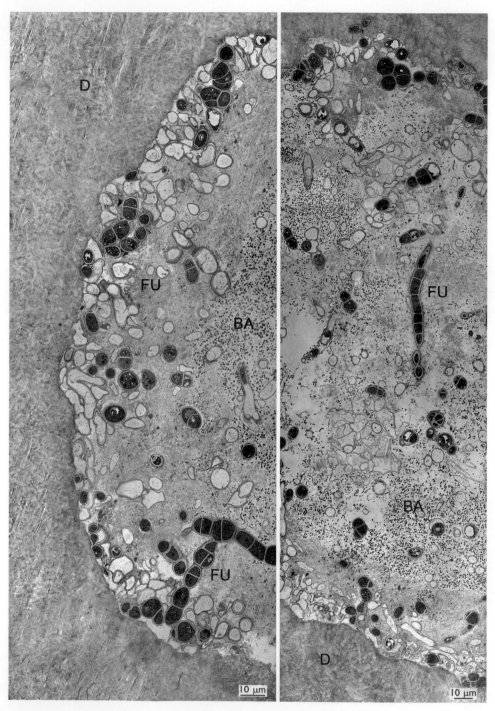

Fig. 4.5 Composite transmission electron micrographs show the presence of bacteria (BA) and fungi (FU) in the accessory canal illustrated in Fig. 4.4. Note the distinct electron lucent cell wall and the larger size of fungal organisms in comparison to that of the bacteria (BA). The fungus (FU) shows several dividing forms some of which form chains (original magnifications: a ×750, b ×600). (From Nair *et al.* [186].)

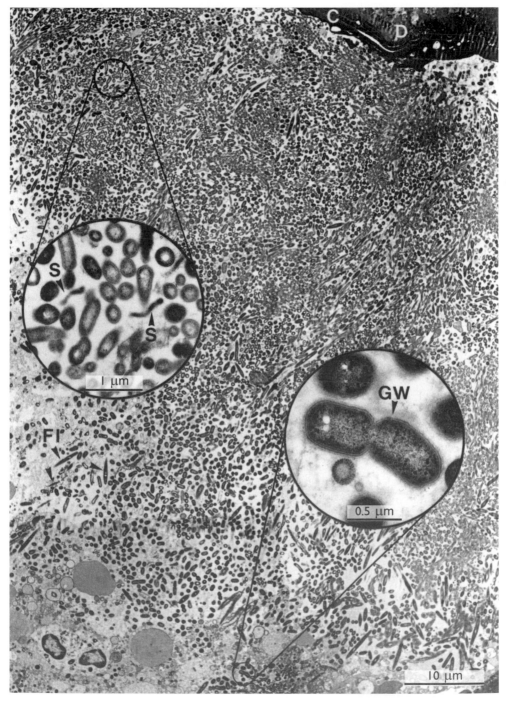

Fig. 4.6 A microbial biofilm at the root tip of a human tooth with secondary acute apical periodontitis of endodontic origin. The mixed bacterial flora consists of numerous dividing cocci, rods (lower inset), filaments (FI) and spirochetes (S, upper inset). Rods often reveal a Gram-negative cell wall (GW, lower inset). C, cementum; D, dentin (original magnifications: ×2680; upper inset ×19,200; lower inset ×36,400). (Adapted from Nair [179].)

Microbial remnants

The current understanding of the endontic microflora is based on various methods such as conventional and correlative microscopy, microbial culturing, biochemical, and molecular genetic techniques. These methods have varying degrees of limitations with respect to sensitivity, specificity, and etiological relevance. Among the molecular methods, the development of the polymerase chain reaction (PCR) [174] and its application in microbiology [218,281] has enabled detection of microbes by amplification of their DNA, when PCR has been targeted at 16S rRNA gene sequences for taxonomic identification. These methods have not only confirmed the microbial species that have been previously detected and grown by culture methods [175,228], but also facilitated the identification of "as-yet-culture-difficult" endodontic organisms [175]. The PCR is a sophisticated technique for accurately replicating and amplifying the DNA, but a valid scientific procedure remains essential [197] without which the resulting data have only limited etiological relevance [183]. Apart from the possible contamination of samples, the molecular technique does not differentiate between viable and nonviable organisms, but can pick up a minuscule amount of microbial DNA that is amplified using the PCR [174], resulting in an exponential accumulation of several million copies of the original DNA fragments. How long DNA from dead microorganisms may persist in the root canal is unknown [298]. Application of PCR methods has enabled the detection and amplification of DNA fragments of *Mycobacterium tuberculosis* from hundreds of years old human remains [75,127,242] and from that of an "extinct bison dated 17,000 years before the present" [230]. The data derived from the molecular technique, therefore, require very careful interpretation in the light of the technique's many advantages and numerous limitations. While the DNA-based molecular method is superior for microbial sensitivity and specificity, it is prone to false positive results due to detection of dead organisms and/or contaminants. Further, a mere observation of the presence of certain microbial remnants is not sufficient to implicate the associated organisms as etiological agents of diseases. Therefore, the onus is on researchers to come up with convincing evidence that the culture-difficult organisms reported using the molecular genetic methods are viable root canal microbes that cause apical periodontitis.

4.3.4 Virulence and pathogenicity

Any metabolically active microbe within the root canal has the potential to initiate inflammation of periradicular tissues. However, it is necessary to differentiate between a mere presence and the ability of the microbe to induce the disease or similar pathological changes in susceptible experimental animals. This is significant in infectious diseases in which the organisms must be present within the body milieu. In apical and marginal periodontitis the microbes, generally living in a biofilm, are stationed in the necrotic pulp or periodontal pocket, which are outside the body milieu. Metabolically active microbes present at those locations release antigenic and other molecules that irritate periodontal tissues both at the apical and marginal sites to cause inflammation, irrespective of them living there with or without virulence and tissue invasiveness. Although the individual species in the endodontic flora are usually of low virulence, their intraradicular survival and pathogenic properties are influenced by a combination of several factors. These include: (i) the ability to build biofilms by interacting with other microorganisms in the biofilm so as to develop synergistically beneficial partners, (ii) the capability to interfere with and evade host defenses, (iii) the release of lipopolysaccharides (LPS) and other microbial modulins, and (iv) the synthesis of enzymes that damage host tissues.

Biofilms

The importance of a mixed endodontic microflora in the development of apical periodontitis has long been recognized through carefully planned studies [70,71,302]. There is clear evidence that interaction among various microbial species [41,71,140,147] plays a significant role in the ecological regulation and eventual development of an endodontic habitat-adapted polymicrobial flora [293,294,298] that live in biofilms. Biofilms are matrix-embedded microbial populations adherent to each other and/or to surfaces or interfaces [49]. Current understanding of biofilms has been based on diverse research approaches that particularly include the application novel scanning confocal laser microscopy, molecular methods to determine gene expression, cell signaling, and culture-independent methods that identify (gene amplification and sequencing) and localize [fluorescent *in situ* hybridization (FISH)] biofilm components. These methods have shown that biofilms are well structured with diverse microbial species existing as organized symbiotic communities in a protective extracellular matrix and traversed by a network of fluid channels reminiscent of a very primitive circulatory system [49]. The ability to organize and live in biofilms with an open architecture has provided several biological advantages to the microbes such as gene transfer, novel gene expression, coordinated gene expression, population size dependent (quorum sensing) and independent cell signaling, limiting physical hazards (dehydration), protection from host defenses, increased resistance to biocides and enhanced virulence. The ability to form biofilms is a survival strategy of most microbes and must be considered as a virulence factor for disease producing organisms.

Microbial interference

The ability of certain microbes to shirk and interfere with the host defenses has been well elaborated (see [295] for a review). Bacterial LPS can signal the endothelial cells to express leukocyte adhesion molecules that initiate extravasation of leukocytes into the area of the infection. It has been reported that *Porphyromonas gingivalis*, an important endodontic and periodontal pathogen, and its LPS do not signal the endothelial cells to express E-selectin. *Porphyromonas gingivalis* therefore has the ability to block the initial step of the inflammatory response, "hide" from the host and multiply. The antigenicity of LPS occurs in several forms that include mitogenic stimulation of B-lymphocytes so as to produce nonspecific antibodies. Gram-negative organisms release membrane particles (blebs) and soluble antigens which may "mop up" effective antibodies so as to make them unavailable to act against the organism itself [163]. *Actinomyces israelii*, a recalcitrant periapical pathogen, is easily killed by PMNs *in vitro* [74]. In tissues, *A. israelii* aggregate to form large cohesive colonies that cannot be killed by host phagocytes [74].

LPS and other microbial modulins

Lipopolysaccharides, also historically known as endotoxin, form an integral part of Gram-negative cell walls. They are released during disintegration of bacteria after death and also during multiplication and growth. The effects of LPS are due to its interaction with endothelial cells and macrophages; LPS not only signals the endothelial cells to express adhesion molecules, but also activates macrophages to produce a number of molecular mediators such as tumor necrosis factor-α (TNF-α) and interleukins (IL) [11]. Exogenous TNF-α administered into experimental animals can induce a lethal shock that is indistinguishable from that induced by LPS. The LPS signal the presence of Gram-negative microorganisms in the area. The impact of LPS in tissues has been aptly stated [313]: "When we sense LPS, we are likely to turn on every defense at our disposal; we will bomb, defoliate, blockade, seal off and destroy all tissues in the area." The presence of LPS has been reported in samples taken from the root canal [57,245] and the pulpal dentinal wall of periapically involved teeth [109]. The Gram-negative organisms of the endodontic flora multiply and also die in the apical root canal, thereby releasing LPS that egresses through apical foramina into the periapex [346], where it initiates and sustains apical periodontitis [56,60].

However, LPS is not the only bacterial degradation product that can induce mammalian cells to produce cytokines. Many proteins, certain carbohydrates and lipids of bacterial origin are now considered as belonging to a novel class of "modulins" that induce the formation of cytokine networks and host tissue disease [103].

Enzymes

Endodontic microbes produce a variety of enzymes, which are not directly toxic but may aid the spread of the organisms in host tissues. Microbial collagenase, hyaluronidase, fibrinolysins and several proteases are examples. Microbes are also known to produce enzymes that degrade various plasma proteins involved in blood coagulation and other body defenses. The ability of some *Porphyromonas* and *Prevotella* species to break down plasma proteins, particularly IgG, IgM [123], and the complement factor C_3 [296] is of particular significance as these molecules are opsonins necessary for both humoral and phagocytic host defenses.

4.4 Host defense

Apical periodontitis is viewed as the consequence of a dynamic encounter between root canal microbes and host defense [180]. The latter involves cells, intercellular mediators and antibodies.

4.4.1 Cellular elements

Several classes of body cells participate in the periapical defense (Fig. 4.7). The majority of them are from the defense systems and include polymorphonuclear leukocytes (PMNs), lymphocytes, plasma cells and monocytes/macrophages. Structural cells include fibroblasts, osteoblasts and epithelial rests [153] that play significant roles. The importance of PMNs and monocyte derivatives in apical periodontitis has been shown experimentally [283]. The intensity of induced murine pulpitis and apical periodontitis can be suppressed by treating the animals with a biological response-modifying drug, PGG glucan that enhances the number and ability of circulating neutrophils and monocytes.

Polymorphonuclear leucocytes

They are the hallmark of acute inflammation; PMNs are nonspecific phagocytes and are well equipped to attack microbes with weapons already stored within them or quickly assembled by them [330]. In response to tissue injury, PMNs extravasate (Fig. 4.8) in great numbers and seek the targets by chemotaxis. They move in the direction of an ascending gradient of the chemotactic molecules so as to congregate at the site of microbial presence (Fig. 4.7a). By the time the PMNs meet the microbes the latter are generally opsonized. The microbes are ingested and isolated in membrane bound phagosomes. The PMNs have two pathways for intracellular killing of microbes. During the initial phases of inflammation there is generally plenty of oxygen in the tissues and the PMNs follow an aerobic route ("respiratory burst") in which the enzyme NADPH oxidase situated on the phagosome-membrane converts molecular O_2 into O_2^--derived free radicals. These are atoms or molecules with unpaired electrons. They are highly unstable, reactive and literally "snatch" electrons from other molecules thereby damaging them. Superoxide (O_2^-) is formed when NADPH oxidase acts on stable O_2. A pair of O_2^- can interact to form a molecule of hydrogen peroxide (H_2O_2). Both the O_2^- and H_2O_2 are mildly microbicidal. The latter in the presence of the enzyme, myeloperoxidase, oxidises halides (Cl^-) to form hypochlorous acid (HOCl), which is highly bactericidal. This pathway is known as the *H_2O_2–halide–myeloperoxidase system*. Under hypoxic conditions (abscess), PMNs shift the process to the anaerobic phagosomal pathway of microbial killing.

The PMNs (Fig. 4.7a) also cause severe damage to the host tissues. Their cytoplasmic granules contain several enzymes that on release degrade the structural elements of tissue cells and extracellular matrices. The zinc-dependent enzymes that are responsible for the breakdown of the extracellular matrices belong to the super family of enzymes called the matrix metalloproteinases (MMP) [177]. However, once launched or released these enzymatic and chemical weapons do not discriminate between hostile enemy and host tissues [330]. The PMNs are very short–living cells (about 3 days) that die in great numbers (Fig. 4.7a) at acute inflammatory sites [234]. Therefore, irrespective of the cause of PMN mobilization, the accumulation and massive death of neutrophils is a major cause for tissue breakdown in acute phases of apical periodontitis.

Lymphocytes

They have several roles in apical periodontitis. Among the three major classes of lymphocytes, designated as T lymphocytes (T cells), B lymphocytes (B cells) and the natural killer (NK) cells, the T and B cells are of particular importance. They are phenotypically identical (Fig. 4.7b) and cannot be distinguished by conventional staining or microscopical examination, but are typed on the basis of surface receptors using monoclonal antibodies against the latter. Cells so identified are given a cluster of differentiation (CD) number.

T cells

The thymus-derived (T) cells constitute about 60–70% of blood circulating lymphocytes. They are multifunctional with specific division of labor so that the various functions are performed by their subpopulations. The nomenclature of T-cells can be confusing. Traditionally, they have been designated after their effect or functions, as for instance the T-cells working with B-cells have long been known as T-helper/inducer ($T_{h/i}$) cells and those with direct toxic and suppressive effects on other cells have been named T-cytotoxic/suppressive ($T_{c/s}$) cells. The $T_{h/i}$ cells are $CD4^+$; and the $T_{c/s}$ cells are $CD8^+$. The $CD4^+$ cells differentiate further into two types known as T_{h1} and T_{h2} cells. The former produce interleukin-2 (IL-2) and interferon-γ (IF-γ), and control the cell-mediated arm of the immune system. The T_{h2} cells secrete

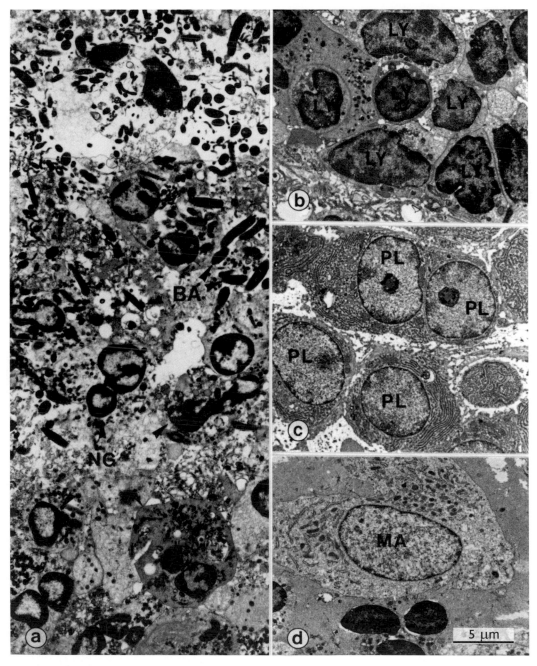

Fig. 4.7   The primary body cells involved in the pathogenesis of apical periodontitis. Neutrophils (NG in a) in combat with bacteria (BA) in secondary acute apical periodontitis. Lymphocytes (LY in b) are the major components of chronic apical periodontitis but their subpopulations cannot be identified on a structural basis. Plasma cells (PL in c) form a significant component of chronic asymptomatic lesions. Note the highly developed rough endoplasmic reticulum of the cytoplasm and the localized condensation of heterochromatin subjacent to the nuclear membrane which gives the typical "cartwheel" appearance in light microscopy. Macrophages (MA in d) are voluminous cells with elongated or U-forming nuclei and cytoplasm with rough endoplasmic reticulum (original magnifications: a–d ×3900).

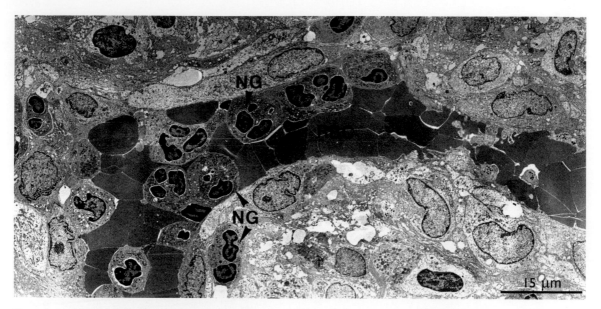

Fig. 4.8 Intravascular neutrophilic granulocytes (NG) marginating, adhering to the endothelial cells, and transmigrating across the blood vessel wall into the inflamed periapical tissues. RBC, red blood cells (original magnification: ×1650).

IL-4, IL-5, IL-6 and IL-10 that regulate the production of antibodies by the plasma cells.

B cells

The lymphocytes directly responsible for antibody production are the bursa-equivalent (B) cells, named after their discovery in the chicken organ called the bursa of Fabricius. They constitute about 10–20% of the lymphocyte population. On receiving signals from antigens and the T_{h2}-cells, some of the B-cells transform into large *plasma cells* (Fig. 4.7c) with characteristic nuclei of "cartwheel" appearance and extensive rough endoplasmic reticulum. Plasma cells are the only cells that can manufacture and secrete antibodies.

Macrophages

These are large mononuclear phagocytes (Fig. 4.7d) [161] that represent the major differentiated cell of the mononuclear phagocytic system [206,331], previously known as the reticuloendothelial system. Depending on their location, they have been known by various names; they produce various types of multinucleate cells such as osteoclasts, odontoclasts, and foreign body giant cells. Macrophages have several func-

tions that include: (i) phagocytic killing of microorganisms, (ii) scavenging of dead cells and tissue components, (iii) removal of small foreign particles, (iv) immunological surveillance by antigen capture, (v) processing and presentation of antigens to immune competent cells and (vi) secretion of a wide variety of biologically active molecules and their regulation.

Extravasation of monocytes is governed by the same factors that are involved in PMN emigration. On reaching the extravascular tissue monocytes undergo transformation into large phagocytic cells, the tissue macrophages. They are long living and slow-moving cells that stay at the inflammatory site for several months. If the first wave of PMN defense has failed to exterminate the enemy the process becomes a chronic inflammation. Thus, macrophages form a major component of the inflammatory cells in later stages of inflammation. They move by chemotaxis and are activated by microorganisms, their products (LPS), chemical mediators or foreign particles. Activated macrophages become larger, show numerous lysosomal and other cytoplasmic granules and have a greater affinity for phagocytosis and intracellular killing of microorganisms. They possess the same biochemical systems for killing of microbes as the PMNs do and can attach to foreign objects [269]. Among the various molecular mediators that are secreted by macrophages, the cytokines

IL-1, TNF-α, interferons (IFN) and growth factors are of particular importance in apical periodontitis. They also contribute serum components and metabolites such as prostaglandins and leukotrienes that are important in inflammation. Antigen presenting *dendritic cells* are also reported in induced murine apical periodontitis [202]. Whether they seed in periapical lesions via general circulation or spread locally from inflamed dental pulp [116] is unknown.

Osteoclasts

A major pathological event of apical periodontitis is the osteoclastic destruction of bone and dental hard tissues. There are reviews on the origin [198], structure [85], regulation [102] and "coupling" [221] of these cells with osteoblasts. The pro-osteoclasts migrate through blood as monocytes to the periradicular tissues and attach themselves to the surface of bone. They remain dormant until signaled for further changes and activity. In the physiological state those signals, involving several cytokines and other mediators, are given by osteoblasts. During apical periodontitis these mediators are released not only by osteoblasts but also by several other cells that stimulate the pro-osteoclasts. The latter begin to proliferate and several daughter cells fuse to form multinucleate osteoclasts that spread over injured and exposed bone surface. The cytoplasmic border of the osteoclasts facing the bony surface becomes ruffled as a result of multiple infolding of the plasma membrane. Bone resorption take place beneath this ruffled border known as the subosteoclastic resorption compartment. At the periphery, the cytoplasmic clear zone is a highly specialized area that regulates the biochemical activities involved in breaking down the bone. The bone destruction happens extracellularly at the osteoclast/bone interface and involves (i) demineralization of the bone by solubilizing the mineral phase in the resorption compartment as a result of ionic lowering of pH in the microenvironment and (ii) enzymatic dissolution of the organic matrix. In the process the enzyme-families, cystine proteinases and MMP, are involved. Root cementum and dentin are also resorbed in apical periodontitis by fusion macrophages designated as odontoclasts. They belong to the same cell population as osteoclasts in view of their ultrastructural and histochemical similarities [240].

Epithelial cells

About one-third to a half of all lesions of apical periodontitis contain proliferating epithelium [79,137, 188,252,261,276,312,348]. During periapical inflammation, the epithelial cell rests [153] are believed to be stimulated by cytokines and growth factors to undergo division and proliferation, a process commonly described as inflammatory hyperplasia. These cells participate in the pathogenesis of radicular cysts by serving as the source of epithelium. However, ciliated epithelial cells are also found in periapical lesions [187,257] particularly in lesions affecting maxillary molars. The maxillary sinus-epithelium was suggested to be a source of those cells [187,189].

4.4.2 Molecular mediators

Several cytokines [46] and eicosanoides are involved in the pathogenesis and progression of apical periodontitis.

Proinflammatory and chemotactic cytokines

They include IL-1, IL-6, IL-8 and tumor necrosis factors (TNF) [204]. The systemic effects IL-1 are identical to those observed in toxic shock. Local effects include enhancement of leukocyte adhesion to endothelial walls, stimulation of lymphocytes, potentiation of neutrophils, activation of the production of prostaglandins and proteolytic enzymes, enhancement of bone resorption and inhibition of bone formation. The IL-1β is the predominant form found in human periapical lesions and their exudates [13,14,141,158]. The IL-1α is primarily involved in apical periodontitis in rats [306,336]. The IL-6 [105] is produced by both lymphoid and nonlymphoid cells under the influence of IL-1, TNF-α and IFN-γ; it down-regulates the production and counters some of the effects of IL-1. The IL-6 has been demonstrated in human periapical lesions [62] and in inflamed marginal periodontal tissues [347]. The IL-8 is a family of chemotactic cytokines [61]. They are produced by monocyte/macrophages and fibroblasts under the influence of IL-1β and TNF-α. Massive infiltration of neutrophils is a characteristic of the acute phases of apical periodontitis for which IL-8 and other chemo-attractants such as bacterial peptides, plasma-derived complement split-factor C5a and leukotriene B$_4$ are important. The TNF have direct cytotoxic effects and general debilitating effects in chronic disease. In addition, the macrophage derived TNF-α [325] and the T-lymphocyte derived TNF-β [233], formerly *lymphotoxin*, have numerous systemic and local effects similar to those of IL-1. The presence of TNF-α has been reported in lesions of human apical periodontitis and root canal exudates of teeth with apical periodontitis [12,13,239].

IFN

These were originally described as antiviral agents and are now classified as cytokines. There are three distinct IFN designated as α, β and γ molecules. The antiviral protein is the IFN-γ produced by virus-infected cells and normal T-lymphocytes under various stimuli whereas the IFN-α/β proteins are produced by a variety of normal cells, particularly macrophages and B-lymphocytes.

Colony stimulating factors

These are cytokines that regulate the proliferation and differentiation of hemopoietic cells. The name originates from the early observation that certain polypeptide molecules promote the formation of granulocyte or monocyte colonies in semisolid medium. Three distinct proteins of this category have been isolated, characterized and designated as cytokines. They are (i) granulocyte-macrophage colony stimulating factor (G-MCF), (ii) granulocyte colony stimulating factor (G-CSF) and (iii) macrophage colony stimulating factor (M-CSF). In general, colony stimulating factors (CSF) stimulate the proliferation of neutrophil and osteoclast precursors in the bone marrow. They are also produced by osteoblasts [221], thus providing one of the communication links between osteoblasts and osteoclasts in bone resorption.

Growth factors

These are proteins that regulate the growth and differentiation of nonhemopoietic cells. Not all growth factors are cytokines, but many posses some cytokine-like actions. Transforming growth factors (TGF) are produced by normal and neoplastic cells that were originally identified by their ability to induce non-neoplastic, surface adherent colonies of fibroblasts in soft agar cultures. This process appears to be similar to neoplastic transformation of normal to malignant cells and therefore the name TGF. Based on their structural relationship to the epidermal growth fac-

tor (EGF), they are classified into TGF-α and TGF-β. The former is closely related to EGF in structure and effects, but is produced primarily by malignant cells and therefore is not significant in apical periodontitis. But TGF-β is synthesized by a variety of normal cells and platelets and is involved in the activation of macrophages, proliferation of fibroblasts, synthesis of connective tissue fibers and matrices, local angiogenesis, healing and downregulation of numerous functions of T-lymphocytes. Therefore, TGF-β is important to counter the adverse effects of the inflammatory host response.

Eicosanoids

Activated and/or injured cells remodel their membrane lipids to generate biologically active compounds that serve as intra- and intercellular signals. Arachidonic acid, a 20-carbon polysaturated fatty acid present in all cell membranes, is released from membrane lipids by a variety of stimuli and is rapidly metabolized to form several C_{20} compounds, known collectively as eicosanoides (Greek εικοσι = twenty). The eicosanoides are thought of as hormones with physiological effects at very low concentrations. They mediate inflammatory response, regulate blood pressure, induce blood clotting, pain and fever, and control several reproductive functions such as ovulation and induction of labor. Prostaglandins (PG) and leukotrienes (LT) are two major groups of eicosanoids involved in inflammation [244].

Prostaglandins

They were first identified in human semen through their ability to lower blood pressure and induce uterine contractions. Prostaglandins were thought to have originated from prostate gland that gave the name. They (e.g., PGE_2, PGD_2, PGF_{2a}, PGI_2) are formed when arachidonic acid is metabolized via the cyclic pathway, which is inhibited by aspirin. The PGE_2 and PGI_2 are potent activators of osteoclasts. Much of the rapid bone loss in marginal and apical periodontitis happens during episodes of acute inflammation when the lesions are dominated by PMNs, which are an important source of PGE_2. High levels of PGE_2 have been shown to be present in acute apical periodontitis lesions [160]. Apical hard tissue resorption can be suppressed by parenteral administration of indomethacin, an inhibitor of cyclooxygenase [319].

Leukotrienes

Arachidonic acid also serves as a precursor to compounds whose formation is not inhibited by aspirin. Leukotrienes (e.g., LTA_4, LTB_4, LTC_4, LTD_4 and LTE_4) are formed when arachidonic acid is oxidized via the linear pathway pathway. The LTB_4 is a powerful chemotactic agent for neutrophils [203] and causes adhesion of PMNs to the endothelial walls. The LTB_4 [320] and LTC_4 [52] have been detected in apical periodontitis with a high concentration of the former in symptomatic lesions [320].

Effector-molecules

A major histopathological change that takes place in apical periodontitis is the degradation of extracellular matrices. The dissolution of the tissue matrices is caused by enzymatic effector-molecules. Four major tissue degradation pathways have been recognized: (i) osteoclastic, (ii) phagocytic, (iii) plasminogen-dependent, and (iv) MMP-dependent [27]. The MMP are responsible for the degradation of much of the tissue matrices built on collagen, fibronectin, laminin, gelatin, and proteoglycan-core-proteins. The biology of MMP has been extensively researched and reviewed [28,29]. The MMP have been reported to be present in lesions of apical periodontitis [259,309].

4.4.3 Antibodies

They are specific weapons of the body that are produced solely by plasma cells. Different classes of immunoglobulins have been found in plasma cells [115,133,173,220,271,286] and extracellularly [133,157,178,324] in human apical periodontitis. The concentration of IgG in apical periodontitis was found to be nearly five times that of noninflamed oral mucosa [89]. Immunoglobulins have also been shown in plasma cells residing in the periapical cyst wall [220,273,286,317] and in the cyst fluid [248,270,317,351]. Their concentration in the cyst fluid was several times higher than that in blood. [248,270]. The specificity of the antibodies present in apical periodontitis may be low as LPS may act as antigens or mitogens. The resulting antibodies may be a mixture of both monoclonal and polyclonal varieties. The latter are nonspecific to its inducer and therefore ineffective. However, the specific monoclonal component may participate in the antimicrobial response and may even intensify the pathogenic pro-

cess by forming antigen–antibody complexes [319]. Intracanal application of an antigen against which the animal was previously immunized resulted in the induction of a transient apical periodontitis [322].

4.5 Pathogenesis: a dynamic encounter

The above outlined dynamic encounter between the microbial and host factors at the periapex results in various categories of lesions of apical periodontitis (Fig. 4.1). The equilibrium at the periapex, in favor of or against the host defense, determines the histological picture of the lesions.

4.5.1 Initial apical periodontitis

Apical periodontitis is generally initiated by microorganisms residing in or invading from the apical root canal into the periapical tissues (Fig. 4.6). A periapical inflammation can also be induced by accidental trauma, injury from instrumentation or irritation from chemicals and endodontic materials, each of which can provoke an intense tissue response of short duration. The process is accompanied by clinical symptoms such as pain, tooth elevation and tenderness to pressure on the tooth. Such initial, symptomatic lesions are viewed as acute apical periodontitis (Fig. 4.1a). The tissue response is generally limited to the apical periodontal ligament and the neighboring spongiosa. It is initiated by the typical neurovascular response of inflammation resulting in hyperemia, vascular congestion, and edema of the periodontal ligament and extravasation of neutrophils. The latter are attracted to the area by chemotaxis, induced initially by tissue injury, bacterial products (LPS) and complement factor C5a. As the integrity of bone, cementum and dentin has not yet been disturbed, the periapical changes at this stage are undetectable radiographically. If noninfectious irritants have induced inflammation, the lesion may subside and the structure of the apical periodontium may be restored [9].

When microbial infection is present, the PMNs not only fight the microorganisms (Fig. 4.7a), but also release leukotrienes and prostaglandins. The former (LTB_4) attract more neutrophils and macrophages into the area and the latter activate osteoclasts. In a few days time the bone surrounding the periapex can be resorbed and a radiolucent area may become detectable [284]. This initial rapid bone resorption can be prevented by indomethacin [319,322] that inhibits cyclooxygenase, thus suppressing prostaglandin synthesis. Neutrophils die at the inflammatory site (Fig. 4.7a) and release enzymes from their cytoplasmic granules that cause destruction of the extracellular matrices and cells. The self-induced destruction of the tissues prevents the spread of infection to other parts of the body and provides space for the infiltration of specialized defense cells. During the acute phase, macrophages also appear at the periapex. Activated macrophages produce a variety of mediators among which the proinflammatory (IL-1, IL-6, and TNF-α) and chemotactic (IL-8) cytokines are of particular importance. These cytokines intensify the local vascular response, osteoclastic bone resorption, effector-mediated degradation of the extracellular matrices and can place the body on a general alert by endocrine action so as to raise the output of acute phase proteins by hepatocytes [139]. They also act in concert with IL-6 to upregulate the production of hemopoietic CSF, which rapidly mobilizes the neutrophils and the promacrophages from bone marrow. The acute response can be intensified, particularly in later stages, by the formation of antigen–antibody complexes [319,322]. The acute primary apical periodontitis has several possible outcomes such as spontaneous healing, further intensification and spreading into the bone (alveolar abscess), open to the exterior (fistulation or sinus tract formation) or becoming chronic.

4.5.2 Chronic apical periodontitis

Persistence of microbial irritants leads to a shift in the PMN-dominated lesion to a macrophage, lymphocyte and plasma cell rich one, encapsulated in a collagenous connective tissue. Such an asymptomatic, radiolucent lesion can be visualized as a "lull phase" following an intense phase in which PMNs die *en masse*; the foreign intruders have been temporarily beaten and held back in the root canal (Fig. 4.9). The macrophage-derived proinflammatory cytokines (IL-1, IL-6, and TNF-α) are powerful lymphocyte stimulators. The quantitative data on the various types of cells residing in chronic periapical lesions may not be representative. Nevertheless, investigations based on monoclonal antibodies suggest a predominant role for T-lymphocytes and macrophages. Activated T-cells produce a variety of cytokines that downregulate the output of proinflammatory cytokines (IL-1, IL-6, and TNF-α), leading to the suppression

of osteoclastic activity and reduced bone resorption. On the other hand, the T-cell derived cytokines may concomitantly upregulate the production of connective tissue growth factors (TGF-β), with stimulatory and proliferative effects on fibroblasts and the microvasculature. The T_{h1} and T_{h2} cell populations may participate in this process [282]. The option to downregulate the destructive process explains the absence or retarded bone resorption and rebuilding of the collagenous connective tissue during the chronic phase of the disease. Consequently, the chronic lesions can remain "dormant" and symptomless for long periods of time without major changes in the radiological status. But the delicate equilibrium prevailing at the periapex can be disturbed by one or more factors that may favor the microorganisms within the root canal. The microbes may advance into the periapex (Fig. 4.6) and the lesion spontaneously becomes acute with clinical manifestations (secondary acute apical periodontitis, periapical exacerbation, Phoenix abscess). As a result, microorganisms can be found extraradicularly during these acute episodes with rapid enlargement of the radiolucent area. This radiological feature is due to apical bone resorption occurring rapidly during the acute phases with relative inactivity during the chronic periods. The progression of the disease, therefore, is not continuous, but happens in discrete leaps after periods of "stability".

Asymptomatic chronic apical periodontitis is also referred to as solid dental or periapical granuloma. Histopathologically the lesion consists of granulomatous tissue with cellular infiltrate, fibroblasts and a well-developed fibrous capsule. Serial sectioning shows [188] that about 45% of all chronic periapical lesions are epithelialized. When the epithelial cells begin to proliferate, they may do so in all directions at random forming an irregular epithelial mass in which vascular and infiltrated connective tissue becomes enclosed. In some lesions the epithelium may grow into the entrance of the root canal forming a plug-like seal at the apical foramen [154,191,276]. The epithelial cells generate an "epithelial attachment" to the root surface or canal wall which in electron microscopy reveals a basal lamina and hemidesmosomal structures [191]. In random histological sections the epithelium in the lesion appears as arcades and rings. The extraepithelial tissue consists predominantly of small blood vessels, lymphocytes, plasma cells and macrophages. Among the lymphocytes T-cells are likely to be more numerous than B-

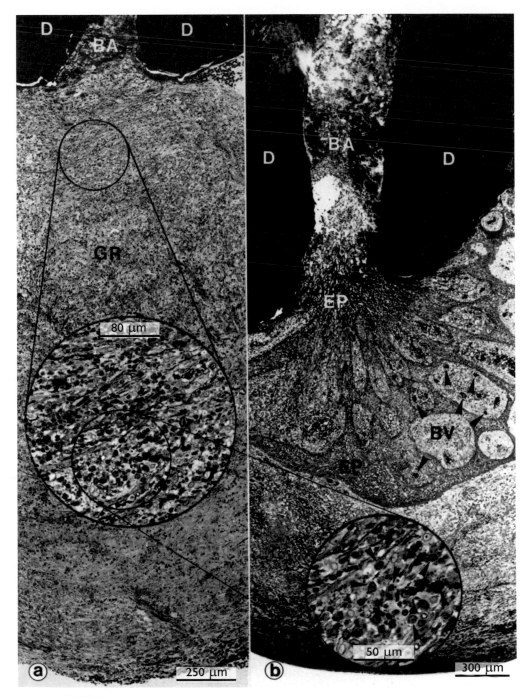

Fig. 4.9 Chronic asymptomatic apical periodontitis without (a) and with (b) epithelium (EP). The root canal contains bacteria (BA in a and b). The lesion in (a) has no acute inflammatory cells, even at the mouth of the root canal with visible bacteria at the apical foramen (BA). Note the collagen-rich maturing granulation tissue (GR) infiltrated with plasma cells and lymphocytes (insets in a and b), D, dentin; BV, blood vessels (original magnifications: a ×80; b ×60; inset in a ×250; inset in b ×400). (From Nair [180].)

cells [53,128,199,321] and CD4+ cells may outnumber CD8+ cells [14,150,156,214] in certain phases of the lesions. The connective tissue capsule of the lesion consists of dense collagenous fibers that are firmly attached to the root surface so that the lesion may be removed *in toto* with the extracted tooth.

4.5.3 Cystic apical periodontitis (radicular cysts)

Periapical cysts are a sequel to chronic apical periodontitis. However, every chronic lesion does not develop into a cyst. Although the reported prevalence of cysts among apical periodontitis lesions varies from 6% to 55% [181] investigations based on meticulous serial sectioning and strict histopathological criteria [188,261,276] show that the actual prevalence of the cysts may be well below 20%. There are two distinct categories of radicular cysts namely, those containing cavities completely enclosed in epithelial lining (Fig. 4.10) and those containing epithelium-lined cavities that are open to the root canals (Fig. 4.11) [188,261]. The latter was originally described as "bay cysts" [261] and has been newly designated as "periapical pocket cysts" [188]. More than half of the cystic lesions are apical true cysts and the remainder are apical pocket cysts [188,261]. In view of the structural difference between the two categories of cysts, the pathogenic pathways leading to the formation of them may differ in certain respects.

Periapical true cyst

Many authors attempted to explain the pathogenesis of apical true cysts [83,152,227,256,308,312,318]. The formation of true cyst has been discussed as taking place in three stages [257].

During the first phase the dormant epithelial cell rests [153,154] are believed to proliferate, probably under the influence of growth factors [82,143,310] that are released by various cells residing in the lesion.

During the second phase an epithelium-lined cavity comes into existence. The two long-standing theories regarding the formation of the cyst cavity are: (i) the "nutritional deficiency theory" is based on the assumption that the central cells of the epithelial strands lose their source of nutrition and undergo necrosis and degeneration. The products in turn attract neutrophilic granulocytes into the necrotic area. Such microcavities containing degen-

erating epithelial cells, infiltrating leukocytes and tissue exudate coalesce to form the cyst cavity lined by stratified squamous epithelium, (ii) the "abscess theory" postulates that the proliferating epithelium surrounds an abscess formed by tissue necrosis and lysis because of the innate nature of epithelial cells to cover exposed connective tissue surfaces.

During the third phase, the cyst grows, the exact mechanism of which has not yet been adequately clarified. Theories based on osmotic pressure [114,315,316] have receded to the background in favor of a molecular basis for the cystogenesis [26,35,97,98,309]. The fact that the apical pocket cyst (Fig. 4.11), with a lumen open to the necrotic root canal, can grow would eliminate osmotic pressure as a potential factor in the development of radicular cysts [180,188]. Although no direct evidence is yet available, the tissue dynamics and the cellular components of radicular cysts suggest possible molecular pathways for cyst expansion. The neutrophils that die in the cyst lumen provide a continuous source of prostaglandins [76], which can diffuse through the porous epithelial wall [257] into the surrounding tissues. The cell population residing in the extraepithelial area contains numerous T-lymphocytes [321] and macrophages produce a battery of cytokines particularly the IL-1β. The prostaglandins and the inflammatory cytokines can activate osteoclasts culminating in bone resorption. The presence of effector molecules (MMP-1 and -2) has also been reported in human periapical cysts [309].

Periapical pocket cyst

The pathogenesis of periapical pocket cyst is not well understood. It is probably initiated by the accumulation of PMNs around the apical foramen in response to the microbial presence in the apical root canal [180,188]. The microabscess so formed can get enclosed by the proliferating epithelium, which on coming in contact with the root-tip forms an epithelial collar with "epithelial attachment" [191]. The latter seals off the infected root canal with the microabscess from the periapical tissue milieu. When the externalized neutrophils die and disintegrate, the space occupied by them becomes a microcystic sac. The presence of microbes in the apical root canal, their products and the necrotic cells in the cyst lumen attract more neutrophils by a chemotactic gradient. However, the pouch-like lumen – biologically outside the periapical milieu – acts as a "death trap" to

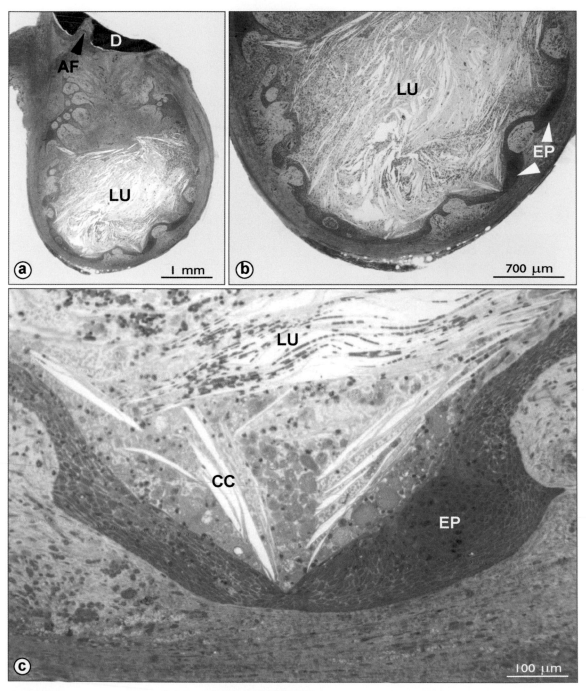

Fig. 4.10   Structure of an apical true cyst. (a) Photomicrograph of an axial section passing through the apical foramen (AF). The lower half of the lesion and the epithelium (EP in b) are magnified in (b and c), respectively. Note the cystic lumen (LU) with cholesterol clefts (CC) completely enclosed in epithelium (EP), with no communication to the root canal (original magnifications: a ×15; b ×30; c ×180). (From Nair [184].)

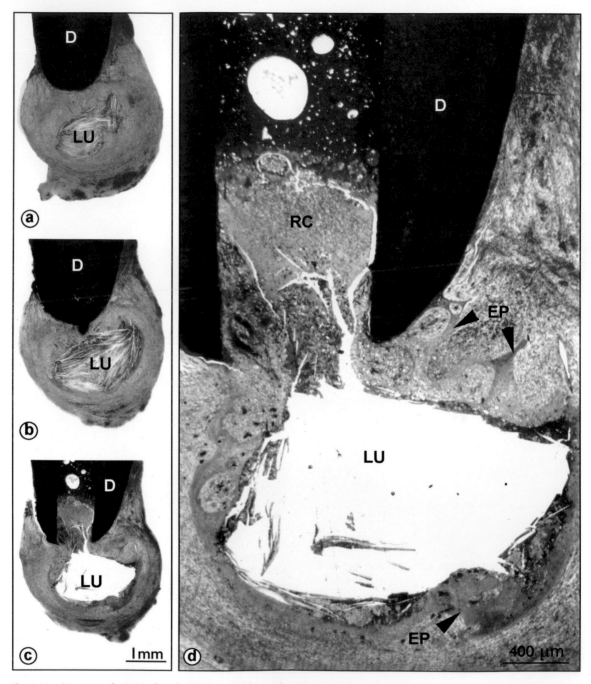

Fig. 4.11 Structure of an apical pocket cyst. (a and b) Axial sections passing peripheral to the root canal give the false impression of a cystic lumen (LU) completely enclosed in epithelium. Sequential section (c) passing through the axial plane of the root canal clearly reveals the continuity of the cystic lumen (LU) with the root canal (RC in d). The apical foramen and cystic lumen (LU) of the section (c) are magnified in (d). Note the pouchlike lumen (LU) of the pocket cyst, with the epithelium (EP) forming a collar at the root apex. D, dentin (original magnifications: a–c ×15; d ×50). (From Nair [184].)

the transmigrating neutrophils. As the necrotic cells accumulate, the sac-like lumen enlarges and may form a voluminous diverticulum of the root canal space extending into the periapical area [180,188]. Bone resorption and degradation of the matrices occurring in association with the enlargement of the pocket cyst are likely to follow a similar molecular pathway as in the case of the periapical true cyst [188]. From the pathogenic, structural, tissue dynamic and host benefit points of view the pouch-like extension of the root canal space has much in common with a marginal periodontal pocket to justify the name periapical pocket cyst [188].

4.6 Persistent apical periodontitis

As intraradicular microorganisms are the essential etiological agents of apical periodontitis [117,292], the treatment of apical periodontitis consists of eradicating the root canal microbes or substantially reducing the microbial load and preventing reinfection by standard obturation [186]. When root canal treatment is undertaken properly, healing of the periapical lesion usually occurs with hard tissue regeneration, which is characterized by a gradual resolution of the radiolucency [88,122,168,169,251,265,266,288,289, 299]. Nevertheless, complete healing of the periapex or reduction of the apical radiolucency may not occur in all root canal treated teeth. Such cases of nonresolving post-treatment periapical radiolucencies usually occur when treatment procedures have not reached a satisfactory standard for the control and elimination of infection. Inadequate aseptic control, poor access cavity preparation, missed canals, insufficient instrumentation, and leaking temporary or permanent fillings are common problems that may lead to post-treatment apical periodontitis [297]. Even when most careful clinical procedures are followed, apical periodontitis may persist in certain cases. This is because of the anatomical complexity of the root canal system [104,212] with regions that cannot be debrided and obturated with existing techniques [186]. In addition, there are causative factors located beyond the root canal system, [74,183,184,190,192,267] within the inflamed periapical tissue, that can interfere with post-treatment healing of the lesion, including compromising host factors associated with certain systemic disease such as diabetes [77].

4.6.1 Microbial causes

Intraradicular microbes

Histological examination of periapical tissues removed by surgery has been a method to detect potential etiological agents of failures in root canal treated teeth. Early investigations [10,30,137,142,250] of apical biopsies had several limitations such as the use of unsuitable specimens, inappropriate methodology and criteria of analysis. Therefore, these studies did not yield relevant information about the reasons for apical periodontitis persisting as asymptomatic radiolucencies even after proper root canal treatment.

In one microscopical analysis [250] of apical specimens of failed cases, there was not even a mention of persisting microbial infection as a potential cause of the failures. A histobacteriological study, [10] using serial step sectioning and special bacterial stains, found bacteria in the root canals of 14% of the 66 specimens examined. Two other studies [30,137] analyzed 230 and 35 endodontic surgical specimens, respectively, by routine paraffin histology. Although bacteria were found in 10% and 15% of the respective biopsies, only in a single specimen, in each study, was intraradicular infection detected. In the remaining biopsies in which bacteria were found, the data also included those specimens in which bacteria were found as "contaminants on the surface of the tissue". In yet another study [142] "bacteria and/or debris" were found in the root canals of 63% of the 86 endodontic surgical specimens, although it is obvious that "bacteria and debris" cannot be equated as etiological agents in endodontic treatment failures. The low reported incidence of intraradicular infections in these studies is primarily due to a methodological inadequacy as microorganisms may go undetected when the investigations are based on random paraffin sections alone. This has been convincingly demonstrated [179,193]. Consequently, early studies on post-treatment apical periodontitis did not consider residual intraradicular infection as an etiological factor.

To identify the etiological agents of asymptomatic post-treatment apical periodontitis by microscopy, the cases must be selected from teeth that have had the best possible root canal treatment and the radiological lesions remain asymptomatic until surgical intervention. The specimens must be anatomically intact block biopsies that include the apical part of the roots and the inflamed soft tissue of the lesions. Such specimens should undergo meticulous investigation by serial sections for light microscopy, or step-serial sections that are analyzed using correlative light and transmission electron microscopy. A study that met these criteria and also included microbial monitoring before and during treatment [193] revealed intra-radicular microorganisms in six of the nine block biopsies (Fig. 4.12). The findings conclusively show that the majority of root canal treated teeth evincing asymptomatic apical periodontitis harbor persistent infection in the apical part of the complex root canal system. However, the proportion of failed cases with intraradicular infection is likely to be much higher in routine endodontic practice than the two-thirds of nine cases reported [193] for several reasons. At the light microscopic level it was possible to detect bacteria in only one of the six cases [193]. Microorganisms were found as a biofilm located within small canals of apical ramifications of the root canal (Fig. 4.12), or in the space between the root filling and the canal wall. This demonstrates the limitation of conventional paraffin technique to detect infections in apical biopsies.

The microbial status of the apical root canal system immediately after endodontic treatment has been unknown. However, in a very recent study, it has been shown that 14 of the 16 instrumented and root canal-treated mandibular molars showed residual infection of mesial roots when the treatment was completed in one visit during which instrumentation, irrigation with NaOCl and obturation were carried out. The infectious agents were mostly located in the uninstrumented recesses of the main canals, isthmuses communicating between them and accessory canals. The microbes in such untouched locations existed primarily as biofilms that were not removed by instrumentation and irrigation with NaOCl. In view of the great anatomical complexity of the root canal system, particularly of molars, [104,212] and the ecological organization of the flora into protected sessile biofilms [50,51] composed of microbial cells embedded in a hydrated exopolysaccharide complex in micro-colonies [179], it is unlikely that an absolutely microorganism-free canal system can be achieved by any of the contemporary procedures for root canal preparation, cleaning and root filling. Then the question arises as to why a large number of apical lesions heal after root canal treatment. It has been shown that some periapical lesions heal even when infection persists in the canals at the time of root filling [265]. Although this may imply that the

organisms may not survive post-treatment, it is more likely that the microbes may be present in quantities and virulence that may be sub-critical to sustain the inflammation of the periapex [186]. In some cases such residual microbes can delay or prevent periapical healing, as was the case with six of the nine biopsies already reported [193].

On the basis of cell wall ultrastructure alone, Gram-positive bacteria were found (Fig. 4.13), an observation in agreement with the results of purely microbiological investigations of root canals of previously root filled teeth with persisting periapical lesions. Of the six specimens that contained intra-radicular infections, four had one or more morphologically distinct types of bacteria and two revealed yeasts (Fig. 4.14). The presence of intracanal fungi in root treated teeth with apical periodontitis has also been confirmed by microbiological techniques [209,333]. These findings clearly associate intra-radicular fungi as a potential nonbacterial, microbial cause of endodontic failures. It has been suggested that intraradicular infection can also remain within the innermost parts of infected dentinal tubules that serve as a reservoir for endodontic reinfection that might interfere with periapical healing [148,149,176,213,260,329].

The microbiology of treated root canals is less well understood than that of untreated infected necrotic dental pulps. This may be as a result of searching for nonmicrobial causes of a purely technical nature for the failure of root canal treatments [297]. Only a small number of species have been found in the root canals of teeth that have undergone proper endodontic treatment that, on follow-up, revealed persisting, asymptomatic periapical radiolucencies. The bacteria found in these cases by culturing have been predominantly Gram-positive cocci, rods and filaments. By culture-based techniques, species belonging to the genera *Actinomyces, Enterococcus,* and *Propionibacterium* (previously *Arachnia*) are frequently isolated and characterized from such root canals [81,93,94,165,166,215,267,299,301]. The presence of *Enterococcus faecalis* in cases of post-treatment apical periodontitis is of particular interest because it is rarely found in infected but untreated root canals [297]; *E. faecalis* is the most consistently reported organism from former cases, with a prevalence ranging from 22% to 77% of cases analyzed [78,93, 165,166,208,215,264,299]. The organism is resistant to most of the intracanal medicaments, and can tolerate [38] a pH up to 11.5, which may be one reason

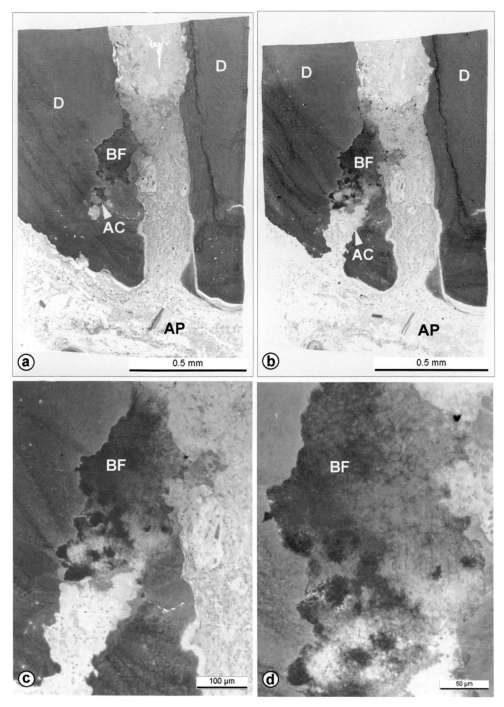

Fig. 4.12 Photomicrographs of axial semithin sections through the surgically removed apical part of a root with persistent apical periodontitis. Note the adhesive biofilm (BF) in the root canal. Consecutive sections (a to b) reveal the emerging widened profile of an accessory canal (AC) that is clogged with biofilm. The accessory canal and biofilm are magnified in (c and d), respectively (original magnifications: a ×75, b ×70, c ×110, d ×300). (Adapted from Nair *et al.* [193].)

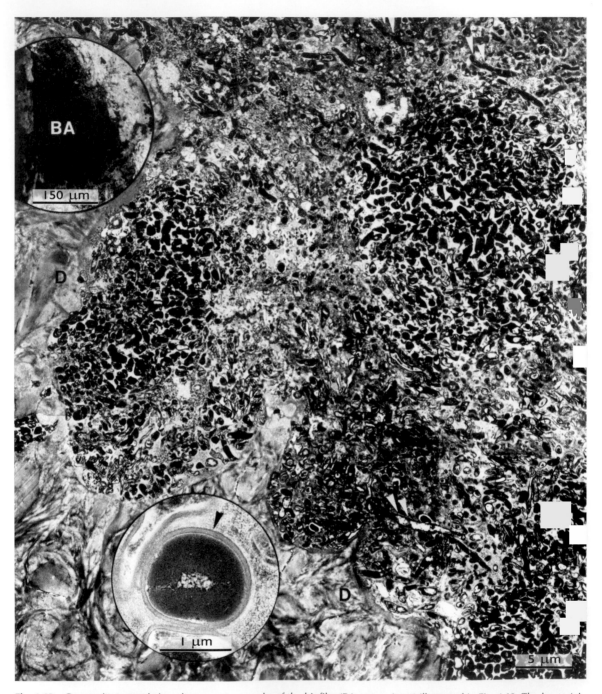

Fig. 4.13 Composite transmission electron micrographs of the biofilm (BA, upper inset) illustrated in Fig. 4.12. The bacterial population is composed of only Gram-positive, filamentous organisms (arrowhead in lower inset). Note the distinctive Gram-positive cell wall. The upper inset is a light microscopic view of the biofilm (BA); D, dentin (original magnifications: ×3400; insets: upper ×135, lower ×21,300). (From Nair *et al.* [193].)

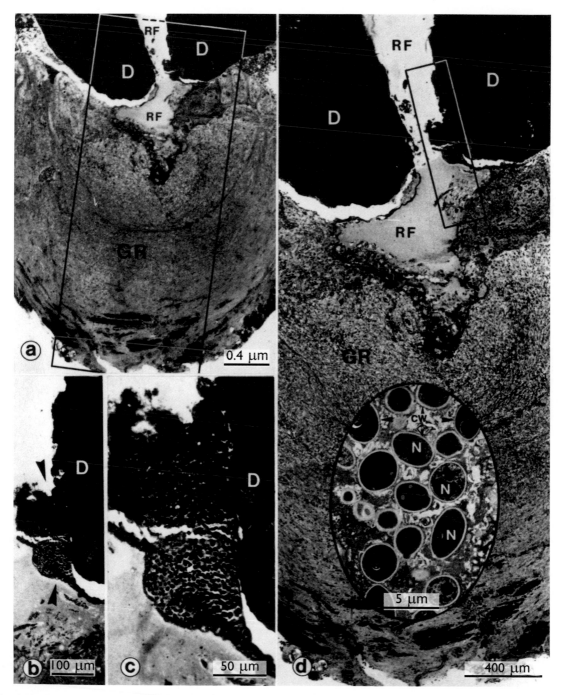

Fig. 4.14 Fungi as a potential cause of endodontic failure. (a) Low-power overview of an axial section of a root-filled (RF) tooth with persisting apical periodontitis (GR); D, dentin. The rectangular demarcated areas in (a) and (d) are magnified in (d) and (b), respectively. Note the two microbial clusters (arrowheads in b) further magnified in (c). The oval inset in (d) is a transmission electron microscopic view of the organisms. Note the electron-lucent cell wall (CW), nuclei (N) and budding forms (BU) (original magnifications: a ×35, b ×130, c ×330, d ×60, oval inset ×3400). (Adapted from Nair *et al.* [193].)

as to why this organism survives antimicrobial treatment with CaOH dressings [23]. This is probably by virtue of its ability to regulate internal pH with an efficient proton pump [68]. *E. faecalis* can survive prolonged starvation [73]; and it can grow as monoinfection in treated canals in the absence of synergistic support from other bacteria [70]. Therefore, *E. faecalis* is held to be a very recalcitrant microbe among the potential etiological agents of post-treatment apical periodontitis. However, the presence of *E. faecalis* in cases of post-treatment apical periodontits has not been a universal observation; one microbial culture study [43] and a molecular based [228] study failed to detect the presence of *E. faecalis*. Further, the prevalence of *E. faecalis* was found to be 22% and 77% respectively of cases analyzed by two molecular techniques [78,264]. In this context the long reported correlation between the prevalence of enterococci in root canals of primary and retreatment cases and that in other oral sites, such as gingival sulcus and tonsils, of the same patients, is worth noting [66]. It has been suggested that enterococci may be opportunistic organisms that populate exposed root filled canals from elsewhere in the mouth [78]. Therefore, in spite of the current focus of attention, it still remains to be shown by controlled studies that *E. faecalis* is the pathogen of significance in most cases of failing endodontic treatment [185].

Microbiological [166,333] and correlative electron microscopic [193] studies have shown the presence of yeasts (Fig. 4.14) in canals of root filled teeth with unresolved apical periodontitis. *Candida albicans* is the most frequently isolated fungus from root filled teeth with apical periodontitis [165,299].

Extraradicular microbes

Actinomycosis. Actinomycosis is a chronic, granulomatous, infectious disease in humans and animals caused by the genera *Actinomyces* and *Propionibacterium* [159]. The etiological agent of bovine actinomycosis, *Actinomyces bovis*, was the first species to be identified. [100]. The disease in cattle, known as "lumpy jaw'"or "big head disease", is characterized by extensive bone rarefaction, swelling of the jaw, suppuration and fistulation. The causative agents were described as nonacid fast, nonmotile, Gram-positive organisms revealing characteristic branching filaments that end in clubs or hyphae. Because of the morphological appearance these organisms were considered fungi and the taxonomy of *Actinomyces*

remained controversial for more than a century. The intertwining filamentous colonies are often called "sulfur granules" because of their appearance as yellow specks in exudates. On careful crushing, the tiny clumps of branching microorganisms with radiating filaments in pus, give a "starburst appearance" which prompted Harz [100] to coin the name *Actinomyces* or "ray fungus". Soon after, *A. israelii* was isolated from humans in pure culture, characterized and its pathogenicity in animals demonstrated [345]. Many researchers, nevertheless, considered the human and bovine isolates as identical. However, *A. bovis* and *A. israelii* are now classified as two distinct bacterial species and in natural infections the former is restricted to animals and the latter to humans.

Human actinomycosis has been clinically divided into cervicofacial, thoracic and abdominal forms, with about 60% of cases in the cervicofacial region, 20% in the abdomen and 15% in the thorax [119,205]. The most common species isolated is *A. israelii* [345], which is followed by *Propionibacterium propionicum* [36], *A. naeslundii* [314], *A. viscosus* [110], and *A. odontolyticus* [15] in descending order.

Periapical actinomycosis (Fig. 4.15) is a cervicofacial form of actinomycosis. The endodontic infections are generally considered a sequel to caries. *A. israelii* is a commensal of the oral cavity and can be isolated from tonsils, dental plaque, periodontal pockets and carious lesions [301]. Most of the publications on periapical actinomycosis are case reports and have been reviewed [34,155,190,241,243,338]. Although periapical actinomycosis is considered to be rare [190], it may not be so infrequent [112,170,241]. The data on the frequency of periapical actinomycosis in apical periodontitis are scarce. A microbiological control study revealed actinomycotic involvement in two of the 79 endodontically treated cases [39]. A histological analysis showed the presence of characteristic actinomycotic colonies (Fig. 4.15) in two of the 45 investigated lesions [190]. Identification and etiological association of the species involved can be established only through laboratory culturing [301] of the organisms, molecular techniques and by experimental induction of the lesion in susceptible animals [74]. However, the strict growth requirements of *A. israelii* make isolation in pure culture difficult. A histopathological diagnosis has generally been reached on the basis of demonstration of typical colonies [190] and by specific immunohistochemical staining of such colonies [95,301]. Today, an unequivocal identification of the organism can be achieved by molecular

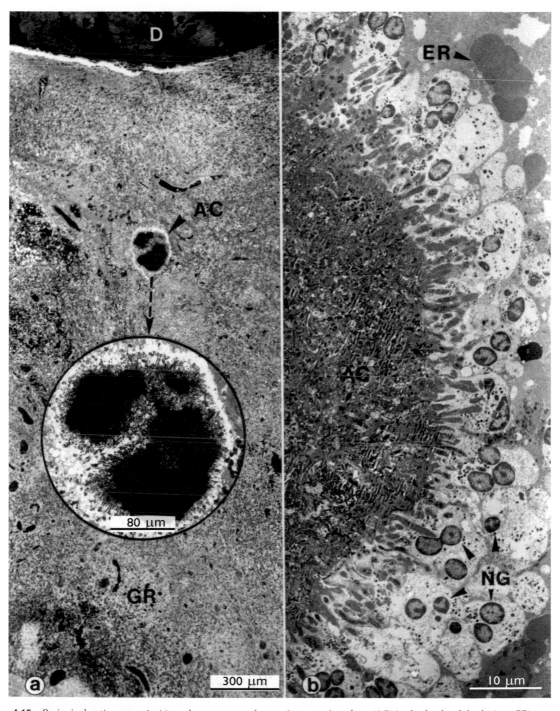

Fig. 4.15 Periapical actinomycosis. Note the presence of an actinomycotic colony (AC) in the body of the lesion (GR) revealing a typical "starburst" appearance (inset in a). The transmission electron microscopic montage (b) shows the peripheral area of the colony with filamentous organisms surrounded by few layers of neutrophilic granulocytes (NG). D, dentin; ER, erythrocytes (original magnifications: a ×70; inset ×250; b ×2200). (Adapted from Nair and Schroeder [190].)

methods. The characteristic light microscopic feature of an actinomycotic colony is the presence of an intensely dark staining, Gram and PAS positive, core with radiating peripheral filaments (Fig. 4.15), that give the typical "star burst" or "ray fungus" appearance. Ultrastructurally, [74,190] the center of the colony consists of a very dense aggregation of branching filamentous organisms held together by an extracellular matrix (Fig. 4.15). Several layers of PMNs usually surround an actinomycotic colony.

The ability of the actinomycotic organisms to establish extraradicularly means that they can perpetuate the inflammation at the periapex even after root canal treatment. Therefore, periapical actinomycosis is important in endodontology [94,95,190,192,267,301]. *A. israelii* and *P. proprionicum* are consistently isolated and characterized from the periapical tissue of teeth, that have not responded to proper endodontic treatment [94,267]. A strain of *A. israelii*, isolated from a case of failed endodontic treatment and grown in pure culture, was inoculated into subcutaneously implanted tissue cages in animals [74]. Typical actinomycotic colonies were formed within the experimental host tissue. This would implicate *A. israelii* as a potential etiological factor of failed endodontic treatments. *Actinomyces* have been shown to possess a hydrophobic cell surface and a Gram-positive cell wall surrounded by a fuzzy outer coat through which fimbriae-like structures protrude [72]. These may help the cells to aggregate into cohesive colonies [74]. The properties that enable these bacteria to establish in the periapical tissues are not fully understood, but appear to involve the ability to build cohesive colonies that enable them to escape the host defense system [74]. The species, *P. propionicum*, is known to be pathogenic and associated with actinomycotic infections, but the pathogenic mechanism has not yet been explained.

Other microbes in inflamed periapical tissue. Apical periodontitis has long been considered to be a dynamic defense enclosure against unrestrained invasion of microorganisms into periradicular tissues [132,180]. It is, therefore, conceivable that microorganisms generally invade extraradicular tissues during expanding and exacerbating phases of the disease process. Based on classical histology [96] there has been a consensus of opinion that a "solid granuloma" may not harbor infectious agents within the inflamed periapical tissue, but microorganisms are consis-

tently present in the periapical tissue of cases with clinical signs of exacerbation, abscesses and draining sinuses. This has been substantiated by more modern correlative light and transmission electron microscopic investigations [179].

However, in the late 1980s, there was a resurgence of the idea of extraradicular microbes in apical periodontitis [113,326,327,337] with the controversial suggestion that extraradicular infections are the cause of many failed endodontic treatments; such cases would not be amenable to root canal treatment but would need apical surgery and/or systemic medications. Several species of bacteria have been reported to be present at extraradicular locations of lesions described as "asymptomatic periapical inflammatory lesions ... refractory to endodontic treatment" [327]. However, five of the eight patients had "long-standing fistulae to the vestibule ..." [327], a clear sign of abscessed apical periodontitis draining by sinus tracts. It is clear that the microbial samples were obtained from periapical abscesses that always contain microbes and not from asymptomatic periapical lesions persisting after proper endodontic treatment. Other reports also show serious methodological issues. In one [113], the 16 periapical specimens studied were collected "during normal periapical curettage, apicectomy or (during the procedure of) retrograde filling". Of the 58 specimens that were investigated in another [337], "29 communicated with the oral cavity through vertical root fractures or fistulas"; further, the specimens were obtained during routine surgery and were "submitted by seven practitioners". An appropriate method is essential and in these studies [113,327,337] unsuitable cases were selected for investigation, or the sampling was not performed with the utmost stringency needed to avoid bacterial contamination [166].

Microbial contamination of periapical samples is generally considered as occurring from the oral cavity and other extraneous sources. Even if such "extraneous contamination" is avoided, contamination of periapical tissue samples with microbes from the infected root canal remains a serious problem. This is because microorganisms generally live in the apical foramen of teeth affected in both primary apical periodontitis [179,216,335] and post-treatment apical periodontitis [192,193], and microbes can be easily dislodged during surgery or the sampling procedures. Tissue samples so contaminated with *intraradicular* microbes may be reported as positive for the presence of an *extraradicular* infection. This is probably the reason for the repeated reporting of microbes in the periapical tissue of asymptomatic post-treatment lesions by culture [2,290] and molecular techniques [84,291] even if strict aseptic sampling procedures could have been used.

The molecular techniques, despite sophistication and high sensitivity, seem less suitable to solve the problem of extraradicular infection. Apart from the unavoidable contamination of the samples with intraradicular microbes, they: (i) do not differentiate between viable and nonviable organisms, (ii) do not distinguish between microbes and their structural elements in phagocytes from extracellular microorganisms in periapical tissues, and (iii) exaggerate the findings by PCR amplification.

Viruses

In recent years a series of publications [235–238,272] reported the presence of certain viruses in inflamed periapical tissues with the suggestion of an etiological relationship to apical periodontitis. It is almost impossible to provide controls for such observations because the reported viruses are present in almost all humans from previous primary infections. The possibility exists that the latent viruses may be activated by the periapical inflammatory process.

In summary, extraradicular infections do occur in: (i) exacerbating apical periodontitis [179], (ii) periapical actinomycosis [94,95,190,267,301], (iii) association with pieces of infected root dentine that may be displaced into the periapex during root canal instrumentation [108,352] or having been cut off from the rest of the root by massive apical resorption [138,329], and (iv) infected periapical cysts, particularly in periapical pocket cysts with cavities open to the root canal [179,188,192]. These situations are quite compatible [23,180] with the long-standing and still valid concept that solid granuloma generally do not harbor microorganisms. Therefore, the primary target of treatment for persistent apical periodontitis should be the microorganisms that grow and live in the complex apical root canal system as biofilms [186].

4.6.2 Nonmicrobial causes

Cystic apical periodontitis

The question as to whether or not periapical cysts heal after conventional root canal treatment has been a long-standing one. Surgeons have been of the opinion that cysts do not heal and must be removed by surgery. Many endodontists, on the other hand, hold the view that the majority of cysts heal after endodontic treatment. This conflict of opinion is probably an outcome of the reported high prevalence of cysts in apical periodontitis and the reported high "success rate" of root canal treatment. There have been several studies on the prevalence of radicular cysts among human apical periodontitis (Table 4.2). The recorded prevalence of cysts among apical periodontitis lesions varies from 6% to 55%. Apical periodontitis cannot be differentially diagnosed into cystic and noncystic lesions based on radiographs alone [16,24,134,144,172,219,224,332]. Correct histopathological diagnosis of periapical cysts is possible only through serial sectioning or step-serial sectioning of the lesions removed *in toto* as has been convincingly shown in a recent study correlating the presence of a radiopaque lamina with histological findings [224]. The vast discrepancy in the reported prevalence of periapical cysts is probably due to the difference in the interpretation of the sections. Histopathological diagnosis based on random or limited number of serial sections, may lead to incorrect categorization of epithelialized lesions as radicular cysts. This was clearly shown in a study using meticulous serial sectioning [188] in which an overall 52% of the lesions ($n = 256$) were found to be epithelialized but only 15% were actually periapical cysts. In routine histopathological diagnosis, the structure of a radicular cyst in relation to the root canal of the affected tooth has not been taken into account. As apical biopsies obtained by curettage do not include root-tips of the diseased teeth, structural reference to the root canals of the affected teeth is not possible. Histopathological diagnostic laboratories that review such histopathological reports sustain the notion that nearly half of all lesions of apical periodontitis are cysts.

An endodontic "success rate" of 85–90% has been recorded by investigators [122,266,285]. However, the histological status of an apical radiolucent lesion at the time of treatment is unknown to the clinician who is also unaware of the differential diagnosis of the "successful" and "failed" cases. Nevertheless, purely based on deductive logic, a great majority of the cystic lesions should heal in order to account for the "high success rate" after endodontic treatment and the reported "high histopathological incidence" of radicular cysts. As endodontic treatment removes

Table 4.2   The prevalence of radicular cysts in lesions of apical periodontitis

Reference	Cysts (%)	Granuloma (%)	Others (%)	Total lesions (n)
Sommer and Kerr (1966) [275]	6	84	10	170
Block et al. (1976) [30]	6	94	–	230
Sonnabend and Oh (1966) [276]	7	93	–	237
Winstock (1980) [343]	8	83	9	9804
Linenberg et al. (1964) [144]	9	80	11	110
Wais (1958) [332]	14	84	2	50
Patterson et al. (1964) [207]	14	84	2	501
Nair et al. (1996) [188]	15	50	35	256
Simon (1980) [261]	17	77	6	35
Stockdale and Chandler (1988) [287]	17	77	6	1108
Lin et al. (1991) [142]	19	–	81	150
Nobuhara and Del Rio (1993) [200]	22	59	19	150
Baumann and Rossman (1956) [16]	26	74	–	121
Mortensen et al. (1970) [172]	41	59	–	396
Bhaskar (1966) [24]	42	48	10	2308
Spatafore et al. (1990) [279]	42	52	6	1659
Lalonde and Leubke (1968) [135]	44	45	11	800
Seltzer et al. (1967) [250]	51	45	4	87
Priebe et al. (1954) [219]	55	45	–	101

much of the infectious material from the root canal and prevents reinfection by obturation, a periapical pocket cyst (Fig. 4.11) may heal after conventional endodontic therapy [188,195,261]. In contrast, a true cyst (Fig. 4.10) is *self-sustaining* [195] by virtue of its tissue dynamics and independence of the presence or absence of irritants in the root canal [261].

The therapeutic significance of the structural difference between apical true cysts and pocket cysts should also be considered. The aim of root canal treatment is the elimination of infection from the root canal and the prevention of reinfection by root filling. Periapical pocket cysts, particularly the smaller ones, may heal after root canal therapy [261]. A true cyst is *self-sustaining* as the lesion is no longer dependent on the presence or absence of root canal infection [188,261]. Therefore, true cysts, particularly the large

ones, are less likely to be resolved by nonsurgical root canal treatment. This has been reported in a long-term radiographic follow-up (Fig. 4.16) of a case and subsequent histological analysis of the surgical block-biopsy [195]. It can be argued that the prevalence of cysts in post-treatment apical periodontitis should be substantially higher than that in primary apical periodontitis. However, this remains to be clarified by research based on a statistically reliable number of specimens. Limited investigations [192,193,195] on 16 histologically reliable block biopsies of post-treatment apical periodontitis revealed two cystic specimens (13%), which is well above the 9% of true cysts observed in a large study [188] on mostly primary apical periodontitis lesions. The two distinct histological categories of periapical cysts and the low prevalence of cystic lesions among apical periodontitis would

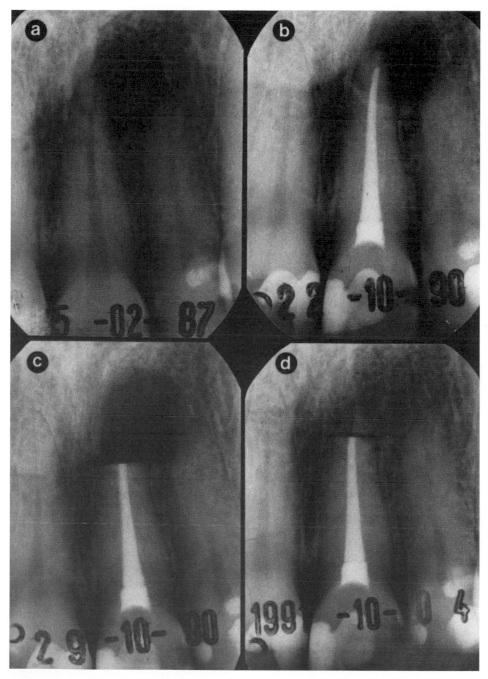

Fig. 4.16 Radiographs (a–d) of a periapically affected maxillary central incisor of a 37-year-old woman over a period of 4 years 9 months. Note the large radiolucent asymptomatic lesion before treatment (a); 3 years 8 months after root filling (b); and immediately after root-end resection (c). The periapical area shows distinct bony healing after 1 year (d). Histopathological examination of the surgical specimen by modern tissue processing and step-serial sectioning technique confirmed that the lesion was a true radicular cyst that also contained cholesterol clefts. (Selected radiographs from Nair *et al.* [195].)

question the rationale of: (i) routine histopathological examination of periapical lesions removed by curettage, which does not provide any relevant information but only satisfies certain health-care formalities, (ii) disproportionate application of apical surgery based on unfounded radiographic diagnosis of apical lesions as cysts, and (iii) the widely held belief that the majority of cysts heal after root canal treatment. Nevertheless, clinicians must recognize the fact that the cysts can sustain post-treatment apical periodontitis, and consider the option of apical surgery, particularly when previous attempts at retreatment have not resulted in healing [184].

Cholesterol crystals

The presence of cholesterol clefts in apical periodontitis has long been observed to be a common histopathological feature, but its etiological significance to failed root canal treatment has not been fully appreciated [182]. Cholesterol [307] is a steroid lipid that is present in abundance in all "membrane-rich" animal cells. Excess blood level of cholesterol is suspected to play a role in arteriosclerosis as a result of its deposition in the vascular walls [349,350]. Deposition of cholesterol crystals in tissues and organs can cause ailments such as otitis media and the "pearly tumor" of the cranium [7]. Accumulation of cholesterol crystals occurs in apical periodontitis [24,33,195,256,328] with clinical significance in endodontics [181,195]. In histopathological sections, such deposits of cholesterol appear as narrow elongated clefts because the crystals dissolve in fat solvents used for tissue processing and leave behind spaces that they occupied as clefts (Fig. 4.17). The incidence of cholesterol clefts in apical periodontitis varies from 18% to 44% of such lesions [33,256,328]. The crystals are believed to be formed from cholesterol released by, (i) disintegrating erythrocytes of stagnant blood vessels within the lesion [33], (ii) lymphocytes, plasma cells and macrophages which die in great numbers and disintegrate in chronic periapical lesions, and (iii) the circulating plasma lipids [256]. All these sources may contribute to the concentration and crystallization of cholesterol in periapical area. Nevertheless, locally dying inflammatory cells may be the major source of cholesterol as a result of its release from disintegrating membranes of such cells in long-standing lesions [195,249].

Cholesterol crystals are intensely sclerogenic [1,20]. They induce granulomatous lesions in various animal species: dogs [45], mice [1,4,5,20,278], and rabbits [106,277,278]. In an experimental study that specifically investigated the potential association of cholesterol crystals and nonresolving apical periodontitis lesions [196], pure cholesterol crystals were placed in Teflon cages that were implanted subcutaneous in guinea pigs. The cage contents were retrieved after 2, 4 and 32 weeks of implantation and processed for light and electron microscopy. The cages revealed delicate soft connective tissue that grew in through perforations in the cage wall. The crystals were densely surrounded by numerous macrophages and multinucleate giant cells forming a well-circumscribed area of tissue reaction (Fig. 4.18). The cells, however, were unable to eliminate the crystals during an observation period of 8 months. The accumulation of macrophages and giant cells around cholesterol crystals suggests that the crystals induced a typical foreign-body reaction [47,194,269].

The macrophages and giant cells that surround cholesterol crystals are not only unable to degrade the crystalline cholesterol, but are major sources of apical inflammatory and bone resorptive mediators. Bone resorbing activity of cholesterol-exposed macrophages due to enhanced expression of IL-1α has been experimentally shown [268]. Accumulation of cholesterol crystals in apical periodontitis (Fig. 4.17) can adversely affect post-treatment healing as has been shown in a long-term longitudinal follow-up of a case in which it was concluded that "the presence of vast numbers of cholesterol crystals ... would be sufficient to sustain the lesion indefinitely" [195]. The evidence from the general literature reviewed [182] is clearly in support of that assumption. Therefore, accumulation of cholesterol crystals in apical periodontitis lesions can prevent healing of periapical tissues after conventional root canal treatment, as root canal retreatment cannot remove the tissue irritating cholesterol crystals that exist outside the root canal system.

Foreign bodies

Foreign materials trapped in periapical tissue during endodontic treatment [131,194] can perpetuate apical periodontitis persisting after root canal treatment. Endodontic clinical materials [131,194] and certain food particles [262] can reach the periapex, induce a foreign body reaction that appears radiolucent and remain asymptomatic for several years [194].

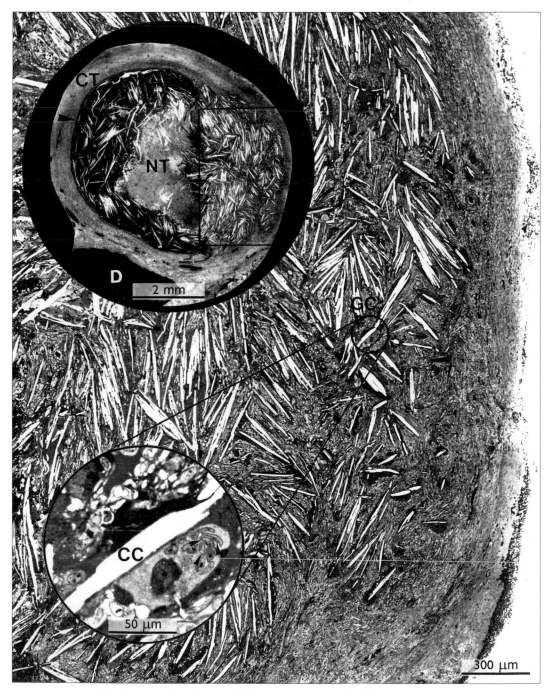

Fig. 4.17 Cholesterol crystals and cystic condition of apical periodontitis as potential causes for endodontic failure. Overview of a histological section (upper inset) of asymptomatic apical periodontitis that persisted after root canal treatment. Note the vast number of cholesterol clefts (CC) surrounded by giant cells (GC) of which a selected one with several nuclei (arrowheads) is magnified in the lower inset. D, dentin; CT, connective tissue; NT, necrotic tissue (original magnifications: ×68; upper inset ×11; lower inset ×412). (From Nair [182].)

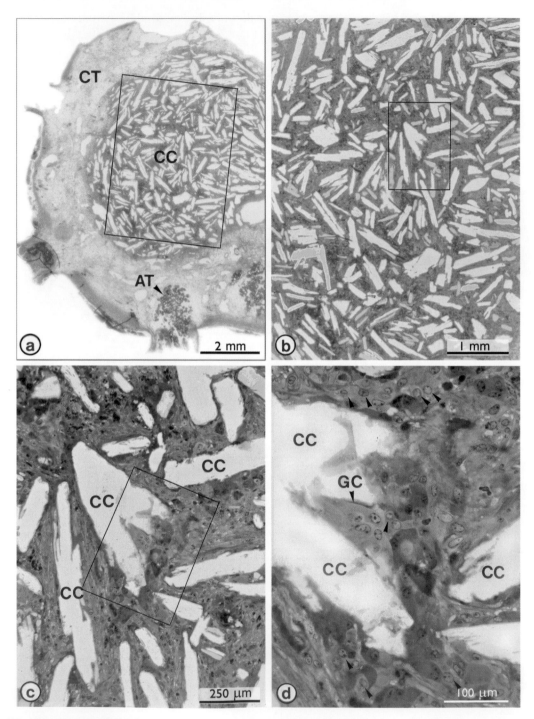

Fig. 4.18 Photomicrograph (a) of guinea-pig tissue reaction to aggregates of cholesterol crystals after 32 weeks. The rectangular demarcated areas in (a–c) are magnified in (b–d), respectively. Note the rhomboid clefts left by cholesterol crystals (CC) surrounded by giant cells (GC) and numerous mononuclear cells (arrowheads in d). AT, adipose tissue; CT, connective tissue (original magnifications: a ×10, b ×21, c ×82 and d ×220). (From Nair [182].)

Gutta-percha. The most frequently used material in root canal filling is gutta-percha. The widely held view that it is biocompatible and well tolerated by human tissues is inconsistent with the clinical observation that extruded gutta-percha is associated with delayed healing of the periapex [122,194,251,266,289]. It has been experimentally shown in guinea-pigs that large pieces of gutta-percha are well encapsulated in collagen, but fine particles of gutta-percha induce an intense, localized tissue response (Fig. 4.19), characterized by the presence of macrophages and giant cells [269]. The congregation of macrophages around the fine particles of gutta-percha is important when healing of apical periodontitis is impaired on teeth root filled to excess. Gutta-percha cones contaminated with tissue irritating materials can induce a foreign body reaction at the periapex. In an investigation of nine lesions of asymptomatic apical periodontitis that were removed as surgical block biopsies and analyzed by correlative light and electron microscopy, one biopsy revealed the involvement of contaminated gutta-percha [194]. The radiolucency grew in size, but remained asymtomatic for a decade of post-treatment follow-up. The lesion was characterized by the presence of vast numbers of multinucleate giant cells with birefringent inclusion bodies (Fig. 4.20). In transmission electron microscope the birefringent bodies were highly electron dense. An X-ray microanalysis of the inclusion bodies using scanning transmission electron microscope (STEM) revealed the presence of magnesium and silicon. These elements are presumably the remnants of a talc-contaminated gutta-percha that protruded into the periapex and had been resorbed during the follow-up period.

Other plant materials. Vegetable food particles, particularly leguminous seeds (pulses), and endodontic clinical materials of plant origin can get lodged in the periapical tissue before and/or during endodontic treatment and cause treatment failures. Oral pulse granuloma is a distinct histopathological entity [124]. The lesions are also referred to as the giant cell hyaline angiopathy [65,124], vegetable granuloma [99] and food-induced granuloma [31]. Pulse granuloma has been reported in lungs [101], stomach walls and peritoneal cavities [258]. Experimental lesions have been induced in animals by intratracheal, intraperitonial and submucous introduction of leguminous seeds [126,305]. Periapical pulse granuloma is associated with teeth damaged by caries and conditions prior to endodontic treatment [262,304]. Pulse gran-

uloma is characterized by the presence of intensely staining iodine and PAS-positive hyaline rings or bodies surrounded by giant cells and inflammatory cells [164,262,304,305]. Leguminous seeds are the most frequently involved vegetable food material in such granulomatous lesions. This indicates that certain components in pulses such as antigenic proteins and mitogenic phytohemagglutinins may be involved in the pathological tissue response [126]. The pulse granuloma is clinically significant because particles of vegetable food materials can reach the periapical tissue via root canals of teeth exposed to the oral cavity by trauma, caries or endodontic procedures [262].

Apical periodontitis developing against particles of predominantly cellulose-containing materials that are used in endodontic practice [129,130,247,339] has been denoted as *cellulose granuloma*. The cellulose in plant materials is a granuloma-inducing agent [126]. Endodontic paper points (Fig. 4.21) and medicated cotton wool can get pushed into the periapical tissue [339] so as to induce a foreign body reaction at the periapex. The resultant clinical situation may be a "prolonged, extremely troublesome and disconcerted course of events" [339]. Presence of cellulose fibers in periapical biopsies with a history of previous endodontic treatment has been reported [129,130,247]. The endodontic paper points and cotton wool consist of cellulose that cannot be degraded by human body cells. They remain in tissues for long periods of time [247] and induce a foreign body reaction around them. The particles, in polarized light, are birefringent due to the regular structural arrangement of the molecules within cellulose [130]. Infected paper points can protrude through the apical foramen (Fig. 4.21) and allow a biofilm to grow around it. This will sustain and even intensify the apical periodontitis after root canal treatment.

Other foreign materials. These include amalgam, endodontic sealers, and calcium salts derived from periapically extruded $Ca(OH)_2$. In a histological and X-ray microanalytical investigation of 29 apical biopsies 31% of the specimens were found to contain amalgam or endodontic sealer components [131].

Scar tissue healing

Unresolved periapical radiolucencies may occasionally be due to healing of the lesion by scar tissue [24,192,210,250] that may be misdiagnosed as a radiological sign of failed endodontic treatment (Fig.

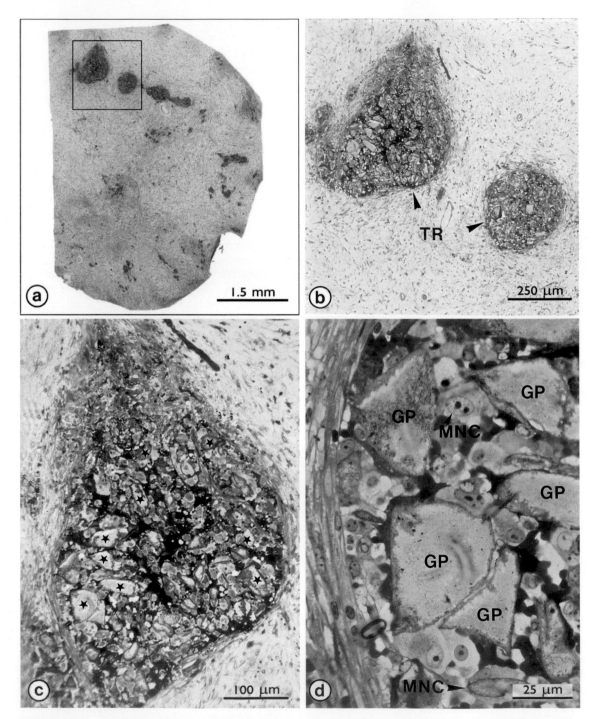

Fig. 4.19 Disintegrated gutta-percha as a potential cause of post-treatment apical periodontitis. As clusters of fine particles (a) they induce intense circumscribed tissue reaction (TR) around them (b). Note that the fine particles of gutta-percha (∗ in c, GP in d) are surrounded by numerous mononuclear cells (MNC) (original magnifications: a ×20, b ×80, c ×200, d ×750). (From Nair [183].)

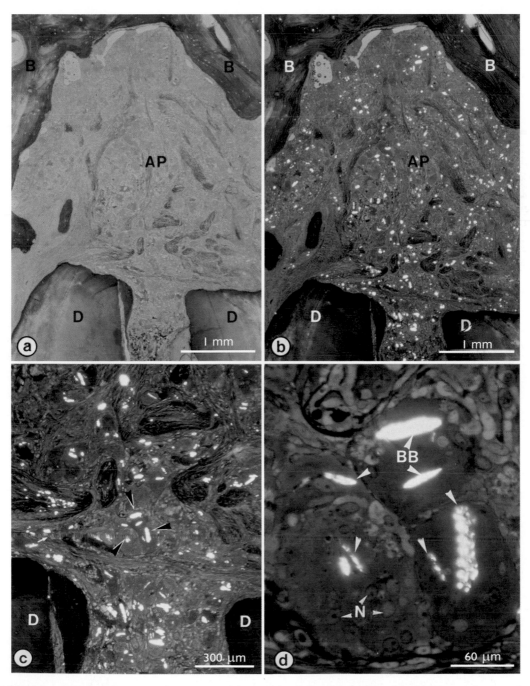

Fig. 4.20 Talc-contaminated gutta-percha as a potential cause of endodontic failure. Note the apical periodontitis (AP) characterized by foreign-body giant cell reaction to gutta-percha cones contaminated with talc (a). The same field when viewed in polarized lights (b). Note the birefringent bodies distributed throughout the lesion (b). The apical foramen is magnified in (c) and the dark arrowheaded cells in (c) are further enlarged in (d). Note the birefringence (BB) emerging from slit-like inclusion bodies in multinucleated (N) giant cells; B, bone; D, dentin (original magnifications: a, b ×25; c ×66; d ×300).

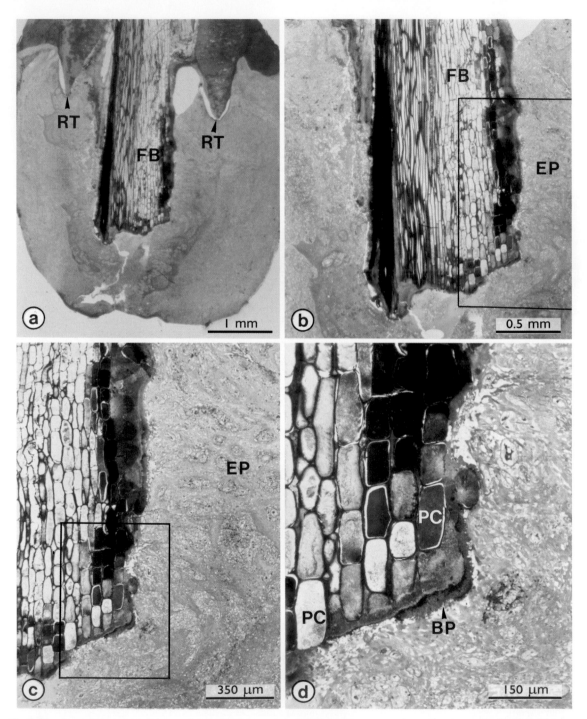

Fig. 4.21 A massive paper-point granuloma affecting a root canal treated human tooth (a). The demarcated area in (b) is magnified in (c) and that in (c) is further magnified in (d). Note the tip of the paper-point (FB) projecting into the lesion and the biofilm (BP) adhering to the surface of the paper-point; RT, root tip; EP, epithelium; PC, plant cell (original magnifications: a ×20, b ×40, c ×60, d ×150).

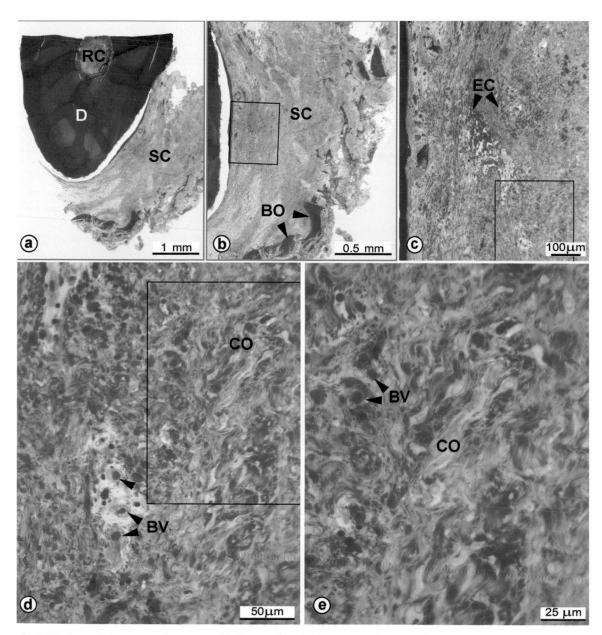

Fig. 4.22 Periapical scar (SC) of a root canal (RC) treated tooth after 5-year follow-up and surgery. The rectangular demarcated areas in (b–d) are magnified in (c–e), respectively. The scar tissue reveals bundles of collagen fibers (CO), blood vessels (BV) and erythrocytes due to hemorrhage. Infiltrating inflammatory cells are notably absent. BO, bone. (Original magnifications: a ×14, b ×35, c ×90, d ×340, e ×560.) (Partially adapted from Nair *et al.* [192].)

4.22). The tissue dynamics of periapical healing after root canal treatment and surgical endodontics are not well known. However, certain deductions can be made from the data available on normal healing and guided regeneration of the marginal periodontium. Various tissue cells participate in the healing process. The pattern of healing depends on several factors, two of which are decisive. They are the regeneration potential and the speed with which the tissue cells bordering the defect react [120,121,201,246]. A periapical scar is likely to develop when precursors of soft connective tissue colonize both the root tip and periapical tissue; this may occur before the appropriate cells, which have the potential to restore various structural components of the apical periodontium are able to do so [192].

4.7 Postsurgical apical periodontitis

Treatment of apical periodontitis persisting after conventional root canal treatment generally consists of root canal retreatment and/or surgical endodontics. The term surgical endodontics covers various procedures, including periapical curettage, root-end resection and root-end filling. However, for further clinical management of teeth with persistent apical lesions, a careful consideration of the potential causes is necessary. Such cases when associated with substandard endodontic procedures respond well with proper root canal retreatment. However, for cases in which root canal retreatment is unlikely to result in periapical healing, as outlined in previous sections, or such treatment may not be possible, surgical endodontics should be the preferred clinical procedure to follow. Several investigators assessed the outcome of surgical endodontics and the works have been extensively reviewed [80,222]. The reported success rates of surgical endodontics range from 25% to 95% [222,353]. This great disparity has been attributed to differences in methods and criteria for evaluation of success [222]. Methods include several critical aspects such as selection of appropriate cases, surgical procedures, period of follow-up, sample size and so on. Direct comparison between such studies is not only difficult, but may lead to the erroneous interpretation that the treatment outcome of surgical endodontics is unpredictable. It is recognized that surgical endodontics has been performed on a large number of cases in which such treatment is not justified [3]. Well-defined case selection and skilled appli-

cation of contemporary surgical techniques resulted in a success rate of 91% after surgical endodontics [353]. This study also showed that a small percentage of surgically treated cases may not show bony healing at the periapex even after proper case selection and skilled surgical procedures. Despite the classical histological reports of the pioneers [231,232], the reasons for postsurgical persistent radiological lesions are currently unknown. In order to identify the potential causative agents of asymptomatic postsurgical apical radiolucencies by microscopy, the cases must be selected from teeth that have had proper root canal treatment, good coronal restoration, the best possible surgical retreatment and the lesions remain asymptomatic. For analysis, the specimens must be anatomically intact block-biopsies that include a certain length of the apical part of the previously treated root and the lesion. Such specimens should undergo thorough investigation by serial or step-serial sections that are analyzed using correlative light and transmission electron microscopy as has been done for apical lesions persisting after conventional root canal treatment [193]. There is no study that meets these criteria.

Taken together, to identify the reasons for postsurgery failures, the problem must be approached in a scientific way. It cannot be achieved by evaluating radiographs, retrospective analysis of literature on prognostic studies, or by conducting surveys and epidemiological type of investigations. An indepth approach denotes rigorous analysis of well-documented cases by careful and painstaking correlative light and transmission electron microscopy.

4.8 Concluding remarks

The essential cause of primary apical periodontitis affecting teeth that have not undergone root canal treatment is infection within the root canal system. Therefore, the aim of endodontic treatment is to eliminate infectious agents or to reduce substantially the microbial load from the root canal and to prevent reinfection by root filling [185,186]. The anatomical complexity of the root canal system [104,212] and the organization of the microbes into biofilms [50,51] make it unlikely that a sterile canal-system can be achieved by contemporary technology [186]. Therefore, healing of the periapex may not occur in all root canal treated teeth.

The etiological spectrum of post-treatment apical periodontitis is broader than that of teeth with primary apical periodontitis. The causes of such persistent apical periodontitis include: (i) intraradicular infection persisting in the complex apical root canal system; (ii) extraradicular infection, generally in the form of periapical actinomycosis; (iii) extruded root canal filling or other exogenous materials that cause a foreign body reaction; (iv) accumulation of endogenous cholesterol crystals that irritate periapical tissues; (v) true cystic lesions, and (vi) scar tissue healing of the periapex. Among these factors, residual microbes in the complex root canal system are the major cause of apical periodontitis persisting post-treatment. Extraradicular actinomycosis, true cysts, foreign-body reaction and scar tissue healing are of rare occurrence. As the primacy of residual intracanal infection in persistent apical periodontitis has been recognized [193], the main target of treatment should be the microorganisms residing within the root canal system.

However, the tissue dynamics of apical periodontitis persisting due to nonmicrobial causes, such as a foreign body reaction and cystic condition, are not dependent on the presence or absence of infectious agents in the root canal. The host cells that accumulate in sites of foreign body reaction and reside in cystic lesions are not only unable to resolve the disease, but are also major sources of inflammatory and bone resorptive cytokines and other mediators. Therefore, initiation of a foreign body reaction in periapical tissues and/or cystic transformation of the lesion delay or prevent post-treatment healing. In well-treated teeth with adequate root filling, a nonsurgical retreatment is unlikely to resolve the problem, as it does not remove the offending agents and disease that exist beyond the root canal [130,131,192–195]. Currently, a clinical differential diagnosis for the existence of these extraradicular agents of persistent apical periodontitis is not possible. Further, the great majority of persistent apical periodontitis is caused by residual infection in the complex apical root canal system [104,212]. It is not guaranteed that root canal retreatment of an otherwise well treated tooth can eradicate the residual intraradicular infection.

Therefore, with cases of asymptomatic, persistent, periapical radiolucencies, clinicians should consider the necessity of removing the extraradicular factors by surgery [353], in order to improve the long-term outcome of treatment. Surgical endodontics provides an opportunity to remove the extraradicular agents

that sustain the apical radiolucency post-treatment and simultaneously allows retrograde access to any potential infection in the apical part of the root canal system that can also be removed or sealed within the canal by a root-end filling [183]. Even after surgical treatment of persistent apical periodontitis, complete hard tissue healing of all treated cases cannot be expected. Currently there are no data on causes that maintain apical radiolucent lesions persisting after surgical endodontics.

4.9 References

1. Abdulla YH, Adams CWM, Morgan RS (1967) Connective tissue reactions to implantation of purified sterol, sterol esters, phosphoglycerides, glycerides and free fatty acids. *Journal of Pathology and Bacteriology* **94**, 63–71.
2. Abou-Rass M, Bogen G (1997) Microorganisms in closed periapical lesions. *International Endodontic Journal* **31**, 39–47.
3. Abramovitz I, Better H, Shacham A, Shlomi B, Metzger Z (2002) Case selection for apical surgery: A retrospective evaluation of associated factors and rational. *Journal of Endodontics* **28**, 527–30.
4. Adams CWM, Bayliss OB, Ibrahim MZM, Webster MW (1963) Phospholipids in atherosclerosis: The modification of the cholesterol granuloma by phospholipid. *Journal of Pathology and Bacteriology* **86**, 431–6.
5. Adams CWM, Morgan RS (1967) The effect of saturated and polyunsaturated lecithins on the resorption of 4–14c-cholesterol from subcutaneous implants. *Journal of Pathology and Bacteriology* **94**, 73–6.
6. Allard U, Nord CE, Sjöberg L, Strömberg T (1979) Experimental infections with *Staphylococcus aureus*, *Streptococcus sanguis*, *Pseudomonas aeruginosa*, and *Bacteroides fragilis* in the jaws of dogs. *Oral Surgery, Oral Medicine, Oral Pathology* **48**, 454–62.
7. Anderson WAD (1996) *Pathology*, 5th edn. St. Louis, MO: CV Mosby.
8. Ando N, Hoshino E (1990) Predominant obligate anaerobes invading the deep layers of root canal dentine. *International Endodontic Journal* **23**, 20–7.
9. Andreasen FM (1985) Transient apical breakdown and its relation to color and sensibility changes after luxation injuries to teeth. *Endodontics and Dental Traumatology* **2**, 9–19.
10. Andreasen JO, Rud J (1972) A histobacteriologic study of dental and periapical structures after endodontic surgery. *International Journal of Oral Surgery* **1**, 272–81.
11. Arden LA (1979) Revised nomenclature for antigen non-specific T cell proliferation and helper factors. *Journal of Immunology* **123**, 2928–9.
12. Artese L, Piattelli A, Quaranta M, Colasante A, Musiani P (1991) Immunoreactivity for interleukin 1β

and tumor necrosis factor-α and ultrastructural features of monocytes/macrophages in periapical granulomas. *Journal of Endodontics* **17**, 483–7.

13. Ataoglu T, Üngör M, Serpek B, Haliloglu S, Ataoglu H, Ari H (2002) Interleukin-1β and tumour necrosis factor-α levels in periapical exudates. *International Endodontic Journal* **35**, 181–5.

14. Barkhordar RA, Hussain MZ, Hayashi C (1992) Detection of interleukin-1 beta in human periapical lesions. *Oral Surgery, Oral Medicine, Oral Pathology* **73**, 334–6.

15. Batty I (1958) *Actinomyces odontolyticus*, a new species of actinomycete regularly isolated from deep carious dentine. *Journal of Pathology and Bacteriology* **75**, 455–9.

16. Baumann L, Rossman SR (1956) Clinical, roentgenologic and histologic findings in teeth with apical radiolucent areas. *Oral Surgery, Oral Medicine, Oral Pathology* **9**, 1330–6.

17. Baumgartner JC, Falkler WA (1991) Bacteria in the apical 5 mm of infected root canals. *Journal of Endodontics* **17**, 380–3.

18. Baumgartner JC, Khemaleelkul SU, Xia T (2003) Identification of spirochetes (treponemas) in endodontic infections. *Journal of Endodontics* **29**, 794–7.

19. Baumgartner JC, Watkins BJ, Bae K-S, Xia T (1999) Association of black-pigmented bacteria with endodontic infections. *Journal of Endodontics* **25**, 413–15.

20. Bayliss OB (1976) The giant cell in cholesterol resorption. *British Journal of Experimental Pathology* **57**, 610–18.

21. Bergenholtz G (1974) Micro-organisms from necrotic pulp of traumatized teeth. *Odontologisk Revy* **25**, 347–58.

22. Bergenholtz G, Lekholm U, Liljenberg B, Lindhe J (1983) Morphometric analysis of chronic inflammatory periapical lesions in root filled teeth. *Oral Surgery, Oral Medicine, Oral Pathology* **55**, 295–301.

23. Bergenholtz G, Spångberg L (2004) Controversies in endodontics. *Critical Reviews in Oral Biology and Medicine* **15**, 99–114.

24. Bhaskar SN (1966) Periapical lesion – types, incidence and clinical features. *Oral Surgery, Oral Medicine, Oral Pathology* **21**, 657–71.

25. Birch RH, Melville TH, Neubert EW (1964) A comparison of root-canal and apical lesion flora. *British Dental Journal* **116**, 350–2.

26. Birek C, Heersche D, Jez D, Brunette DM (1983) Secretion of bone resorbing factor by epithelial cells cultured from porcine rests of Malassez. *Journal of Periodontal Research* **18**, 75–81.

27. Birkedal-Hansen H (1993) Role of matrix metalloproteinases in human periodontal diseases. *Journal of Periodontology* **64**, 474–84.

28. Birkedal-Hansen H, Moore WG, Bodden MK, Windsor LJ, Birkedal-Hansen B, Decarlo A, *et al.* (1993) Matrix metalloproteinases: A review. *Critical Review of Oral Biology and Medicine* **4**, 197–250.

29. Birkedal-Hansen H, Werb Z, Welgus HG, Van Wart HE (1992) *Matrix metalloproteinases and inhibitors.* Stuttgart: Gustav Fischer.

30. Block RM, Bushell A, Rodrigues H, Langeland K (1976) A histopathologic, histobacteriologic, and radiographic study of periapical endodontic surgical specimens. *Oral Surgery, Oral Medicine, Oral Pathology* **42**, 656–78.

31. Brown AMS, Theaker JM (1987) Food induced granuloma – an unusual cause of a submandibular mass with observations on the pathogenesis of hyalin bodies. *British Journal of Maxillofacial Surgery* **25**, 433–6.

32. Brown LR, Rudolph CE (1957) Isolation and identification of microorganisms from unexposed canals of pulp-involved teeth. *Oral Surgery, Oral Medicine, Oral Pathology* **10**, 1094–9.

33. Browne RM (1971) The origin of cholesterol in odontogenic cysts in man. *Archives of Oral Biology* **16**, 107–13.

34. Browne RM, O'Riordan BC (1966) Colony of actinomyces-like organism in a periapical granuloma. *British Dental Journal* **120**, 603–6.

35. Brunette DM, Heersche JNM, Purdon AD, Sodek J, Moe HK, Assuras JN (1979) In vitro cultural parameters and protein and prostaglandin secretion of epithelial cells derived from porcine rests of Malassez. *Archives of Oral Biology* **24**, 199–203.

36. Buchanan BB, Pine L (1962) Characterization of a propionic acid producing actinomycete, *Actinomyces propionicus*, sp nov. *Journal of General Microbiology* **28**, 305–23.

37. Burke GWJ, Knighton HT (1960) The localization of microorganisms in inflamed dental pulps of rats following bacteremia. *Journal of Dental Research* **39**, 205–14.

38. Byström A, Claesson R, Sundqvist G (1985) The antibacterial effect of camphorated paramonochlorophenol, camphorated phenol and calcium hydroxide in the treatment of infected root canals. *Endodontics and Dental Traumatology* **1**, 170–5.

39. Byström A, Happonen RP, Sjögren U, Sundqvist G (1987) Healing of periapical lesions of pulpless teeth after endodontic treatment with controlled asepsis. *Endodontics and Dental Traumatology* **3**, 58–63.

40. Byström A, Sundqvist G (1981) Bacteriologic evaluation of the efficacy of mechanical root canal instrumentation in endodontic therapy. *Scandinavian Journal of Dental Research* **89**, 321–8.

41. Carlsson J (1990) Microbiology of plaque associated periodontal disease. In: Lindhe J, editor. *Textbook of clinical periodontology*, pp. 129–152. Copenhagen: Munksgaard.

42. Carlsson J, Frölander F, Sundqvist G (1977) Oxygen tolerance of anaerobic bacteria isolated from necrotic dental pulps. *Acta Odontologica Scandinavica* **35**, 139–45.

43. Cheung GS, Ho MW (2001) Microbial flora of root canal-treated teeth associated with asymptomatic periapical radiolucent lesions. *Oral Microbiology and Immunology* **16**, 332–7.

44. Chirnside IM (1957) A bacteriological and histological study of traumatised teeth. *New Zealand Dental Journal* **53**, 176–91.

45. Christianson OO (1939) Observations on lesions produced in arteries of dogs by injection of lipids. *Archives of Pathology* **27**, 1011–20.

46. Cohen S, Bigazzi PE, Yoshida T (1974) Similarities of T cell function in cell-mediated immunity and antibody production. *Cellular Immunology* **12**, 150–9.

47. Coleman DL, King RN, Andrade JD (1974) The foreign body reaction: a chronic inflammatory response. *Journal of Biomedical Materials Research* **8**, 199–211.

48. Costerton JW, Geesy GG, Cheng GK (1978) How bacteria stick. *Scientific American* **238**, 86–95.

49. Costerton JW, Lewandowski DE, Caldwell DE, Krober DR, Lappin-Scott H (1995) Microbial biofilms. *Annual Reviews of Microbiology* **49**, 711–45.

50. Costerton JW, Stewart PS (2000) Biofilms and device-related infections. In Nataro PJ, Balser MJ, Cunningham-Rundels S, editors. *Persistent bacterial infections*, pp. 423–39. Washington, DC: ASM Press.

51. Costerton W, Veeh R, Shirtliff M, Pasmore M, Post C (2003) The application of biofilm science to the study and control of chronic bacterial infections. *Journal of Clinical Investigations* **112**, 1466–77.

52. Cotti F, Torabinejad M (1994) Detection of leukotriene C4 in human periradicular lesions. *International Endodontic Journal* **27**, 82–6.

53. Cymerman JJ, Cymerman DH, Walters J, Nevins AJ (1984) Human T-lymphocyte subpopulations in chronic periapical lesions. *Journal of Endodontics* **10**, 9–11.

54. Dahle UR, Tronstad L, Olsen I (1993) Observation of an unusually large spirochete in endodontic infection. *Oral Microbiology and Immunology* **8**, 251–3.

55. Dahle UR, Tronstad L, Olsen I (1996) Characterization of new periodontal and endodontic isolates of spirochetes. *European Journal of Oral Sciences* **104**, 41–7.

56. Dahlén G (1980) Studies on lipopolysaccharides from oral Gram-negative anaerobic bacteria in relation to apical periodontitis. Dr. Odont Thesis. Göteborg: University of Göteborg.

57. Dahlén G, Bergenholtz G (1980) Endotoxic activity in teeth with necrotic pulps. *Journal of Dental Research* **59**, 1033–40.

58. Dahlén G, Fabricius L, Heyden G, Holm SE, Möller ÅJR (1982) Apical periodontitis induced by selected bacterial strains in root canals of immunized and non-immunized monkeys. *Scandinavian Journal of Dental Research* **90**, 207–16.

59. Dahlén G, Fabricius L, Holm SE, Möller ÅJR (1982) Circulating antibodies after experimental chronic infection in the root canal of teeth in monkeys. *Scandinavian Journal of Dental Research* **90**, 338–44.

60. Dahlén G, Magnusson BC, Möller Å (1981) Histological and histochemical study of the influence of lipopolysaccharide extracted from *Fusobacterium nucleatum* on the periapical tissues in the monkey *Macaca fascicularis*. *Archives of Oral Biology* **26**, 591–8.

61. Damme JV (1994) Interleukin-8 and related chemotactic cytokines. In: Thomson AW, editor. *The cytokine handbook*, 2nd edn, pp. 185–221. London: Academic Press.

62. De Sá AR, Pimenta FJGS, Dutra WO, Gomez RS (2003) Immunolocalization of interleukin 4, interleukin 6, and lymphotoxin α in dental granuloma. *Oral Surgery, Oral Medicine, Oral Pathology, Oral Radiology, Endodontics* **96**, 356–60.

63. Delivanis PD, Fan VSC (1984) The localization of blood-borne bacteria in instrumented unfilled and overinstrumented canals. *Journal of Endodontics* **10**, 521–4.

64. Dubrow H (1976) Silver points and gutta-percha and the role of root canal fillings. *Journal of the American Dental Association* **93**, 976–80.

65. Dunlap CL, Barker BF (1977) Giant cell hyalin angiopathy. *Oral Surgery, Oral Medicine, Oral Pathology* **44**, 587–91.

66. Engström B (1964) The significance of enterococci in root canal treatment. *Odontologisk Revy* **15**, 87–106.

67. Engström B, Frostell G (1961) Bacteriological studies of the non-vital pulp in cases with intact pulp cavities. *Acta Odontologica Scandinavica* **19**, 23–39.

68. Evans M, Davies JK, Sundqvist G, Figdor D (2002) Mechanisms involved in the resistance of *Enterococcus faecalis* to calcium hydroxide. *International Endodontic Journal* **35**, 221–8.

69. Fabricius L (1982) Oral bacteria and apical periodontitis. An experimental study in monkeys. Dr. Odont. Thesis. Göteborg: University of Göteborg.

70. Fabricius L, Dahlén G, Holm SC, Möller ÅJR (1982) Influence of combinations of oral bacteria on periapical tissues of monkeys. *Scandinavian Journal of Dental Research* **90**, 200–6.

71. Fabricius L, Dahlén G, Öhman AE, Möller ÅJR (1982) Predominant indigenous oral bacteria isolated from infected root canal after varied times of closure. *Scandinavian Journal of Dental Research* **90**, 134–44.

72. Figdor D, Davies J (1997) Cell surface structures of *Actinomyces israelii*. *Australian Dental Journal* **42**, 125–8.

73. Figdor D, Davies JK, Sundqvist G (2003) Starvation survival, growth and recovery of *Enterococcus faecalis* in human serum. *Oral Microbiology and Immunology* **18**, 234–9.

74. Figdor D, Sjögren U, Sorlin S, Sundqvist G, Nair PNR (1992) Pathogenicity of *Actinomyces israelii* and *Arachnia propionica*: Experimental infection in guinea pigs and phagocytosis and intracellular killing by human polymorphonuclear leukocytes *in vitro*. *Oral Microbiology and Immunology* **7**, 129–36.

75. Fletcher HA, Donoghue HD, Holton J, Pap I, Spigelman M (2003) Widespread occurrence of *Mycobacterium tuberculosis* DNA from 18th–19th century Hungarians. *American Journal Physiological Anthropology* **120**, 144–52.

76. Formigli L, Orlandini SZ, Tonelli P, *et al.* (1995) Osteolytic processes in human radicular cysts: Morphological and biochemical results. *Journal of Oral Pathology and Medicine* **24**, 216–20.

77. Fouad AF, Burleson J (2003) The effect of diabetes mellitus on endodontic treatment outcome: data from an electronic patient record. *Journal of the American Dental Association* **134**, 43–51.

78. Fouad AF, Zerella J, Barry J, Spångberg LS (2005) Molecular detection of *Enterococcus* species in root canals of therapy-resistant endodontic infections. *Oral Surgery, Oral Medicine, Oral Pathology, Oral Radiology, Endodontics* **99**, 112–18.

79. Freeman N (1931) Histopathological investigation of dental granuloma. *Journal of Dental Research* **11**, 176–200.

80. Friedman S (1998) Treatment outcome and prognosis of endodontic therapy. In Ørstavik D, Pitt Ford TR, editors. *Essential endodontology*; pp. 368–401. Oxford: Blackwell.

81. Fukushima H, Yamamoto K, Hirohata K, Sagawa H, Leung KP, Walker CB (1990) Localization and identification of root canal bacteria in clinically asymptomatic periapical pathosis. *Journal of Endodontics* **16**, 534–8.

82. Gao Z, Flaitz CM, Mackenzie IC (1996) Expression of keratinocyte growth factor in periapical lesions. *Journal of Dental Research* **75**, 1658–663.

83. Gardner AF (1962) A survey of periapical pathology: Part one. *Dental Digest* **68**, 162–7.

84. Gatti JJ, Dobeck JM, Smith C, Socransky SS, Skobe Z (2000) Bacteria of asymptomatic periradicular endodontic lesions identified by DNA–DNA hybridization. *Endodontics and Dental Traumatology* **16**, 197–204.

85. Gay CV (1992) Osteoclast ultrastructure and enzyme histochemistry: functional implications. In Rifkin BR, Gay CV, editors. *Biology and physiology of the osteoclast*, pp. 129–150. Boca Raton, FL: CRC Press.

86. Gier RE, Mitchell DF (1968) Anachoretic effect of pulpitis. *Journal of Dental Research* **47**, 564–70.

87. Glick M, Trope M, Bagasra O, Pliskin ME (1991) Human immunodeficiency virus infection of fibroblasts of dental pulp in seropositive patients. *Oral Surgery, Oral Medicine, Oral Pathology, Oral Radiology, Endodontics* **71**, 733–6.

88. Grahnén H, Hansson L (1961) The prognosis of pulp and root canal therapy: A clinical and radiographic follow-up examination. *Odontologisk Revy* **12**, 146–65.

89. Greening AB, Schonfeld SE (1980) Apical lesions contain elevated immunoglobulin G levels. *Journal of Endodontics* **12**, 867–9.

90. Grossman LI (1967) Origin of microorganisms in traumatized, pulpless, sound teeth. *Journal of Dental Research* **46**, 551–3.

91. Haapasalo M (1989) *Bacteroides* spp in dental root canal infections. *Endodontics and Dental Traumatology* **5**, 1–10.

92. Hampp EG (1957) Isolation and identification of spirochetes obtained from unexposed canals of pulp-involved teeth. *Oral Surgery, Oral Medicine, Oral Pathology* **10**, 1100–4.

93. Hancock H, Sigurdsson A, Trope M, Moiseiwitsch J (2001) Bacteria isolated after unsuccessful endodontic treatment in a North American population. *Oral Surgery, Oral Medicine, Oral Pathology* **91**, 579–86.

94. Happonen RP (1986) Periapical actinomycosis: a follow-up study of 16 surgically treated cases. *Endodontics and Dental Traumatology* **2**, 205–9.

95. Happonen RP, Söderling E, Viander M, Linko-Kettunen L, Pelliniemi LJ (1985) Immunocytochemical demonstration of *Actinomyces* species and *Arachnia propionica* in periapical infections. *Journal of Oral Pathology* **14**, 405–13.

96. Harndt E (1926) Histo-bakteriologische Studie bei Parodontitis chronika granulomatosa. *Korrespondenz-Blatt für Zahnärzte* **50**, 330–5, 365–70, 399–404, 426–33.

97. Harris M, Goldhaber P (1973) The production of a bone resorbing factor by dental cysts in vitro. *British Journal of Oral Surgery* **10**, 334–8.

98. Harris M, Jenkins MV, Bennett A, Wills MR (1973) Prostaglandin production and bone resorption by dental cysts. *Nature* **145**, 213–15.

99. Harrison JD, Martin IC (1986) Oral vegetable granuloma: Ultrastructural and histological study. *Journal of Oral Pathology* **23**, 346–50.

100. Harz CO (1879) *Actinomyces bovis,* ein neuer Schimmel in den Geweben des Rindes. *Deutsche Zeitschrift für Thiermedizin, Leipzig* **5** (2 Supplement), 125–40.

101. Head MA (1956) Foreign body reaction to inhalation of lentil soup: giant cell pneumonia. *Journal of Clinical Pathology* **9**, 295–9.

102. Heersche JN (1992) Systemic factors regulating osteoclast function. In: Rifkin BR, Gay CV, editors. *Biology and physiology of the osteoclast*, pp. 151–70. Boca Raton, FL: CRC Press.

103. Henderson B, Poole S, Wilson M (1996) Bacterial modulins: a novel class of virulence factors which cause host tissue pathology by inducing cytokine synthesis. *Microbiological Reviews* **60**, 316–41.

104. Hess W (1921) Formation of root canal in human teeth. *Journal of the National Dental Association* **3**, 704–34.

105. Hirano T (1994) Interleukin-6. In: Thomson AW, editor. *The cytokine handbook*, 2nd edn, pp. 145–68. London: Academic Press.

106. Hirsch EF (1938) Experimental tissue lesions with mixtures of human fat, soaps and cholesterol. *Archives of Pathology* **25**, 35–9.

107. Holdeman LV, Cato EP, Moore WEC (1977) *Anaerobe laboratory manual*. Blacksburg, VA: Virginia Polytechnic Institute and State University.

108. Holland R, De Souza V, Nery MJ, de Mello W, Bernabé PFE, Filho JAO (1980) Tissue reactions following apical plugging of the root canal with infected dentin chips. *Oral Surgery, Oral Medicine, Oral Pathology* **49**, 366–9.

109. Horiba N, Maekawa Y, Matsumoto T, Nakamura H (1990) A study of the distribution of endotoxin in the dentinal wall of infected root canals. *Journal of Endodontics* **16**, 331–4.

110. Howell A, Jordan HV, Georg LK, Pine L (1965) *Odontomyces viscosus* gen nov spec nov. A filamentous

microorganism isolated from periodontal plaque in hamsters. *Sabouraudia* **4**, 65–7.

111. Hungate RE (1950) The anaerobic mesophilic cellulolytic bacteria. *Bacteriological Reviews* **14**, 1–49.

112. Hylton RP, Samules HS, Oatis GW (1970) Actinomycosis: Is it really rare? *Oral Surgery, Oral Medicine, Oral Pathology* **29**, 138–47.

113. Iwu C, MacFarlane TW, MacKenzie D, Stenhouse D (1990) The microbiology of periapical granulomas. *Oral Surgery, Oral Medicine, Oral Pathology* **69**, 502–5.

114. James WW (1926) Do epithelial odontomes increase in size by their own tension? *Proceedings of the Royal Society of Medicine* **19**, 73–7.

115. Jones OJ, Lally ET (1980) Biosynthesis of immunoglobulin isotopes in human periapical lesions. *Journal of Endodontics* **8**, 672–7.

116. Jontell M, Okiji T, Dhalgren U, Bergenholtz G (1998) Immune defense mechanisms of the dental pulp. *Critical Reviews in Oral Biology and Medicine* **9**, 179–200.

117. Kakehashi S, Stanley HR, Fitzgerald RJ (1965) The effects of surgical exposures of dental pulps in germ-free and conventional laboratory rats. *Oral Surgery, Oral Medicine, Oral Pathology* **20**, 340–9.

118. Kantz WE, Henry CA (1974) Isolation and classification of anaerobic bacteria from intact pulp chambers of non vital teeth in man. *Archives of Oral Biology* **19**, 91–6.

119. Kapsimalis P, Garrington GE (1968) Actinomycosis of the periapical tissues. *Oral Surgery, Oral Medicine, Oral Pathology* **26**, 374–80.

120. Karring T, Nyman S, Gottlow J, Laurell L (1993) Development of the biological concept of guided tissue regeneration – animal and human studies. *Periodontology 2000* **1**, 26–35.

121. Karring T, Nyman S, Lindhe J (1980) Healing following implantation of periodontitis affected roots into bone tissue. *Journal of Clinical Periodontology* **7**, 96–105.

122. Kerekes K, Tronstad L (1979) Long-term results of endodontic treatment performed with standardized technique. *Journal of Endodontics* **5**, 83–90.

123. Kilian M (1981) Degradation of human immunoglobulins A1, A2 and G by suspected principal periodontal pathogens. *Infection and Immunity* **34**, 757–65.

124. King OH (1978) "Giant cell hyaline angiopathy": Pulse granuloma by another name? Proceedings of the 32nd Annual Meeting of the American Academy of Oral Pathologists, Fort Lauderdale.

125. Klevant FJH, Eggink CO (1983) The effect of canal preparation on periapical disease. *International Endodontic Journal* **16**, 68–75.

126. Knoblich R (1969) Pulmonary granulomatosis caused by vegetable particles. So-called lentil pulse granuloma. *American Review of Respiratory Diseases* **99**, 380–389.

127. Konomi N, Lebwohl E, Mowbray K, Tattersall I (2002) Detection of mycobacterial DNA in Andean mummies. *Journal of Clinical Microbiology* **40**, 4738–40.

128. Kopp W, Schwarting R (1989) Differentiation of T-lymphocyte subpopulations, macrophages, HLA-DR-restricted cells of apical granulation tissue. *Journal of Endodontics* **15**, 72–5.

129. Koppang HS, Koppang R, Solheim T, Aarnes H, Stølen SØ (1987) Identification of cellulose fibers in oral biopsies. *Scandinavian Journal of Dental Research* **95**, 165–73.

130. Koppang HS, Koppang R, Solheim T, Aarnes H, Stølen SØ (1989) Cellulose fibers from endodontic paper points as an etiologic factor in postendodontic periapical granulomas and cysts. *Journal of Endodontics* **15**, 369–72.

131. Koppang HS, Koppang R, Stølen SØ (1992) Identification of common foreign material in postendodontic granulomas and cysts. *Journal of the Dental Association of South Africa* **47**, 210–16.

132. Kronfeld R (1939) *Histopathology of the teeth and their surrounding structures*. Philadelphia, PA: Lea & Febiger.

133. Kuntz DD, Genco RJ, Guttuso J, Natiella JR (1977) Localization of immunoglobulins and the third component of complement in dental periapical lesions. *Journal of Endodontics* **3**, 68–73.

134. Lalonde ER (1970) A new rationale for the management of periapical granulomas and cysts. An evaluation of histopathological and radiographic findings. *Journal of the American Dental Association* **80**, 1056–9.

135. Lalonde ER, Luebke RG (1968) The frequency and distribution of periapical cysts and granulomas. *Oral Surgery, Oral Medicine, Oral Pathology* **25**, 861–8.

136. Langeland K (1993) Erkrankungen der Pulpa und des Periapex. In: Guldener PHA, Langeland K, editors. *Endodontie*, 2nd edn, pp. 59, 66, 70. Stuttgart: Georg Thieme.

137. Langeland MA, Block RM, Grossman LI (1977) A histopathologic and histobacteriologic study of 35 periapical endodontic surgical specimens. *Journal of Endodontics* **3**, 8–23.

138. Laux M, Abbott P, Pajarola G, Nair PNR (2000) Apical inflammatory root resorption: a correlative radiographic and histological assessement. *International Endodontic Journal* **33**, 483–93.

139. Lerner UH (1994) Regulation of bone metabolism by the kallikrein–kinin system, the coagulation cascade, and acute phase reactions. *Oral Surgery, Oral Medicine, Oral Pathology* **78**, 481–93.

140. Lew M, Keudel KC, Milford AF (1971) Succinate as a growth factor for *Bacteroides melaninogenicus*. *Journal of Bacteriology* **108**, 175–8.

141. Lim CG, Torabinejad M, Kettering J, Linkhardt TA, Finkelman RD (1994) Interleukin 1β in symptomatic and asymptomatic human periradicular lesions. *Journal of Endodontics* **20**, 225–7.

142. Lin LM, Pascon EA, Skribner J, Gängler P, Langeland K (1991) Clinical, radiographic, and histologic study of endodontic treatment failures. *Oral Surgery, Oral Medicine, Oral Pathology* **71**, 603–11.

143. Lin LM, Wang SL, Wu-Wang C, Chang KM, Leung C (1996) Detection of epidermal growth fac-

tor in inflammatory periapical lesions. *International Endodontic Journal* **29**, 179–84.

144. Linenberg WB, Waldron CA, DeLaune GF (1964) A clinical, roentgenographic, and histopathologic evaluation of periapical lesions. *Oral Surgery, Oral Medicine, Oral Pathology* **17**, 467–72.

145. Listgarten MA (1976) Structure of the microflora associated with periodontal health and disease in man. A light and electron microscopic study. *Journal of Periodontology* **47**, 1–18.

146. Listgarten MA, Lewis DW (1967) The distribution of spirochetes in the lesion of acute necrotizing ulcerative gingivitis: An electron microscopical and statistical study. *Journal of Periodontology* **38**, 379–86.

147. Loesche WJ, Gusberti F, Mettraux G, Higgins T, Syed S (1983) Relationship between oxygen tension and subgingival bacterial flora in untreated human periodontal pockets. *Infection and Immunity* **42**, 659–67.

148. Love RM, Jenkinson HF (2002) Invasion of dentinal tubules by oral bacteria. *Critical Reviews in Oral Biology and Medicine* **13**, 171–83.

149. Love RM, McMillan MD, Jenkinson HF (1997) Invasion of dentinal tubules by oral streptococci is associated with collagen regeneration mediated by the antigen I/II family of polypeptides. *Infection and Immunity* **65**, 5157–64.

150. Lukic A, Arsenijevic N, Vujanic G, Ramic Z (1990) Quantitative analysis of the immunocompetent cells in periapical granuloma: correlation with the histological characteristics of the lesion. *Journal of Endodontics* **16**, 119–22.

151. Macdonald JB, Hare GC, Wood AWS (1957) The bacteriologic status of the pulp chambers in intact teeth found to be nonvital following trauma. *Oral Surgery, Oral Medicine, Oral Pathology* **10**, 318–22.

152. Main DMG (1970) The enlargement of epithelial jaw cysts. *Odontologisk Revy* **21**, 29–49.

153. Malassez ML (1884) Sur l'existence de masses épithéliales dans le ligament alvéolodentaire chez l'homme adulte et à l'état normal. *Comptes Rendus des Séauces de la Société de Biologie et de ses filiales* **36**, 241–4.

154. Malassez ML (1885) Sur la role débris épithélaux paradentaris: In: *Travaux de l'année 1885, Laboratorie d'histologie du Collége de France*, Paris: Masson. Librairie de l'Académie de Médicine, pp. 21–121.

155. Martin IC, Harrison JD (1984) Periapical actinomycosis. *British Dental Journal* **156**, 169–70.

156. Marton IJ, Kiss C (1993) Characterization of inflammatory cell infiltrate in dental periapical lesions. *International Endodontic Journal* **26**, 131–6.

157. Matsumoto Y (1985) Monoclonal and oligoclonal immunoglobulins localized in human dental periapical lesion. *Microbiology and Immunology* **29**, 751–7.

158. Matsuo T, Ebisu S, Nakanishi T, Yonemura K, Harada Y, Okada H (1994) Interleukin-1α and interleukin-1β in periapical exudates of infected root canal: correlations with the clinical findings of the involved teeth. *Journal of Endodontics* **20**, 432–5.

159. McGhee JR, Michalek SM, Cassel GH (1982) *Dental microbiology*. Philadelphia, PA: Harper & Row.

160. McNicholas S, Torabinejad M, Blankenship J (1991) The concentration of prostaglandin E2 in human periradicular lesions. *Journal of Endodontics* **17**, 97–100.

161. Metchinkoff E (1968) *Lectures on the comparative pathology of inflammation*. New York: Dover.

162. Miller WD (1890) *The micro-organisms of the human mouth*. Philadelphia, PA: White Dental Mfg Co.

163. Mims CA (1988) *The pathogenesis of infectious disease*, 3rd edn. London: Academic Press.

164. Mincer HH, McCoy JM, Turner JE (1979) Pulse granuloma of the alveolar ridge. *Oral Surgery, Oral Medicine, Oral Pathology* **48**, 126–30.

165. Molander A, Reit C, Dahlén G, Kvist T (1998) Microbiological status of root filled teeth with apical periodontitis. *International Endodontic Journal* **31**, 1–7.

166. Möller ÅJR (1966) Microbiological examination of root canals and periapical tissues of human teeth. Thesis, Akademiförlaget. Göteborg: University of Göteborg.

167. Möller ÅJR, Fabricius L, Dahlén G, Öhman AE, Heyden G (1981) Influence on periapical tissues of indigenous oral bacteria and necrotic pulp tissue in monkeys. *Scandinavian Journal of Dental Research* **89**, 475–84.

168. Molven O (1976) The frequency, technical standard and results of endodontic therapy. *Norske Tannlaegeforenings Tidende* **86**, 142–7.

169. Molven O, Halse A (1988) Success rates for gutta-percha and Klorperka N-Ø root fillings made by undergraduate students: radiographic findings after 10–17 years. *International Endodontic Journal* **21**, 243–50.

170. Monteleone L (1963) Actonomycosis. *Journal of Oral Surgery, Anesthesia and Hospital Dental Service* **21**, 313–18.

171. Moore WEC (1966) Techniques for routine culture of fastidious anaerobes. *International Journal of Systematic Bacteriology* **16**, 173–90.

172. Mortensen H, Winther JE, Birn H (1970) Periapical granulomas and cysts. *Scandinavian Journal of Dental Research* **78**, 241–50.

173. Morton TH, Clagett JA, Yavorsky JD (1977) Role of immune complexes in human periapical periodontitis. *Journal of Endodontics* **3**, 261–8.

174. Mullis KB, Faloona FA (1987) Specific synthesis of DNA in vitro via a polymerase-catalyzed chain reaction. *Methods in Enzymology* **155**, 335–50.

175. Munson MA, Pitt-Ford T, Chong B, Weightman A, Wade WG (2002) Molecular and cultural analysis of the microflora associated with endodontic infections. *Journal of Dental Research* **81**, 761–6.

176. Nagaoka S, Miyazaki Y, Liu HJ, Iwamoto Y, Kitano M, Kawagoe M (1995) Bacterial invasion into dentinal tubules in human vital and nonvital teeth. *Journal of Endodontics* **21**, 70–3.

177. Nagase H, Barrett AJ, Woessner JF (1992) Nomenclature and glossary of the matrix metalloproteinases. In: Birkedal-Hansen H, Werb Z, Welgus HG, Van Wart

HE, editors. *Matrix metalloproteinases and inhibitors.* pp. 421–4. Stuttgart: Gustav Fischer.

178. Naidorf IJ (1975) Immunoglobulins in periapical granulomas: a preliminary report. *Journal of Endodontics* **1**, 15–17.

179. Nair PNR (1987) Light and electron microscopic studies of root canal flora and periapical lesions. *Journal of Endodontics* **13**, 29–39.

180. Nair PNR (1997) Apical periodontitis: a dynamic encounter between root canal infection and host response. *Periodontology 2000* **13**, 121–48.

181. Nair PNR (1998) New perspectives on radicular cysts: Do they heal? *International Endodontic Journal* **31**, 155–60.

182. Nair PNR (1999) Cholesterol as an aetiological agent in endodontic failures – a review. *Australian Endodontic Journal* **25**, 19–26.

183. Nair PNR (2003) Non-microbial etiology: foreign body reaction maintaining post-treatment apical periodontitis. *Endodontic Topics* **6**, 96–113.

184. Nair PNR (2003) Non-microbial etiology: periapical cysts sustain post-treatment apical periodontitis. *Endodontic Topics* **6**, 114–34.

185. Nair PNR (2004) Pathogenesis of apical periodontitis and the causes of endodontic failures. *Critical Reviews in Oral Biology and Medicine* **15**, 348–81.

186. Nair PNR, Henry S, Cano V, Vera J (2005) Microbial status of apical root canal system of human mandibular first molars with primary apical periodontitis after 'one-visit' endodontic treatment. *Oral Surgery, Oral Medicine, Oral Pathology, Oral Radiology, Endodontics* **99**, 231–52.

187. Nair PNR, Pajarola G, Luder HU (2002) Ciliated epithelium lined radicular cysts. *Oral Surgery, Oral Medicine, Oral Pathology, Oral Radiology, Endodontics* **94**, 485–93.

188. Nair PNR, Pajarola G, Schroeder HE (1996) Types and incidence of human periapical lesions obtained with extracted teeth. *Oral Surgery, Oral Medicine, Oral Pathology* **81**, 93–102.

189. Nair PNR, Schmid-Meier E (1986) An apical granuloma with epithelial integument. *Oral Surgery, Oral Medicine, Oral Pathology* **62**, 698–703.

190. Nair PNR, Schroeder HE (1984) Periapical actinomycosis. *Journal of Endodontics* **10**, 567–70.

191. Nair PNR, Schroeder HE (1985) Epithelial attachment at diseased human tooth-apex. *Journal of Periodontal Research* **20**, 293–300.

192. Nair PNR, Sjögren U, Figdor D, Sundqvist G (1999) Persistent periapical radiolucencies of root filled human teeth, failed endodontic treatments and periapical scars. *Oral Surgery, Oral Medicine, Oral Pathology* **87**, 617–27.

193. Nair PNR, Sjögren U, Kahnberg KE, Krey G, Sundqvist G (1990) Intraradicular bacteria and fungi in root-filled, asymptomatic human teeth with therapy-resistant periapical lesions: a long-term light and electron microscopic follow-up study. *Journal of Endodontics* **16**, 580–8.

194. Nair PNR, Sjögren U, Krey G, Sundqvist G (1990) Therapy-resistant foreign-body giant cell granuloma at the periapex of a root-filled human tooth. *Journal of Endodontics* **16**, 589–95.

195. Nair PNR, Sjögren U, Schumacher E, Sundqvist G (1993) Radicular cyst affecting a root-filled human tooth: a long-term post-treatment follow-up. *International Endodontic Journal* **26**, 225–33.

196. Nair PNR, Sjögren U, Sundqvist G (1998) Cholesterol crystals as an etiological factor in non-resolving chronic inflammation: an experimental study in guinea pigs. *European Journal of Oral Sciences* **106**, 644–50.

197. Ng YL, Spratt D, Sriskantharaja S, Gulabivala K (2003) Evaluation protocols for field decontamination before bacterial sampling of root canals for contemporary microbiology techniques. *Journal of Endodontics* **29**, 317–20.

198. Nijweide PJ, De Grooth R (1992) Ontogeny of the osteoclast. In: Rifkin BR, Gay CV, editors. *Biology and physiology of the osteoclast*, pp. 81–104. Boca Raton, FL: CRC Press.

199. Nilsen R, Johannessen A, Skaug N, Matre R (1984) In situ characterization of mononuclear cells in human dental periapical lesions using monoclonal antibodies. *Oral Surgery, Oral Medicine, Oral Pathology* **58**, 160–5.

200. Nobuhara WK, Del Rio CE (1993) Incidence of periradicular pathoses in endodontic treatment failures. *Journal of Endodontics* **19**, 315–18.

201. Nyman S, Lindhe J, Karring T, Rylander H (1982) New attachment following surgical treatment of human periodontal disease. *Journal of Clinical Periodontology* **9**, 290–6.

202. Okiji T, Kawashima N, Kosaka T, Kobayashi C, Suda H (1994) Distribution of Ia antigen-expressing nonlymphoid cells in various stages of induced periapical lesions in rat molars. *Journal of Endodontics* **20**, 27–31.

203. Okiji T, Morita I, Sunada I, Murota S (1991) The role of leukotriene B4 in neutrophil infiltration in experimentally-induced inflammation of rat tooth pulp. *Journal of Dental Research* **70**, 34–7.

204. Oppenheim JJ (1994) Foreword. In: Thomson AW, editor. *The cytokine handbook*, 2nd edn, pp. xvii–xx. London: Academic Press.

205. Oppenheimer S, Miller GS, Knopt K, Blechman H (1978) Periapical actinomycosis. *Oral Surgery, Oral Medicine, Oral Pathology* **46**, 101–6.

206. Papadimitriou JM, Ashman RB (1989) Macrophages: current views on their differentiation, structure and function. *Ultrastructural Pathology* **13**, 343–72.

207. Patterson SS, Shafer WG, Healey HJ (1964) Periapical lesions associated with endodontically treated teeth. *Journal of the American Dental Association* **68**, 191–4.

208. Peciuliene V, Balciuniene I, Eriksen H, Haapasalo M (2000) Isolation of *Enterococcus faecalis* in previously root filled canals in a Lithuanian population. *Journal of Endodontics* **26**, 593–5.

209. Peciuliene V, Reynaud A, Balciuniene I, Haapasalo M (2001) Isolation of yeasts and enteric bacteria in root-

filled teeth with chronic apical periodontitis. *International Endodontic Journal* **34**, 429–34.

210. Penick EC (1961) Periapical repair by dense fibrous connective tissue following conservative endodontic therapy. *Oral Surgery, Oral Medicine, Oral Pathology* **14**, 239–42.

211. Perez F, Calas P, de Falguerolles A, Maurette A (1993) Migration of a *Streptococcus sanguis* strain through the root dentinal tubules. *Journal of Endodontics* **19**, 297–301.

212. Perrini N, Castagnola L (1998) *W. Hess & O. Keller's anatomical plates: studies on the anatomical structure of root canals in human dentition by a method of making the tooth substance transparent (1928)*. Lainate: Altini Communicazioni Grafiche.

213. Peters LB, Wesselink PR, Moorer WR (1995) The fate and the role of bacteria left in root dentinal tubules. *International Endodontic Journal* **28**, 95–9.

214. Piattelli A, Artese L, Rosini S, Quarenta M, Musiani P (1991) Immune cells in periapical granuloma: morphological and immunohistochemical characterization. *Journal of Endodontics* **17**, 26–9.

215. Pinheiro ET, Gomes BPFA, Ferraz CCR, Sousa ELR, Teixeira FB, Souza-Filho FJ (2003) Microorganisms from canals of root filled teeth with periapical lesions. *International Endodontic Journal* **36**, 1–11.

216. Pitt Ford TR (1982) The effects on the periapical tissues of bacterial contamination of the filled root canal. *International Endodontic Journal* **15**, 16–22.

217. Poertzel E, Petschelt A (1986) Bakterien in der Wurzelkanalwand bei Pulpagangrän. *Deutsche Zahnärztliche Zeitschrift* **41**, 772–7.

218. Pollard DR, Tyler SD, Ng CW, Rozee KR (1989) A polymerase chain reaction (PCR) protocol for the specific detection of chlamydia spp. *Molecular Cell Probes* **3**, 383–9.

219. Priebe WA, Lazansky JP, Wuehrmann AH (1954) The value of the roentgenographic film in the differential diagnosis of periapical lesions. *Oral Surgery, Oral Medicine, Oral Pathology* **7**, 979–83.

220. Pulver WH, Taubman MA, Smith DJ (1978) Immune components in human dental periapical lesions. *Archives of Oral Biology* **23**, 435–43.

221. Puzas JE, Ishibe M (1992) Osteoblast/osteoclast coupling. In: Rifkin BR, Gay CV, editors. *Biology and physiology of the osteoclast*, pp. 337–56.

222. Rahbaran S, Gilthorpe MS, Harrison SD, Gulabivala K (2001) Comparison of clinical outcome of periapical surgery in endodontic and oral surgery units of a teaching dental hospital: a retrospective study. *Oral Surgery, Oral Medicine, Oral Pathology, Oral Radiology, Endodontics* **91**, 700–9.

223. Rickert UG, Dixon CM (1931) The controlling of root surgery. In: *Transactions of the eighth international dental congress*, Paris. Section IIIa, pp. 15–22.

224. Ricucci D, Mannocci F, Pitt Ford TR (2006) A study of periapical lesions correlating the presence of a radiopaque lamina with histological findings. *Oral Surgery, Oral Medicine, Oral Pathology, Oral Radiology, Endodontics* **101**, 389–94.

225. Robinson HBG, Boling LR (1941) The anachoretic effect in pulpitis. Bacteriologic studies. *Journal of the American Dental Association* **28**, 268–82.

226. Rôças I, Siqueira J, Andrade A, Uzeda M (2003) Polymerase chain reaction detection of treponema denticola in endodontic infections within root canals. *International Dental Journal* **34**, 280–4.

227. Rohrer A (1927) Die Aetiologie der Zahnwurzelzysten. *Deutsche Monatszeitschrift für Zahnheilkunde* **45**, 282–94.

228. Rolph HJ, Lennon A, Riggio MP, Saunders WP, MacKenzie D, Coldero L, *et al.* (2001) Molecular identification of microorganisms from endodontic infections. *Journal of Clinical Microbiology* **39**, 3282–9.

229. Rosebury T, Reynolds JB (1964) Continuous anaerobiosis for cultivation of spirochetes. *Proceedings of the Society for Experimental Biology and Medicine* **117**, 813–15.

230. Rothschild BM, Martin LD, Lev G, *et al.* (2001) *Mycobacterium tuberculosis* complex DNA from an extinct bison dated 17,000 years before the present. *Clinical Infectious Diseases* **33**, 305–11.

231. Rud J, Andreasen JO (1972) A study of failures after endodontic surgery by radiographic, histologic and stereomicroscopic methods. *International Journal of Oral Surgery* **1**, 311–28.

232. Rud J, Andreasen JO, Möller-Jensen JE (1972) Radiographic criteria for the assessment of healing after endodontic surgery. *International Journal of Oral Surgery* **1**, 195–214.

233. Ruddle NH (1994) Tumour necrosis factor-beta (lymphotoxin-alpha). In: Thomson AW, editor. *The cytokine handbook*, 2nd edn, pp. 305–19. London: Academic Press.

234. Ryan GB, Majno G (1977) Acute inflammation. *American Journal of Pathology* **86**, 185–276.

235. Sabeti M, Simon JH, Nowzari H, Slots J (2003) Cytomegalovirus and Epstein–Barr virus active infection in periapical lesions of teeth with intact crowns. *Journal of Endodontics* **29**, 321–3.

236. Sabeti M, Simon JH, Slots J (2003) Cytomegalovirus and Epstein–Barr virus are associated with symptomatic periapical pathosis. *Oral Microbiology and Immunology* **18**, 327–8.

237. Sabeti M, Slots J (2004) Herpesviral-bacterial coinfection in periapical pathosis. *Journal of Endodontics* **30**, 69–72.

238. Sabeti M, Valles Y, Nowzari H, Simon JH, Kermani-Arab V, Slots J (2003) Cytomegalovirus and Epstein–Barr virus DNA transcription in endodontic symptomatic lesions. *Oral Microbiology and Immunology* **18**, 104–8.

239. Safavi KE, Rossomando ER (1991) Tumor necrosis factor identified in periapical tissue exudates of teeth with apical periodontitis. *Journal of Endodontics* **17**, 12–14.

240. Sahara N, Okafugi N, Toyoki A, Ashizawa Y, Deguchi T, Suzuki K (1994) Odontoclastic resorption of the superficial nonmineralized layer of predentine

in the shedding of human deciduous teeth. *Cell and Tissue Research* **277**, 19–26.

241. Sakellariou PL (1996) Periapical actinomycosis: report of a case and review of the literature. *Endodontics and Dental Traumatology* **12**, 151–4.

242. Salo WL, Aufderheide AC, Buikstra J, Holcomb TA (1994) Identification of *Mycobacterium tuberculosis* DNA in a pre-Columbian Peruvian mummy. *Proceedings of the National Academy of Sciences in USA* **91**, 2091–4.

243. Samanta A, Malik CP, Aikat BW (1975) Periapical actinomycosis. *Oral Surgery, Oral Medicine, Oral Pathology* **39**, 458–62.

244. Samuelsson B (1983) Leukotrienes: mediators of immediate hypersensitivity reactions and inflammation. *Science* **220**, 268–75.

245. Schein B, Schilder H (1975) Endotoxin content in endodontically involved teeth. *Journal of Endodontics* **1**, 19–21.

246. Schroeder HE (1986) *The periodontium*, vol. V/5, *Handbook of microscopic anatomy*. Berlin: Springer.

247. Sedgley CM, Messer H (1993) Long-term retention of a paper-point in the periapical tissues: a case report. *Endodontics and Dental Traumatology* **9**, 120–3.

248. Selle G (1974) Zur Genese von Kieferzysten anhand vergleichender Untersuchungen von Zysteninhalt und Blutserum. *Deutsche Zahnärztliche Zeitschrift* **29**, 600–10.

249. Seltzer S (1988) *Endodontology*, 2nd edn. Philadelphia, PA: Lea & Febiger.

250. Seltzer S, Bender IB, Smith J, Freedman I, Nazimov H (1967) Endodontic failures – an analysis based on clinical, roentgenographic, and histologic findings. Parts I and II. *Oral Surgery, Oral Medicine, Oral Pathology* **23**, 500–30.

251. Seltzer S, Bender IB, Turkenkopf S (1963) Factors affecting successful repair after root canal treatment. *Journal of the American Dental Association* **67**, 651–62.

252. Seltzer S, Soltanoff W, Bender IB (1969) Epithelial proliferation in periapical lesions. *Oral Surgery, Oral Medicine, Oral Pathology* **27**, 111–21.

253. Sen BH, Piskin B, Demirci T (1995) Observation of bacteria and fungi in infected root canals and dentinal tubules by SEM. *Endodontics and Dental Traumatology* **11**, 6–9.

254. Shah HN, Collins MD (1988) Proposal for classification of *Bacteroides asaccharolyticus, Bacteroides gingivalis*, and *Bacteroides endodontalis* in a new genus, *Porphyromonas*. *International Journal of Systematic Bacteriology* **38**, 128–31.

255. Shah HN, Collins MD (1990) *Prevotella*, a new genus to include *Bacteroides melaninogenicus* and related species formerly classified in the genus *Bacteroides*. *International Journal of Systematic Bacteriology* **40**, 205–8.

256. Shear M (1963) The histogenesis of the dental cyst. *Dental Practitioner and Dental Record* **13**, 238–43.

257. Shear M (1992) *Cysts of the oral regions*, 3rd edn. Oxford: Wright.

258. Sherman FE, Moran TJ (1954) Granulomas of stomach. Response to injury of muscle and fibrous tissue of wall of human stomach. *American Journal of Clinical Pathology* **24**, 415–21.

259. Shin SJ, Lee JI, Baek SH, Lim SS (2002) Tissue levels of matrix metalloproteinases in pulps and periapical lesions. *Journal of Endodontics* **28**, 313–15.

260. Shovelton DS (1964) The presence and distribution of micro-organisms within non-vital teeth. *British Dental Journal* **117**, 101–7.

261. Simon JHS (1980) Incidence of periapical cysts in relation to the root canal. *Journal of Endodontics* **6**, 845–8.

262. Simon JHS, Chimenti Z, Mintz G (1982) Clinical significance of the pulse granuloma. *Journal of Endodontics* **8**, 116–19.

263. Siqueira J, Rôças I (2003) PCR-based identification of *Treponema maltophilum*, *T. amylovorum*, *T. medium* and *T. lecithinolyticum* in primary root canal infections. *Archives of Oral Biology* **48**, 495–502.

264. Siqueira JF, Rôças IN (2004) Polymerase chain reaction-based analysis of microorganisms associated with failed endodontic treatment. *Oral Surgery, Oral Medicine, Oral Pathology, Oral Radiology, Endodontics* **97**, 85–94.

265. Sjögren U, Figdor D, Persson S, Sundqvist G (1997) Influence of infection at the time of root filling on the outcome of endodontic treatment of teeth with apical periodontitis. (Published erratum appears in *Int Endod J* 1998, **31**: 148.) *International Endodontic Journal* **30**, 297–306.

266. Sjögren U, Hägglund B, Sundqvist G, Wing K (1990) Factors affecting the long-term results of endodontic treatment. *Journal of Endodontics* **16**, 498–504.

267. Sjögren U, Happonen RP, Kahnberg KE, Sundqvist G (1988) Survival of *Arachnia propionica* in periapical tissue. *International Endodontic Journal* **21**, 277–82.

268. Sjögren U, Mukohyama H, Roth C, Sundqvist G, Lerner UH (2002) Bone-resorbing activity from cholesterol-exposed macrophages due to enhanced expression of interleukin-1α. *Journal of Dental Research* **81**, 11–16.

269. Sjögren U, Sundqvist G, Nair PNR (1995) Tissue reaction to gutta-percha of various sizes when implanted subcutaneously in guinea pigs. *European Journal of Oral Sciences* **103**, 313–21.

270. Skaug N (1974) Proteins in fluids from non-keratinizing jaw cysts: 4. Concentrations of immunoglobulins (IgG, IgA and IgM) and some non-immunoglobulin proteins: relevance to concepts of cyst wall permeability and clearance of cyst proteins. *Journal of Oral Pathology* **3**, 47–61.

271. Skaug N, Nilsen R, Matre R, Bernhoft C-H, Christine A (1982) *In situ* characterization of cell infiltrates in human dental periapical granulomas 1. Demonstration of receptors for Fc region of IgG. *Journal of Oral Pathology* **11**, 47–57.

272. Slots J, Sabeti M, Simon JH (2003) Herpes virus in periapical pathosis: An etiopathologic relationship?

Oral Surgery, Oral Medicine, Oral Pathology, Oral Radiology, Endodontics **96**, 327–31.

273. Smith G, Matthews JB, Smith AJ, Browne RM (1987) Immunoglobulin-producing cells in human odontogenic cysts. *Journal of Oral Pathology* **16**, 45–8.

274. Socransky S, Macdonald JB, Sawyer S (1959) The cultivation of *Treponema microdentium* as surface colonies. *Archives of Oral Biology* **1**, 171–2.

275. Sommer RF, Ostrander F, Crowley M (1966) *Clinical endodontics*, 3rd edn. Philadelphia, PA: W.B. Saunders.

276. Sonnabend E, Oh CS (1966) Zur Frage des Epithels im apikalen Granulationsgewebe (Granulom) menschlicher Zähne. *Deutsche Zahnärztliche Zeitschrift* **21**, 627–43.

277. Spain D, Aristizabal N (1962) Rabbit local tissue response to triglycerides, cholesterol and its ester. *Archives of Pathology* **73**, 94–7.

278. Spain DM, Aristizabal N, Ores R (1959) Effect of estrogen on resolution of local cholesterol implants. *Archives of Pathology* **68**, 30–3.

279. Spatafore CM, Griffin JA, Keyes GG, Wearden S, Skidmore AE (1990) Periapical biopsy report: an analysis over a 10-year period. *Journal of Endodontics* **16**, 239–41.

280. Spinner JR (1947) Vom Chemismus der Pulpagangrän. Ein akutes Problem der konservierenden Zahnheilkunde. *Zahnärztliches Welt* **2**, 305–13.

281. Spratt DA, Weightman AJ, Wade WG (1999) Diversity of oral asaccharolytic *Eubacterium* species in periodontitis: identification of novel polytypes representing uncultivated taxa. *Oral Microbiology and Immunology* **14**, 56–9.

282. Stashenko P, Teles R, D'Souza R (1998) Periapical inflammatory responses and their modulation. *Critical Reviews in Oral Biology and Medicine* **9**, 498–521.

283. Stashenko P, Wang CY, Riley E, Wu Y, Ostroff G, Niederman R (1995) Reduction of infection-stimulated periapical bone resorption by the biological response modifier PGG glucan. *Journal of Dental Research* **74**, 323–30.

284. Stashenko P, Yu SM, Wang CY (1992) Kinetics of immune cell and bone resorptive responses to endodontic infections. *Journal of Endodontics* **18**, 422–6.

285. Staub HP (1963) Röntgenologische Erfolgstatistik von Wurzelbehandlungen. Dr. med. dent. Thesis. Zurich: University of Zurich.

286. Stern MH, Dreizen S, Mackler BF, Levy BM (1981) Antibody producing cells in human periapical granulomas and cysts. *Journal of Endodontics* **7**, 447–52.

287. Stockdale CR, Chandler NP (1988) The nature of the periapical lesion – a review of 1108 cases. *Journal of Dentistry* **16**, 123–9.

288. Storms JL (1969) Factors that influence the success of endodontic treatment. *Journal of Canadian Dental Association* **35**, 83–97.

289. Strindberg LZ (1956) The dependence of the results of pulp therapy on certain factors. An analytic study based on radiographic and clinical follow-up examinations. *Acta Odontologica Scandinavica* **14**, 1–175.

290. Sunde PT, Olsen I, Debelian GJ, Tronstad L (2002) Microbiota of periapical lesions refractory to endodontc therapy. *Journal of Endodontics* **28**, 304–10.

291. Sunde PT, Tronstad L, Eribe ER, Lind PO, Olsen I (2000) Assessment of periradicular microbiota by DNA–DNA hybridization. *Endodontics and Dental Traumatology* **16**, 191–6.

292. Sundqvist G (1976) Bacteriological studies of necrotic dental pulps. Dr. Odont. Thesis. Umeå: University of Umeå.

293. Sundqvist G (1992) Associations between microbial species in dental root canal infections. *Oral Microbiology and Immunology* **7**, 257–62.

294. Sundqvist G (1992) Ecology of the root canal flora. *Journal of Endodontics* **18**, 427–30.

295. Sundqvist G (1994) Taxonomy, ecology and pathogenicity of the root canal flora. *Oral Surgery, Oral Medicine, Oral Pathology* **78**, 522–30.

296. Sundqvist G, Carlsson J, Herrman B, Tärnvik A (1985) Degradation of human immunoglobulins G and M and complement factor C3 and C5 by black pigmented *Bacteroides*. *Journal of Medical Microbiology* **19**, 85–94.

297. Sundqvist G, Figdor D (1998) Endodontic treatment of apical periodontitis. In: Ørstavik D, Pitt Ford TR, editors. *Essential endodontology*, pp. 242–77. Oxford: Blackwell.

298. Sundqvist G, Figdor D (2003) Life as an endodontic pathogen: ecological differences between the untreated and root-filled root canals. *Endodontic Topics* **6**, 3–28.

299. Sundqvist G, Figdor D, Persson S, Sjögren U (1998) Microbiologic analysis of teeth with failed endodontic treatment and the outcome of conservative re-treatment. *Oral Surgery, Oral Medicine, Oral Pathology* **85**, 86–93.

300. Sundqvist G, Johansson E, Sjögren U (1989) Prevalence of black pigmented *Bacteroides* species in root canal infections. *Journal of Endodontics* **15**, 13–19.

301. Sundqvist G, Reuterving CO (1980) Isolation of *Actinomyces israelii* from periapical lesion. *Journal of Endodontics* **6**, 602–6.

302. Sundqvist GK, Eckerbom MI, Larsson AP, Sjögren UT (1979) Capacity of anaerobic bacteria from necrotic dental pulps to induce purulent infections. *Infection and Immunity* **25**, 685–93.

303. Szajkis S, Tagger M (1983) Periapical healing in spite of incomplete root canal debridement and filling. *Journal of Endodontics* **9**, 203–9.

304. Talacko AA, Radden BG (1988) Oral pulse granuloma: clinical and histopathological features. *International Journal of Oral and Maxillofacial Surgery* **17**, 343–6.

305. Talacko AA, Radden BG (1988) The pathogenesis of oral pulse granuloma: an animal model. *Journal of Oral Pathology* **17**, 99–105.

306. Tani-Ishii N, Wang CY, Stashenko P (1995) Immunolocalization of bone-resorptive cytokines in rat pulp

and periapical lesions following surgical pulp exposure. *Oral Microbiology and Immunology* **10**, 213–19.

307. Taylor E (1988) *Dorland's illustrated medical dictionary*, 27th edn. Philadelphia, PA: W.B. Saunders.
308. Ten Cate AR (1972) Epithelial cell rests of Malassez and the genesis of the dental cyst. *Oral Surgery, Oral Medicine, Oral Pathology* **34**, 956–64.
309. Teronen O, Salo T, Laitinen J *et al.* (1995) Characterization of interstitial collagenases in jaw cyst wall. *European Journal of Oral Sciences* **103**, 141–7.
310. Thesleff I (1987) Epithelial cell rests of Malassez bind epidermal growth factor intensely. *Journal of Periodontal Research* **22**, 419–21.
311. Thilo BE, Baehni P, Holz J (1986) Dark-field observation of bacterial distribution in root canals following pulp necrosis. *Journal of Endodontics* **12**, 202–5.
312. Thoma KH (1917) A histo-pathological study of the dental granuloma and diseased root apex. *Journal of the National Dental Association* **4**, 1075–90.
313. Thomas L (1974) *The lives of a cell*. Toronto: Bantam.
314. Thompson L, Lovestedt SA (1951) An Actinomyces-like organism obtained from the human mouth. *Proceedings of the Staff Meetings of Mayo Clinic* **26**, 169–75.
315. Toller PA (1948) Experimental investigations into factors concerning the growth of cysts of the jaw. *Proceedings of the Royal Society of Medicine* **41**, 681–8.
316. Toller PA (1970) The osmolarity of fluids from cysts of the jaws. *British Dental Journal* **129**, 275 8.
317. Toller PA, Holborow EJ (1969) Immunoglobulins and immunoglobulin-containing cells in cysts of the jaws. *Lancet* **2**, 178–81.
318. Torabinejad M (1983) The role of immunological reactions in apical cyst formation and the fate of the epithelial cells after root canal therapy: a theory. *International Journal of Oral Surgery* **12**, 14–22.
319. Torabinejad M, Clagett J, Engel D (1979) A cat model for evaluation of mechanism of bone resorption; induction of bone loss by simulated immune complexes and inhibition by indomethacin. *Calcified Tissue International* **29**, 207–14.
320. Torabinejad M, Cotti E, Jung T (1992) Concentration of leukotriene B4 in symptomatic and asymptomatic periapical lesions. *Journal of Endodontics* **18**, 205–8.
321. Torabinejad M, Kettering J (1985) Identification and relative concentration of B and T lymphocytes in human chronic periapical lesions. *Journal of Endodontics* **11**, 122–5.
322. Torabinejad M, Kriger RD (1980) Experimentally induced alterations in periapical tissues of the cat. *Journal of Dental Research* **59**, 87–96.
323. Torneck CD (1966) Reaction of rat connective tissue to polyethylene tube implants. Part I. *Oral Surgery, Oral Medicine, Oral Pathology* **21**, 379–87.
324. Torres JOC, Torabinejad M, Matiz RAR, Mantilla EG (1994) Presence of secretory IgA in human periapical lesions. *Journal of Endodontics* **20**, 87 9.
325. Tracey KJ (1994) Tumour necrosis factor-alpha. In: Thomson AW, editor *The cytokine handbook*, 2nd edn, pp. 289–304. London: Academic Press.

326. Tronstad L, Barnett F, Cervone F (1990) Periapical bacterial plaque in teeth refractory to endodontic treatment. *Endodontics and Dental Traumatology* **6**, 73–7.
327. Tronstad L, Barnett F, Riso K, Slots J (1987) Extraradicular endodontic infections. *Endodontics and Dental Traumatology* **3**, 86–90.
328. Trott JR, Chebib F, Galindo Y (1973) Factors related to cholesterol formation in cysts and granulomas. *Journal of the Canadian Dental Association* **38**, 76–8.
329. Valderhaug J (1974) A histologic study of experimentally induced periapical inflammation in primary teeth in monkeys. *International Journal of Oral Surgery* **3**, 111–23.
330. Van Dyke TE, Vaikuntam J (1994) Neutrophil function and dysfunction in periodontal disease. In: Williams RC, Yukna RA, Newman MG, editors. *Current opinions in periodontology*, 2nd edn, pp. 19–27. Philadelphia, PA: Current Science.
331. Van Furth R, Cohn ZA, Hirsch JG, Humphry JH, Spector WG, Langevoort HL (1972) The mononuclear phagocyte system: a new classification of macrophages, monocytes and their precursors. *Bulletin of the World Health Organization* **46**, 845–52.
332. Wais FT (1958) Significance of findings following biopsy and histologic study of 100 periapical lesions. *Oral Surgery, Oral Medicine, Oral Pathology* **11**, 650–3.
333. Waltimo TMT, Sirén EK, Torkko HLK, Olsen I, Haapasalo M (1997) Fungi in therapy-resistant apical periodontitis. *International Endodontic Journal* **30**, 96–101.
334. Waltimo TR, Sen BH, Meurman JH, Ørstavik D, Haapasalo M (2003) Yeasts in apical periodontitis. *Critical Reviews in Oral Biology and Medicine* **14**, 128–37.
335. Walton RE, Ardjmand K (1992) Histological evaluation of the presence of bacteria in induced periapical lesions in monkeys. *Journal of Endodontics* **18**, 216–21.
336. Wang CY, Stashenko P (1993) The role of interleukin-1α in the pathogenesis of periapical bone destruction in a rat model system. *Oral Microbiology and Immunology* **8**, 50–6.
337. Wayman BE, Murata M, Almeida RJ, Fowler CB (1992) A bacteriological and histological evaluation of 58 periapical lesions. *Journal of Endodontics* **18**, 152–5.
338. Weir JC, Buck WH (1982) Periapical actinomycosis. *Oral Surgery, Oral Medicine, Oral Pathology* **54**, 336–40.
339. White EW (1968) Paper point in mental foramen. *Oral Surgery, Oral Medicine, Oral Pathology* **25**, 630–2.
340. World Health Organization (1995) *Application of the international classification of diseases to dentistry and stomatology*, 3rd edn. Geneva: WHO.
341. Wilson M (1996) Susceptibility of oral bacterial biofilms to antimicrobial agents. *Journal of Medical Microbiology* **44**, 79–87.

342. Winkler TF (1975) Review of the literature: a histologic study of bacteria in periapical pathosis. *Pharmacology and Therapeutics in Dentistry* **2**, 157–81.

343. Winstock D (1980) Apical disease: an analysis of diagnosis and management with special reference to root lesion resection and pathology. *Annals of the Royal College of Surgeons of England* **62**, 171–9.

344. Wittgow WC, Sabiston CB (1975) Microorganisms from pulpal chambers of intact teeth with necrotic pulps. *Journal of Endodontics* **1**, 168–71.

345. Wolff M, Israel J (1891) Ueber Reinkultur des Actinomyces und seine Ubertragbarkeit auf Thiere. *Archives der Pathologishe Anatomie Physiologie und Klinishe Medizin (Virchow)* **126**, 11–59.

346. Yamasaki M, Nakane A, Kumazawa M, Hashioka K, Horiba N, Nakamura H (1992) Endotoxin and Gram-negative bacteria in the rat periapical lesions. *Journal of Endodontics* **18**, 501–4.

347. Yamazaki K, Nakajima T, Gemmell E, Polak B, Seymour GJ, Hara K (1994) IL-4 and IL-6-producing cells in human periodontal disease tissue. *Journal of Oral Pathology and Medicine* **23**, 347–53.

348. Yanagisawa W (1980) Pathologic study of periapical lesions. I. Periapical granulomas: clinical, histologic and immunohistopathologic studies. *Journal of Oral Pathology* **9**, 288–300.

349. Yeagle PL (1988) *The biology of cholesterol.* Boca Raton, FL: CRC Press.

350. Yeagle PL (1991) *Understanding your cholesterol.* San Diego, CA: Academic Press.

351. Ylipaavalniemi P (1977) Cyst fluid concentrations of immunoglobulins alpha2-macroglobulin and alpha1-antitrypsin. *Proceedings of the Finnish Dental Society* **73**, 185–8.

352. Yusuf H (1982) The significance of the presence of foreign material periapically as a cause of failure of root treatment. *Oral Surgery, Oral Medicine, Oral Pathology* **54**, 566–74.

353. Zuolo ML, Ferreira MOF, Gutmann JL (2000) Prognosis in periradicular surgery: a clinical prospective study. *International Endodontic Journal* **33**, 91–8.

Chapter 5
Microbiology of Apical Periodontitis

José F. Siqueira Jr

5.1 Introduction

In essence, endodontic infection is the infection of the dental root canal system and is the major etiologic agent of apical periodontitis (Fig. 5.1). Although chemical and physical factors can induce periradicular inflammation, a large body of scientific evidence indicates that microorganisms are essential to the progression and perpetuation of apical periodontitis [142,200,366]. The root canal infection usually develops after pulp necrosis, which can occur as a sequel to caries, trauma, periodontal disease, or operative procedures. These events create pathways by which oral microorganisms can gain access to the root canal

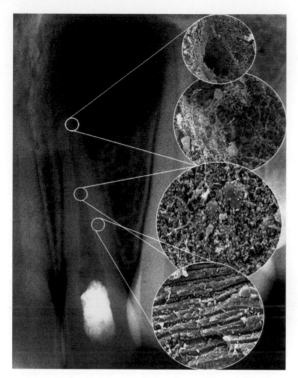

Fig. 5.1 Microorganisms colonizing the root canal system are the major causative agents of apical periodontitis lesions.

system. A necrotic pulp lacks an active circulation and thereby can no longer protect itself against invasion and colonization by oral microorganisms. After endodontic infection is established, microorganisms will enter in contact with the periradicular tissues via the apical foramen and accessory foraminas. As a consequence of the encounter between microorganisms and host defenses, inflammatory changes take place in the periradicular tissues and give rise to diverse forms of apical periodontitis. Even though fungi and most recently archaea and viruses have been found in association with apical periodontitis, bacteria are the major microorganisms implicated in the etiology of this disease. Thus, the main focus of this chapter will be on bacteria, but specific discussions on fungi, archaea and viruses and their participation in apical periodontitis will appear wherever appropriate.

Because apical periodontitis can be regarded as an infectious disorder caused by microorganisms colonizing the root canal system, successful treatment of this disease is contingent on effective elimination of the endodontic microbiota. The cardinal principle

of any healthcare profession is the thorough understanding of the disease's etiology, which provides a framework for effective treatment. In this context, a thorough understanding of the microbiological aspects of apical periodontitis is of utmost importance for endodontic practice of high quality and founded on solid scientific basis.

5.2 Microbial causation of apical periodontitis

The first recorded observation of bacteria in the root canal dates back to the seventeenth century by the Dutch amateur microscope builder Antony van Leeuwenhoek (1632–1723). He wrote in 1697: "The crown of this tooth was nearly all decayed, while its roots consisted of two branches, so that the very roots were uncommonly hollow and the holes in them were stuffed with a soft matter. I took this stuff out of the hollows in the roots and mixed it with clean rain water, and set it before the magnifying glass so as to see if there were as many living creatures in it as I had aforetime discovered; and I must confess that the whole stuff seemed to me to be alive" [54]. However, it took almost 200 years before his observation was confirmed and a cause-and-effect relationship between bacteria and apical periodontitis was suggested.

In 1894, Willoughby Dayton Miller, an American dentist who developed his seminal experiments in oral microbiology inspired by Robert Koch, in Berlin, Germany, published a milestone study reporting on the association between bacteria and apical periodontitis, after the analysis of material collected from root canals [195]. By means of bacterioscopy of the canal samples, he was able to find bacterial cells in the three basic morphologies, i.e., cocci, bacilli, and spirilla (Fig. 5.2). He wrote: "We assume, in a general way, that bacteria must in some manner be connected with these processes [pulp diseases]. ... There are, then, as I have already pointed out, different species of bacteria in the diseased pulp that have not yet been cultivated on artificial media, and of whose pathogenesis we know nothing definite. Their great numbers in some pulps, and especially the repeated occurrence of spirochaetes, justify the supposition that, under certain circumstances, they may play an important role in suppurative processes."

Miller raised the hypothesis that bacteria were the causative factors of diseases of endodontic origin and

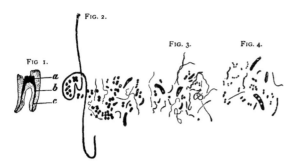

Fig. 5.2 Drawings from Miller's classic paper showing different bacterial forms in a root canal sample observed by microscopy.

that the microbiota was clearly different in the coronal, middle and apical parts of the root canal. He recognized that some bacteria from root canal samples that he had seen under light microscopy could not be cultivated using the technology available at that time. Most of those bacteria were conceivably anaerobic bacteria. Nonetheless, in spite of the considerable technologic advances in the last century regarding bacterial cultivation, it is widely recognized that a large number of microbial species still remain uncultivated [5,121,122,224,252,254–256].

Miller's findings, although pioneering, only suggested a causal relationship between microorganisms and endodontic diseases. Two events occurring simultaneously do not necessarily imply a cause-and-effect relationship. It was not until approximately 70 years after Miller's classic findings that the causal relationship between microorganisms and apical periodontitis was demonstrated by a classic study in germ-free rats from Kakehashi *et al.* [142]. They investigated the response of the dental pulps of conventional and germ-free rats after exposure to their own oral cavities. Histologic evaluation was performed at intervals ranging from 1 to 42 days postoperatively. They reported that in conventional animals, without exception, all older specimens showed complete pulp necrosis with apical inflammatory lesions. On the other hand, in germ-free animals the dental pulps repaired themselves by dentinal bridge formation, which was already evident at 14 days and by 21 and 28 days was completely sealing the exposure area, regardless of the angle or severity of the exposure. In every instance, the pulp tissue remained vital beneath the newly formed hard tissue.

Another classic study confirmed the important role played by bacteria in the etiology of apical peri-

odontitis. Sundqvist, in 1976 [366], used modern anaerobic cultivation techniques to evaluate the bacteriology of pulps of human intact teeth that became devitalized after trauma. His findings revealed that whereas the necrotic pulps of teeth without apical periodontitis lesions were aseptic, those showing periradicular bone destruction were almost always infected. Anaerobic bacteria predominated, comprising more than 90% of the isolates. Sundqvist's findings also served to demonstrate that the necrotic pulp tissue itself and stagnant tissue fluid in the root canal cannot induce and maintain a periradicular inflammatory disease. Previous studies that had not observed bacteria in necrotic pulps associated with apical periodontitis did not use anaerobic culturing procedures. Thus, the failure in isolating bacteria in necrotic pulps associated with apical periodontitis does not necessarily mean that they were absent. It is highly likely that bacteria were present in the root canals but limitations of earlier bacteriologic methods did not allow their detection.

Strong evidence about the causal relationship between microorganisms and apical periodontitis was also provided by Möller *et al.* [200]. In a study using monkey's teeth, they demonstrated that only devitalized pulps that were infected induced apical periodontitis lesions whereas devitalized and uninfected pulps did not show any pathological changes in the periradicular tissues. In addition to corroborating the importance of microorganisms for the development of apical periodontitis, this study also confirmed that the necrotic pulp tissue, in the absence of infection, does not induce and perpetuate a periradicular inflammatory disease.

Epidemiological studies using sophisticated culture and molecular biology techniques have collectively shown that approximately 300 different microbial species can be found in infected root canals, usually in combinations of 10–30 species [341]. Theoretically, any one of these species would have the potential to be an endodontic pathogen. The question now is no longer whether microorganisms are involved with causation of apical periodontitis, but which species are [314].

5.2.1 Guidelines for establishing specific microbial causation

Determining the specific etiologic agent of a given disease is of paramount importance for treatment but it has always been a big challenge for infectious disease specialists. Several criteria have been proposed to ascribe a disease to a microorganism but many are loose, vague and have not stood the test of time. New criteria have arisen or old ones have been revised, but they are far from reaching a consensus among microbiologists. In this text, the most accepted guidelines (which are by no means free from criticism) will be addressed as well as their application to determine specific microbial causation of apical periodontitis.

For more than a century, Koch's postulates have been widely used to establish the causal relationship between a given microbial species and a certain infectious disease. Koch's postulates can be summarized as follows [155]:

- The microorganism must occur in every case of the disease in question and under circumstances that can account for the pathological changes and clinical course of the disease.
- The microorganism must be able to grow in pure culture on artificial medium.
- After isolation from the diseased host and growth in pure culture, the microorganism must be able to induce a similar disease in experimental animals.
- The microorganisms should be isolated again from the experimentally inoculated host.

Using these criteria, Koch established microbial etiology for many diseases, but he was himself aware of their shortcomings and did not believe that every postulate must be fulfilled to prove disease causation [78]. The main limitations of Koch's postulates are the following:

- They place considerable emphasis on the pathogenicity as a trait that resides particularly in the microorganism and do not take into consideration the susceptibility of the host.
- They emphasize the ability to cultivate the causative microorganism in pure culture. There are some diseases for which the causative bacterium has not yet been able to be cultured in laboratory artificial media. In reality, it is currently assumed that over one-half of the bacteria making up the microbiota of different body sites resist cultivation [60,159,231,362].
- They imply that all strains of a given species are equally virulent. Nowadays, it is a common finding that different clonal types within a species can vary remarkably in virulence [71,72,210].
- A presupposition that only a single species causes each disease. There are some diseases, including

apical periodontitis, that have a polymicrobial etiology.
- The requirement that the suspected microorganism, after reinoculation into an animal, produces the signs and symptoms of the disease. Several human pathogens either do not cause the disease in animals or cause a disease with different characteristics from the human form of the disease [196,282].

Based on these limitations, one can realize that a given microorganism that fails to fulfill Koch's postulates may still represent the etiologic agent of a disease.

Several modifications of Koch's postulates or even new criteria have been proposed to establish the specific microbial causation of infectious diseases. Socransky and Socransky and Haffajee [354,355] have proposed some criteria to establish the causal relationship between microorganisms and marginal periodontitis. Some of these criteria might be adapted to apical periodontitis.

- *Association.* The suspected pathogen should be found more frequently and in higher number in cases of the infection than in individuals without overt disease or with different forms of disease. While in periodontal diseases researchers must distinguish pathogens within a normal microbiota, in endodontic infections this problem does not exist since the root canal system does not possess a normal microbiota. As long as the pulp is intact and vital it is a sterile tissue as any connective tissue elsewhere in the body. Infection only occurs after the pulp has been compromised or undergone necrosis. Theoretically, any microbial species colonizing the necrotic pulp can participate in the pathogenesis of apical periodontitis lesions.
- *Elimination.* The elimination of a species should be accompanied by a remission of disease. One should try to eliminate the suspected pathogen, even when it is occurring in mixed infections, from root canals associated with apical periodontitis and determine if the disease resolves. Even though this approach might be of interest, it poses certain difficulties in that root canal therapy never eliminates only one selected species at a time. To mount an approach to experimentally eliminate each individual species separately would be a great challenge, and should obviously use animal models.
- *Host response.* If a microbial species gains access to connective tissues and causes damage, it seems

likely that the host will mount a specific immunologic response, producing antibodies and/or a cellular immune response that is directed specifically at that species. A few studies have reported on the production of specific antibodies against a number of putative endodontic pathogens in apical periodontitis lesions [14,150]. This indicates that the host mounts a humoral immune response against specific endodontic bacteria. While the occurrence of a cellular immune response in apical periodontitis lesions has been demonstrated [360], there are no definite reports regarding its specificity against putative endodontic pathogens.

- *Virulence*. Virulence factors may also provide valuable clues to pathogenicity. Potentially damaging products released and/or properties possessed by certain species may be suggestive that the species could play a role in disease process. Putative endodontic pathogens have a potential array of virulence factors as demonstrated *in vitro*, but if they produce the same factors *in vivo* it is still uncertain. In the laboratory, after primary isolation, bacteria may be subject to repeated subculturing procedures. As a consequence, such bacteria may undergo adaptation to the new environment, culture media, and may no longer exhibit the characteristics they displayed under *in vivo* conditions. Studies have reported the detection of virulence factors within infected root canals, including lipopolysaccharide, enzymes, and metabolites, and tried to establish association with signs and symptoms of disease [110,119,183]. However, it remains to be clarified which species within the root canal specifically produce these factors.

- *Animal pathogenicity*. Experimentally induced disease in animals can be manipulated to favor selection of single or subsets of species that may or may not induce the disease. These models usually suggest a possible etiologic role of a species or a set of species in the pathogenesis of the animal's disease that may have some analogy in the human disease. While there are several studies that evaluated the pathogenicity of putative endodontic pathogens by subcutaneous inoculation in small animals [13,304,375], a few studies have evaluated the pathogenicity of such species and their combinations after inoculation into root canals of animals [47,65]. Results from both study designs have supported that a selected group of cultivated bacteria are potential endodontic pathogens.

- *Risk factor analysis*. Technologic developments can permit the development of prospective studies in which the risk of disease progression conferred by the presence of a microorganism at given levels may be assessed. Because of obvious ethical reasons, this criterion is only applicable to experimental root canal infections in animal models. There is a paucity of information regarding this issue. Animal studies have shown that there is a shift in the root canal microbiota from predominantly Gram-positive and facultative in the first days to increasingly Gram-negative and anaerobic after a short period of time (from weeks to months) [66,379]. These changes were reported to occur during the period of rapid lesion expansion [379]. Again, results from these studies have indicated that a restricted set of species may be implicated in the pathogenesis of apical periodontitis.

Molecular biology methods have been recently used to decipher the diversity of the endodontic microbiota and many fastidious species and even uncultivated phylotypes have been disclosed [341]. Given the significant impact that molecular methods for microbial identification have had on clinical microbiology, Fredricks and Relman [78] proposed some "molecular guidelines" for establishing microbial disease causation. These criteria assume special importance as many microbial species remain uncultivated and it would be difficult or even impossible to ascribe any role for them with regard to disease causation on the basis of Koch's postulates. Their set of "molecular guidelines" for disease causation is based on nucleic acid sequence detection of a suspected pathogen:

- A nucleic acid sequence belonging to a putative pathogen should be present in most cases of an infectious disease.
- Fewer or no copy numbers of pathogen-associated nucleic acid sequences should occur in health tissues.
- With resolution of disease, the copy number of pathogen-associated nucleic acid sequences should decrease or become undetectable. With clinical relapse, the opposite should occur.
- When sequence detection predates disease, or sequence copy number correlates with severity of disease or pathology, the sequence-disease association is more likely to be a causal relationship.
- The nature of the microorganism inferred from the available sequence should be consistent with

the known biological characteristics of that group of microorganisms.

- Tissue-sequence correlates should be sought at the cellular level: efforts should be made to demonstrate specific *in situ* hybridization of microbial sequence to areas of tissue pathology and to visible microorganisms or to areas where microorganisms are presumed to be located.
- These sequence-based forms of evidence for microbial causation should be reproducible.

It is fair to assume that it is not entirely possible and perhaps not even required to fulfill every criterion for evidence of causation in order to consider a microorganism as a pathogen in a given infectious disorder. In fact, a preponderance of scientific evidence supporting the significance of a given microorganism in a disease may suffice for many infectious diseases [351].

Although neither a single microorganism nor a specific microbial mixture has fulfilled all of these different criteria, results from epidemiological studies carried out in different geographical locations suggest that a restricted group of bacterial species usually forming a mixed consortium is associated with the pathogenesis of apical periodontitis. At this point in time, no single species has been assigned as the "major" endodontic pathogen. Even advanced molecular techniques have failed to detect a single species involved with all cases of infection or at least with all cases of a particular form of apical periodontitis. However, it is conceivable that some species are more significant than others. This is particularly indicated by the prevalence in which the species occurs in association with disease, production of a demonstrable array of virulence factors, at least *in vitro* and ideally *in vivo*, pathogenicity in animal models, and association with other human diseases. Regardless of the possibility that some species can occur as mere bystanders in the endodontic microbial consortium, we have no basis to exclude any of the microorganisms as having a role, even if their pathogenicity capacity has not been proven or a specific virulence factor has not been disclosed, which is particularly true for newly described species or as-yet-uncultivated phylotypes. Thus, it is not possible to exclude any species found in infected root canals from having at least an ecological role and thereby participating somehow in the disease process [221]. Many of the most prevalent species found in endodontic infections are potentially pathogenic, particularly in mixed infections,

and may be implicated in the pathogenesis of other human diseases, mainly in the oral cavity. Therefore, these most frequently detected species have been considered as putative endodontic pathogens.

Evidence suggests that a consortium, not a single species, possesses the physiological requirements necessary to cause damage to the periradicular tissues. In addition, it is becoming apparent that different compositions of the root canal microbiota can possess equal ability to elicit tissue injury. Specific mixtures of species that are implicated in the pathogenesis of apical periodontitis are still unknown, but it is conceivable that the most frequently isolated species may make a major contribution to the ecology of the community colonizing the root canal system and consequently to the degree of pathogenicity of the consortium.

Of the more than 700 microbial species inhabiting the oral cavity, perhaps a restricted set of 20–40 species have been more frequently detected in infected root canals and may be responsible for the majority of apical periodontitis lesions in uncompromised patients. Other additional species may be implicated in diseases in a small percentage of the cases. Particularly in failed cases (persistent or secondary infections), the number of microbial species involved may be even smaller. Thus, some groups of bacteria are probably more involved in the etiology of some forms of apical periodontitis, usually composing a mixed consortium.

5.2.2 Requirements for endodontic pathogens

The following requisites should be fulfilled for a given microorganism to establish itself in the root canal system and further participate in the pathogenesis of apical periodontitis lesions:

- The microorganism must be present in sufficient numbers to initiate and maintain the periradicular inflammatory disease.
- The microorganism must possess an array of virulence factors, which should be expressed during root canal infection.
- The microorganism must be spatially located in the root canal system in such a way that it or its virulence factors can gain access to the periradicular tissues.
- The root canal environment must permit the survival and growth of the microorganism and

provide signals or cues that stimulate the expression of virulence genes.

- Inhibiting microorganisms must be absent or present in low numbers in the root canal environment.
- The host must mount a defense strategy at the periradicular tissues, which inhibits the spread of the infection but also results in tissue damage.

5.3 Mechanisms of microbial pathogenicity

The ability of microorganisms to cause disease is regarded as *pathogenicity*. *Virulence* denotes the degree of pathogenicity of a microorganism, and *virulence factors* are the microbial products, structural components or strategies that contribute to pathogenicity. Bacteria can exert their pathogenicity by wreaking havoc on host tissues through direct and/or indirect mechanisms. Direct harmful effects caused by bacteria usually involve secreted products, including enzymes (proteinases, hyaluronidase, chondroitin sulfatase, acid phosphatase, etc.), exotoxins and metabolites (butyrate, propionate, ammonium, polyamines, indole, volatile sulfured compounds, etc.) [314]. Furthermore, bacterial structural components, including peptidoglycan, teichoic and lipoteichoic acids, fimbriae, flagella, outer membrane proteins, exopolysaccharides, and lipopolysaccharide, may act by stimulating the development of host immune reactions capable not only of defending the host against infection but also of causing severe tissue destruction [116,388]. For instance, inflammatory and noninflammatory host cells can be stimulated by bacterial components to release chemical mediators such as cytokines and prostaglandins, which are involved in the induction of bone resorption characteristically observed in chronic apical periodontitis lesions [361]. Bacterial DNA is also efficient in activating macrophages and dendritic cells and in triggering release of proinflammatory cytokines [158]. Another example of indirect damage caused by bacteria refers to purulent exudate formation in the acute apical abscess. Host defense mechanisms against bacteria egressing from the root canal appear to be the most important factor involved in pus formation associated with abscesses. Formation of oxygen-derived free radicals, such as superoxide and hydrogen peroxide, alongside the release of lysosomal enzymes by polymorphonuclear neutrophils, gives rise to destruction of the connective extracellular matrix, leading to pus formation [387]. Therefore, bacteria can exert indirect destructive effects, which seem to be more significant in the tissue damage associated with acute and chronic apical periodontitis lesions. Few, if any, of the putative endodontic pathogens are individually capable of inducing all of the events involved in the pathogenesis of the different forms of apical periodontitis. Probably, the process requires an integrated and orchestrated interaction of the selected members of the mixed endodontic microbiota.

The isolate location of the root canal microbiota indicates that to exert its pathogenicity the bacteria must either invade the periradicular tissues or their products and/or structural components must penetrate the tissue and be able to elicit a defense response in the host. It is assumed that the oral microbiota contains only a few pathogenic species, and most of them have low virulence. This is consistent with the chronic slowly progressive nature of most forms of apical periodontitis. Frank invasion of the periradicular tissues is rather uncommon and, when it occurs, bacteria are usually rapidly eliminated. In some instances, which will depend on several factors, massive invasion of the periradicular tissues by bacteria may result in abscess formation. The presence of more virulent species or strains, or a more virulent mixed consortium, can predispose to abscess formation.

5.3.1 Genetic control of virulence

Bacterial ability to induce disease is genetically determined and influenced by environmental factors. In a number of bacterial species, virulence genes are found in large contiguous blocks in chromosomal DNA, termed *pathogenicity islands* [96]. Pathogenicity islands carry one or more virulence factor and are present in the genome (chromosome or plasmid) of pathogenic bacteria but absent from the genome of related nonpathogens [103]. Islands range in size from 10 to 200 kb and often have different guanine plus cytosine content, suggesting their acquisition by horizontal transfer of DNA [72,196]. Some virulence plasmids of certain bacteria have been referred to as "archipelagos" of pathogenicity islands, and smaller elements (1–10 kb) "islets" [72]. Together with pathogenicity islands, phage insertions, plasmids and transposons provide the genetic basis of pathogenicity of many medical pathogens, and endodontic pathogens are probably no exceptions.

Virulence depends on coordinated expression of several genes whose products mediate attachment to host surfaces or other microorganisms, the capability to survive in a hostile environment by evading host defense mechanisms and scavenging nutrients, the invading ability, the production of exotoxins and enzymes that can damage host tissues, and so forth. Bacteria can also express new gene products in response to changing environments, which enable them to modify their behavior and to survive during different stages of the infectious process. Since many virulence genes are encoded on mobile genetic elements, they have the ability to spread to other microorganisms, including nonpathogenic strains of the same or closely related species.

Nearly all virulence factors are tightly regulated, with their expression linked to diverse environmental signals or cues. Some biochemical and physical parameters that affect virulence factor regulation include starvation, population density, pH, temperature, iron availability, oxygen tension, and redox potential. Therefore, on receiving the appropriate environmental signals, different sets of virulence genes can be turned on or turned off. This affords a given microorganism the ability to adapt to different and varying environmental conditions.

Stress conditions, such as starvation, can be responsible for inducing the virulence apparatus in certain pathogens [166,189]. Periods of starvation are commonly experienced by living bacteria in their natural environments. It is clear now that bacteria activate complex molecular regulatory mechanisms in response to starvation [166,189]. Once starvation genes are expressed, bacteria shift their behavior in order to survive in conditions of nutrient depletion. The major induced mechanisms include control of the energy generation during starvation and enhancement of the scavenging ability of the scarce nutrient. These mechanisms may allow bacteria to survive in root-canal-treated teeth and induce persistent apical periodontitis lesions even in well-treated root canals.

5.3.2 Bacterial intercommunication and "quorum-sensing" systems

Evidence indicates that bacteria living in communities can communicate with one another, capacitating them to behave collectively as a group. This intercellular communication phenomenon is referred to as *quorum sensing* and has been described in both Gram-positive and Gram-negative bacteria [10,57,230,413]. Quorum sensing involves the production, release and subsequent detection of chemical signaling molecules called autoinducers. As a bacterial population producing and releasing autoinducers multiplies, the extracellular concentration of autoinducer increases with increasing cell number. When the autoinducer reaches a crucial threshold level, the group responds with a population-wide alteration in gene expression [230]. Linking alterations in gene expression to the presence of autoinducer gives bacteria a means to perform specific behaviors and functions only when living in groups. Such behavior provides some advantages to a bacterial population, affording adaptability to and protection against dangerous environments. Quorum sensing systems are now known to regulate virulence, production of secondary metabolites, and biofilm formation. For instance, some opportunistic pathogens express virulence factors in response to sensing their own cell density.

Some oral (and endodontic) pathogens have been demonstrated to produce quorum sensing signal molecules [79,243,409,419]. It is entirely possible that quorum sensing systems are involved in bacterial adaptability to the root canal environment and coordinate community activity resulting in enhanced pathogenicity.

5.4 Virulence factors

Virulence factors comprise structural cellular components and released products. Most of the microbial virulence factors have primary functions other than causing host tissue damage. They have a structural or physiological role and that of a virulence factor is merely coincidental and consequential. Different virulence factors usually act in combination at various stages of infection, and a single factor may have several functions in different stages. Virulence factors can be involved in attachment to host surfaces, tissue and host cell invasion, spread in the host, direct and indirect tissue damage, and survival strategies, including evasion of host defense responses. It is unlikely that a single virulence factor will be responsible for tissue damage associated with apical periodontitis lesions. A given factor may be sometimes essential, but is unlikely to be sufficient for disease pathogenesis.

5.4.1 Lipopolysaccharide

Richard Pfeiffer, one of the Koch's students, found that *Vibrio cholerae* synthesized not only a heat-labile exotoxin but also a heat-resistant substance only released after cell disintegration [259]. He named his discovery endotoxin, which was subsequently revealed to be a misnomer: endotoxins reside on the surface of bacteria, not inside. Even though the terms lipopolysaccharides (LPS) and endotoxin have been used interchangeably, it has been recommended that the term LPS be reserved for purified bacterial extracts that are free of contaminants (mainly protein) and the term endotoxin be used to refer to macromolecular complexes of LPS, protein and phospholipids.

LPS is an amphipathic molecule that along with certain proteins is the dominating constituent in the outer leaflet of the outer membrane of most Gram-negative bacteria. One bacterial cell can contain approximately 3.5×10^6 LPS molecules occupying an area of 4.9 μm^2. As the surface of an *Escherichia coli* cell amounts to 6.7 μm^2, it appears that about three-quarters of the bacterial surface consists of LPS, the remaining area being filled by proteins [258].

Chemically, LPS consists of a hydrophilic polysaccharide, subdivided into the O-polysaccharide specific chain (O-antigen) and the core oligosaccharide, and a hydrophobic glycolipid component, termed lipid A [257]. Whilst the lipid A is embedded in the outer membrane, the core and the O-antigen portions extend outward from the bacterial surface. The long polysaccharide chains of LPS can allow the fixation of the complement system at a site distant from the bacterial cell membrane, protecting the bacterium from the lethal lytic effect of that host defense system. The LPS molecule is virtually not toxic when it is incorporated into the bacterial outer membrane, but after release from the cell wall, its toxic moiety, lipid A, is exposed to host defense cells and can evoke an inflammatory response. Lipid A is set free from the outer membrane during bacterial multiplication or after death, when LPS is then released either as a free form, or as a complex of LPS with bacterial surface proteins (endotoxin).

The major inflammatory effects ascribed to LPS depend upon its interaction with host cells and the macrophage appears to be a key cell involved in host response to LPS. After release from the bacteria, LPS is initially bound to a plasma protein called LPS-binding protein (LBP) and is then delivered to CD14,

a cell receptor for LPS on the surface of macrophages [298]. Subsequent activation of the macrophage is a result of a signal triggered by a signal-transducing receptor called Toll-like receptor (TLR)-4 [2]. Thus, in this system, LBP component acts as the carrier of LPS, CD14 is the recognizing receptor, and the TLR-4 functions as the signal-transducing component. Engagement of the receptor activates transcription factors, which induce activation of genes encoding several cytokines and enzymes of the respiratory burst.

LPS can induce:

- Activation of macrophages/monocytes with consequent synthesis and release of proinflammatory cytokines (IL-1β, IL-6, IL-8, TNF-α), prostaglandins, nitric oxide, and oxygen-derived free radicals [116,388,412]. These substances are chemical mediators of inflammation and most of them can stimulate bone resorption.
- Activation of the complement system via both classical and alternative pathway. O-antigen triggers the alternative pathway by binding to C3 [137], while lipid A binds C1q and activates the classical pathway [417]. Some products of complement activation are chemotactic to inflammatory cells (C5a), act as opsonins (C3b) and can increase vascular permeability (C3a and C5a).
- Activation of the Hageman factor [26,204,244], the first step of the intrinsic clotting system, triggering the coagulation cascade or the production of bradykinin, an important chemical mediator of inflammation;
- Induction of the expression of leukocyte adhesion molecules on endothelial cells [90,120,135,216].
- LPS may be mitogenic to B lymphocytes and epithelial cells [220].
- LPS can stimulate naive B cells in the absence of T-cell help. At low concentrations, LPS stimulates specific antibody production. At high concentrations, this molecule can cause unspecific polyclonal activation of B cells [130].
- Stimulation of osteoclast differentiation and bone resorption, particularly via interactions with TLR-4 on osteoblast-lineage cells [424]. LPS induces RANKL expression in osteoblasts and stimulates these cells to secrete interleukin (IL)-1, IL-6, prostaglandin E$_2$ (PGE$_2$), and TNF-α, each known to induce osteoclast activity and differentiation [127,213,271].

Concentration of LPS in infected canals is obviously expected to be directly proportional to the load (number of cells) of Gram-negative bacteria [46]. Studies have revealed that the content of endotoxin or LPS in infected root canals is higher in teeth with symptomatic apical periodontitis, teeth with periradicular bone destruction, or teeth with persistent exudation than in those without them [46,119,129,285,286]. Murakami *et al.* [208] detected *Porphyromonas endodontalis* LPS in samples from infected root canals or in the pus samples of acute abscesses of about 90% of the patients tested. They suggested that *P. endodontalis* LPS can play an integral role as a potent stimulator of inflammatory cytokines that are involved in the formation of acute abscesses [208]. Dahlén *et al.* [48] inoculated *Fusobacterium nucleatum* LPS into the root canals of monkeys and reported the occurrence of inflammatory reaction in the periradicular tissues of all the experimental teeth with resorption of both bone and teeth. Dwyer and Torabinejad [58] evaluated both histologically and radiographically the periradicular tissues of cats after deposition of *Escherichia coli* endotoxin solutions in the root canals and concluded that endotoxin may have a role in the induction and perpetuation of periradicular inflammatory lesions. Such results were similar to those obtained by Pitts *et al.* [246] after inoculation of *Salmonella minnesota* endotoxin solution in the root canals of dogs.

Not all Gram-negative bacteria produce LPS. For instance, some treponemes possess lipooligosaccharides (with a carbohydrate portion much shorter), and lipoproteins in the outer membrane. Treponemal lipooligosaccharides and lipoproteins may have similar bioactivity to LPS [39,118,273,282].

5.4.2 Peptidoglycan

The cell wall of almost every bacterium contains peptidoglycan (except for cell wall-less mycoplasmas), which is largely responsible for protecting the cell against osmotic lysis. Peptidoglycan is a complex polymer that, as the name implies, consists of two parts: a glycan portion and a tetrapeptide portion. Due to cross-linkages, peptidoglycan forms a strong, multilayered sheet that entirely surrounds the bacterial cell. In Gram-positive bacteria, there are as many as 40–100 sheets of peptidoglycan, comprising up to 50% of the cell wall material. In Gram-negative bacteria, there appears to be only one or two sheets, comprising 5–10% of the cell wall material.

Peptidoglycan has long been recognized to have potent immunomodulatory actions. Peptidoglycan fragments released during infection, possibly in combination with lipoteichoic acid can exert the same biological activities as LPS [388,403]. Peptidoglycan may induce diverse biological effects [28], which may play a role in the pathogenesis of apical periodontitis lesions. These effects include activation of macrophages/monocytes with consequent release of the proinflammatory cytokines, such as IL-1β, IL-6, TNF-α, granulocyte-macrophage colony-stimulating factor (GM-CSF), and G-CSF, and activation of the complement system via the alternative pathway [28,388,403]. Signaling of peptidoglycan is mediated mainly through TLR-2 [287].

5.4.3 Teichoic and lipoteichoic acids

Anionic polymers such as teichoic and lipoteichoic acids (LTAs) are major components of the cell wall of Gram-positive bacteria, accounting for up to 50% of dry weight. Teichoic acids consist of chains of glycerol or ribitol covalently linked by phosphodiester bonds and are attached to peptidoglycan. LTAs are polymers of glycerol phosphate covalently attached to a glycolipid in the cytoplasmic membrane and protruding through the peptidoglycan layer. LTA may serve to anchor the cell wall to the underlying membrane and to regulate the activity of autolytic wall enzymes. Both teichoic and lipoteichoic acids are antigenic and often constitute the major antigens of Gram-positive bacteria. LTA can be released after cell wall lysis, which can be induced by lysozyme, cationic peptides from leukocytes, or beta-lactam antibiotics [85]. They can activate macrophages/monocytes and induce the release of proinflammatory cytokines, such as IL-1β, IL-6, IL-8, and TNF-α [388,403]. LTA exerts its effects by signaling via TLR-2 [287]. LTA may also activate the complement system [85]. All these effects may indirectly account for the induction of tissue damage. Because LTA resembles LPS in certain respects, it can be considered as the Gram-positive counterpart of LPS.

5.4.4 Outer membrane proteins

Approximately 50% of the dry mass of the outer membrane of Gram-negative bacteria consists of proteins. Apart from their structural role, outer membrane proteins (OMPs) have also been demonstrated to have other functions, such as porin activity. Porins are OMPs that form trimers that span the outer membrane and contain a central pore with a diameter of approximately 1 nm. Porins are usually permeable to molecules with molecular masses less than 600 Da. They have been shown to stimulate macrophages and lymphocytes to release a range of proinflammatory and immunomodulatory cytokines including IL-1, IL-4, IL-6, IL-8, TNF-α, GM-CSF, and IFN-γ [116]. A recent study demonstrated that more than one-half of the sera from patients with apical periodontitis lesions showed strong reactions to *Porphyromonas gingivalis* cell components, especially RagB, which is a major outer membrane protein of this species [126]. It was suggested that outer membrane proteins can be a possible virulence factor in apical periodontitis lesions.

5.4.5 Outer membrane vesicles

The release of membranous material from the outer surface of Gram-negative bacteria has been reported for a number of pathogenic bacteria. This material has been referred to as vesicles or blebs. Vesicles are thought to be formed by extrusion of the outer membrane, arising from an imbalance between the growth of the outer membrane and other underlying cellular structures. In addition to containing LPS, outer membrane vesicles have a capacity to entrap contents of the periplasmic space, particularly lytic enzymes that break down large and impermeable molecules favoring their uptake as well as enzymes that confer resistance to antibiotics. Therefore, vesicles may afford bacteria a formidable virulence potential.

5.4.6 Lipoproteins

Lipoproteins are usually present in the cell wall of Gram-negative bacteria and are responsible for anchoring the outer membrane to the peptidoglycan layer. This protein is present in about 700,000 copies per cell. Lipoproteins have been demonstrated to have cytokine-stimulating ability. They may stimulate the release of IL-1β, IL-6, IL-12, and TNF-α by macrophages [116].

5.4.7 Fimbriae

Fimbriae are rod-shaped proteic structures originating in the cytoplasmic membrane and are composed of a single protein subunit termed fimbrillin. Fimbriae in most bacteria have approximately the same size (3–25 μm long) and are shorter than pili [181]. In fact, fimbriae is the correct term for rod-like surface adhesins, while pili are longer, more flexible rod-like structures involved in conjugation. Distribution and numbers of fimbriae vary significantly, with some species showing 10 fimbriae per cell and others showing up to 1000 [117]. Fimbriae are found mainly on Gram-negative bacteria, albeit they can also be present on certain streptococci and actinomycetes. Their main function in bacterial pathogenicity is to enable the bacterium to adhere to host surfaces or to other microorganisms by means of specific receptors. A given bacterium may be able to elaborate a number of fimbriae with different specificities. This enables the bacterium to adhere to particular host cell receptors. In addition to promoting adhesion, fimbriae have been demonstrated to elicit the release of cytokines by macrophages, including IL-1α, IL-1β, IL-6, IL-8, and TNF-α [104].

5.4.8 Exopolysaccharides (capsule and slime layer)

Production of exopolysaccharides is a common characteristic of bacterial cells growing in their natural environment. Exopolysaccharides form highly hydrated, water insoluble gels. They may be formed by either homo- or heteropolysaccharides. Exopolysaccharides may have some important roles when it comes to bacterial pathogenicity. They may allow bacterial adhesion to host surfaces and may also serve as metabolic substrate in periods of starvation. In addition, exopolysaccharides can play a crucial role in bacterial virulence by hindering phagocytosis or inhibiting complement activation and complement-mediated killing. Several bacterial species produce a capsule with a chemical structure that mimics host tissue, camouflaging the microorganism from the immune system. Whilst exopolysaccharides are usually poor immunogens, they can stimulate cytokine synthesis by macrophages, including IL-1β, IL-6, IL-8, and TNF-α [116], thus contributing to the damage to host tissues. Encapsulated bacteria have an increased ability to cause abscesses [31].

5.4.9 Bacterial DNA

Bacterial DNA differs from mammalian DNA because of the presence of DNA motifs containing a central unmethylated CG dinucleotide (CpG).

While CpG motifs are unmethylated and usually fairly abundant in bacterial DNA, they are methylated and highly suppressed in mammalian DNA. Moreover, the base context of CpG nucleotides in the human genome is not random, with CpGs being most frequently preceded by a C or followed by a G, which is unfavorable for immune stimulation [158]. Because of this, cells of the innate immune system can sense bacterial DNA and interpret its presence as infectious danger [114]. Indeed, macrophages and dendritic cells can be directly stimulated by bacterial DNA to produce a variety of cytokines, such as IL-1β, TNF-α, IL-6, IL-1ra, IL-18, monocyte chemoattractant protein-1, and IFN-γ. Also, bacterial DNA has been demonstrated to be a potent B-cell mitogen [158]. TLR-9 is involved in initiation of cellular activation by CpG DNA [2]. Similar to LPS, CpG DNA modulates osteoclastogenesis in bone marrow cell/osteoblast co-cultures. On TLR-9 ligation, CpG DNA increases in osteoblasts the expression of TNF-α and macrophage-colony stimulating factor (M-CSF) [425]. Thus, CpG DNA interacts with osteoblastic TLR-9 and elicits intracellular events leading to the increased expression of molecules regulating osteoclastogenesis.

Isolated DNA from some oral bacteria stimulates murine macrophages and human gingival fibroblasts to produce TNF-α and IL-6 in a dose-dependent manner [218]. Thus, DNA from putative oral pathogens possesses immunostimulatory properties in regard to cytokine secretion by macrophages and fibroblasts. These stimulatory effects are due to the unmethylated CpG motifs within bacterial DNA and differ between distinct bacterial strains. It is possible that bacterial DNA can contribute to the pathogenesis of apical periodontitis.

5.4.10 Enzymes

Most bacterial pathogens produce a battery of enzymes. Some of them are hydrolytic enzymes that degrade extracellular matrix components and thus disrupt host tissue structure. It might be argued that the enzymes produced by bacterial pathogens might not be necessary to the pathogenesis of disease since similar enzymes can be derived from the host cells, usually in higher amounts. However, in addition to allegedly inducing direct tissue damage, hydrolytic enzymes allow bacteria to invade the host tissues. This can play a role during spread of the infection through anatomical spaces during an acute apical abscess. Also, hydrolytic enzymes can be involved with acquisition of nutrients and evasion of host defenses.

Proteinases (or proteases) are enzymes either secreted extracellularly or expressed on the bacterial cell surface that are capable of hydrolyzing peptide bonds of proteins. They are candidates for contribution to the pathogenesis of apical periodontitis lesions through several mechanisms, including direct damage by degrading components of the extracellular matrix of the connective tissue; indirect damage by activating host matrix metalloproteinases; and subversion of the host defense mechanisms by inactivation of proteins such as immunoglobulins and complement components [181,247,371]. In addition to having direct and indirect harmful effects as well as protective activities against host defenses, bacterial proteinases can play a pivotal role in the acquisition of nutrients in the form of peptides and amino acids [133].

Some proteinases can degrade or inactivate human plasma proteins involved in host defense against infection. Immunoglobulins and the complement system play important roles in the combat of invading microorganisms. In addition to providing nutrients for the bacteria, the ability of several oral species, including *P. endodontalis*, *P. gingivalis*, *Prevotella intermedia*, *Prevotella nigrescens*, and *Prevotella loescheii*, to degrade immunoglobulins [131,132,153,367], and of *P. endodontalis*, *P. gingivalis* and *P. intermedia* to degrade complement factor C3 [367,376] may be of particular importance in bacterial evasion from phagocytosis, since IgG and C3b are important opsonins. *P. gingivalis* can also degrade the proteinase inhibitors α-2-macroglobulins and α-1-antitrypsin [34], which may be important for the spread of the infection since the proteinase inhibitors play an important role for the preservation of the integrity of the tissues surrounding the site of infection.

Several other enzymes can play a role in bacterial pathogenicity. *Hyaluronidase* is involved in the hydrolysis of hyaluronic acid, a constituent of the ground substance of the connective tissue. This enzyme can also be important for bacterial spread through tissues. Hashioka *et al.* [110] observed that bacteria with hyaluronidase activity were isolated from root canals with acute or subacute clinical symptoms. *Chondroitin sulfatase* and *acid phosphatase* are other enzymes that can be involved with degradation of components of the extracellular matrix of the connective tissue. *DNases* reduce the viscosity of debris from dead host cells (like in abscesses) and may thus allow the spread of bacteria within an area where extensive damage to host tissue has occurred. *Fibrinolysin* is produced by many hemolytic streptococci and activates a proteolytic enzyme of plasma, which then dissolves coagulated plasma and probably promotes the spread of the infection through tissues.

5.4.11 Exotoxins

Many Gram-positive and Gram-negative bacteria produce exotoxins of considerable medical importance. They are heat-labile polypeptides excreted by living cells and are highly antigenic and usually highly toxic. Leukotoxin is the most documented exotoxin known to play a role in the pathogenesis of periodontal diseases. Leukotoxin is cell-specific and binds to neutrophils, monocytes and a subset of lymphocytes, forming pores in the plasmatic membranes of these target cells. As a result of pore formation induced by the toxin, the cell loses the ability to sustain osmotic homeostasis and dies. Relatively few oral bacteria, including *Aggregatibacter actinomycetemcomitans*, *Fusobacterium necrophorum*, and *Campylobacter rectus*, are recognized to produce exotoxins [84,214]. Of these, only the latter has been frequently observed in endodontic infections [324].

5.4.12 Metabolic end-products

Several end-products of the bacterial metabolism are released to the extracellular environment and may be toxic to host cells and cause degradation of constituents of the extracellular matrix of the connective tissue [91,389]. Furthermore, some end-products of bacterial metabolism, such as butyrate, may cause inhibition of T-cell proliferation and induce the production of proinflammatory cytokines by monocytes [61]. The composition of the bacterial consortium within infected root canals will certainly dictate the type of metabolites present as well as their concentration. On the one hand, some compounds may be consumed by other species and be degraded further. On the other hand, metabolites can be left to accumulate and reach toxic levels to the periradicular tissues. Accumulation of metabolic end-products of bacteria in the infected root canal may thus represent an additional pathogenic mechanism of the root canal microbiota. Many of these end-products, such as short-chain fatty acids, polyamines and particular-

ly volatile sulfur compounds, are responsible for the foul smell typical of anaerobic infections.

5.4.13 Flagella

Bacterial flagella are relatively long projections extending outward from the cytoplasmic membrane that confer motility to bacteria. The flagellum consists of a single filament composed of many subunits of the protein flagellin. The filament of the bacterial flagellum is attached to the cell by a hook and a basal body, which has a set of rings that attach to the cytoplasmic membrane and a rod that passes through the rings to anchor the flagellum to the cell. The flagellum can rotate at speeds of up to 1200 rpm, thus enabling bacterial cells to move at speeds of 100 μm/s [6]. In some bacteria, the flagella originate from the end of the cell: polar flagella. Unlike polar flagella that emanate from an end of the cell, peritrichous flagella surround the cell. Although the basic structure of the bacterial flagellum appears to be similar for all bacteria, there are some structural variations that reflect bacterial diversity. For instance, the flagella of spirochetes do not extend from the cell but rather are inserted subterminally at each pole of the cell, wrap around the protoplasmic cylinder, and usually are long enough to overlap near the middle of the cell body. They are termed periplasmic flagella and are located between the protoplasmic cylinder and the outer sheath. The rotation of the periplasmic axial filament propels the cell by propagating a helical wave along the length of the cell so that it moves with a corkscrew motion. The periplasmic flagella of oral treponemes, in addition to being required for motility, have strong influences on the helical morphology of the cell.

Main examples of oral bacteria that possess flagella and have motility include treponemes (periplasmic flagella), *C. rectus* and some other *Campylobacter* species (single polar flagellum), *Selenomonas* species (up to 16 lateral flagella forming a tuft), *Centipeda periodontii* (peritrichous flagella), some *Eubacterium* species (like *E. yurii*, which has a single polar flagellum), and species of the genera *Bacillus* and *Clostridium* (most having peritrichous flagella).

5.5 The oral microbiota

The oral cavity has a resident microbiota, which exists, for the most part, in harmony with the host

[188]. Under certain circumstances, disease can arise as a consequence of the breakdown of this harmonious relationship, which is usually a consequence of significant disturbances to the habitat leading to instability of the microbial communities. Microorganisms causing disease in this way are opportunistic pathogens and many species inhabiting the oral cavity behave in this manner [186].

The mouth is continuously bathed with saliva and the volume of saliva within the oral cavity typically ranges from 0.77 to 1.07 ml. The total viable counts of bacteria in saliva average about 10^8 [357]. The different habitats in the oral cavity provide microorganisms with a warm (34–36°C) and moist environment, with a pH of between 6.7 and 7.3 [185]. These conditions are highly conducive to the survival and growth of many microbial species. However, one should be mindful that these conditions exert a rather selective pressure for those species that can adapt themselves to the physicochemical characteristics of the oral environment. It becomes clear when one takes into account that the more than 700 oral species are still a minuscule fraction of the estimated one billion or more bacterial species living on Earth [59,146], which potentially could have colonized the oral cavity [357].

There are a number of distinct surfaces for microbial colonization in the 215 cm^2 surface area of the oral cavity [44]. In this context, the teeth make up about 20% of the available surface. The consortia that establish on each surface vary in composition, both quantitatively and qualitatively, reflecting intrinsic differences in the ecological determinants of these sites [188]. Habitats that provide distinct ecological conditions include mucosal surfaces of the cheek, gingiva, palate, and dorsum of the tongue, as well as supragingival and subgingival plaques.

The oral cavity harbors one of the highest accumulations of microorganisms in the body. Even though viruses, archaea, fungi and protozoa can be found as constituents of the oral microbiota, bacteria are by far the most dominant inhabitants of the oral cavity. There are an estimated 10 billion bacterial cells in the mouth [196]. A high diversity of bacterial species is evident from culture studies, but application of molecular biology methods to the analysis of the bacterial diversity has revealed a still broader and more diverse spectrum of extant oral bacteria. Taken as a whole, bacteria detected from the oral cavity fall into 12 separate phyla, namely Obsidian Pool OP11, TM7, *Chloroflexi*, *Deinococcus*, *Acidobacteria*, *Synergistes*

(including phylotypes previously assigned to the phylum *Deferribacteres*), *Spirochaetes*, *Fusobacteria*, *Actinobacteria*, *Firmicutes*, *Proteobacteria*, and *Bacteroidetes* [145,171,231,232]. Data based on culture-dependent and culture-independent approaches have revealed that there are presently 771 bacterial taxa in the oral cavity: 273 are named bacterial species, 412 phylotypes are known by 16S rRNA gene sequence only, and 86 are unnamed, partially characterized, strains [154]. Thus, over 50% of the oral bacteria remain to be cultivated and fully characterized. This raises the interesting possibility that uncultivated and as-yet-uncharacterized species that have remained invisible to studies using traditional identification methods, but actually make up a large fraction of the living oral microbiota, can play an important ecological role as well as participate in the etiology of oral diseases.

In fact, the introduction of molecular biology approaches in oral microbiological research has brought about a significant body of new knowledge with regard to the oral microbiota in health and disease. The development of molecular bacterial identification methods has made it possible to study the role that fastidious and even uncultivated bacteria play in oral diseases. Consequently, this has resulted in a better understanding of the etiology of many oral diseases. Endodontists should keep abreast of the advances in knowledge of microbial diversity in the oral cavity, not only because endodontic pathogens are not exclusive of endodontic infections, but also to better understand the need for a redefinition of the endodontic microbiota with the use of more sensitive and specific new technology. The following sections summarize some of the most recent contributions of molecular biology methods to oral microbiology.

5.5.1 Caries

Dental caries is a result of the interaction between oral microorganisms, the diet, the dentition and the oral environment. Acid production by bacteria in dental plaque is crucial to pathogenesis of the disease. It is well known that species of *Streptococcus*, *Lactobacillus*, and *Actinomyces* are closely associated with the etiopathogenesis of different forms and stages of caries [29,186]. However, nearly all investigations into the microbial pathogenesis of caries have been conducted by cultivation of bacteria. Recently, molecular biology approaches have been used in an

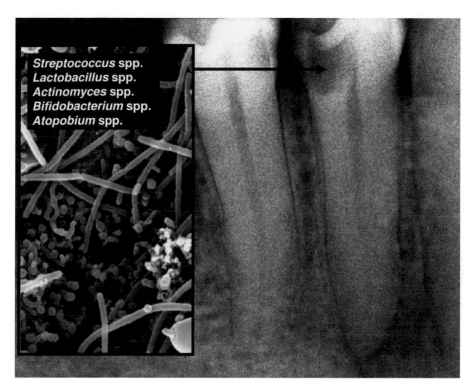

Streptococcus spp.
Lactobacillus spp.
Actinomyces spp.
Bifidobacterium spp.
Atopobium spp.

Fig. 5.3 Bacteria in caries lesions. Data from molecular studies have confirmed the role of some bacterial groups in causation of caries, but have also found novel bacterial phylotypes in association with disease.

attempt to unraveling the bacterial diversity associated with carious lesions.

Molecular studies demonstrate that the diversity and complexity of the microbiota associated with caries are far greater than anticipated (Fig. 5.3). Many taxa identified in caries lesions have still to be cultivated and the role of these taxa in the disease process is not known. Overall, about 40–60% of the microbiota occurring in carious lesions consists of as-yet-uncultivated species [1,207]. Molecular studies revealed that *Actinomyces gerencseriae*, *Bifidobacterium* species, *Streptococcus mutans*, *Veillonella* species, *Streptococcus salivarius*, *Streptococcus constellatus*, *Streptococcus parasanguinis*, and *Lactobacillus fermentum* are associated with caries [21]. *A. gerencseriae* and other *Actinomyces* species appear to be associated with caries initiation, while novel phylotypes of *Bifidobacterium* and *Atopobium* may represent important pathogens in deep caries [1,21].

Lactobacilli have been demonstrated to predominate in carious dentin, with *Prevotella* species also abundant. Other taxa present in a number of dentinal caries lesions or occurring in abundance include *Selenomonas* species, *Dialister* species, *F. nucleatum*, *Eubacterium* species, members of the *Lachnospiraceae* family, *Olsenella* species, *Bifidobacterium* species, *Propionibacterium* species, and *Pseudoramibacter alactolyticus* [38]. Most of the bacterial species found in carious dentine have also been detected in infected root canals, clearly indicating that, in addition to being involved with pulpal damage, these dentinal lesions might well be the primary source of bacteria for endodontic infections.

5.5.2 Halitosis

Bacteria colonizing the dorsum of the tongue have been implicated as a major source of oral malodor in subjects with halitosis [176]. Many oral bacteria can produce volatile sulfur compounds, especially methyl-mercaptan (CH_3SH) and hydrogen sulfide (H_2S) [238,239], which may be the major contributing substances to malodor. Other bacterial products, including short-chain fatty acids such as butyric, propionic and valeric acids as well as polyamines such as cadaverine and putrescine, can also contribute to the complex mixture of odorous molecules found in the exhaled air.

Limitations inherent to cultivation techniques have hampered the knowledge on the bacterial composition of the tongue associated with halitosis. It has been shown that about 60% of the total number of bacteria detected on the tongue dorsum remains uncultivated [145]. The tongue dorsum appears to possess a unique microbiota: about one-third of the bacterial population is found only on the tongue and not in or on the surfaces of other oral sites. While *S. salivarius* is by far the predominant species in healthy subjects, this species is typically absent from subjects with halitosis. Other species/phylotypes most associated with health are *Rothia mucilaginosa* and *Eubacterium* clone FTB41. Species most associated with halitosis include *Atopobium parvulum*, *Dialister* clone BS095, *Eubacterium sulci*, TM7 clone DR034, *Solobacterium moorei*, and *Streptococcus* clone BW009. It appears that an overgrowth of oral bacterial species, especially proteolytic anaerobic bacteria, can cause or contribute to the oral malodor. Subjects without malodor tend to harbor more saccharolytic streptococcal species, especially *S. salivarius* [176].

5.5.3 Periodontal diseases

Periodontal diseases result from the subgingival presence of complex bacterial biofilms (Fig. 5.4), although specific etiologic agents have not been unequivocally identified [202]. Important advances in understanding the infectious agents of periodontal diseases have occurred in the past three decades. The application of molecular identification approaches to the study of the microbiota associated with different forms of periodontal diseases has confirmed results from cultivation studies with regard to the participation of some species but has also enabled identification of new bacterial species or phylotypes possibly implicated in the etiology of these diseases [30,95,108,160,161,231,279].

Socransky *et al.* [356] attempted to define subgingival bacterial communities by using whole genomic probes and the checkerboard DNA–DNA hybridization technique for bacterial identification in large numbers of plaque samples. After data analysis by different clustering and ordination techniques, five major bacterial complexes were consistently observed. One group (termed "the red complex") consisted of the cultivated species *Tannerella forsythia*, *P. gingiva-*

lis, and *Treponema denticola* and was strikingly related to the severity of periodontal disease.

Comprehensive studies using broad-range polymerase chain reaction (PCR) and 16S rRNA gene clone library have determined the bacterial diversity in the subgingival plaque and reported that about 50–60% of the microbiota is made up of as-yet-uncultivated phylotypes [161,231]. Several phylotypes belonging to the phyla OP11 and TM7, both previously associated with extreme natural environments and for which there are no cultivated representatives, have been detected in association with periodontal diseases [231]. Indeed, TM7 bacteria (particularly the oral clone I025) have been detected in an extremely high number of samples from periodontitis patients [30]. It has also been revealed that there are at least 57 oral spirochetal species, all of them falling into the genus *Treponema*, of which about 80% remain uncultivated [52]. The genera *Synergistes*, *Megasphaera*, *Desulfobulbus*, and *Lachnospira* have been found to be represented in subgingival samples exclusively by as-yet-uncultivated phylotypes, which are also predominant within the genera *Selenomonas*, *Veillonella*, and *Peptostreptococcus* [161].

At the species level, there are several candidates as additional putative periodontal pathogens, i.e., bacteria commonly detected in disease, but not or rarely in health. These new putative pathogens include several uncultivated phylotypes, such as *Synergistes* clones D084, BH017 and W090, *Peptostreptococcus* clones BS044 and CK035, *Bacteroidetes* clone AU126, *Dialister* clone GBA27, *Megasphaera* clones BB166 and MCE3_141, *Desulfobulbus* oral clones CH031 and R004, and *Selenomonas* clones D0042 and EY047 [160,161]. Named and cultivated species other than the members of the "red complex", that have also been recently suggested to be candidate periodontal pathogens on the basis of molecular studies, include *Dialister pneumosintes*, *Filifactor alocis*, *Prevotella denticola*, *Cryptobacterium curtum*, *Treponema medium*, *Treponema socranskii*, *Eubacterium saphenum*, *Catonella morbi*, and *Selenomonas sputigena* [160,161,231]. Interestingly, *P. endodontalis*, a putative endodontic pathogen, has also been often detected in diseased subjects and rarely in healthy subjects [160,231].

Knowledge of the infectious etiologic agents of periodontal diseases keeps expanding as microorganisms other than bacteria, namely archaea [168] and herpesviruses [353], have also been found in asso-

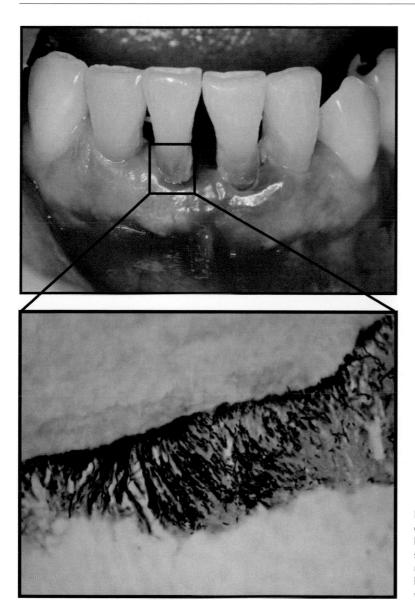

Fig. 5.4 Periodontal diseases are caused by subgingival complex bacterial biofilms. Several bacterial species/phylotypes and even other microorganisms, such as archaea and herpesviruses have been implicated with disease causation.

ciation with periodontal diseases. A causative role for archaea and herpesviruses has been suspected.

A significant revolution in the knowledge of the oral microbiota in health and disease has taken place over recent years after the advent of new technology for microbial identification. In this context, endodontic infections are far from being an exception. Bacterial diversity in the different types of endodontic infections will be discussed further below in this chapter.

5.6 Microbial ecology and the root canal ecosystem

Ecology is the study of the interrelationships between organisms and their environments. Some other concepts assume special importance to the understanding of the endodontic microbial ecology. Initially, individual microorganisms proliferate to form *populations*. Such populations often occur as microcolonies in the environment. Populations interact with one another to form *communities*. A community consists of a unified assemblage of populations that coexist and interact at a given *habitat*. The community and habitat are part of a larger system called *ecosystem*, which can be defined as a functional self-supporting system that includes the microorganisms in a community and their environment. This leads to a hierarchy from ecosystem to community to population to the single individual (cell). Populations perform functions that contribute to the overall community and maintain the ecological balance of the ecosystem. Each population occupies a functional role (*niche*) within the community. There are a limited number of niches within the community for which populations must compete. More competent populations occupy the niches and displace those less competent. Highly structured and spatially organized microbial communities have properties that are more than the sum of the component populations.

A root canal system with a necrotic pulp provides a space for microbial colonization and affords microorganisms a moist, warm, nutritious and anaerobic environment, which is by and large protected from the host defenses because of the lack of microcirculation in the necrotic pulp tissue. Intuitively, the root canal system might be considered a rather lush environment for microbial growth and it might be realized that colonization should not be a difficult task for virtually all oral bacterial species. More than 700 different microbial species have been reported to occur in the oral cavity and about 75–100 species can make up one individual's oral microbiota. Theoretically, these species share similar opportunities to invade and colonize root canals. Nonetheless, the restricted set of species found in infected root canals argues otherwise. Even without the significant presence of host defense factors, the root canal system provides a rather stringent environment in which to live. Selective pressures must occur in the root canal system that favor the establishment of some species and inhibit others [56,372,374].

Of the ecological factors that influence the establishment of a colonizing microbiota in a given environment, the following are considered important:

- oxygen tension and redox potential (*Eh*);
- available nutrients;
- microbial interactions;
- host defense factors;
- temperature;
- pH.

5.6.1 Oxygen tension, redox potential, and available nutrients

The root canal infection is a dynamic process and different bacterial species apparently dominate at different phases of the infectious process. Shifts in the composition of the microbiota are largely due to changes in environmental conditions, particularly in regard to oxygen tension, redox potential and nutrient availability. In the earliest stages of root canal infection, the number of bacterial species and the bacterial density (number of cells) colonizing the root canal system are low. If caries is the path of bacterial invasion of the pulp, the species in the front of the carious lesions are arguably the first to reach the pulp tissue. Early colonizers or pioneer species set the stage for further colonization by other species. For instance, in the very initial phases of pulpal infectious process, facultative bacteria have been shown to predominate [66]. After a few days or weeks, oxygen is depleted within the root canal as a result of pulp necrosis and consumption by facultative bacteria. Further oxygen supply is interrupted because of loss of blood circulation in the necrotic pulp tissue. An anaerobic milieu with consequent low redox potential develops, which is highly conducive to the survival and growth of obligate anaerobic bacteria. With the passage of time, anaerobic conditions become even more pronounced, particularly in the apical third of the root canal.

The selective physical environment of the root canal system is characterized by an apparent excellent access to nutrients, which however may be in limited availability depending on the spatial location of a given bacterial population in the environment and the stage of infection. It is possible to speculate that the majority of nutrients are derived from the host. However, certain essential nutrients to some species are not provided by the host and must be delivered by other species in the infected site (discussed below in Section 5.6.2 "Microbial interactions"). Because the root canal system may not be that rich in nutrients, there must be a fierce bacterial competition for the amounts available. Oral bacterial species have different nutritional demands and competence in acquiring or scavenging nutrients. As a consequence, bacterial species that can best utilize and compete for nutrients in the root canal system will succeed in colonization.

In the root canal system, microorganisms can utilize the following as sources of nutrients: (1) the necrotic pulp tissue, containing remnants of dead pulp cells and other degenerated constituents of the pulp connective tissue; (2) components (usually glycoproteins) of tissue fluids and exudate that seep into the root canal system via apical and lateral foramens as well as saliva that may coronally penetrate in the root canal; and (3) products of the metabolism of other microorganisms (discussed below). Because the largest amount of nutrients is available in the main canal, which is the most voluminous part of the root canal system, most of the infecting microbiota, particularly fastidious species, is expected to be located in this region.

The dynamics of nutrient utilization by microbial species can also influence shifts in the infecting microbiota of the root canal system. Saccharolytic species often dominate the early stages of the infectious process, but are soon outnumbered by asaccharolytic species, which will dominate later stages [374]. For a better understanding, an analogy can be done based on studies related to the utilization of nutrients present in serum [381]. In the initial phases of an infectious process, the low amount of carbohydrates available in serum is rapidly consumed by saccharolytic bacteria. In an intermediary phase, carbohydrates are split off from glycoproteins and their content is totally consumed. Proteins are also hydrolyzed and some amino acid fermentation takes place. This reflects a shift from a saccharolytic microbiota to a proteolytic one. Species from the genera *Prevotella*, *Eubacterium*, *Veillonella*, and *Fusobacterium* can predominate in this phase. In a final phase, progressive protein degradation and extensive amino acid fermentation can be observed, with *Peptostreptococcus*, *Prevotella*, *Porphyromonas*, *Eubacterium* and *F. nucleatum* predominating over other species [381].

Given the small volume of a necrotic pulp, which is progressively degraded, the necrotic pulp tissue can be regarded as a finite source of nutrients to bacteria. However, the induction of periradicular inflammation guarantees a sustainable source of nutrients, particularly in the form of proteins and glycoproteins present in the exudate that seep into the canal. At this stage of the infectious process, bacteria that have a proteolytic capacity, or can establish a cooperative interaction with those that can utilize this substrate in the metabolism, start dominating. Thus, the root canal environment in untreated teeth affords bacteria a shifting pattern of nutrient availability and type

over time, which will be reflected in the composition of the microbiota.

Absence of high concentrations of carbohydrates in the necrotic root canal leads to colonization of a largely asaccharolytic microbiota. Thus, apart from a few species, the great majority of the predominant species found in the root canal system of teeth evincing apical periodontitis lesions are asaccharolytic or weakly saccharolytic, and ferment peptides and amino acids to obtain energy. However, the amount of substrate that can be readily fermented by bacteria, such as small peptides and amino acids, may be limited. Degradation of intact proteins seems to be a crucial step in providing the polypeptides necessary for energy generation by nonproteinase and peptidase-producing, amino acid fermenting bacteria (such as *F. nucleatum*, *C. rectus*, *Eubacterium* species, *Peptostreptococcus micros*, and *Streptococcus intermedius*) [134]. Therefore, bacteria that produce proteolytic enzymes can play an important ecological role in the environment, by degrading macromolecular compounds such as glycoproteins and proteins to release nutrients not only to their own catabolism but also to be utilized by other species. Examples of putative endodontic pathogens that possess strong proteolytic activity include species of the genera *Porphyromonas*, *Prevotella*, *Actinomyces*, and *Capnocytophaga*, as well as *T. denticola* and *T. forsythia* [118,133,184,272,367]. In addition to providing nutrients, proteolytic and other hydrolytic enzymes are important virulence factors since they have tissue-destructive ability and can impair host defenses by degrading immunoglobulins and complement (protecting not only themselves but also other species in the community).

5.6.2 Microbial interactions

The establishment of the endodontic microbiota can also be influenced by ecological relationships between the species that invade the root canal system. Because endodontic infections are usually mixed infections, different bacterial species are in close proximity with one another and interactions become inevitable. These interactions can be positive, negative or neutral. Whilst positive and negative interactions are common at high population densities and when populations are actively growing, neutralism is more likely to occur at low population densities so that microorganisms are less likely to come into contact and to compete with each other. Neutralism is unlikely to occur in infected root canals.

Positive interactions enhance the survival capacity of the interacting microorganisms. Sometimes different species coexist in habitats where neither could exist alone. Examples of positive interactions that can occur in the root canal microbiota include mutualism and commensalism. Mutualism is an interrelationship between two species that benefits both. Commensalism is a unidirectional relationship between microorganisms in which one species benefits and the other is unaffected. It is common in situations where the unaffected microorganisms modify the habitat in such a way that another species benefits. For example, removal of oxygen from the root canal system carried out by the metabolism of facultative bacteria sets the stage for the establishment of obligate anaerobic latecomers.

Negative interactions act as feedback mechanisms that limit population densities. Examples that can occur in the endodontic microbiota include competition and amensalism. Competition occurs when two species are striving for the same resource. It usually focuses on available nutrients and space for colonization. Competition can prevent two different species from occupying the same ecological niche in a community. One will succeed in occupation of a given niche and the other will fail. Amensalism (antagonism) occurs when one species produces a substance (bacteriocin or metabolic end-products) that inhibits another species. Pioneer species in a habitat gain a competitive edge as a result of their ability to inhibit the establishment of competitive latecomers. The simplest way to avoid inhibition factors released by one bacterial species is to find sites that are not colonized by antagonistic species. In addition, another method is to counterattack the antagonistic species by producing inhibitory or killing factors against them.

In the endodontic ecosystem, the metabolism of some bacterial species can influence the survival of other species. Metabolic products can either be metabolized by others or accumulate in the environment, reaching toxic levels to many species. A typical example is ammonia resulting from the catabolism of amino acids. Whilst ammonia can be utilized as an important nitrogen source for many bacteria, it can be toxic in high concentrations [370]. Short-chain fatty acids and sulfur compounds, if left to accumulate in high concentrations, can also inhibit the growth of some species.

In a mixed community, different microbial populations have to find a way to live in harmony with one another and to behave collectively so that the whole community can benefit from interactions. The association of microbial species within a community is not random, but dictated by mutual nutritional and functional interests as well as by specific affinities, including coaggregation. This is highly dependent on positive interactions that can be mediated by one species providing growth conditions favorable to another, e.g., by altering the redox potential, protecting from host defenses or even by releasing products of the metabolism that turn out to be an essential substrate for other species. Cooperation between microbial species can also be necessary to break down complex substrates. Therefore, positive interactions increase the probability of certain species to be found together in a given habitat. There are several examples of positive interactions involving endodontic bacteria:

- The respiratory metabolism of *C. rectus* depends on formate and hydrogen as electron donors and fumarate, nitrate, or oxygen as electron acceptors [370]. This makes this species dependent on formate- or hydrogen-producing bacteria, such as *Eubacterium* species, *Peptostreptococcus* species and *F. nucleatum*. Proteolytic bacteria, such as *Prevotella* species and *Porphyromonas* species can degrade proteins to provide amino acids which can also serve as electron acceptors to *C. rectus*. Thus, in a community, *C. rectus* is expected to be associated with these bacteria.
- Most strains of black-pigmented anaerobic rods show specific nutritional requirements for vitamin K and hemin. In addition to being obtained when hemoglobin is broken down, a hemin-related compound can be provided to black-pigmented bacteria by *C. rectus* [92]. Vitamin K can be provided by some bacterial species, such as *Veillonella parvula*, *Propionibacterium* species, and *Eubacterium* species [83,249]. *T. denticola*, *Eikenella corrodens*, *Fusobacterium* species, *Eubacterium* species, and *Peptostreptococcus* species produce succinate, which may substitute the requirement of hemin or vitamin K as growth factor for some black-pigmented bacteria [192].
- Oral *Treponema* species can utilize isobutyrate produced by black-pigmented bacteria, *Fusobacterium* species or *Eubacterium* species [186].
- *Pseudoramibacter alactolyticus* may depend on the production of acetate by other bacteria, such as streptococci and *Actinomyces* species [370].
- *Veillonella* species utilize lactate secreted by Gram-positive facultatives such as streptococci [193].

- *T. denticola* depends on bacterial interactions for its growth in serum. *P. intermedia*, *Eubacterium nodatum*, *V. parvula*, and *F. nucleatum* are found to enhance growth of *T. denticola* in co-cultures. Mechanisms involved in growth stimulation may include the ability of *P. intermedia* and *E. nodatum* to cleave the protein-core of serum glycoproteins, making these molecules accessible for degradation by *T. denticola*. *V. parvula* may provide peptidase activities complementary to those of *T. denticola* [382].

As can be inferred from Fig. 5.5, a complex array of interbacterial nutritional interactions can take place into infected root canals, in which the growth of some species can be dependent on the metabolism of other species.

Several approaches can be used to define positive and negative associations between bacterial species. One approach commonly used for the endodontic microbiota determines which bacterial species are frequently detected together and which are rarely detected in the same samples. Based on this approach, several positive interactions have been reported for intracanal bacteria: *F. nucleatum* is positively associated with *P. micros*, *P. endodontalis*, *S. sputigena*, and *C. rectus* [369]. Strong positive associations exist between *P. intermedia* and *P. micros* [241,369]. *P. endodontalis* can be positively correlated with *F. nucleatum*, *P. alactolyticus*, and *Campylobacter* species [369]. *Propionibacterium propionicum* is positively associated with *Actinomyces species* [369]. Positive associations have also been found between *P. intermedia* and *Prevotella oralis*, and *Actinomyces odontolyticus* and *P. micros* [241]. Significant associations were identified between *T. maltophilum*, *T. forsythia*, and *P. gingivalis* [141]. *D. pneumosintes* has been found in positive association with *T. denticola*, *P. endodontalis*, *F. nucleatum*, *F. alocis*, *P. micros*, *C. rectus*, *P. intermedia*, *Treponema pectinovorum*, and *Treponema vincentii* [329]. Several positive associations have been disclosed for newly recognized candidate endodontic pathogens (unpublished data) (Fig. 5.6).

Coaggregation is the cell-to-cell recognition of genetically distinct partner cell types and has been observed to occur between several different oral species [156]. Coaggregations differ from agglutinations and aggregations in that the latter two interactions occur between genetically identical cells [157]. A given pair of species can attach to each other by means of specific receptor–adhesin interactions, which are usually lectin-like interactions (attachment of a specific protein on the surface of one species to a specific carbohydrate on the surface of the other). Coaggregation can even occur between non-coaggregating species and, in this case, it is mediated by cellular constituents, such as outer membrane vesicles, of a third species. Coaggregation can favor colonization of host surfaces and also facilitate metabolic interactions between the partners.

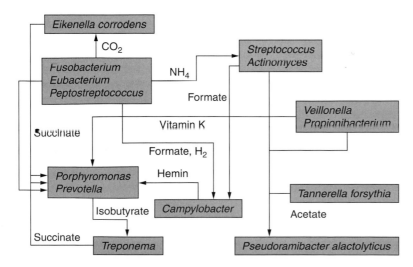

Fig. 5.5 Nutritional relationships that can occur between bacteria in endodontic mixed consortia.

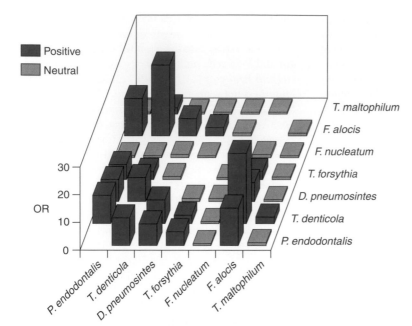

Fig. 5.6 Associations between newly recognized putative endodontic pathogens. Data were based on odds ratio calculation and values >2 indicate a positive association.

5.6.3 Host defense factors, temperature, and pH

Host defense factors. The root canal microbiota is by and large protected from the host defenses because of its anatomical location and the presence of necrotic pulp tissue, which make bacteria relatively inaccessible to host defense cells and molecules. However, a multitude of host factors are produced in the tissue response, the nature and effects of which are discussed in Chapter 3.

Temperature. Although there are no clear reports on the temperature level within the root canal, it is likely to range from 30 to 38°C. This temperature range discriminates whole classes of potential colonizers such as thermophiles and psychrophiles. It remains questionable, however, whether temperature changes and differences within the root canal are important determinants for infection and disease.

pH. The pH in the necrotic pulp ranges from 6.4 to 7.0 [383], but it can rise slightly as a result of the metabolism of proteins by intracanal bacteria. Some putative endodontic pathogens grow better at slightly alkaline pH values and present marked alterations in the enzyme profile under such conditions. For instance, trypsin-like activity in *P. gingivalis* is maxi-

mal at pH 8.0 [187]. Bacteria vary in regard to their pH tolerance, with most species best growing within a range of 6 to 9 pH [6]. Fungi generally exhibit a slightly wider pH range, growing within a range of 5 to 9 pH [6]. Microorganisms that are known to thrive under pH conditions near neutrality are considered neutralophiles. Intracanal pH may be incompatible with growth of some acidophiles and alkaliphiles, though most of these organisms can adapt themselves to neutral pH conditions.

5.6.4 Climax community

It is now clear that a dynamic microbial community installs in the root canal system and that microbial succession occurs over time [66,379]. The pioneer community influences the pattern of microbial succession within the root canal. This involves the progressive development of a pioneer community composed of a few species through some stages in which the number of microbial species gradually increases. With the passage of time, the microbial community becomes more complex and community members may be joined by or replaced by other species. The spatial organization of bacterial populations within the root canal system is unlikely to be at random. Microbial associations based on mutual interests between species are highly likely to dictate population arrangements within a community in such a way that microbial species that are metabolically interdependent are disposed close to each other. Determined groups of anaerobic bacteria start dominating the endodontic microbiota just a few days or weeks following pulpal necrosis. Eventually, a stable situation and a high level of community organization may be reached, with microbial populations existing in harmony and equilibrium with their environment. This is referred to as the *climax community* [186,357]. A multitude of niches (metabolic functions) then takes place in the consortium. In a climax community, the metabolic efficiency of the whole is usually far greater than that of the sum of the individual populations.

In spite of species diversity, the climax community is characterized by a remarkable degree of stability or balance between the component members. Dying cells are constantly being replaced. When the environment is perturbed, self-regulatory mechanisms enter the scene to restore the original equilibrium. While most environments are variable and are constantly exposed to some types of perturbation, the root canal milieu does not appear to be subject to significant variations, especially in advanced stages of infection. Obviously, minor environmental changes can even spontaneously occur. However, minor perturbations do not provoke significant changes in an established, climax community.

In an organized microbial community, inhabitants usually share resources and interrelated activities. Microorganisms living in a consortium show different phenotypical behavior depending on the environmental conditions. Most members of a microbial community can regulate their catabolic and anabolic pathways according to nutrient limitation or surplus. Communication of microbial cells is necessary for optimum community development and is carried out by secretion of diffusible signaling molecules (quorum-sensing systems) and perhaps by the exchange of genetic information.

Inasmuch as the climax contains many niches, physiologically different microbial species can coexist indefinitely provided they are functionally compatible. Environmental conditions within the root canal system are not uniform and differences will be reflected in the composition of the infecting microbial community and in the establishment of different ecological niches. Organization of microcolonies in the endodontic microbial community may be dictated by the ecological determinants occurring in different parts of the root canal system. Environmental conditions can vary along the entire extent of the root canal, with differences being more pronounced at the two ends (coronal and apical) of the system. Oxygen and nutrient gradients arguably set up in root canals exposed to the oral environment [359]. In the coronal region of the canal, given the proximity with the oral cavity, the oxygen tension is higher than in other regions of the canal. As a consequence, facultatives and aerotolerant anaerobes can be more commonly found in this area. Anaerobic conditions in the apical third are highly conducive to the establishment of a microbiota dominated almost exclusively by obligately anaerobic bacteria [66]. Similarly, bacteria located in the most coronal aspects of the canal can utilize carbohydrates from the host diet and saliva, which can seep into the canal via coronal exposure. Bacteria in the most apical area of the root canal system utilize protein- and glycoprotein-rich tissue fluids and exudate which penetrate in the canals via apical and lateral foramens. Therefore, the dominance of different bacterial groups in different parts of the root canal system can be predicted based on oxygen and nutrient requirements.

Results from morphological and ecological studies suggest that a microbial climax community may develop in the root canal system [201,212,318,369] (Fig. 5.7). The precise time required for a climax community to develop within the root canal system is unknown. Although speculative, it is highly likely that most root canal infections, if untreated, will

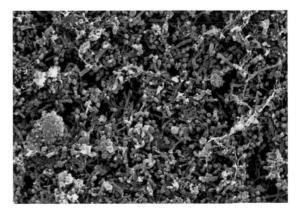

Fig. 5.7 Scanning electron micrograph showing dense colonization of the root canal walls by different bacterial morphotypes. In a consortium like this, a climax community (original magnification ×2500).

sooner or later reach a degree of community organization and stability typical of a climax community entity. It is entirely possible that in most teeth with associated apical periodontitis lesions a climax community is already installed in the root canal system. Theoretically, it is fair to assume that the larger the periradicular bone destruction the higher the probability for a climax community to be established in the root canal. As a climax community can be difficult to be eradicated, this could help explain why teeth with large lesions have a significantly lower success rate after conventional treatment [373].

5.7 Patterns of microbial colonization

The knowledge of the pattern of microbial location and organization within the root canal system assumes special importance in the understanding of the disease process and in the establishment of effective antimicrobial therapeutic strategies. Primary endodontic infections are caused by oral bacteria, which are usually opportunistic pathogens. Theoretically, any of the more than 700 bacterial species from the oral microbiota may invade a root canal containing necrotic pulp tissue and establish an infectious process. Nonetheless, evidences suggest that some bacterial species are related to some forms of apical periodontitis and thereby are considered putative endodontic pathogens. Most of the knowledge of the structure of the endodontic microbiota comes from morphologic studies, which do not usually provide information as to the bacterial identity. Consequently, it is difficult to delineate the role of the visualized bacteria in the consortium. Thus, as each bacterial cell observed in the root canal system might be an endodontic pathogen, findings from morphologic studies should be used to understand the topography of the root canal infection and to establish therapeutic measures in an attempt to completely eradicate the root canal infection or at least to reduce the bacterial load to thresholds that are compatible with periradicular tissue healing.

Studies using light and/or electron microscopy have been carried out to disclose microorganisms in the root canal system and to investigate the structure of the root canal microbiota in teeth with apical periodontitis [201,212,291,318]. Morphologically, the root canal microbiota consists of cocci, rods, filaments, and spirochetes (Fig. 5.8). Fungal cells can also be sporadically found [291,318] (Fig. 5.9). Most of the

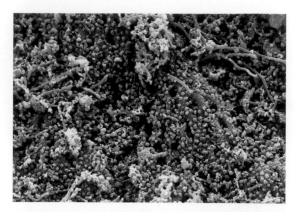

Fig. 5.8   Mixed bacterial population colonizing the root canal wall. Cocci are the predominant forms, but rods, filaments, and spirilla are also observed. In some areas, coccoid cells are relatively apart from each other (original magnification ×2200). (Reproduced from Siqueira *et al.* [318] with permission.)

endodontic microbiota remains suspended in the fluid phase of the main root canal. In addition, dense bacterial aggregates or coaggregates can be seen adhered to the root canal walls, sometimes forming multilayered bacterial condensations that resemble biofilm-like communities [212,318] (Fig. 5.10). Planktonic bacterial cells in the fluid phase of the root canal may either be newcomers or released from the aggregates adhering to the root canal walls, as occurs in biofilms elsewhere in nature, even though shearing forces are not expected to occur in the root canal.

A commonly observed finding is that the pattern of colonization is not uniform among different teeth, not even in the same root canal. Whereas most of the root canal walls are usually heavily colonized, with what resembles biofilm structures, there are areas in which colonization is slight [318]. This is apparently independent of the root canal third and can be a reflex of diverse ecological factors operating in each area.

Bacteria forming dense accumulations on the root canal walls are often seen penetrating the dentinal tubules (Figs 5.11 and 5.12). The diameter of dentinal tubules is large enough to permit penetration of most oral bacteria. It has been reported that dentinal tubule infection can occur in about 50–80% of the teeth evincing apical periodontitis lesions [102]. Albeit a shallow penetration is more common, bacterial cells can be observed reaching approximately 300 µm in some teeth [318] (Fig. 5.13). While some

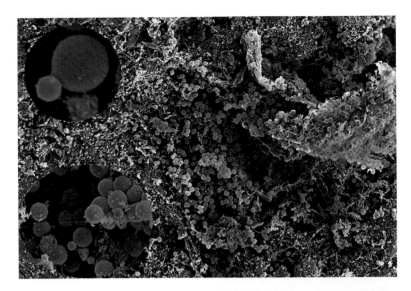

Fig. 5.9 Heavy colonization of yeast cells in the root canal of an extracted tooth associated with apical periodontitis. Note that some cells are in the stage of budding. A daughter cell is growing on the surface of the mother cell (insets) (original magnification ×300; insets, bottom ×2700, and top ×3500). (Reproduced from Siqueira and Sen [337] with permission.)

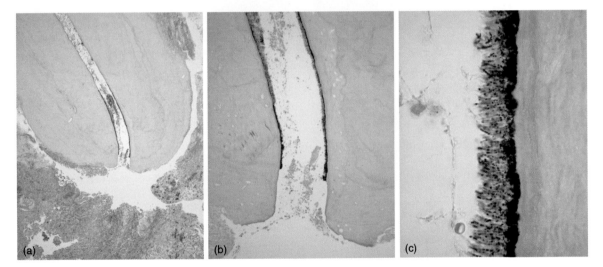

(a) (b) (c)

Fig. 5.10 Biofilm formation on the root canal walls of an extracted tooth with attached apical periodontitis lesion. The section has been stained with a Taylor-modified Brown and Brenn method for bacterial identification. Bacteria are seen lining the walls of the root canal in a biofilm-like structure (a, b). High magnification in (c) displays aggregation of numerous coccoid and filamentous organisms. (Courtesy of Dr Domenico Ricucci and reproduced from Svensäter G, Bergenholtz G (2004) Biofilms in endodontic infections. *Endodontic Topics* **9**, 27–36, with permission.)

tubules can be heavily infected, adjacent tubules can be free of infection (Fig. 5.14). This has been observed even in regions where the entire root canal wall is heavily colonized. Most of the bacteria invading dentinal tubules are cocci, but rods can also be seen inside tubules. Motility does not appear to be a necessary bacterial attribute to dentinal invasion, since most bacteria that have been so far identified

in tubules are nonmotile species. Dividing cells can be observed frequently within tubules during *in situ* investigations [318] (Fig. 5.14), indicating that bacteria can derive nutrients within tubules, probably from degrading odontoblastic processes, denatured collagen, bacterial cells that die during the course of infection and intracanal fluids that enter the tubules by capillarity.

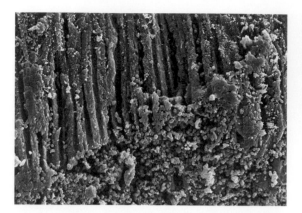

Fig. 5.11 Dense bacterial aggregates colonizing the root canal walls. Some bacterial cells are seen invading dentinal tubules (original magnification ×1800).

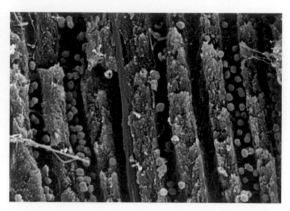

Fig. 5.13 Cocci in dentinal tubules approximately 300 μm from the main root canal (original magnification ×5000). (Reproduced from Siqueira *et al.* [318] with permission.)

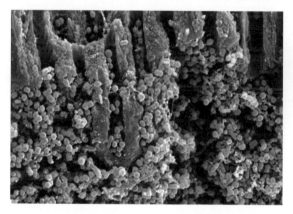

Fig. 5.12 Heavy infection of the root canal walls mainly by cocci, but some small rods are also seen. Cocci are penetrating into dentinal tubules (original magnification ×3500). (Reproduced from Siqueira *et al.* [318] with permission.)

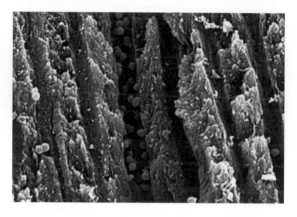

Fig. 5.14 Dentin infection. Some tubules can be heavily infected, while adjacent tubules can be free of infection. Dividing cells are seen within tubules (original magnification ×5500).

Several putative endodontic pathogens have been shown to be capable of penetrating dentinal tubules. Siqueira *et al.* [301] observed that *P. endodontalis*, *P. gingivalis*, *F. nucleatum*, *Actinomyces israelii*, *Propionibacterium acnes*, and *Enterococcus faecalis* invaded dentinal tubules *in vitro*, but to different depths (Fig. 5.15). Streptococci are amongst the most commonly identified bacteria that invade dentin [179,237]. These bacteria may recognize components present within dentinal tubules, such as collagen type I, which stimulate bacterial adhesion and intratubular growth [178]. In a clinical study, Peters *et al.* [240] isolated and identified bacteria present in root dentin at different depths. A larger number of cells and species were detected in dentinal layers closer to the pulp. Bacteria were also found in more than one-half of the infected teeth in the deep dentin close to the cementum. The most common isolates belonged to the genera *Prevotella*, *Porphyromonas*, *Fusobacterium*, *Veillonella*, *Peptostreptococcus*, *Eubacterium*, *Actinomyces*, *Lactobacillus*, and *Streptococcus*. Matsuo *et al.* [190], using immunohistological analysis, disclosed bacteria in dentinal tubules of about 70% of extracted infected teeth with apical periodontitis.

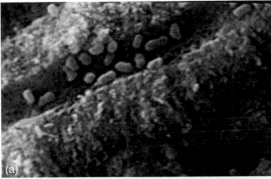

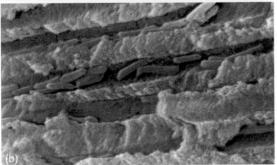

Fig. 5.15 *In vitro* bacterial penetration within dentinal tubules. (a) *Propionibacterium acnes* (original magnification ×4900). (b) *Actinomyces israelii* (original magnification ×4500). (Reproduced from Siqueira *et al.* [301] with permission.)

The most commonly found species were *F. nucleatum*, *P. alactolyticus*, *E. nodatum*, *Lactobacillus casei*, and *P. micros*. Yeasts, particularly *Candida albicans*, also have the ability to invade dentinal tubules [319,401] (Fig. 5.16). Microorganisms located into tubules may pose a treatment problem, because of difficulties in their elimination during intracanal procedures [102].

5.8 Types of endodontic infections

Endodontic infections can be classified according to their anatomical location (intraradicular or extraradicular infection) and the time participating microorganisms gained entry into the root canal (primary, secondary, or persistent infection) [314]. The composition of the microbiota may vary depending on the different types of infection and different forms of apical periodontitis. Delineation of the various types of endodontic infections favors the understanding of the pathological processes involving different clinical conditions and may help establish proper therapeutic measures for these conditions.

5.8.1 Intraradicular infections

As the name suggests, this infection is caused by microorganisms colonizing the root canal system. It can be subdivided into three categories according

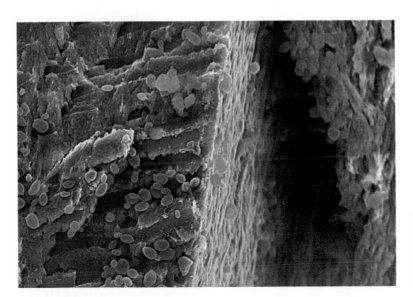

Fig. 5.16 Cells of *Candida albicans* invading dentinal tubules at the root canal wall. Many cells are in budding process (original magnification ×1100). (Reproduced from Siqueira *et al.* [319] with permission.)

to the time microorganisms entered the root canal system.

(a) Primary intraradicular infection

Primary intraradicular infection is caused by microorganisms that initially invade and colonize the necrotic pulp tissue. It has also been referred to as initial infection or "virgin" infection. Primary infections are characterized by a mixed consortium composed of 10–30 species per canal [341]. The number of bacterial cells in an infected canal varies from 10^3 to 10^8 [281,366,396]. The involved microbiota is conspicuously dominated by anaerobic bacteria, particularly Gram-negative species belonging to the genera *Tannerella, Dialister, Porphyromonas, Prevotella, Fusobacterium, Campylobacter,* and *Treponema.* However, Gram-positive anaerobes from the genera *Peptostreptococcus, Eubacterium, Filifactor, Actinomyces,* and *Pseudoramibacter,* as well as facultative or microaerophilic streptococci can also be commonly found in primary intraradicular infections.

(b) Secondary intraradicular infection

Secondary intraradicular infections are caused by microorganisms that were not present in the primary infection, but that were introduced into the root canal system at some time after professional intervention. The moment can be during treatment, between appointments, or even after the conclusion of the endodontic treatment. In any circumstance, if penetrating microorganisms succeed in surviving and colonizing the root canal system, a secondary infection is established. Species commonly associated with secondary infections include *Pseudomonas aeruginosa, Staphylococcus* species, *E. coli,* other enteric rods, *Candida* species, and *E. faecalis,* all of them not usually found in primary infections [99,250,251,315,345,398].

The main causes of microbial introduction in the canal *during treatment* include: remnants of dental plaque, calculus or caries on the tooth crown; leaking rubber dam; contamination of endodontic instruments, as for instance, after touch with the fingers; contamination of irrigant solutions or other solutions of intracanal use (such as saline solution, distilled water, citric acid, etc.). Microorganisms can enter the root canal system *between appointments,* following: leakage through the temporary restorative material; breakdown, fracture or loss of the temporary resto-

ration; fracture of the tooth structure; and in teeth left open for drainage. Microorganisms can penetrate the root canal system even *after completion of the root canal filling* in the following situations: leakage through the temporary or permanent restorative material; breakdown, fracture or loss of the temporary/permanent restoration; fracture of the tooth structure; recurrent decay exposing the root canal filling material; or delay in placement of permanent restorations [315].

(c) Persistent intraradicular infection

Persistent intraradicular infections are caused by microorganisms that in some way resisted intracanal antimicrobial procedures and that are able to endure periods of nutrient deprivation in a prepared canal. It is also termed recurrent infection. Involved microorganisms are remnants of a primary or secondary infection.

The microbiota associated with persistent infections is usually composed of fewer species than primary infections, and Gram-positive facultative bacteria, particularly *E. faecalis,* are predominant [198,332,373]. Fungi can also be found, in frequencies significantly higher when compared with primary infections [337].

Persistent and secondary infections are for the most part clinically indistinguishable and can be responsible for several clinical problems, including persistent exudation, persistent symptoms, interappointment exacerbations, and failure of the endodontic treatment, characterized by persistence of the apical periodontitis lesion (Fig. 5.17).

5.8.2 Extraradicular infection

Extraradicular infection is characterized by microbial invasion of the inflamed periradicular tissues, and is almost invariably a sequel to the intraradicular infection. Extraradicular infection can be dependent on or independent of the intraradicular infection. The most common form of extraradicular infection dependent on the intradicular infection is the acute apical abscess (Fig. 5.18). The most common form of extraradicular infection that can be independent of the intraradicular infection is the apical actinomycosis, caused by *Actinomyces* species or *P. propionicum* (Fig. 5.19). The question as to whether the extraradicular infection is dependent on or independent of the intraradicular infections assumes special

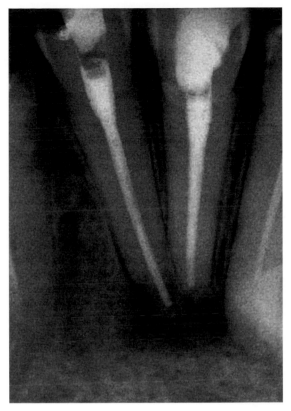

Fig. 5.17 Persistence of apical periodontitis lesions in root-filled teeth. Persistent or secondary intraradicular infections are the main causative agents of endodontic treatment failure.

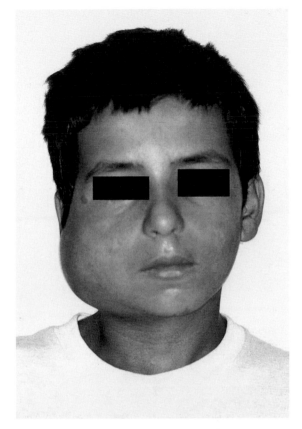

Fig. 5.18 Acute apical abscess. Cases like this represent the most common form of extraradicular infection dependent on the intradicular infection.

relevance from a therapeutic standpoint, since the former can be successfully managed by root canal therapy while the latter can only be handled by periradicular surgery.

5.9 Primary endodontic infections

In spite of the large number of species that can colonize the oral cavity, only a limited set of bacterial species is consistently selected out of the oral microbiota for growth and survival within root canals containing necrotic pulp tissue. Taken together, data from studies using culture-dependent or culture-independent identification approaches have suggested that a select group of bacterial species can be considered as candidate endodontic pathogens, based on both frequency of detection and potential pathogenicity.

Studies using culture-dependent approaches have definitely demonstrated the essential role of microorganisms in causation of the different forms of apical periodontitis. Furthermore, several putative endodontic pathogens have been recognized. More recently, with the advent of molecular biology tools, significant technical hurdles of culture methods have been deftly overcome [339]. Not only have molecular methods confirmed findings from most culture studies, but a great deal of new information has been added to the knowledge of candidate endodontic pathogens. This new technology has enabled the recognition of new putative pathogens, which had never been previously found in endodontic infections [341]. Moreover, many species that had already been considered as putative pathogens due to their frequencies as reported by culture-dependent methods have been found in even higher prevalence values by molecu-

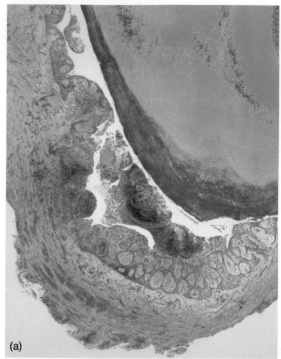

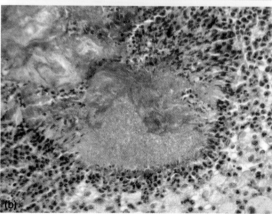

Fig. 5.19 Apical actinomycosis. (a) Bacterial aggregate in an epithelialized periapical lesion, suggestive of actinomycosis. (b) Higher magnification of the actinomycotic aggregate, which is surrounded by inflammatory cells. (Courtesy of Dr Domenico Ricucci.)

lar approaches, strengthening their association with causation of apical periodontitis.

Modern culture and molecular biology techniques have clearly revealed the polymicrobial nature of endodontic infections with a conspicuous dominance of obligate anaerobic bacteria in primary infections. In addition, bacterial profiles of the endodontic microbiota also vary from individual to individual [336], suggesting that apical periodontitis has a heterogeneous etiology, where multiple bacterial combinations can play a role in disease causation.

5.9.1 Microbial composition and diversity

In 1894, Miller wrote: "It must strike every one that the results of the culture experiments do not tally with those of the microscopical examination. While a careful microscopical examination of the diseased pulp almost invariably revealed a mixed infection, the pure cultures show, in the majority of cases, either only cocci or only bacilli." One of Miller's possible explanations for this finding was the following: "many species of bacteria occurring in the diseased pulp, vibriones, spirochaetes, the stiff pointed bacilli and threads, have not been found cultivable on artificial media anyway; and possibly there are still other uncultivable pulp-bacteria" [195]. He was absolutely right. And it was not until the development of sophisticated methods for anaerobic cultivation and further breakthroughs in microbial identification represented by molecular biology technology that many of the endodontic bacteria were brought to light.

Table 5.1 shows bacteria that have been detected in primary intraradicular infections in association with different forms of apical periodontitis by using a highly sensitive and specific molecular biology assay. The most prevalent and significant species or groups are discussed below.

The black-pigmented Gram-negative anaerobic rods formerly known as *Bacteroides melaninogenicus* have been reclassified: the saccharolytic species were transferred to the genus *Prevotella* and the asaccharolytic species to the genus *Porphyromonas* [295,296]. Some bile-sensitive nonpigmented *Bacteroides* species were also transferred to the genus *Prevotella* [139]. *Prevotella* species, especially *P. intermedia*, *P. nigrescens*, *Prevotella tannerae*, *Prevotella multissacharivorax*, *Prevotella baroniae*, and *P. denticola*, have been frequently isolated from or detected in infections of endodontic origin [7,15,19,40,55,82,89, 100,151,280,294,368,405,415]. Of the *Porphyromonas* species of human origin, only *P. endodontalis* (the specific epithet "endodontalis" referring to its original isolation from endodontic infections) and *P. gingivalis* have been consistently isolated from or detected in endodontic infections. They seem to play

Table 5.1   Prevalence of bacteria detected in primary endodontic infections of teeth with different forms of apical periodontitis (%)

Taxa[a]	Chronic apical periodontitis	Acute apical periodontitis	Acute apical abscess	Total
Treponema denticola	57	75	77	68
Dialister invisus	81	60	53	66
Porphyromonas endodontalis	61	50	68	61
Tannerella forsythia	54	58	64	58
Pseudoramibacter alactolyticus	76	60	32	56
Dialister pneumosintes	57	33	64	55
Filifactor alocis	57	30	42	46
Porphyromonas gingivalis	32	50	59	45
Propionibacterium propionicum	29	50	37	36
Treponema socranskii	39	42	25	35
Streptococcus species	29	10	41	31
Peptostreptococcus micros	27	20	32	28
Catonella morbi	33	30	16	26
Treponema parvum	52	20	0	26
Treponema maltophilum	33	50	0	24
Veillonella parvula	33	10	21	24
Olsenella uli	33	40	5	24
Lactobacillus species	38	20	11	24
Fusobacterium nucleatum	18	0	41	23
Campylobacter rectus	30	33	12	23
Campylobacter gracilis	21	17	24	21
Synergistes clone BA121	33	20	5	20
Eikenella corrodens	14	10	26	18
Enterococcus faecalis	33	10	5	18
Prevotella nigrescens	11	10	27	16
Synergistes clone BH017	29	10	5	16
Treponema lecithinolyticum	33	10	0	16
Prevotella intermedia	11	0	27	15
Centipeda periodontiii	13	14	15	14
Treponema pectinovorum	14	0	22	14
Granulicatella adiacens	19	10	11	14
Synergistes clone W090	24	20	0	14

[a] Species/phylotypes detected in more than 10% of the total cases. Taxa detected in less than 10% of the samples included: *Treponema vincentii, Treponema amylovorum, Treponema medium, Treponema putidum, Actinomyces israelii, Actinomyces radicidentis, Olsenella profusa, Olsenella EI15, Actinobaculum EL030, Desulfobulbus R004,* TM7 clone I025, *Prevotella pallens, Atopobium parvulum, Synergistes* F3_33, and fungi

an important role in the etiology of different forms of apical periodontitis lesions, including acute apical abscesses [89,100,180,294,307,312,368,390].

An important periodontal pathogen, *T. forsythia* (formerly *Bacteroides forsythus*), a Gram-negative obligate anaerobe that had never been detected in root canals by culture, was for the first time report-

ed to occur in primary endodontic infections in a study using the PCR technique [45]. Ensuing studies using PCR technology and other molecular biology approaches have confirmed that *T. forsythia* is a common member of the microbiota associated with different types of endodontic infections, including abscesses [76,140,260,307,313,323,394] (Fig. 5.20).

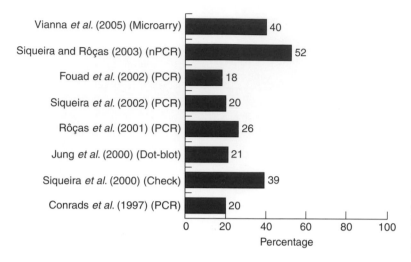

Fig. 5.20 Prevalence of *Tannerella forsythia* in primary endodontic infections as determined by different studies using molecular biology techniques.

Dialister species represent another example of bacteria that have been consistently detected in endodontic infections only after the advent of molecular biology techniques. *D. pneumosintes* and the recently described *Dialister invisus* have been frequently present in the microbiota associated with asymptomatic and symptomatic primary endodontic infections [206,261,268,278,280,316,329,340].

F. nucleatum is one of the most commonly encountered Gram-negative species in endodontic infections. Currently, it consists of five subspecies (*fusiforme, nucleatum, polymorphum, vincentii,* and *animalis*) and is very heterogeneous [41]. *F. nucleatum* has been frequently isolated from or detected in primarily infected root canals as well as in endodontic abscesses [19,50,76,140,165,369,407]. However, the frequency of its subspecies has yet to be accurately established. Different clonal types of *F. nucleatum* can be found in the same infected canal [203]. A study using the checkerboard DNA–DNA hybridization method reported the occurrence of *Fusobacterium periodonticum* in acute abscesses of endodontic origin [313].

Although spirochetes have been frequently observed in samples taken from endodontic infections by microscopy, they had never been identified to the species level. The application of molecular diagnostic methods to the identification of spirochetes has demonstrated that occurrence of these spiral bacteria in infections of endodontic origin has been overlooked by technical hurdles of culture techniques. All oral spirochetes fall into de genus *Treponema* [52]. Thus far, 10 species have been cultured and validly named.

They can be classified into two groups according to the fermentation of carbohydrates: the saccharolytic species include *T. pectinovorum, T. socranskii, T. amylovorum, T. lecithinolyticum, T. maltophilum,* and *T. parvum,* and the asaccharolytic species include *T. denticola, T. medium, T. putidum,* and *T. vincentii.* All these species have been recently disclosed in primary endodontic infections by studies using molecular biology methods for bacterial identification [17,74,141,263,269,306,310,311,325,326, 333,394] (Fig. 5.21). The most predominant treponemes in endodontic infections are *T. denticola* and *T. socranskii* [17,263,306,333]. The species *T. parvum, T. maltophilum* and *T. lecithinolyticum* have been moderately prevalent [17,141,325,333].

Even though anaerobic Gram-negative bacteria have been found to be the most common microorganisms in primary endodontic infections, several Gram-positive rods have also been frequent members of the endodontic microbial consortium. Of these, *P. alactolyticus* has been frequently isolated from or detected in samples from endodontic infections, in prevalence values as high as the most commonly found Gram-negative species [327,335,369]. *Filifactor alocis* (formerly *Fusobacterium alocis*) is an obligately anaerobic Gram-positive rod that had been only occasionally isolated from root canal infections by culture [369], but recent molecular studies detected this species in about one-half of the cases of primary endodontic infections [328]. *Slackia exigua, Mogibacterium timidum, E. saphenum,* and *Eubacterium infirmum* have also been reported to occur in infected root canals in relatively high prevalence [77,109]. *Actinomyces*

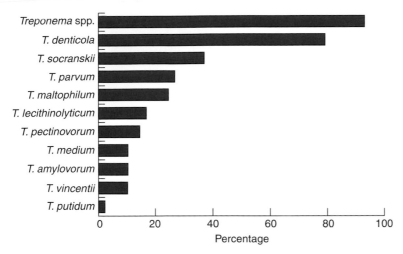

Fig. 5.21 Prevalence of oral *Treponema* species in primary endodontic infections. Data according to references [263,269,306,310,311,325,326,333].

species, particularly *A. gerencseriae* and *A. israelii*, which have been associated with failure of the endodontic treatment by causing apical actinomycosis, have been found in about 10% of the infected canals [321,369], though even higher prevalence rates have been reported for members of this genus [378,416]. *P. propionicum*, another species that can participate in apical actinomycosis, has also been commonly detected in samples from primary endodontic infections [344]. *Olsenella* species comprise small nonmotile Gram-positive obligately anaerobic rods, which represent another example of bacteria that have been detected in endodontic infections only after the introduction of molecular biology methods [76,206]. Amongst the *Olsenella* clade, *O. uli* has been the most commonly found species in endodontic infections [36,267].

Gram-positive cocci, specifically peptostreptococci and streptococci, are frequently present in primary endodontic infections. *Peptostreptococcus* species, particularly *P. micros*, have been isolated from or detected in about one-third of the primarily infected canals and their prevalence in symptomatic infections has also been relatively high [40,88,151,330,369,407]. Members of the *Streptococcus anginosus* group have been reported to be the most prevalent streptococci, but *S. gordonii*, *S. mitis*, and *S. sanguinis* can also be often detected [321,369]. *E. faecalis*, which is often found in association with root-canal-treated teeth, has not been so frequent in primary infections [266,321].

Campylobacter species, including *C. rectus* and *C. gracilis*, are Gram-negative anaerobic rods that

have been detected in primary endodontic infections, but in low to moderate prevalence values [167,250,307,324,369]. Other bacteria detected more sporadically in primary infections include: *V. parvula*, *E. corrodens*, *Neisseria mucosa*, *Centipeda periodontii*, *Gemella morbillorum*, *Capnocytophaga gingivalis*, *Corynebacterium matruchotii*, *Bifidobacterium dentium*, and anaerobic lactobacilli [307,313,334,369].

Some bacteria that are not normal inhabitants of the oral cavity have been occasionally found in primary root canal infections. They include *P. aeruginosa* and *E. coli*, and may be more commonly found in secondary root canal infections. Their entry into the root canal may occur during professional intervention as a result of a breach in the aseptic chain.

A. actinomycetemcomitans, which is implicated in the etiology of periodontal diseases, particularly the localized aggressive periodontitis (previously localized juvenile periodontitis) [355], has been a rare finding in root canal infections [317]. This suggests that this capnophilic species is not favored in the root canal environment and thus does not participate in the pathogenesis of apical periodontitis lesions.

Data from recent molecular studies have indicated that new bacterial phylotypes (species for which only a 16S rRNA gene sequence is known) can participate in endodontic infections. For instance, oral *Synergistes* clones BA121, E3_33, BH017 and W090, which had been originally assigned to the *Flexistipes* or *Deferribacteres* groups [87,231], have been commonly detected in samples from asymptomatic and symptomatic endodontic infections [268,340,343]. The great majority of *Synergistes* bacteria remain uncultivated and this can be the primary reason for the fact that their presence in endodontic infections has been overlooked by culture studies. Similarly, clone I025 from the TM7 candidate phylum, which has no as-yet-cultivated representative, has also been detected in primary endodontic infections [268,340]. Results from 16S rRNA gene clone libraries have also shown the occurrence of uncultivated phylotypes related to the genera *Dialister, Solobacterium, Olsenella, Eubacterium, Megasphaera*, and *Cytophaga* as well as phylotypes related to the family *Lachnospiraceae* [206,270,278,280]. One study [280] found some as-yet-uncultivated phylotypes among the most prevalent bacteria in primary intraradicular infections, including *Lachnospiraceae* oral clone 55A-34, *Megasphaera* oral clone CS025 and *Veillonella* oral clone BP1-85. Three phylotypes: *Prevotella* oral clone PUS9.180, *Eubacterium* oral clone BP1-89, and *Lachnospiraceae* oral clone MCE7_60, were exclusively detected in symptomatic teeth [280]. Detection of as-yet-uncultivated phylotypes in samples from endodontic infections suggests that they can be previously unrecognized bacteria that play a role in the pathogenesis of different forms of apical periodontitis.

Current evidence reveals that endodontic bacteria fall into eight of the 12 phyla that have oral representatives, namely *Bacteroidetes, Firmicutes, Spirochaetes, Fusobacteria, Actinobacteria, Proteobacteria, Synergistes*, and TM7 [206,278,280,340] (Fig. 5.22). Noteworthy is the high prevalence of uncultivated species – about 40–55% of the endodontic microbiota is composed of bacteria that have yet to be cultivated and fully characterized [206,280]. The genera, representative species and some other characteristics of bacteria found in endodontic infections are shown in Table 5.2.

In addition to bacteria, other microorganisms have also been sporadically found in primary endodontic infections. They include fungi, archaea, and viruses.

Fungi. Fungi are eukaryotic microorganisms that occur in two basic forms: molds (multicellular filamentous fungi consisting of branching cylindrical tubules) and yeasts (unicellular fungi with cells being spherical or oval in shape). Fungi have been only occasionally found in primary root canal infections [62,165,199,320], even though a recent molecular study [16] has reported the occurrence of *Candida*

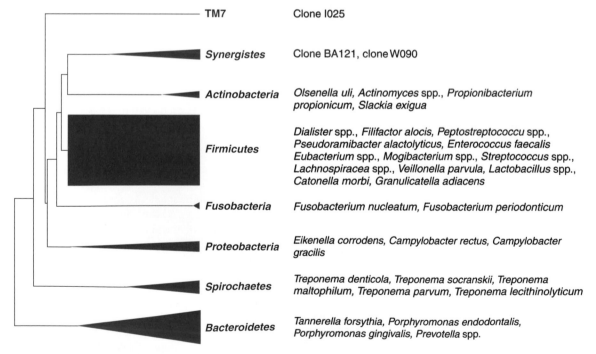

Fig. 5.22 Bacterial phyla that have representatives in endodontic infections. On the right, example species or phylotypes for each phylum are presented.

Table 5.2 Bacterial genera and respective common representatives occurring in endodontic infections

Genus	Common representatives	Pathogenicity[a,b]
Gram-negative		
Anaerobic rods		
Dialister	*D. invisus, D. pneumosintes*, uncultivated phylotypes[c]	++
Porphyromonas	*P. endodontalis, P. gingivalis*	+++
Tannerella	*T. forsythia*	+++
Prevotella	*P. intermedia, P. nigrescens, P. tannerae, P. multissacharivorax, P. baroniae, P. denticola*, uncultivated phylotypes[c]	++/+++
Fusobacterium	*F. nucleatum, F. periodonticum*, uncultivated phylotypes[c]	++
Campylobacter	*C. rectus, C. gracilis, C. curvus, C. showae*	++
Synergistes	Uncultivated phylotypes[c]	?
Catonella	*C. morbi*	+
Selenomonas	*S. sputigena, S. noxia*, uncultivated phylotypes[c]	++
Centipeda	*C. periodontii*	+
Anaerobic cocci		
Veillonella	*V. parvula*, uncultivated phylotypes[c]	+
Megasphaera	Uncultivated phylotypes[c]	?
Anaerobic spirilla		
Treponema	*T. denticola, T. socranskii, T. parvum, T. maltophilum, T. lecithinolyticum*	++/+++
Facultative rods		
Capnocytophaga	*C. gingivalis, C. ochracea*	+
Eikenella	*E. corrodens*	++
Haemophilus	*H. aphrophilus*	+
Facultative cocci		
Neisseria	*N. mucosa, N. sicca*	+
Gram-positive		
Anaerobic rods		
Actinomyces	*A. israelii, A. gerencseriae, A. meyeri, A. odontolyticus*	+/++
Pseudoramibacter	*P. alactolyticus*	+
Filifactor	*F. alocis*	+
Eubacterium	*E. infirmum, E. saphenum, E. nodatum, E. brachy, E. minutum*	+/++
Mogibacterium	*M. timidum, M. pumilum, M. neglectum, M. vescum*	+
Propionibacterium	*P. acnes, P. propionicum*	++
Eggerthella	*E. lenta*	+
Olsenella	*O. uli, O. profusa*	+
Bifidobacterium	*B. dentium*	+
Slackia	*S. exigua*	+
Atopobium	*A. parvulum, A. minutum, A. rimae*	+
Solobacterium	*S. moorei*, uncultivated phylotypes[c]	+
Lactobacillus	*L. catenaformis*	+
Anaerobic cocci		
Peptostreptococcus	*P. micros, P. anaerobius*, uncultivated phylotypes[c]	++
Finegoldia	*F. magna*	++
Peptoniphilus	*P. asaccharolyticus, P. lacrimalis*	+
Anaerococcus	*A. prevotii*	+

continued

Table 5.2   Bacterial genera and respective common representatives occurring in endodontic infections (*continued*)

Genus	Common representatives	Pathogenicity[a,b]
Streptococcus	*S. anginosus, S. constellatus, S. intermedius*	++
Gemella	*G. morbillorum*	++
Facultative rods		
Actinomyces	*A. naeslundii*	+
Corynebacterium	*C. matruchotii*	+
Lactobacillus	*L. salivarius, L. acidophilus, L. paracasei*	+
Facultative cocci		
Streptococcus	*S. mitis, S. sanguinis, S. gordonii, S. oralis*	+/++
Enterococcus	*E. faecalis*	+
Granulicatella	*G. adiacens*	+

[a] Data according to pathogenicity tests in animals and/or to association with other human diseases.
[b] Except for some species and strains, data on anaerobic bacteria refer to mixed infections.
[c] For uncultivated phylotypes, Gram-staining patterns, cell morphology and relationship to oxygen are estimates based on the general features of the genus.

albicans in 21% of the samples from primary root canal infections.

Archaea. Archaea represent one of the three primary evolutionary domains of life, distinct in their phylogenetic relations to members of the domains *Bacteria* and *Eucarya.* Archaea comprise a highly diverse group of prokaryotes, distinct from bacteria. To date, no member of the *Archaea* domain has been described as a human pathogen. Methanogenic archaea have been detected in samples from subgingival plaque associated with periodontal disease [168]. Although one study failed to disclose archaea in necrotic root canals [342], in another investigation methanogenic archaea were found in 25% of the canals of teeth with chronic apical periodontitis [395]. Archaeal diversity was limited to a *Methanobrevibacter oralis*-like phylotype and the size of the archaeal population accounted for up to 2.5% of the total prokaryotic community (i.e., bacteria plus archaea).

Viruses. Viruses are not cells but particles structurally composed of a nucleic acid molecule (DNA or RNA) and a protein coat. They are inert in the extracellular environment and, as obligate intracellular parasites, are totally dependent on living cells to perform life functions. When viruses enter (infect) living cells, the viral nucleic acid molecule has the ability of directing the replication of the complete virus and the viral nucleic acid assumes control of the metabolic activities of the host cell. Because viruses require viable host cells to infect and use the cell's machinery to replicate the viral genome, they cannot survive in the root canal containing necrotic pulp tissue. The presence of viruses in the root canal has been reported only for noninflamed vital pulps of patients infected with the human immunodeficiency virus (HIV) [86]. On the other hand, herpesviruses, specifically human cytomegalovirus (HCMV) and Epstein–Barr virus (EBV), have been detected in apical periodontitis lesions [274-277,352], where living cells are present in abundance. It has been hypothesized that HCMV and EBV may be implicated in the pathogenesis of apical periodontitis as a direct result of virus infection and replication or as a result of virally induced impairment of local host defenses, which might give rise to overgrowth of pathogenic bacteria in the very apical part of the root canal [352]. Bacterial challenge emanating from the canals may cause an influx of herpesvirus-infected cells into the periradicular tissues. Reactivation of HCMV and/or EBV by tissue injury induced by bacteria may evoke impairment of host immune response in the periradicular microenvironment, changing the potential of local defense cells to mount an adequate response against infectious agents. Moreover, herpesvirus-infected inflammatory cells are stimulated to release proinflammatory cytokines [197,404]. HCMV and EBV transcripts have been found in high frequencies in the presence of symptoms [275,276], in lesions exhibiting elevated occurrence of anaerobic bacteria [277], and in cases of large periradicular bone destruction [276,277].

5.9.2 Symptomatic infections

Although it has been suggested that some Gram-negative anaerobic bacteria can be closely associated with the etiology of symptomatic apical periodontitis lesions [88,93,262,366,390,420], several studies have found rather similar frequencies of the same species in asymptomatic cases [15,76,100,140,307,313]. It would appear that factors other than the mere presence of a given putative pathogenic species can influence the development of symptoms. These factors include [314,331]:

- *Presence of virulent clonal types.* Clonal types of a given pathogenic bacterial species can significantly differ in their virulence ability [8,71,94,210,223]. A disease ascribed to a given pathogenic species is in fact caused by specific virulent clonal types of that species. Therefore, the possibility exists that the presence of virulent clonal types of candidate endodontic pathogens in the root canal may be a predisposing factor for pain.
- *Microbial synergism or additism.* Most of the presumed endodontic pathogens only show virulence or are significantly more virulent when in association with other species [13,69,147,304,375,418]. This is because of synergic or additive microbial interactions, which can influence virulence and play a role in symptom causation. It is entirely possible that the microbiota associated with symptomatic cases contains more virulent bacterial combinations.
- *Number of microbial cells.* The microbial load is well recognized as an important factor for a microorganism to cause disease. It is possible that the number of cells of a given species that is found in both symptomatic and asymptomatic infections is larger in the former.
- *Environmental cues.* A virulent clonal type of a given pathogenic species does not always express its virulence factors throughout its lifetime. A great deal of evidence indicates that the environment exerts an important role in inducing the turning on or the turning off of microbial virulence genes [10,72,152,413]. This is a crucial part of bacterial adaptation process to the environment and allows for establishment, optimal growth and survival in

the environment [73]. Microorganisms can sense environmental changes and then respond by expression of gene products, allowing them to effectively adapt to the varying environment. Throughout the different stages of the infectious process, different sets of virulence genes are turned on and off in response to different environmental cues [73]. Studies have demonstrated that environmental cues can influence gene/protein expression and consequently the behavior (including virulence) of some putative oral (and endodontic) pathogens, including *P. gingivalis*, *F. nucleatum*, *P. intermedia*, and oral treponemes [79,148,149,421,422]. If the root canal environmental conditions may be conducive to the expression of virulence genes, microbial virulence can be enhanced and symptoms can arise.

- *Host resistance.* It is well known that different individuals present different patterns of resistance to infections, and such differences can certainly become evident during an individual's lifetime [196]. Hypothetically, individuals who have reduced ability to cope with infections may be more prone to develop clinical symptoms.
- *Concomitant herpesvirus infection.* This is a factor that may be coupled with diminished host resistance. Active infections of apical periodontitis lesions by HCMV and/or EBV may be associated with symptomatology [275,276] (Fig. 5.23). Thus, active herpesvirus infections in apical periodontitis lesions may initiate or contribute to symptoms [352].

The changes in the microbiota from asymptomatic cases to symptomatic ones are not at all understood. Cross-sectional studies suggest microbial succession between these stages [336]. The possibility exists that, at a given moment during the endodontic infectious process, the microbiota reaches a certain degree of pathogenicity that elicits acute inflammation at the periradicular tissues with consequent development of pain and sometimes swelling. The structure of the endodontic bacterial communities in symptomatic teeth has been shown to be significantly different from that of asymptomatic teeth [336]. Differences are represented by different dominant species in the communities and higher number of species in symptomatic cases. Therefore, a shift in the structure of the microbial community is likely to occur before appearance of symptoms. Such a shift is probably a result of the arrival of new pathogenic species or

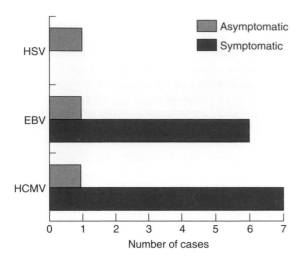

Fig. 5.23 Prevalence of herpesviruses in asymptomatic and symptomatic apical periodontitis lesions. Data according to Sabeti *et al.* [275].

of variations and rearrangements in the number of members of the bacterial consortium. Differences in the type and load of dominant species and the resulting bacterial interactions may be responsible for differences in the pathogenicity degree of the whole bacterial consortium. These findings confirmed that there is no key pathogen involved with symptomatic infections but, along with the factors mentioned above, the occurrence of certain specific bacterial combinations in infected root canals may be a decisive factor in causation of symptoms.

5.10 Persistent/secondary endodontic infections

Given the essential role played by microorganisms in the causation of periradicular inflammatory diseases, endodontic treatment should focus on both elimination of microbial cells colonizing the root canal system (through antiseptic means) and prevention of introduction of new microorganisms in the canal (through aseptic means). If microorganisms are allowed to remain in the root canal system at the time of filling, there is an increased risk of adverse outcome of the endodontic treatment [67,349,397]. Nonetheless, microbial persistence in the canal will not always lead to treatment failure. If the root canal filling succeeds in providing a proper apical and

coronal seal, residual microorganisms can be entombed within the root canal system, can have their access to the periradicular tissues denied, and can have acquisition of nutrients from tissue fluids prevented. In these instances, chances of treatment success are high. Thus, there are some requirements for residual microorganisms to survive in well-filled root canals and then to cause treatment failure.

The huge majority of root-canal-treated teeth with persistent apical periodontitis have been demonstrated to harbor an intraradicular infection [172,173]. This indicates that microorganisms can in some way acquire nutrients within filled root canals. Because virtually all microleakage studies have demonstrated that no root canal filling technique or material succeeds in promoting a fluid-tight coronal and apical seal of the root canal [98], residual microorganisms can derive nutrients from saliva (coronally seeping into the canal) or from the periradicular inflammatory exudate (apically or laterally seeping into the canal) [308]. Even though most necrotic pulp tissue is removed during chemomechanical procedures, remaining microorganisms can also utilize necrotic tissue remnants as nutrient source. Tissue remnants can be localized in isthmuses, irregularities, dentinal tubules, and lateral canals, which very often remain unaffected by instruments and irrigants [303,402,426]. In addition, even in the main root canal some dentinal walls can remain untouched after instrumentation [303,414], with different instrumentation techniques leaving at least 35% of the root canal surface area untouched [242]. Although pulp tissue remnants comprise only a temporary source of nutrients, they can maintain microbial survival before a sustainable source of nutrients is established by apical or coronal leakage.

Even if we consider that microorganisms in filled root canals may have a source of substrate, it seems worth pointing out that nutrients may not be available at all times, and when the source is established, the quantity is usually low. Indeed, an instrumented and filled root canal has a low amount, if any, of necrotic pulpal tissue remnants and a limited room for fluid seepage into the canal. As a consequence, availability of nutrients is low and residual microorganisms must be able to endure starvation, otherwise they die. Most anaerobic bacterial species commonly found in untreated root canals are not able to survive in a barren environment like a filled root canal. Nevertheless, some species, such as *E. faecalis*, have displayed the ability to withstand long periods of nutrient deprivation and to flourish again when the source of nutrients is re-established [70,289].

Remaining microorganisms must also survive the antimicrobial effects of endodontic filling materials. Most endodontic sealers have antimicrobial activity [3,42,144,302,305], which is however not pronounced and usually decreases after setting [222,297,358]. Theoretically, microorganisms in the very apical part of the canal, within dentinal tubules, embedded in necrotic tissue remnants or forming biofilm-like structures on uninstrumented canal walls may be protected from lethal effects of filling materials.

Free access of microorganisms to the periradicular tissues through the apical foramen or foraminas is necessary for them to wreak havoc on host tissues. Microleakage channels or voids by which periradicular tissue fluids can seep into the filled canal can also provide an avenue for communication between remaining intraradicular microorganisms and the periradicular tissues.

Acquiring nutrients, enduring starvation, surviving antimicrobial effects of materials and having access to the periradicular tissues may still not be sufficient for residual microorganisms to induce a persistent apical periodontitis lesion. After all, remaining microorganisms must ultimately reach sufficient numbers and be virulent enough to induce and/or sustain periradicular inflammation. If microorganisms are sequestered into the root canal system, they cannot be reached by host defenses and therefore can cause a persistent intraradicular infection. If remaining microorganisms are in the vicinity of the apical foramen or even within the apical periodontitis lesion, the development of a persistent infection will depend on the ability of those microorganisms to evade or overcome the host defenses. In the latter situation, an extraradicular infection can settle in and be the cause of treatment failure.

As one can realize, it is a difficult task for remaining microorganisms to cause endodontic failures in well-treated root canals. However, one should be mindful that this is not an impossible task. The ability of microorganisms to adapt to a modified environment, survive in adverse conditions, and cause persistent infections should never be underestimated.

5.10.1 Microbial composition and diversity

Unlike primary infections, a more restricted group of microbial species has been found in persistent or secondary intraradicular infections. *E. faecalis* and *C. albicans* have been more frequently detected in persistent or secondary infections associated with the unsatisfactory outcome of the endodontic treatment (Table 5.3). These species have been demonstrated to be resistant to commonly used endodontic medicaments [33,64,101,300,400,408], and special therapeutic strategies may be necessary to deal with infections involving these microorganisms. *Streptococcus* species have also been commonly found in persistent/secondary intraradicular infections [35,245,264,332,373]. Recent findings from molecular studies have also suggested that some anaerobic species commonly found in primary infections,

Table 5.3   Data from studies of microorganisms associated with root-canal-treated teeth evincing apical periodontitis lesions

Study	Identification method	Samples positive for the presence of microorganisms	*Enterococcus faecalis*	Fungi
Engström, 1964 [63]	Culture	39%	24%	–
Möller, 1966 [199]	Culture	57%	29%	3%
Molander et al., 1998 [198]	Culture	68%	47%	4%
Sundqvist et al., 1998 [373]	Culture	44%	38%	8%
Peciuliene et al., 2000 [235]	Culture	80%	70%	–
Peciuliene et al., 2001 [236]	Culture	83%	64%	18%
Hancock et al., 2001 [105]	Culture	63%	30%	3%
Cheung and Ho, 2001 [37]	Culture	67%	0%	17%
Rolph et al., 2001 [270]	Broad-range PCR	91%	0%	–
Pinheiro et al., 2003 [245]	Culture	85%	53%	4%
Siqueira and Rôças, 2004 [332]	Species-specific PCR	100%	77%	9%
Rôças et al., 2004 [264]	Species-specific PCR	100%	64%	0%

such as *T. forsythia, P. alactolyticus, P. propionicum, F. alocis, D. pneumosintes,* and *D. invisus,* can also be involved in persistent/secondary intraradicular infections [332,340] (Table 5.4). Persistent/secondary infections by *P. aeruginosa,* enteric rods and staphylococci leading to prolonged endodontic therapy have been reported [99,251,315]. These bacteria are highly likely to be secondary invaders that can gain entry into the root canal due to a breach in the aseptic chain during intracanal intervention.

E. faecalis is a facultatively anaerobic Gram-positive coccus that can be a normal inhabitant of the oral cavity. This species has been found in low prevalence values in cases of primary endodontic infections [24,63,266,321,368], and analysis of the prevalence of *E. faecalis* in these infections revealed that this species is more frequently detected in asymptomatic cases than in symptomatic ones [266] (Fig. 5.24). Unlike primary infections, *E. faecalis* has been frequently found in root-canal-treated teeth evincing persistent apical periodontitis lesions in prevalence

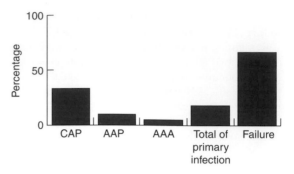

Fig. 5.24 Prevalence of *Enterococcus faecalis* in endodontic infections associated with different forms of periradicular diseases. AAP, acute apical periodontitis; AAA, acute apical abscess; CAP, chronic apical periodontitis. Data according to Rôças [266].

Table 5.4 Microorganisms detected in root-canal-treated teeth associated with apical periodontitis lesions. Data from molecular biology studies [332, 340]

Target species	Total[a]
Enterococcus faecalis	17/22 (77%)
Pseudoramibacter alactolyticus	12/22 (55%)
Propionibacterium propionicum	11/22 (50%)
Filifactor alocis	10/21 (48%)
Dialister pneumosintes	10/22 (46%)
Streptococcus spp.	5/22 (23%)
Tannerella forsythia	5/22 (23%)
Dialister invisus	3/22 (14%)
Campylobacter rectus	3/21 (14%)
Porphyromonas gingivalis	3/21 (14%)
Treponema denticola	3/21 (14%)
Fusobacterium nucleatum	2/21 (10%)
Prevotella intermedia	2/21 (10%)
Candida albicans	2/22 (9%)
Campylobacter gracilis	1/21 (5%)
Actinomyces radicidentis	1/21 (5%)
Porphyromonas endodontalis	1/21 (5%)
Peptostreptococcus micros	1/22 (5%)
Synergistes oral clone BA121	1/22 (5%)
Olsenella uli	1/22 (5%)

[a] Number of positive cases/number of examined cases.

values ranging from 30 to about 90% of the cases [63,105,198,235,245,264,266,288,332,373,411,423] (Table 5.3). Quantitative real-time PCR analysis has revealed that *E. faecalis* may constitute a median 0.98% (range 0.14–100%) of the overall bacterial load in root-canal-treated teeth [288]. Root-canal-treated teeth are about nine times more likely to harbor *E. faecalis* than cases of primary infections [266] (Fig. 5.24). This suggests that this species can be inhibited by other members of a mixed bacterial consortium commonly present in primary infections but that the bleak environmental conditions within filled root canals do not prevent its survival.

E. faecalis has some definite and candidate virulence factors, which may be involved in disease causation. They include cytolysin, lytic enzymes such as gelatinase and hyaluronidase, aggregation substance, pheromones, and lipoteichoic acid [43,136,143,205,290]. It remains to be clarified which of these factors, if any, play a role in the pathogenesis of persistent apical periodontitis lesions. However, the major involvement of *E. faecalis* with asymptomatic persistent apical periodontitis diseases supports the assumption that enterococci are in general not highly virulent microorganisms, and their emergence as pathogens can be much more related to its persistence than to high virulence [248].

For a given microorganism to survive in a filled root canal, it has to resist intracanal procedures of disinfection and to endure periods of starvation. Studies have revealed that *E. faecalis* has the ability to penetrate far into dentinal tubules [101,301] (Fig. 5.25). This property can enable this species to escape from

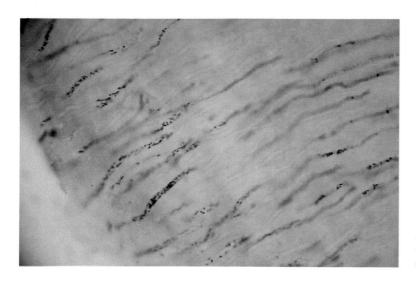

Fig. 5.25 Dentinal tubule infection by *Enterococcus faecalis* in dog's teeth after experimental infection. Notice that cells invaded the entire extent of some tubules up to the cementum.

the action of endodontic instruments and irrigants used during chemomechanical preparation [101,300]. In addition, *E. faecalis* has been shown to be able to form biofilms in root canals, and this ability can be important for bacterial resistance to and persistence after intracanal antimicrobial procedures [53]. *E. faecalis* is also resistant to calcium hydroxide [33], a commonly used intracanal medicament, and the ability to resist high pH values seems to be related to a functioning proton pump, which drives protons into the cell to acidify the cytoplasm [64]. Unlike most putative endodontic pathogens that are frequently found in primary infections, *E. faecalis* may colonize root canals in single infections [373] and such a relative independence of living without deriving nutrients from other bacteria can be extremely important for its establishment in filled root canals. Finally, environmental cues can also regulate gene expression in *E. faecalis*, affording this bacterium the ability to adapt to varying environmental conditions [136]. Indeed, it has been shown that *E. faecalis* can enter a viable but nonculturable (VBNC) state [174], which is a survival mechanism adopted by many bacteria when exposed to adverse environmental conditions, including low nutrient concentrations, low or high temperatures, high salinity and extreme pH [175]. In VBNC state bacteria lose the ability to grow in bacteriological media but maintain viability and pathogenicity and sometimes are able to resume division when favorable environmental conditions are restored. VBNC enterococcal cells appear as slightly elongated and are endowed with a wall more resistant to mechani-

cal disruption than dividing cells [299]. Figdor *et al.* [70] reported that *E. faecalis* has the ability to survive in environments with scarcity of nutrients and to flourish when the nutrient source is reestablished. In an *ex vivo* study, Sedgley *et al.* [289] demonstrated that *E. faecalis* has the capacity to recover from a prolonged starvation state in root-canal-treated teeth – when inoculated into root canals, this bacterium maintained viability for 12 months without additional nutrients. Thus, viable *E. faecalis* entombed at the time of root filling may provide a long-term nidus for subsequent infection. Taken together, all these properties help explain the significantly high prevalence of *E. faecalis* in root-canal-treated teeth.

Although fungi have been occasionally found in primary intraradicular infections, they seem to be more frequent in root-canal-treated teeth. Detection frequencies for *Candida* species in persistent/secondary infections range from 3 to 18% of the cases [37,62,198,199,236,245,332,373] (Table 5.3). Fungi can gain access to root canals via contamination during endodontic therapy or can overgrow after inefficient intracanal antimicrobial procedures, which can cause an imbalance in the microbiota [337]. *C. albicans* is by far the fungal species most commonly isolated from or detected in root-canal-treated teeth. This species has been considered as a dentinophilic microorganism due to its ability to colonize and invade dentin [292,293,319] (Fig. 5.26). In addition to the invading ability, *C. albicans* is also resistant to some intracanal medicaments, such as calcium hydroxide [399,400], which can also account

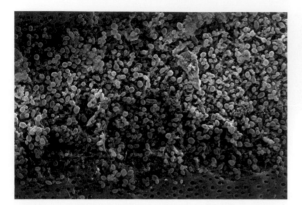

Fig. 5.26 Colonization of the dentinal root canal walls by *Candida albicans* (original magnification ×600).

for its presence in persistent root canal infections. *C. albicans* possesses virulence attributes that may play a role in disease causation. Mechanisms allegedly involved in its pathogenicity include (a) adaptability to a variety of environmental conditions, (b) adhesion to a variety of surfaces, including dentin, (c) production of hydrolytic enzymes, (d) morphological transition, (e) biofilm formation, and (f) evasion from and immunomodulation of the host defense [337].

5.11 Extraradicular infections

Apical periodontitis lesions are formed in response to intraradicular infection and by and large comprise an effective barrier against spread of the infection to the alveolar bone and to other body sites (Fig. 5.27). In most situations, apical inflammatory lesions succeed in preventing microorganisms from gaining access to the periradicular tissues. Nevertheless, in some specific circumstances, microorganisms can overcome this barrier and establish an extraradicular infection. The most common form of extraradicular infection is the acute apical abscess, characterized by purulent inflammation in the periradicular tissues in response to a massive egress of virulent bacteria from the root canal. There is, however, another form of extraradicular infection which, unlike the acute abscess, is usually characterized by absence of overt symptoms. Here microorganisms are established in the periradicular tissues, either by adherence to the apical external root surface in the form of biofilm-like structures [217,385] or by formation of cohesive

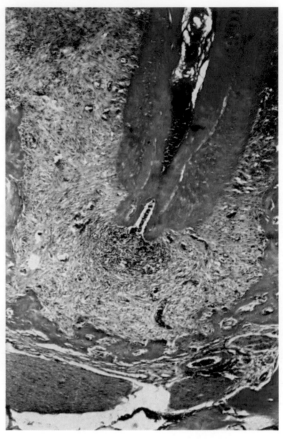

Fig. 5.27 Host defense against endodontic infection. A dense wall composed of defense cells is observed at the apical foramen of this rat tooth associated with apical periodontitis.

colonies within the body of the inflammatory lesion [211]. Extraradicular microorganisms have been discussed as one of the etiologies of persistence of apical periodontitis lesions in spite of diligent root canal treatment [386].

Conceivably, the extraradicular infection can be dependent on, or independent of the intraradicular infection [322]. For instance, the acute apical abscess is for the most part clearly dependent on the intraradicular infection: once the intraradicular infection is properly controlled by root canal treatment or tooth extraction and drainage of pus is achieved, the extraradicular infection is handled by the host defenses and usually subsides. Nonetheless, it should be appreciated that in some rare cases, bacteria that have participated in acute apical abscesses may persist in the periradicular tissues following resolution of the acute response and establish a persistent extraradicular infection associated with a chronic periradicular inflammation. This would then characterize an example of extraradicular infection independent of the intraradicular infection.

Studies using cultivation [364,384,406] or molecular methods [81,363,365] for microbial identification have reported the extraradicular occurrence of a complex microbiota associated with apical periodontitis lesions that do not respond favorably to the root canal treatment. Anaerobic bacteria have been reported to be the dominant microorganisms in several of those lesions [363,364]. Because the studies did not evaluate the bacteriological conditions of the apical part of the root canal, it is difficult to ascertain whether the extraradicular infections were dependent on or independent of an intraradicular infection.

The presence of bacterial colonies outside the root canal usually characterizes a borderline between the intraradicular infection and the inflamed periradicular tissues. Even so, their presence outside the canal may indicate an extraradicular infection, which can be dependent on the intraradicular infection in the sense that if the latter is eradicated or effectively controlled, the former can be handled and eliminated by the host.

In fact, most oral microorganisms are opportunistic pathogens and only a few species have the ability to challenge and overcome host defense mechanisms, acquire nutrients and thrive in the inflamed periradicular tissues and, then, establish an extraradicular infection. Of the several species of putative oral pathogens that have been detected in recalcitrant apical periodontitis lesions, some may have an apparatus of virulence that theoretically can allow them to invade and to survive in a hostile environment, such as the inflamed periradicular tissues. For instance, it is currently recognized that some *Actinomyces* species and *P. propionicum* can participate in extraradicular infections and cause a pathological entity called apical actinomycosis, which is successfully treated only by periradicular surgery [107,322,346]. Some other putative oral pathogens, such as *Treponema* species, *P. endodontalis*, *P. gingivalis*, *T. forsythia*, *Prevotella* species, and *F. nucleatum*, have also been detected in persistent chronic apical periodontitis lesions by culture, immunological or molecular studies [9,81,348,363,384]. Most of these species possess an array of virulence traits that may allow them to avoid

or overcome the host defenses in the periradicular tissues [27,68,118,391].

The incidence of extraradicular infections in untreated teeth is conceivably low [212,309] (Fig. 5.28), which is congruent with the high success rate of nonsurgical root canal treatment [347]. Even in root-canal-treated teeth with recalcitrant lesions, in which a higher incidence of extraradicular bacteria has been reported, a high rate of healing following retreatment [347] indicates that the major cause of endodontic disease is located within the root canal system, i.e., a persistent or secondary intraradicular infection. This has been confirmed by studies investigating the microbiological conditions of root canals associated with persistent apical periodontitis [198,245,265,332,373]. Based on this, one may assume that most of the extraradicular infections observed in root-canal-treated teeth could have been fostered by an intraradicular infection.

There are some situations that permit intraradicular bacteria to reach the periradicular tissues and establish an extraradicular infection [338]. This may be (a) a result of direct advance of some bacterial species that are able to overcome host defenses concentrated near the apical foramen or that manage to penetrate into the lumen of pocket (bay) cysts (Fig. 5.29), which is in direct communication with the apical foramen; (b) due to bacterial persistence in the periradicular lesion after remission of acute abscesses; (c) a sequel to apical extrusion of debris during root canal instrumentation (particularly after overinstrumentation). Bacteria embedded in dentinal chips can be physically protected from the host defense cells and therefore can persist in the periradicular tissues and sustain inflammation. The virulence and the quantity of the involved bacteria as well as the host's ability to deal with infection will be the decisive factors dictating whether an extraradicular infection will develop or not.

5.12 The focal infection theory

Focal infection connotes an infectious disorder caused by microorganisms or their products that have disseminated from a distant body site (focus of infection) [229]. Microorganisms from an infected oral site might spontaneously or after dental procedures enter blood circulation and cause disease in remote human sites. The relationship of oral infections and systemic diseases is not a new issue. Hippocrates,

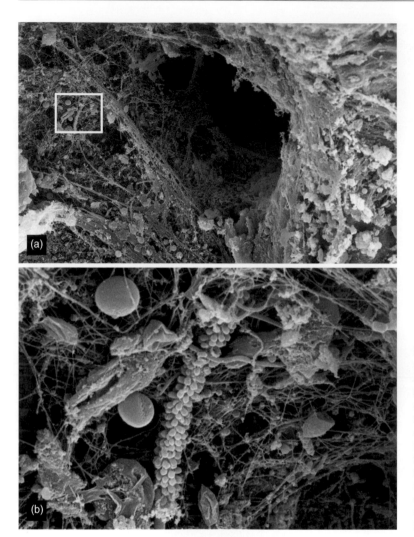

Fig. 5.28 (a) Scanning electron micrograph showing extensive bacterial colonization in the very apical part of the canal, near and at the apical foramen (original magnification ×550). (b) Inset, a fully developed "corn cob" is visualized in the tissue meshwork adjacent to the apical foramen, suggesting an extraradicular infection (original magnification ×4000). However, this occurrence is rare in untreated teeth. (Reproduced from Siqueira and Lopes [309] with permission.)

in 400BC, had reported that a patient was cured of arthritis after tooth extraction.

In a paper published in 1891, Miller described several human diseases, including nonoral diseases, which had been traced to the action of oral microorganisms [194]. He did not necessarily recommend extracting teeth considered to be a focus of infection, and indeed suggested treatment of infected root canals. Conservative dentistry suffered a severe attack at the beginning of the twentieth century, after spread of the concept of oral sepsis into the medical literature by the British physician William Hunter, in 1900 [124]. Hunter believed that oral sepsis was responsible for several infectious diseases in the body, including gastritis, middle ear suppurations, tonsilli-

tis, endocarditis, meningitis, nephritis, osteomyelitis, and other septic conditions [125]. In 1900, he wrote: "... the more I study it [oral sepsis as a cause of medical diseases] the more impressed I am, at once with its importance, and with the extraordinary neglect with which it is treated alike by physicians and surgeons. ... I confess I think it urgent, in the interests of the many sufferers from gastritis as well as in the interests of those suffering from pyogenic conditions generally, that some similar steps be taken with regard to the mouth – the chief channel of access, in my judgement, of all pyogenic infections" [124]. In 1911, he stressed the oral sepsis concept still more emphatically and attacked American dentists: "It is an all-important matter of sepsis and antisepsis that

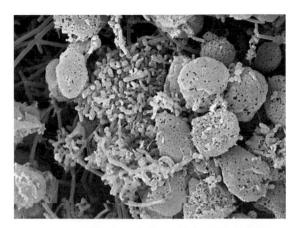

Fig. 5.29   Large bacterial colony being attacked by phagocytes within the lumen of a pocket (bay) cyst (original magnification ×3300). (Reproduced from Siqueira [308] with permission.)

concerns every branch of the medical profession, and concerns very closely the public health of the community. ... My clinical experience satisfies me that if oral sepsis could be successfully excluded, the other channels by which medical sepsis gains entrance into the body might almost be ignored. ... No one has probably had more reason than I have had to admire the sheer ingenuity and mechanical skill constantly displayed by the dental surgeon. Such are the fruits of this baneful so called 'conservative dentistry'. ... [T]he title that would best describe the dentistry here referred to would be that of 'septic dentistry'. Conservative it is, but only in one sense. It conserves the sepsis which it produces by the gold work it places over and around the teeth, by the satisfaction which it gives the patient, by the pride which the dentist responsible for it feels in his 'high-class American' work, and by his inability or unwillingness to recognise the septic effects which it produces" [125].

As a result of the focal infection theory, tooth extraction was favored over conservative, particularly endodontic treatment options for decades. Fortunately, improvements in dental treatment (including root canal therapy) accompanied by advances in biological research giving scientific support to treatment modalities significantly contributed to rescue the fate of the dental profession.

Nevertheless, a revived interest in the focal infection theory has been generated in the past few decades thanks to reports from epidemiological studies suggesting the involvement of oral microorganisms with systemic diseases [191,377]. Although there is a plethora of focal infections having the oral cavity as suspected focus, the most documented examples are bacterial endocarditis [23], brain abscess [169], and orthopedic joint infections [229]. Oral bacteria have also been implicated in aspiration pneumonia [284], preterm low birth weight [219], and coronary heart disease [20]. Infected root canals and apical periodontitis lesions have long been suggested to be potential foci of infection. Once again the focal infection concept is knocking on our doors. Fortunately, this time it can be evaluated and discussed on a scientific basis and has to go through the scrutiny of scientific methods.

To cause a focal disease, bacteria have obviously to travel from the focus of infection to a distant body site. This occurs via bacteremia, a condition in which viable bacteria are present in the blood circulation. There is no evidence showing that bacteremia spontaneously arises from infected root canals associated with a chronic apical periodontitis lesion. On the other hand, bacteremia can occur in cases of acute apical abscesses and during the treatment of infected root canals or periradicular surgery [11,12,22,49,170,209]. It is more probable that a bacteremia occurs if root canal procedures are performed beyond the apical foramen than when maintained within the confines of the root canal system [22]. Bender *et al.* [22] reported that the incidence of bacteremia was none if the instrumentation remained within the canal and 15% if it extended beyond the apical foramen. Even so, the bacteremia following endodontic procedures was demonstrated to last no longer than 10 minutes due to clearance of microorganisms from within the circulation. Using improved anaerobic cultivation methods, Baumgartner *et al.* [11,12] revealed that nonsurgical root canal treatment resulted in a lower incidence of bacteremia (3%, as a result of overinstrumentation) than surgical flap reflection (83%), periradicular curettage (33%) or tooth extraction (100%). In a study that performed intentional instrumentation beyond the apex, a 34–54% incidence of bacteremia was detected [138].

However, it has been recently demonstrated that bacteremia can occur even if instrumentation is maintained within the root canal system. Debelian *et al.* [50] investigated the incidence of bacteremia following endodontic treatment of teeth with apical periodontitis lesions. In the treatment of one-half of the patients, the first three reamers (sizes 15, 20, and 25) were used to a level 2 mm beyond the root apex, while in the other half, instrumentation ended inside the root canal, 1 mm short of the apex. Bacteremia was observed in 54% of the cases where instrumentation through the foramen occurred, and in 31% of the cases where instrumentation was confined to the canals. No statistically significant difference was found when the frequency of bacteremias in the two groups was compared. This may be explained by the fact that all instrumentation techniques induce apical extrusion of debris, some more than others, even when instrumentation is confined to the interior of the canal [4,123,177,253]. If debris is infected, bacteria are launched into the periradicular tissues and then can gain entry into the circulation. In a study where instrumentation was accomplished short of the apical foramen and patency files were not utilized [283], culture analysis revealed detectable bacteremia in 30% of the patients who had no positive preoperative control blood sample.

Therefore, there is no doubt that root canal procedures can induce bacteremia. The questions now are how frequently and at what magnitude (number of bacterial cells in the blood) bacteremia occurs, how long it persists and whether endodontic bacteria are able to cause disease at distant sites. It is very difficult to prove that a given oral microorganism is the causative agent of a focal infection. Although it has been demonstrated that the microbial species present in the blood of patients undergoing root canal treatment are of the same clonal types as those present in their root canals [51], such findings only mean that root canal treatment can cause bacteremia, but not that microorganisms from the root canal cause disease in remote sites of the body. For bacteria present in the bloodstream to reach other body sites and induce disease, they must (a) survive the host defenses in the blood vessels as well as in the distant body site, (b) encounter predisposing conditions in the distant body site for their attachment and further colonization, (c) reach sufficient numbers to induce disease, and (d) possess an array of virulence factors that can inflict direct or indirect damage to the host tissues.

It is apparent from well-conducted studies that oral bacteria are rarely a cause of systemic disease [229]. For instance, periodontal pathogens are very rarely a cause of endocarditis, with 102 reported cases due to *A. actinomycetemcomitans*, two due to *P. oralis*, one due to *Prevotella bivia*, one due to black-pigmented anaerobic bacteria, and five due to *Veillonella* species [228,234]. Except for *A. actinomycetemcomitans*,

which has been infrequently found in endodontic infections [317], the other species have been isolated from infected root canals or apical abscesses. As a matter of fact, obligate anaerobic bacteria from the oral cavity do not appear to survive well in other body locations and viridans group streptococci, considered the principal oral culprits in endocarditis, are not primary pathogens but rather opportunistic bacteria that usually require altered biologic tissue to induce disease [228].

Culture-independent procedures for bacterial identification have revealed previously unsuspected degrees of diversity in the oral microbiota [159,231]. Since many oral (and endodontic) bacteria remain to be cultivated and then fully characterized, their pathogenicity and involvement in causation of disease have yet to be elucidated. A study using molecular technology revealed a large amount of bacterial DNA in blood specimens from healthy individuals [215] and many of the DNA sequences detected were from uncultivated and unknown bacteria. The presence of bacterial DNA in the blood has important implications for a possible role of previously uncharacterized bacterial species in some diseases, sometimes distant from the focus of infection. It would appear that to date no molecular study has been performed to detect the occurrence of uncultivated bacterial phylotypes from the oral cavity in bacteremias following endodontic procedures. In addition, no study has evaluated the presence of those phylotypes in remote diseases in the body. Therefore, future research is warranted to ascertain whether uncultivated bacteria from the oral cavity can be involved in focal diseases.

The establishment of a causal link between oral disease and disorders in remote parts of the body depends on some important factors. Perhaps one of the most important factors is to determine if the microorganism associated with the medical disorder is the same as the suspected oral microorganism, including species, biotype, serotype, and genotype. In addition, the onset of the medical disease should follow the onset of the oral disease. In cases where the dental procedure is suspected to cause bacteremia, the onset of the medical disease should be within the incubation period [350].

Although there is no definitive evidence that bacteria from infected root canals cause systemic diseases after bacteremia, there is a potential risk in some special patients. Consequently, it would be prudent to avoid certain situations that could predispose to bacteremias, such as over-instrumentation. Over-instrumentation induces damage to the periradicular tissues, affecting cells, extracellular matrix and vessels. When over-instrumentation occurs during preparation of infected root canals, large numbers of bacteria can also be carried into the periradicular tissues. Bacteria introduced in the periradicular tissues can then enter injured vessels and a bacteremia ensues. It has been postulated that lymphatics, and not blood vessels (where the pressure gradient is outward and not inward after trauma), may be the primary means of entry of oral bacteria into the blood [229]. In addition to a higher risk of bacteremia, as alluded to earlier, bacteria propelled to the periradicular tissues may cause postoperative pain or even failure of root canal treatment due to an extra-radicular infection [338]. For all these reasons, over-instrumentation should be avoided.

The focal infection theory has remained controversial due to the lack of indisputable evidence regarding the causal relationship between endodontic infections and other medical conditions. A recent cross-sectional study [80] revealed that there was no association between root-canal-treated teeth and coronary heart disease nor between teeth with apical periodontitis and coronary heart disease. Nonsurgical endodontics is perhaps the least likely of dental treatment procedures to produce a significant bacteremia in either incidence or magnitude [229]. One should bear in mind that bacteremia can occur naturally as a result of normal daily activities, including toothbrushing and mastication [97]. Because of the 1000–8000 times greater chance of any bacteremia originating from normal daily activities, it is equally impossible to determine if the bacteremia emanated from the endodontic intervention or a time before or after it [229]. Whatever the origin, bacteremias are usually transient. Even so, in the absence of clear evidence regarding the effects of bacteremia in some compromised patients and before elucidation of the speculative involvement of uncultivated bacteria, empirical consensus indicates that antibiotic prophylaxis should be performed in patients at risk to develop infective endocarditis. Furthermore, antibiotic prophylaxis should also be considered for immunosuppressed patients, individuals with indwelling catheters or patients with orthopedic prosthetic devices, who may have some benefit from antibiotic prophylaxis, although there is not clear evidence in this regard [228].

5.13 Systemic antibiotics for endodontic infections

A hundred years ago infectious diseases were the major recognized causes of death in the world. The advent of antibiotics resulted in a significant decline in the incidence of life-threatening infections and heralded a new era in the therapy of infectious diseases. Over time, however, microbial evolutionary responses to the selective pressure exerted by antibiotics have resulted in microbial species resistant to virtually every known antibiotic agent [111]. The rapid emergence of resistant microbial strains comes as a consequence of the astonishing power of natural selection among microorganisms. If a given member of a microbial community possesses genes of resistance against a certain antibiotic and the community is persistently exposed to the drug, the resistant microorganism is selected to emerge and multiply at the expense of the susceptible portion of the community. The emergence of multidrug-resistant strains of several bacterial species capable of causing life-threatening infections is of particular concern [111,182,233,380,410]. Antibiotic resistance among obligately anaerobic bacteria is increasing, with resistance to penicillins, clindamycin, and cephalosporins noted at community hospitals and major medical centers [112,113].

Among oral bacteria, resistance has been found in *F. nucleatum* strains for penicillin, amoxicillin and metronidazole, in *P. intermedia* for tetracycline and amoxicillin, and in *A. actinomycetemcomitans* for amoxicillin and azithromycin [393]. Erythromycin has presented decreased activity against nonpigmented *Prevotella* and *Fusobacterium* [115,163]. Production of beta-lactamase by oral bacteria has also been reported, with the most prominent beta-lactamase-producing bacteria belonging to the anaerobic genus *Prevotella* [25,32,75,106,392]. Kuriyama *et al.* [163] revealed that beta-lactamase was detected in 36% of the black-pigmented *Prevotella* and 32% of the non-pigmented *Prevotella* species isolated from pus samples of oral abscesses. Other enzyme-producing oral anaerobic species include strains of *F. nucleatum*, *P. acnes*, *Actinomyces* species, and *Peptostreptococcus* species [32,75,106,392]. Facultative bacteria, such as *Capnocytophaga* species and *Neisseria* species, have also been detected among the enzyme-producers [106].

Overuse and misuse of antibiotics have been considered as the major cause responsible for the emergence of multidrug-resistant strains. Improper use of antibiotics includes use in cases with no infection, erroneous choice of the agent, dosage and/or duration of therapy, and excessive use in prophylaxis [226,227]. Antibiotics are used in clinical practice far more often than necessary. Whilst antibiotic therapy is actually warranted in about 20% of the individuals who are seen for clinical infectious disease, antibiotics are prescribed up to 80% of the time. To complicate matters further, in up to 50% of cases recommended agents, doses or duration of therapy are not correct [182].

The appalling rise in the frequency of multidrug resistance among leading pathogens should cause great concern and incite a commitment to act carefully and responsibly. A single erroneous use of antibiotics can be a significant contribution to the current scenario of increasing microbial resistance. Diseases that were effectively treated in the past with a given antibiotic may now require the use of another drug, usually more expensive and potentially more toxic, to achieve effective antimicrobial treatment. Unfortunately, in many cases the new drug may not even be effective.

Antibiotics are defined as naturally occurring substances of microbial origin or similar synthetic (or semi-synthetic) substances that have antimicrobial activity in low concentrations, by inhibiting the growth of or killing selective microorganisms. The purpose of antibiotic therapy is to aid the host defenses in controlling and eliminating microorganisms that temporarily have overwhelmed the host defense mechanisms [226]. Based on the discussion above, it becomes clear that the most important decision-making in antibiotic therapy is not so much what antibiotic should be employed, but whether antibiotics should be used at all [225]. One should bear in mind that antibiotics are very useful drugs classically used to treat or help to treat infectious disease and for prophylaxis in some well-selected cases. The future of infectious disease treatment will certainly depend on how responsible we are now in prescribing these drugs to our patients.

The vast majority of infections of endodontic origin are treated without the need for antibiotics. Due to the absence of blood circulation in a necrotic pulp, antibiotics cannot reach and then eliminate microorganisms present in the root canal system. Thus, the source of infection is unaffected by systemic antibiotic therapy. On the other hand, antibiotics can help impede spread of the infection and the development

of secondary infections in medically compromised patients. Therefore, antibiotic therapy can be a valuable adjunct for the management of some cases of endodontic infection. The rare but selective occasions in which antibiotics are indicated in endodontic practice include:

- Acute apical abscesses associated with systemic involvement, including fever, malaise, and lymphadenopathy.
- Spreading infections resulting in cellulitis, progressive diffuse swelling and/or trismus.
- Acute apical abscesses (even with localized swelling) in medically compromised patients who are at increased risk of a secondary infection at a distant site following bacteremia.
- Prophylaxis for medically compromised patients during routine endodontic therapy with procedures expected to cause significant bacteremia.
- Some cases of persistent exudation not resolved after revision of intracanal procedures.
- Replantation of avulsed teeth.

Acute apical abscess in a healthy patient without systemic involvement and displaying localized swelling is no indication for systemic antibiotic therapy. Such cases are better treated by incision for drainage and root canal intervention to control the intraradicular infection.

Given the circumstances in which antibiotics are prescribed, patients under systemic antibiotic therapy must be monitored daily. The best practical guide for determining the duration of antibiotic therapy is clinical improvement of the patient. When clinical evidence indicates that the infection is certain to resolve or is resolved, antibiotics should be administered for no longer than 1 or 2 days more.

Selection of antibiotics in clinical practice is either empirical or based on the results of microbial susceptibility test. For diseases with known microbial causes, empirical therapy may be used. This is especially applicable to infections of endodontic origin, because culture-dependent antimicrobial tests can take too long to provide results about the susceptibility of endodontic anaerobic bacteria to antibiotics (7–14 days). Therefore, it is preferable to opt for an antimicrobial agent whose spectrum of action includes the most commonly detected bacteria. Most of the root canal microbiota is susceptible to penicillins [18,128,151], which make them the drugs of first choice to be used in infections of endodontic origin. Since the use of antibiotics is restricted to severe infections or to prophylaxis, it seems prudent to use amoxicillin, a semi-synthetic penicillin with broad spectrum of antimicrobial activity. In even more serious cases, including life-threatening conditions, association of amoxicillin with clavulanic acid or metronidazole may be required to achieve optimum antimicrobial effects as a result of the extended spectrum of action to include penicillin-resistant strains. In patients allergic to penicillins or in cases refractory to amoxicillin therapy, clindamycin is indicated. Clindamycin has a strong antimicrobial activity against oral anaerobes [162,164].

The risk/benefit ratio should be always weighted before prescription of antibiotics. Appropriately selected patients will benefit from systemically administered antibiotics. A restrictive and conservative use of systemic antibiotics is highly recommended in endodontic practice. Indiscriminate use of antibiotics is contrary to sound clinical practice. This may cause a selective pressure and consequent overgrowth of intrinsically resistant bacteria. This again predisposes to secondary infections and super-infections, and can render drugs ineffective against potentially fatal medical infectious diseases.

5.14 References

1. Aas JA, Dardis SR, Griffen AL, Stokes LN, Lee AM, Dewhirst FE, *et al* (2003) Molecular analysis of bacteria associated with caries in permanent teeth. *Journal of Dental Research* **83**, IADR Abstract No. 25715.
2. Akira S (2003) Mammalian toll-like receptors. *Current Opinion in Microbiology* **15**, 5–11.
3. al-Khatib ZZ, Baum RH, Morse DR, Yesilsoy C, Bhambhani S, Furst ML (1990) The antimicrobial effect of various endodontic sealers. *Oral Surgery, Oral Medicine, Oral Pathology* **70**, 784–90.
4. al-Omari MA, Dummer PM (1995) Canal blockage and debris extrusion with eight preparation techniques. *Journal of Endodontics* **21**, 154–8.
5. Amann RI, Ludwig W, Schleifer KH (1995) Phylogenetic identification and in situ detection of individual microbial cells without cultivation. *Microbiological Reviews* **59**, 143–69.
6. Atlas RM (1997) *Principles of microbiology*, 2nd edn. Dubuque, NM: WCB Publishers.
7. Bae KS, Baumgartner JC, Shearer TR, David LL (1997) Occurrence of *Prevotella nigrescens* and *Prevotella intermedia* in infections of endodontic origin. *Journal of Endodontics* **23**, 620–3.
8. Baker PJ, Dixon M, Evans RT, Roopenian DC (2000) Heterogeneity of *Porphyromonas gingivalis* strains in the induction of alveolar bone loss in mice. *Oral Microbiology and Immunology* **15**, 27–32.
9. Barnett F, Stevens R, Tronstad L (1990) Demonstration of *Bacteroides intermedius* in periapical tissue using indirect immunofluorescence microscopy. *Endodontics and Dental Traumatology* **6**, 153–6.
10. Bassler BL (1999) How bacteria talk to each other: regulation of gene expression by quorum sensing. *Current Opinion in Microbiology* **2**, 582–7.
11. Baumgartner JC, Heggers JP, Harrison JW (1976) The incidence of bacteremias related to endodontic procedures. I. Nonsurgical endodontics. *Journal of Endodontics* **2**, 135–40.
12. Baumgartner JC, Heggers JP, Harrison JW (1977) Incidence of bacteremias related to endodontic procedures. II. Surgical endodontics. *Journal of Endodontics* **3**, 399–402.
13. Baumgartner JC, Falkler WA Jr, Beckerman T (1992) Experimentally induced infection by oral anaerobic microorganisms in a mouse model. *Oral Microbiology and Immunology* **7**, 253–6.
14. Baumgartner JC, Falkler WA Jr, Bernie RS, Suzuki JB (1992) Serum IgG reactive with oral anaerobic microorganisms associated with infections of endodontic origin. *Oral Microbiology and Immunology* **7**, 106–10.
15. Baumgartner JC, Watkins BJ, Bae KS, Xia T (1999) Association of black-pigmented bacteria with endodontic infections. *Journal of Endodontics* **25**, 413–15.
16. Baumgartner JC, Watts CM, Xia T (2000) Occurrence of *Candida albicans* in infections of endodontic origin. *Journal of Endodontics* **26**, 695–8.
17. Baumgartner JC, Khemaleelakul SU, Xia T (2003) Identification of spirochetes (treponemes) in endodontic infections. *Journal of Endodontics* **29**, 794–7.
18. Baumgartner JC, Xia T (2003) Antibiotic susceptibility of bacteria associated with endodontic abscesses. *Journal of Endodontics* **29**, 44–7.
19. Baumgartner JC, Siqueira JF Jr, Xia T, Rôças IN (2004) Geographical differences in bacteria detected in endodontic infections using polymerase chain reaction. *Journal of Endodontics* **30**, 141–4.
20. Beck J, Gracia R, Heiss G, Vokonas PS, Offenbacher S (1996) Periodontal disease and cardiovascular disease. *Journal of Periodontology* **67**, 1123–37.
21. Becker MR, Paster BJ, Leys EJ, Moeschberger ML, Kenyon SG, Galvin JL, *et al.* (2002) Molecular analysis of bacterial species associated with childhood caries. *Journal of Clinical Microbiology* **40**, 1001–9.
22. Bender IB, Seltzer S, Yermish M (1960) The incidence of bacteremia in endodontic manipulation. *Oral Surgery, Oral Medicine, Oral Pathology* **13**, 353–60.
23. Berbari E, Cockerill FR III, Steckelberg JM (1997) Infective endocarditis due to unusual or fastidious microorganisms. *Mayo Clinic Proceedings* **72**, 532–42.
24. Bergenholtz G (1974) Micro-organisms from necrotic pulp of traumatized teeth. *Odontologisk Revy* **25**, 347–58.
25. Bernal LA, Guillot E, Paquet C, Mouton C (1998) beta-Lactamase-producing strains in the species *Prevotella intermedia* and *Prevotella nigrescens*. *Oral Microbiology and Immunology* **13**, 36–40.
26. Bjornson HS (1984) Activation of Hageman factor by lipopolysaccharides of *Bacteroides fragilis*, *Bacteroides*

vulgatus, and *Fusobacterium mortiferum. Reviews of Infectious Diseases* **6** (Suppl 1), S30–3.

27. Bolstad AI, Jensen HB, Bakken V (1996) Taxonomy, biology, and periodontal aspects of *Fusobacterium nucleatum. Clinical Microbiology Reviews* **9**, 55–71.

28. Boneca IG (2005) The role of peptidoglycan in pathogenesis. *Current Opinion in Microbiology* **8**, 46–53.

29. Bowden GHW (2000) The microbial ecology of dental caries. *Microbial Ecology in Health and Disease* **12**, 138–48.

30. Brinig MM, Lepp PW, Ouverney CC, Armitage GC, Relman DA (2003) Prevalence of bacteria of division TM7 in human subgingival plaque and their association with disease. *Applied and Environmental Microbiology* **69**, 1687–94.

31. Brook I (1986) Encapsulated anaerobic bacteria in synergistic infections. *Microbiological Reviews* **50**, 452–7.

32. Brook I, Frazier EH, Gher ME Jr (1996) Microbiology of periapical abscesses and associated maxillary sinusitis. *Journal of Periodontology* **67**, 608–10.

33. Byström A, Claesson R, Sundqvist G (1985) The antibacterial effect of camphorated paramonochlorophenol, camphorated phenol and calcium hydroxide in the treatment of infected root canals. *Endodontics and Dental Traumatology* **1**, 170–5.

34. Carlsson J, Herrmann BF, Hofling JF, Sundqvist GK (1984) Degradation of the human proteinase inhibitors alpha-1-antitrypsin and alpha-2-macroglobulin by *Bacteroides gingivalis. Infection and Immunity* **43**, 644–8.

35. Chavez de Paz L, Svensäter G, Dahlén G, Bergenholtz G (2005) Streptococci from root canals in teeth with apical periodontitis receiving endodontic treatment. *Oral Surgery, Oral Medicine, Oral Pathology, Oral Radiology and Endodontics* **100**, 232–41.

36. Chavez de Paz LE, Molander A, Dahlén G (2004) Gram-positive rods prevailing in teeth with apical periodontitis undergoing root canal treatment. *International Endodontic Journal* **37**, 579–87.

37. Cheung GS, Ho MW (2001) Microbial flora of root canal-treated teeth associated with asymptomatic periapical radiolucent lesions. *Oral Microbiology and Immunology* **16**, 332–7.

38. Chhour KL, Nadkarni MA, Byun R, Martin FE, Jacques NA, Hunter N (2005) Molecular analysis of microbial diversity in advanced caries. *Journal of Clinical Microbiology* **43**, 843–9.

39. Choi BK, Lee HJ, Kang JH, Jeong GJ, Min CK, Yoo YJ (2003) Induction of osteoclastogenesis and matrix metalloproteinase expression by the lipooligosaccharide of Treponema denticola. *Infection and Immunity* **71**, 226–33.

40. Chu FC, Tsang CS, Chow TW, Samaranayake LP (2005) Identification of cultivable microorganisms from primary endodontic infections with exposed and unexposed pulp space. *Journal of Endodontics* **31**, 424–9.

41. Citron DM (2002) Update on the taxonomy and clinical aspects of the genus Fusobacterium. *Clinical Infectious Diseases* **35** (Suppl 1), S22–7.

42. Cobankara FK, Altinoz HC, Ergani O, Kav K, Belli S (2004) In vitro antibacterial activities of root-canal sealers by using two different methods. *Journal of Endodontics* **30**, 57–60.

43. Coburn PS, Gilmore MS (2003) The *Enterococcus faecalis* cytolysin: a novel toxin active against eukaryotic and prokaryotic cells. *Cellular Microbiology* **5**, 661–9.

44. Collins LMC, Dawes C (1987) The surface area of the adult human mouth and thickness of the salivary film covering the teeth and oral mucosa. *Journal of Dental Research* **66**, 1300–2.

45. Conrads G, Gharbia SE, Gulabivala K, Lampert F, Shah HN (1997) The use of a 16s rDNA directed PCR for the detection of endodontopathogenic bacteria. *Journal of Endodontics* **23**, 433–8.

46. Dahlén G, Bergenholtz G (1980) Endotoxic activity in teeth with necrotic pulps. *Journal of Dental Research* **59**, 1033–40.

47. Dahlén G, Fabricius L, Heyden G, Holm SE, Möller AJ (1982) Apical periodontitis induced by selected bacterial strains in root canals of immunized and nonimmunized monkeys. *Scandinavian Journal of Dental Research* **90**, 207–16.

48. Dahlén G, Magnusson BC, Möller A (1981) Histological and histochemical study of the influence of lipopolysaccharide extracted from *Fusobacterium nucleatum* on the periapical tissues in the monkey *Macaca fascicularis. Archives of Oral Biology* **26**, 591–8.

49. Debelian GJ, Olsen I, Tronstad L (1994) Systemic diseases caused by oral microorganisms. *Endodontics and Dental Traumatology* **10**, 57–65.

50. Debelian GJ, Olsen I, Tronstad L (1995) Bacteremia in conjunction with endodontic therapy. *Endodontics and Dental Traumatology* **11**, 142–9.

51. Debelian GJ, Eribe ER, Olsen I, Tronstad L (1997) Ribotyping of bacteria from root canal and blood of patients receiving endodontic therapy. *Anaerobe* **3**, 237–43.

52. Dewhirst FE, Tamer MA, Ericson RE, Lau CN, Levanos VA, Boches SK, *et al.* (2000) The diversity of periodontal spirochetes by 16S rRNA analysis. *Oral Microbiology and Immunology* **15**, 196–202.

53. Distel JW, Hatton JF, Gillespie MJ (2002) Biofilm formation in medicated root canals. *Journal of Endodontics* **28**, 689–93.

54. Dobell C (1932) *Antony van Leeuwenhoek and his "little animals".* London: Staples Press.

55. Dougherty WJ, Bae KS, Watkins BJ, Baumgartner JC (1998) Black-pigmented bacteria in coronal and apical segments of infected root canals. *Journal of Endodontics* **24**, 356–8.

56. Drucker DB, Natsiou I (2000) Microbial ecology of the dental root canal. *Microbial Ecology in Health and Disease* **12**, 160–9.

57. Dunny GM, Leonard BA (1997) Cell–cell communication in Gram-positive bacteria. *Annual Reviews in Microbiology* **51**, 527–64.

58. Dwyer TG, Torabinejad M (1980) Radiographic and histologic evaluation of the effect of endotoxin on the periapical tissues of the cat. *Journal of Endodontics* **7**, 31–5.

59. Dykhuizen DE (1998) Santa Rosalia revisited: why are there so many species of bacteria? *Antonie Van Leeuwenhoek* **73**, 25–33.

60. Eckburg PB, Bik EM, Bernstein CN, Purdom E, Dethlefsen L, Sargent M, Gill SR, Nelson KE, Relman DA (2005) Diversity of the human intestinal microbial flora. *Science* **308**, 1635–8.

61. Eftimiadi C, Stashenko P, Tonetti M, Mangiante PE, Massara R, Zupo S, *et al.* (1991) Divergent effect of the anaerobic bacteria by-product butyric acid on the immune response: suppression of T-lymphocyte proliferation and stimulation of interleukin-1 beta production. *Oral Microbiology and Immunology* **6**, 17–23.

62. Egan MW, Spratt DA, Ng YL, Lam JM, Moles DR, Gulabivala K (2002) Prevalence of yeasts in saliva and root canals of teeth associated with apical periodontitis. *International Endodontic Journal* **35**, 321–9.

63. Engström B (1964) The significance of enterococci in root canal treatment. *Odontologisk Revy* **15**, 87–106.

64. Evans M, Davies JK, Sundqvist G, Figdor D (2002) Mechanisms involved in the resistance of *Enterococcus faecalis* to calcium hydroxide. *International Endodontic Journal* **35**, 221–8.

65. Fabricius L, Dahlén G, Holm SE, Möller AJR (1982) Influence of combinations of oral bacteria on periapical tissues of monkeys. *Scandinavian Journal of Dental Research* **90**, 200–6.

66. Fabricius L, Dahlén G, Ohman AE, Möller AJR (1982) Predominant indigenous oral bacteria isolated from infected root canals after varied times of closure. *Scandinavian Journal of Dental Research* **90**, 134–44.

67. Fabricius L, Dahlén G, Sundqvist G, Happonen RP, Möller AJR (2006) Influence of residual bacteria on periapical tissue healing after chemomechanical treatment and root filling of experimentally infected monkey teeth. *European Journal of Oral Sciences* **114**, 278–85.

68. Fenno JC, McBride BC (1998) Virulence factors of oral treponemes. *Anaerobe* **4**, 1–17.

69. Feuille F, Ebersole JL, Kesavalu L, Steffen MJ, Holt SC (1996) Mixed infection with *Porphyromonas gingivalis* and *Fusobacterium nucleatum* in a murine lesion model: potential synergistic effects on virulence. *Infection and Immunity* **64**, 2095–100.

70. Figdor D, Davies JK, Sundqvist G (2003) Starvation survival, growth and recovery of *Enterococcus faecalis* in human serum. *Oral Microbiology and Immunology* **18**, 234–9.

71. Finlay BB, Falkow S (1989) Common themes in microbial pathogenicity. *Microbiological Reviews* **53**, 210–30.

72. Finlay BB, Falkow S (1997) Common themes in microbial pathogenicity revisited. *Microbiology and Molecular Biology Reviews* **61**, 136–69.

73. Forng, R-Y, Champagne C, Simpson W, Genco CA (2000) Environmental cues and gene expression in *Porphyromonas gingivalis* and *Actinobacillus actinomycetemcomitans*. *Oral Diseases* **6**, 351–65.

74. Foschi F, Cavrini F, Montebugnoli L, Stashenko P, Sambri V, Prati C (2005) Detection of bacteria in endodontic samples by polymerase chain reaction assays and association with defined clinical signs in Italian patients. *Oral Microbiology and Immunology* **20**, 289–95.

75. Fosse T, Madinier I, Hitzig C, Charbit Y (1999) Prevalence of beta-lactamase-producing strains among 149 anaerobic Gram-negative rods isolated from periodontal pockets. *Oral Microbiology and Immunology* **14**, 352–7.

76. Fouad AF, Barry J, Caimano M, Clawson M, Zhu Q, Carver R, *et al.* (2002) PCR-based identification of bacteria associated with endodontic infections. *Journal of Clinical Microbiology* **40**, 3223–31.

77. Fouad AF, Kum KY, Clawson ML, Barry J, Abenoja C, Zhu Q, *et al.* (2003) Molecular characterization of the presence of *Eubacterium* spp and *Streptococcus* spp in endodontic infections. *Oral Microbiology and Immunology* **18**, 249–55.

78. Fredricks DN, Relman DA (1996) Sequence-based identification of microbial pathogens: a reconsideration of Koch's postulates. *Clinical Microbiology Reviews* **9**, 18–33.

79. Frias J, Olle E, Alsina M (2001) Periodontal pathogens produce quorum sensing signal molecules. *Infection and Immunity* **69**, 3431–4.

80. Frisk F, Hakeberg M, Ahlqwist M, Bengtsson C (2003) Endodontic variables and coronary heart disease. *Acta Odont Scand* **61**, 257–62.

81. Gatti JJ, Dobeck JM, Smith C, White RR, Socransky SS, Skobe Z (2000) Bacteria of asymptomatic periradicular endodontic lesions identified by DNA–DNA hybridization. *Endodontics and Dental Traumatology* **16**, 197–204.

82. Gharbia SE, Haapasalo M, Shah HN, Kotiranta A, Lounatmaa K, Pearce MA, *et al.* (1994) Characterization of *Prevotella intermedia* and *Prevotella nigrescens* isolates from periodontic and endodontic infections. *Journal of Periodontology* **65**, 56–61.

83. Gibbons RJ, Engle LP (1964) Vitamin K compounds in bacteria that are obligate anaerobes. *Science* **146**, 1307–9.

84. Gillespie MJ, Smutko J, Haraszthy GG, Zambon JJ (1993) Isolation and partial characterization of the *Campylobacter rectus* cytotoxin. *Microbial Pathogenesis* **14**, 203–15.

85. Ginsburg I (2002) Role of lipoteichoic acid in infection and inflammation. *Lancet Infectious Diseases* **2**, 171–9.

86. Glick M, Trope M, Bagasra O, Pliskin ME (1991) Human immunodeficiency virus infection of fibroblasts of dental pulp in seropositive patients. *Oral Surgery, Oral Medicine, Oral Pathology* **71**, 733–6.

87. Godon J J, Morinière J, Moletta M, Gaillac M, Bru V, Delgènes J-P (2005) Rarity associated with specific ecological niches in the bacterial world: the 'Synergistes' example. *Environmental Microbiology* **7**, 213–24.

88. Gomes BP, Lilley JD, Drucker DB (1996) Clinical significance of dental root canal microflora. *Journal of Dentistry* **24**, 47–55.

89. Gomes BP, Jacinto RC, Pinheiro ET, Sousa EL, Zaia AA, Ferraz CC, *et al.* (2005) *Porphyromonas gingivalis*, *Porphyromonas endodontalis*, *Prevotella intermedia* and *Prevotella nigrescens* in endodontic lesions

detected by culture and by PCR. *Oral Microbiology and Immunology* **20**, 211–15.

90. Grandel U, Grimminger F (2003) Endothelial responses to bacterial toxins in sepsis. *Critical Reviews in Immunology* **23**, 267–99.

91. Grenier D, Mayrand D (1985) Cytotoxic effects of culture supernatants of oral bacteria and various organic acids on Vero cells. *Canadian Journal of Microbiology* **31**, 302–4.

92. Grenier D, Mayrand D (1986) Nutritional relationships between oral bacteria. *Infection and Immunity* **53**, 616–20.

93. Griffee MB, Patterson SS, Miller CH, Kafrawy AH, Newton CW (1980) The relationship of *Bacteroides melaninogenicus* to symptoms associated with pulpal necrosis. *Oral Surgery, Oral Medicine, Oral Pathology* **50**, 457–61.

94. Griffen AL, Lyons SR, Becker MR, Moeschberger ML, Leys EJ (1999) *Porphyromonas gingivalis* strain variability and periodontitis. *Journal of Clinical Microbiology* **37**, 4028–33.

95. Griffen AL, Kumar PS, Leys EJ (2003) *A quantitative, molecular view of oral biofilm communities in health and disease suggests a role for uncultivated species.* Polymicrobial diseases, American Society for Microbiology conferences, Lake Tahoe, Nevada, p. 13.

96. Groisman EA, Ochman H (1996) Pathogenicity islands: bacterial evolution in quantum leaps. *Cell* **87**, 791–4.

97. Guntheroth WG (1984) How important are dental procedures as a cause of infective endocarditis? *American Journal of Cardiology* **54**, 797–801.

98. Gutmann JL (1992) Clinical, radiographic, and histologic perspectives on success and failure in endodontics. *Dental Clinics of North America* **36**, 379–92.

99. Haapasalo M, Ranta H, Ranta KT (1983) Facultative Gram-negative enteric rods in persistent periapical infections. *Acta Odontologica Scandinavica* **41**, 19–22.

100. Haapasalo M, Ranta H, Ranta K, Shah H (1986) Black-pigmented *Bacteroides* spp. in human apical periodontitis. *Infection and Immunity* **53**, 149–53.

101. Haapasalo M, Ørstavik D (1987) In vitro infection and disinfection of dentinal tubules. *Journal of Dental Research* **66**, 1375–9.

102. Haapasalo M, Endal U, Zandi H, Coil JM (2005) Eradication of endodontic infection by instrumentation and irrigation solutions. *Endodontic Topics* **10**, 77–102.

103. Hacker J, Blum-Oehler G, Mühldorfer I, Tschäpe H (1997) Pathogenicity islands of virulent bacteria: structure, function and impact on microbial evolution. *Molecular Microbiology* **23**, 1089–97.

104. Hamada S, Amano A, Kimura S, Nakagawa I, Kawabata S, Morisaki I (1998) The importance of fimbriae in the virulence and ecology of some oral bacteria. *Oral Microbiology and Immunology* **13**, 129–38.

105. Hancock HH 3rd, Sigurdsson A, Trope M, Moiseiwitsch J (2001) Bacteria isolated after unsuccessful endodontic treatment in a North American population. *Oral Surgery, Oral Medicine, Oral Pathology, Oral Radiology and Endodontics* **91**, 579–86.

106. Handal T, Olsen I, Walker CB, Caugant DA (2004) Beta-lactamase production and antimicrobial susceptibility of subgingival bacteria from refractory periodontitis. *Oral Microbiology and Immunology* **19**, 303–8.

107. Happonen RP (1986) Periapical actinomycosis: a follow-up study of 16 surgically treated cases. *Endodontics and Dental Traumatology* **2**, 205–9.

108. Harper-Owen R, Dymock D, Booth V, Weightman AJ, Wade WG (1999) Detection of unculturable bacteria in periodontal health and disease by PCR. *Journal of Clinical Microbiology* **37**, 1469–73.

109. Hashimura T, Sato M, Hoshino E (2001) Detection of *Slackia exigua, Mogibacterium timidum* and *Eubacterium saphenum* from pulpal and periradicular samples using the Polymerase Chain Reaction (PCR) method. *International Endodontic Journal* **34**, 463–70.

110. Hashioka K, Suzuki K, Yoshida T, Nakane A, Horiba N, Nakamura H (1994) Relationship between clinical symptoms and enzyme-producing bacteria isolated from infected root canals. *Journal of Endodontics* **20**, 75–7.

111. Hayward CMM, Griffin GE (1994) Antibiotic resistance: the current position and the molecular mechanisms involved. *British Journal of Hospital Medicine* **52**, 473–8.

112. Hecht DW, Vedantam G, Osmolski JR (1999) Antibiotic resistance among anaerobes: What does it mean? *Anaerobe* **5**, 421–9.

113. Hecht DW (2004) Prevalence of antibiotic resistance in anaerobic bacteria: worrisome developments. *Clinical Infectious Diseases* **39**, 92–7.

114. Heeg K, Sparwasser T, Lipford GB, Hacker H, Zimmermann S, Wagner H (1998) Bacterial DNA as an evolutionary conserved ligand signalling danger of infection to immune cells. *European Journal of Clinical Microbiology and Infectious Diseases* **17**, 464–9.

115. Heimdahl A, von Konow L, Satoh T, Nord CE (1985) Clinical appearance of orofacial infections of odontogenic origin in relation to microbiological findings. *Journal of Clinical Microbiology* **22**, 299–302.

116. Henderson B, Poole S, Wilson M (1996) Bacterial modulins: a novel class of virulence factors which cause host tissue pathology by inducing cytokine synthesis. *Microbiological Reviews* **60**, 316–41.

117. Holt SC, Kesavalu L, Walker S, Genco CA (1999) Virulence factors of *Porphyromonas gingivalis*. *Periodontology 2000* **20**, 168–238.

118. Holt SC, Ebersole JL (2005) *Porphyromonas gingivalis, Treponema denticola* and *Tannerella forsythia*: the "red complex", a prototype polybacterial pathogenic consortium in periodontitis. *Periodontology 2000* **38**, 72–122.

119. Horiba N, Maekawa Y, Abe Y, Ito M, Matsumoto T, Nakamura H (1991) Correlations between endotoxin and clinical symptoms or radiolucent areas in infected root canals. *Oral Surgery, Oral Medicine, Oral Pathology* **71**, 492–5.

120. Huang K, Fishwild DM, Wu HM, Dedrick RL (1995) Lipopolysaccharide-induced E-selectin expression requires continuous presence of LPS and is inhib-

ited by bactericidal/permeability-increasing protein. *Inflammation* **19**, 389–404.

121. Hugenholtz P, Pace NR (1996) Identifying microbial diversity in the natural environment: a molecular phylogenetic approach. *Trends in Biotechnology* **14**, 190–7.

122. Hugenholtz P, Goebel BM, Pace NR (1998) Impact of culture-independent studies on the emerging phylogenetic view of bacterial diversity. *Journal of Bacteriology* **180**, 4765–74.

123. Hulsmann M, Peters OA, Dummer PMH (2005) Mechanical preparation of root canals: shaping goals, techniques and means. *Endodontic Topics* **10**, 30–76.

124. Hunter W (1900) Oral sepsis as a cause of disease. *British Medical Journal* **2**, 215–16.

125. Hunter W (1911) The rôle of sepsis and antisepsis in medicine. *Lancet* **14**, 79–86.

126. Imai M, Murakami Y, Nagano K, Nakamura H, Yoshimura F (2005) Major outer membrane proteins from *Porphyromonas gingivalis*: strain variation, distribution, and clinical significance in periradicular lesions. *European Journal of Oral Sciences* **113**, 391–9.

127. Ito HO, Shuto T, Takada H, Koga T, Aida Y, Hirata M, Koga T (1996) Lipopolysaccharides from *Porphyromonas gingivalis*, *Prevotella intermedia* and *Actinobacillus actinomycetemcomitans* promote osteoclastic differentiation in vitro. *Archives of Oral Biology* **41**, 439–44.

128. Jacinto RC, Gomes BP, Ferraz CC, Zaia AA, Filho FJ (2003) Microbiological analysis of infected root canals from symptomatic and asymptomatic teeth with periapical periodontitis and the antimicrobial susceptibility of some isolated anaerobic bacteria. *Oral Microbiology and Immunology* **18**, 285–92.

129. Jacinto RC, Gomes BP, Shah HN, Ferraz CC, Zaia AA, Souza-Filho FJ (2005) Quantification of endotoxins in necrotic root canals from symptomatic and asymptomatic teeth. *Journal of Medical Microbiology* **54**, 777–783.

130. Janeway CA, Travers P (1997) *Immunobiology. The immune system in health and disease*, 3rd edn. London: Current Biology.

131. Jansen HJ, van der Hoeven JS, van den Kieboom CW, Goertz JH, Camp PJ, Bakkeren JA (1994) Degradation of immunoglobulin G by periodontal bacteria. *Oral Microbiology and Immunology* **9**, 345–51.

132. Jansen HJ, Grenier D, Van der Hoeven JS (1995) Characterization of immunoglobulin G-degrading proteases of *Prevotella intermedia* and *Prevotella nigrescens*. *Oral Microbiology and Immunology* **10**, 138–45.

133. Jansen HJ, van der Hoeven JS, Walji S, Goertz JH, Bakkeren JA (1996) The importance of immunoglobulin-breakdown supporting the growth of bacteria in oral abscesses. *Journal of Clinical Periodontology* **23**, 717–23.

134. Jansen HJ, van der Hoeven JS (1997) Protein degradation by *Prevotella intermedia* and *Actinomyces meyeri* supports the growth of non-protein-cleaving oral bacteria in serum. *Journal of Clinical Periodontology* **24**, 346–53.

135. Jersmann HP, Hii CS, Ferrante JV, Ferrante A (2001) Bacterial lipopolysaccharide and tumor necrosis factor alpha synergistically increase expression of human endothelial adhesion molecules through activation of NF-kappaB and p38 mitogen-activated protein kinase signaling pathways. *Infection and Immunity* **69**, 1273–9.

136. Jett BD, Huycke MM, Gilmore MS (1994) Virulence of enterococci. *Clinical Microbiology Reviews* **7**, 462–78.

137. Joiner KA, Goldman R, Schmetz M, Berger M, Hammer CH, Frank MM, *et al.* (1984) A quantitative analysis of C3 binding to O-antigen capsule, lipopolysaccharide, and outer membrane protein of E. coli O111B4. *Journal of Immunology* **132**, 369–75.

138. Jostes JL (1999) Anaerobic bacteremia and fungemia in patients undergoing endodontic therapy: an overview. *Oral Surgery, Oral Medicine, Oral Pathology, Oral Radiology and Endodontics* **88**, 483.

139. Jousimies-Somer H, Summanen P (2002) Recent taxonomic changes and terminology update of clinically significant anaerobic gram-negative bacteria (excluding spirochetes). *Clinical Infectious Diseases* **35** (Suppl 1), S17–21.

140. Jung IY, Choi BK, Kum KY, Roh BD, Lee SJ, Lee CY, *et al.* (2000) Molecular epidemiology and association of putative pathogens in root canal infection. *Journal of Endodontics* **26**, 599–604.

141. Jung IY, Choi B, Kum KY, Yoo YJ, Yoon TC, Lee SJ, *et al.* (2001) Identification of oral spirochetes at the species level and their association with other bacteria in endodontic infections. *Oral Surgery, Oral Medicine, Oral Pathology, Oral Radiology and Endodontics* **92**, 329–34.

142. Kakehashi S, Stanley HR, Fitzgerald RJ (1965) The effects of surgical exposures of dental pulps in germfree and conventional laboratory rats. *Oral Surgery, Oral Medicine, Oral Pathology* **20**, 340–9.

143. Kayaoglu G, Ørstavik D (2004) Virulence factors of *Enterococcus faecalis*: relationship to endodontic disease. *Critical Reviews in Oral Biology and Medicine* **15**, 308–20.

144. Kayaoglu G, Erten H, Alacam T, Ørstavik D (2005) Short-term antibacterial activity of root canal sealers towards *Enterococcus faecalis*. *International Endodontic Journal* **38**, 483–8.

145. Kazor CE, Mitchell PM, Lee AM, Stokes LN, Loesche WJ, Dewhirst FE, *et al.* (2003) Diversity of bacterial populations on the tongue dorsa of patients with halitosis and healthy patients. *Journal of Clinical Microbiology* **41**, 558–63.

146. Keller M, Zengler K (2004) Tapping into microbial diversity. *Nature Reviews in Microbiology* **2**, 141–50.

147. Kesavalu L, Holt SC, Ebersole JL (1998) Virulence of a polymicrobic complex, *Treponema denticola* and *Porphyromonas gingivalis*, in a murine model. *Oral Microbiology and Immunology* **13**, 373–7.

148. Kesavalu L, Holt SC, Ebersole JL (1999) Environmental modulation of oral treponeme virulence in a murine model. *Infection and Immunity* **67**, 2783–9.

149. Kesavalu L, Holt SC, Ebersole JL (2003) In vitro environmental regulation of Porphyromonas gingivalis growth and virulence. *Oral Microbiology and Immunology* **18**, 226–33.

150. Kettering JD, Torabinejad M, Jones SL (1991) Specificity of antibodies present in human periapical lesions. *Journal of Endodontics* **17**, 213–16.

151. Khemaleelakul S, Baumgartner JC, Pruksakorn S (2002) Identification of bacteria in acute endodontic infections and their antimicrobial susceptibility. *Oral Surgery, Oral Medicine, Oral Pathology, Oral Radiology and Endodontics* **94**, 746–55.

152. Kievit TR, Iglewski BH (2000) Bacterial quorum sensing in pathogenic relationships. *Infection and Immunity* **68**, 4839–49.

153. Kilian M (1981) Degradation of immunoglobulins A1, A2, and G by suspected principal periodontal pathogens. *Infection and Immunity* **34**, 757–65.

154. Klein EA, Aas JA, Barbuto SM, Boumenna T, Dewhirst FE, Paster BJ (2005) The breadth of bacterial diversity in the human oral cavity. *Journal of Dental Research* **84**, IADR Abstract No. 2609. http://www.dentalresearch.org.

155. Koch R (1884) Die Aetiologie der Tuberkulose. *Mitt Kaiser Gesundh* **2**, 1–88.

156. Kolenbrander PE, Andersen RN, Blehert DS, Egland PG, Foster JS, Palmer RJ Jr (2002) Communication among oral bacteria. *Microbiology and Molecular Biology Reviews* **66**, 486–505.

157. Kolenbrander PE, Egland PG, Diaz PI, Palmer RJ Jr (2005) Genome-genome interactions: bacterial communities in initial dental plaque. *Trends in Microbiology* **13**, 11–15.

158. Krieg AM, Hartmann G, Yi A-K (2000) Mechanism of action of CpG DNA. *Current Topics in Microbiology and Immunology* **247**, 1–21.

159. Kroes I, Lepp PW, Relman DA (1999) Bacterial diversity within the human subgingival crevice. *Proceedings of the National Academy of Sciences USA* **96**, 14547–52.

160. Kumar PS, Griffen AL, Barton JA, Paster BJ, Moeschberger ML, Leys EJ (2003) New bacterial species associated with chronic periodontitis. *Journal of Dental Research* **82**, 338–44.

161. Kumar PS, Griffen AL, Moeschberger ML, Leys EJ (2005) Identification of candidate periodontal pathogens and beneficial species by quantitative 16S clonal analysis. *Journal of Clinical Microbiology* **43**, 3944–55.

162. Kuriyama T, Karasawa T, Nakagawa K, Saiki Y, Yamamoto E, Nakamura S (2000) Bacteriologic features and antimicrobial susceptibility in isolates from orofacial odontogenic infections. *Oral Surgery, Oral Medicine, Oral Pathology, Oral Radiology and Endodontics* **90**, 600–8.

163. Kuriyama T, Karasawa T, Nakagawa K, Yamamoto E, Nakamura S (2001) Incidence of beta-lactamase production and antimicrobial susceptibility of anaerobic gram-negative rods isolated from pus specimens of orofacial odontogenic infections. *Oral Microbiology and Immunology* **16**, 10–15.

164. Lakhssassi N, Elhajoui N, Lodter JP, Pineill JL, Sixou M (2005) Antimicrobial susceptibility variation of 50 anaerobic periopathogens in aggressive periodontitis: an interindividual variability study. *Oral Microbiology and Immunology* **20**, 244–52.

165. Lana MA, Ribeiro-Sobrinho AP, Stehling R, Garcia GD, Silva BK, Hamdan JS, *et al.* (2001) Microorganisms isolated from root canals presenting necrotic pulp and their drug susceptibility in vitro. *Oral Microbiology and Immunology* **16**, 100–5.

166. Lazazzera BA (2000) Quorum sensing and starvation: signals for entry into stationary phase. *Current Opinion in Microbiology* **3**, 177–82.

167. Le Goff A, Bunetel L, Mouton C, Bonnaure-Mallet M (1997) Evaluation of root canal bacteria and their antimicrobial susceptibility in teeth with necrotic pulp. *Oral Microbiology and Immunology* **12**, 318–22.

168. Lepp PW, Brinig MM, Ouverney CC, Palm K, Armitage GC, Relman DA (2004) Methanogenic Archaea and human periodontal disease. *Proceedings of the National Academy of Sciences USA* **101**, 6176–81.

169. Li X, Tronstad L, Olsen I (1999) Brain abscesses caused by oral infection. *Endodontics and Dental Traumatology* **15**, 95–101.

170. Li X, Kolltveit KM, Tronstad L, Olsen I (2000) Systemic diseases caused by oral infection. *Clinical Microbiology Reviews* **13**, 547–58.

171. Lillo A, Ashley FP, Palmer RM, Munson MA, Kyriacou L, Weightman AJ, *et al.* (2006) Novel subgingival bacterial phylotypes detected using multiple universal polymerase chain reaction primer sets. *Oral Microbiology and Immunology* **21**, 61–8.

172. Lin LM, Pascon EA, Skribner J, Gangler P, Langeland K (1991) Clinical, radiographic, and histologic study of endodontic treatment failures. *Oral Surgery, Oral Medicine, Oral Pathology* **71**, 603–11.

173. Lin LM, Skribner JE, Gaengler P (1992) Factors associated with endodontic treatment failures. *Journal of Endodontics* **18**, 625–7.

174. Lleo MM, Bonato B, Tafi MC, Signoretto C, Boaretti M, Canepari P (2001) Resuscitation rate in different enterococcal species in the viable but nonculturable state. *Journal of Applied Microbiology* **91**, 1095–102.

175. Lleo MM, Bonato B, Tafi MC, Signoretto C, Pruzzo C, Canepari P (2005) Molecular vs culture methods for the detection of bacterial faecal indicators in groundwater for human use. *Letters in Applied Microbiology* **40**, 289–94.

176. Loesche WJ, Kazor C (2002) Microbiology and treatment of halitosis. *Periodontology 2000* **28**, 256–79.

177. Lopes HP, Elias CN, Silveira GEL, Araújo-Filho WR, Siqueira JF Jr (1997) Extrusão de material do canal via forame apical. *Revista Paulista de Odontologia* **19**, 34–6.

178. Love RM, McMillan MD, Jenkinson HF (1997) Invasion of dentinal tubules by oral streptococci is associated with collagen recognition mediated by the antigen I/II family of polypeptides. *Infection and Immunity* **65**, 5157–64.

179. Love RM, Jenkinson HF (2002) Invasion of dentinal tubules by oral bacteria. *Critical Reviews in Oral Biology and Medicine* **13**, 171–83.

180. Machado de Oliveira JC, Siqueira JF Jr, Alves GB, Hirata R Jr, Andrade AF (2000) Detection of *Porphyromonas endodontalis* in infected root canals by

16S rRNA gene-directed polymerase chain reaction. *Journal of Endodontics* **26**, 729–32.

181. Madianos PN, Bobetsis YA, Kinane DF (2005) Generation of inflammatory stimuli: how bacteria set up inflammatory responses in the gingiva. *Journal of Clinical Periodontology* **32** (Suppl. 6), 57–71.

182. Madigan MT, Martinko JM, Parker J (2000) *Brock biology of microorganisms*, 9th edn. Upper Saddle River, NJ: Prentice-Hall.

183. Maita E, Horiuchi H (1990) Polyamine analysis of infected root canal contents related to clinical symptoms. *Endodontics and Dental Traumatology* **6**, 213–17.

184. Makinen KK, Makinen PL (1996) The peptidolytic capacity of the spirochete system. *Medical Microbiology and Immunology* **185**, 1–10.

185. Marcotte H, Lavoie MC (1998) Oral microbial ecology and the role of salivary immunoglobulin A. *Microbiology and Molecular Biology Reviews* **62**, 71–109.

186. Marsh P, Martin MV (1999) *Oral microbiology*, 4th edn. Oxford: Wright.

187. Marsh PD, McKee AS, McDermid AS (1993) Continuous culture studies. In Shah HN, Mayrand D, Genco RJ, editors. *Biology of the species* Porphyromonas gingivalis, pp. 105–23. Boca Raton, FL: CRC Press.

188. Marsh PD (2003) Are dental diseases examples of ecological catastrophes? *Microbiology* **149**, 279–94.

189. Matin A (1992) Physiology, molecular biology and applications of the bacterial starvation response. *Journal of Applied Bacteriology* **73** (Symposium suppl), 49S–57S.

190. Matsuo T, Shirakami T, Ozaki K, Nakanishi T, Yumoto H, Ebisu S (2003) An immunohistological study of the localization of bacteria invading root pulpal walls of teeth with periapical lesions. *Journal of Endodontics* **29**, 194–200.

191. Mattila KJ, Nieminen MS, Valtonen VV, Rasi VP, Kesäniemi YA, Syrjälä SL, *et al.* (1989) Association between dental health and acute myocardial infarction. *British Medical Journal* **298**, 779–81.

192. Mayrand D, McBride BC (1980) Ecological relationships of bacteria involved in a simple, mixed anaerobic infection. *Infection and Immunity* **27**, 44–50.

193. Mikx FH, van der Hoeven JS (1975) Symbiosis of *Streptococcus mutans* and *Veillonella alcalescens* in mixed continuous cultures. *Archives of Oral Biology* **20**, 407–410.

194. Miller WD (1891) The human mouth as a focus of infection. *Dental Cosmos* **33**, 689–713.

195. Miller WD (1894) An introduction to the study of the bacterio-pathology of the dental pulp. *Dental Cosmos* **36**, 505–28.

196. Mims C, Nash A, Stephen J (2001) *Mims' pathogenesis of infectious diseases*, 5th edn. San Diego, CA: Academic Press.

197. Mogensen TH, Paludan SR (2001) Molecular pathways in virus-induced cytokine production. *Microbiology and Molecular Biology Reviews* **65**, 131–50.

198. Molander A, Reit C, Dahlén G, Kvist T (1998) Microbiological status of root-filled teeth with apical periodontitis. *International Endodontic Journal* **31**, 1–7.

199. Möller AJR (1966) Microbial examination of root canals and periapical tissues of human teeth. *Odontologisk Tidskrift* **74** (suppl), 1–380.

200. Möller AJR, Fabricius L, Dahlén G, Öhman AE, Heyden G (1981) Influence on periapical tissues of indigenous oral bacteria and necrotic pulp tissue in monkeys. *Scandinavian Journal of Dental Research* **89**, 475–84.

201. Molven O, Olsen I, Kerekes K (1991) Scanning electron microscopy of bacteria in the apical part of root canals in permanent teeth with periapical lesions. *Endodontics and Dental Traumatology* **7**, 226–9.

202. Moore WEC, Moore LVH (1994) The bacteria of periodontal diseases. *Periodontology 2000* **5**, 66–77.

203. Moraes SR, Siqueira JF Jr, Rôças IN, Ferreira MC, Domingues RM (2002) Clonality of *Fusobacterium nucleatum* in root canal infections. *Oral Microbiology and Immunology* **17**, 394–6.

204. Morrison DC, Cochrane CG (1974) Direct evidence for Hageman factor (factor XII) activation by bacterial lipopolysaccharides (endotoxins). *Journal of Experimental Medicine* **140**, 797–811.

205. Mundy LM, Sahm DF, Gilmore M (2000) Relationships between enterococcal virulence and antimicrobial resistance. *Clinical Microbiology Reviews* **13**, 513–22.

206. Munson MA, Pitt-Ford T, Chong B, Weightman A, Wade WG (2002) Molecular and cultural analysis of the microflora associated with endodontic infections. *Journal of Dental Research* **81**, 761–6.

207. Munson MA, Banerjee A, Watson TF, Wade WG (2004) Molecular analysis of the microflora associated with dental caries. *Journal of Clinical Microbiology* **42**, 3023–9.

208. Murakami Y, Hanazawa S, Tanaka S, Iwahashi H, Yamamoto Y, Fujisawa S (2001) A possible mechanism of maxillofacial abscess formation: involvement of *Porphyromonas endodontalis* lipopolysaccharide via the expression of inflammatory cytokines. *Oral Microbiology and Immunology* **16**, 321–5.

209. Murray CA, Saunders WP (2000) Root canal treatment and general health: a review of the literature. *International Endodontic Journal* **33**, 1–18.

210. Musser JM (1996) Molecular population genetic analysis of emerged bacterial pathogens: selected insights. *Emerging Infectious Diseases* **2**, 1–17.

211. Nair PNR, Schroeder HE (1984) Periapical actinomycosis. *Journal of Endodontics* **10**, 567–70.

212. Nair PNR (1987) Light and electron microscopic studies of root canal flora and periapical lesions. *Journal of Endodontics* **13**, 29–39.

213. Nair SP, Meghji S, Wilson M, Reddi K, White P, Henderson B (1996) Bacterially induced bone destruction: mechanisms and misconceptions. *Infection and Immunity* **64**, 2371–80.

214. Narayanan SK, Nagaraja TG, Chengappa MM, Stewart GC (2002) Leukotoxins of Gram-negative bacteria. *Veterinary Microbiology* **84**, 337–56.

215. Nikkari S, McLaughlin IJ, Bi W, Dodge DE, Relman DA (2001) Does blood of healthy subjects contain bacterial ribosomal DNA? *Journal of Clinical Microbiology* **39**, 1956–9.

216. Noel RF Jr, Sato TT, Mendez C, Johnson MC, Pohlman TH (1995) Activation of human endothelial cells by viable or heat-killed gram-negative bacteria requires soluble CD14. *Infection and Immunity* **63**, 4046–53.
217. Noiri Y, Ehara A, Kawahara T, Takemura N, Ebisu S (2002) Participation of bacterial biofilms in refractory and chronic periapical periodontitis. *Journal of Endodontics* **28**, 679–83.
218. Nonnenmacher C, Dalpke A, Zimmermann S, Flores-De-Jacoby L, Mutters R, Heeg K (2003) DNA from periodontopathogenic bacteria is immunostimulatory for mouse and human immune cells. *Infection and Immunity* **71**, 850–6.
219. Offenbacher S, Jared HL, O'Reilly PG, Wells SR, Salvi GE, Lawrence HP, Socransky SS, Beck JD (1998) Potential pathogenic mechanisms of periodontitis associated pregnancy complications. *Annals of Periodontology* **3**, 233–50.
220. Okahashi N, Koga T, Nishihara T, Fujiwara T, Hamada S (1988) Immunobiological properties of lipopolysaccharides isolated from *Fusobacterium nucleatum* and *F. necrophorum*. *Journal of General Microbiology* **134**, 1707–15.
221. Olsen I, Dahlén G (2004) Salient virulence factors in anaerobic bacteria, with emphasis on their importance in endodontic infections. *Endodontic Topics* **9**, 15–26.
222. Ørstavik D (1981) Antibacterial properties of root canal sealers, cements and pastes. *International Endodontic Journal* **14**, 125–33.
223. Özmeriç N, Preus HR, Olsen I (2000) Genetic diversity of *Porphyromonas gingivalis* and its possible importance to pathogenicity. *Acta Odontologica Scandinavica* **58**, 183–7.
224. Pace NR (1997) A molecular view of microbial diversity and the biosphere. *Science* **276**, 734–40.
225. Pallasch TJ (1979) Antibiotics in endodontics. *Dental Clinics of North America* **23**, 737–46.
226. Pallasch TJ (1996) Pharmacokinetic principles of antimicrobial therapy. *Periodontology 2000* **10**, 5–11.
227. Pallasch TJ, Slots J (1996) Antibiotic prophylaxis and the medically compromised patient. *Periodontology 2000* **10**, 107–38.
228. Pallasch TJ (2003) Antibiotic prophylaxis. *Endodontic Topics* **4**, 46–59.
229. Pallasch TJ, Wahl MJ (2003) Focal infection: new age or ancient history? *Endodontic Topics* **4**, 32–45.
230. Parsek MR, Greenberg EP (2005) Sociomicrobiology: the connections between quorum sensing and biofilms. *Trends in Microbiology* **13**, 27–33.
231. Paster BJ, Boches SK, Galvin JL, Ericson RE, Lau CN, Levanos VA, Sahasrabudhe A, Dewhirst FE (2001) Bacterial diversity in human subgingival plaque. *Journal of Bacteriology* **183**, 3770–83.
232. Paster BJ, Falkler WA Jr, Enwonwu CO, Idigbe EO, Savage KO, Levanos VA, *et al*. (2002) Prevalent bacterial species and novel phylotypes in advanced noma lesions. *Journal of Clinical Microbiology* **40**, 2187–91.
233. Patel R (2003) Clinical impact of vancomycin-resistant enterococci. *Journal of Antimicrobial Chemotherapy* **51**(Suppl 3), iii13–21.

234. Paturel L, Casalta JP, Habib G, Nezri M, Raoult D (2004) *Actinobacillus actinomycetemcomitans* endocarditis. *Clinical Microbiology and Infection* **10**, 98–118.
235. Peciuliene V, Balciuniene I, Eriksen HM, Haapasalo M (2000) Isolation of *Enterococcus faecalis* in previously root-filled canals in a Lithuanian population. *Journal of Endodontics* **26**, 593–5.
236. Peciuliene V, Reynaud AH, Balciuniene I, Haapasalo M (2001) Isolation of yeasts and enteric bacteria in root-filled teeth with chronic apical periodontitis. *International Endodontic Journal* **34**, 429–34.
237. Perez F, Calas P, de Falguerolles A, Maurette A (1993) Migration of a *Streptococcus sanguis* strain through the root dentinal tubules. *Journal of Endodontics* **19**, 297–301.
238. Persson S, Claesson R, Carlsson J (1989) The capacity of subgingival microbiotas to produce volatile sulfur compounds in human serum. *Oral Microbiology and Immunology* **4**, 169–72.
239. Persson S, Edlund MB, Claesson R, Carlsson J (1990) The formation of hydrogen sulfide and methyl mercaptan by oral bacteria. *Oral Microbiology and Immunology* **5**, 195–201.
240. Peters LB, Wesselink PR, Buijs JF, van Winkelhoff AJ (2001) Viable bacteria in root dentinal tubules of teeth with apical periodontitis. *Journal of Endodontics* **27**, 76–81.
241. Peters LB, Wesselink PR, van Winkelhoff AJ (2002) Combinations of bacterial species in endodontic infections. *International Endodontic Journal* **35**, 698–702.
242. Peters OA, Schönenberger K, Laib A (2001) Effects of four Ni-Ti preparation techniques on root canal geometry assessed by micro computed tomography. *International Endodontic Journal* **34**, 221–30.
243. Petersen FC, Pecharki D, Scheie AA (2004) Biofilm mode of growth of *Streptococcus intermedius* favored by a competence-stimulating signaling peptide. *Journal of Bacteriology* **186**, 6327–31.
244. Pettinger WA, Young R (1970) Endotoxin-induced kinin (bradykinin) formation: activation of Hageman factor and plasma kallikrein in human plasma. *Life Sciences* **9**, 313–22.
245. Pinheiro ET, Gomes BP, Ferraz CC, Sousa EL, Teixeira FB, Souza-Filho FJ (2003) Microorganisms from canals of root-filled teeth with periapical lesions. *International Endodontic Journal* **36**, 1–11.
246. Pitts DL, Williams BL, Morton TH Jr (1982) Investigation of the role of endotoxin in periapical inflammation. *Journal of Endodontics* **8**, 10–18.
247. Potempa J, Banbula A, Travis J (2000) Role of bacterial proteinases in matrix destruction and modulation of host responses. *Periodontology 2000* **24**, 153–92.
248. Poyart C, Quesnes G, Trieu-Cuot P (2000) Sequencing the gene encoding manganese-dependent superoxide dismutase for rapid species identification of enterococci. *Journal of Clinical Microbiology* **38**, 415–18.
249. Ramotar K, Conly JM, Chubb H, Louie TJ (1984) Production of menaquinones by intestinal anaerobes. *Journal of Infectious Diseases* **150**, 213–18.
250. Ranta H, Haapasalo M, Ranta K, Kontiainen S, Kerosuo E, Valtonen V, *et al*. (1988) Bacteriology of odontogenic apical periodontitis and effect of penicil-

lin treatment. *Scandinavian Journal of Infectious Diseases* **20**, 187–92.

251. Ranta K, Haapasalo M, Ranta H (1988) Monoinfection of root canal with *Pseudomonas aeruginosa*. *Endodontics and Dental Traumatology* **4**, 269–72.

252. Rappe MS, Giovannoni SJ (2003) The uncultured microbial majority. *Annual Reviews in Microbiology* **57**, 369–94.

253. Reddy SA, Hicks ML (1998) Apical extrusion of debris using two hand and two rotary instrumentation techniques. *Journal of Endodontics* **24**, 180–3.

254. Relman DA (1999) The search for unrecognized pathogens. *Science* **284**, 1308–10.

255. Relman DA (2002) New technologies, human–microbe interactions, and the search for previously unrecognized pathogens. *Journal of Infectious Diseases* **186** (Suppl 2), S254–8.

256. Relman DA (2002) Mining the natural world for new pathogens. *American Journal of Tropical Medicine and Hygiene* **67**, 133–4.

257. Rietschel ET, Brade H (1992) Bacterial endotoxins. *Scientific American* **267**, 26–33.

258. Rietschel ET, Kirikae T, Schade U, Mamat U, Schmidt G, Loppnow H, *et al.* (1994) Bacterial endotoxin: molecular relationships of structure to activity and function. *FASEB Journal* **8**, 217–25.

259. Rietschel ET, Cavaillon JM (2003) Richard Pfeiffer and Alexandre Besredka: creators of the concept of endotoxin and anti-endotoxin. *Microbes and Infection* **5**, 1407–14.

260. Rôças IN, Siqueira JF Jr, Santos KR, Coelho AM (2001) "Red complex" (*Bacteroides forsythus*, *Porphyromonas gingivalis*, and *Treponema denticola*) in endodontic infections: a molecular approach. *Oral Surgery, Oral Medicine, Oral Pathology, Oral Radiology and Endodontics* **91**, 468–71.

261. Rôças IN, Siqueira JF Jr (2002) Identification of *Dialister pneumosintes* in acute periradicular abscesses of humans by nested PCR. *Anaerobe* **8**, 75–8.

262. Rôças IN, Siqueira JF Jr, Andrade AFB, Uzeda M (2002) Identification of selected putative oral pathogens in primary root canal infections associated with symptoms. *Anaerobe* **8**, 200–8.

263. Rôças IN, Siqueira JF Jr, Andrade AF, Uzeda M (2003) Oral treponemes in primary root canal infections as detected by nested PCR. *International Endodontic Journal* **36**, 20–6.

264. Rôças IN, Jung IY, Lee CY, Siqueira JF Jr (2004) Polymerase chain reaction identification of microorganisms in previously root-filled teeth in a South Korean population. *Journal of Endodontics* **30**, 504–8.

265. Rôças IN, Siqueira JF Jr, Aboim MC, Rosado AS (2004) Denaturing gradient gel electrophoresis analysis of bacterial communities associated with failed endodontic treatment. *Oral Surgery, Oral Medicine, Oral Pathology, Oral Radiology and Endodontics* **98**, 741–9.

266. Rôças IN, Siqueira JF Jr, Santos KR (2004) Association of *Enterococcus faecalis* with different forms of periradicular diseases. *Journal of Endodontics* **30**, 315–20.

267. Rôças IN, Siqueira JF Jr (2005) Species-directed 16S rRNA gene nested PCR detection of *Olsenella* species in association with endodontic diseases. *Letters in Applied Microbiology* **41**, 12–16.

268. Rôças IN, Siqueira JF Jr (2005) Detection of novel oral species and phylotypes in symptomatic endodontic infections including abscesses. *FEMS Microbiology Letters* **250**, 279–85.

269. Rôças IN, Siqueira JF Jr (2005) Occurrence of two newly named oral treponemes – *Treponema parvum* and *Treponema putidum* – in primary endodontic infections. *Oral Microbiology and Immunology* **20**, 372–5.

270. Rolph HJ, Lennon A, Riggio MP, Saunders WP, MacKenzie D, Coldero L, *et al.* (2001) Molecular identification of microorganisms from endodontic infections. *Journal of Clinical Microbiology* **39**, 3282–9.

271. Roodman GD (1993) Role of cytokines in the regulation of bone resorption. *Calcified Tissue International* **53** (suppl. 1), S94–8.

272. Rosen G, Naor R, Rahamim E, Yishai R, Sela MN (1995) Proteases of *Treponema denticola* outer sheath and extracellular vesicles. *Infection and Immunity* **63**, 3973–9.

273. Rosen G, Sela MN, Naor R, Halabi A, Barak V, Shapira L (1999) Activation of murine macrophages by lipoprotein and lipooligosaccharide of *Treponema denticola*. *Infection and Immunity* **67**, 1180–6.

274. Sabeti M, Simon JH, Nowzari H, Slots J (2003) Cytomegalovirus and Epstein–Barr virus active infection in periapical lesions of teeth with intact crowns. *Journal of Endodontics* **29**, 321–3.

275. Sabeti M, Simon JH, Slots J (2003) Cytomegalovirus and Epstein–Barr virus are associated with symptomatic periapical pathosis. *Oral Microbiology and Immunology* **18**, 327–8.

276. Sabeti M, Valles Y, Nowzari H, Simon JH, Kermani-Arab V, Slots J (2003) Cytomegalovirus and Epstein–Barr virus DNA transcription in endodontic symptomatic lesions. *Oral Microbiology and Immunology* **18**, 104–8.

277. Sabeti M, Slots J (2004) Herpesviral–bacterial coinfection in periapical pathosis. *Journal of Endodontics* **30**, 69–72.

278. Saito D, de Toledo Leonardo R, Rodrigues JLM, Tsai SM, Hofling JF, Gonçalves RB (2006) Identification of bacteria in endodontic infections by sequence analysis of 16S rDNA clone libraries. *Journal of Medical Microbiology* **55**, 101–7.

279. Sakamoto M, Huang Y, Umeda M, Ishikawa I, Benno Y (2002) Detection of novel oral phylotypes associated with periodontitis. *FEMS Microbiology Letters* **217**, 65–9.

280. Sakamoto M, Rôças IN, Siqueira JF Jr, Benno Y (2006) Molecular analysis of bacteria in asymptomatic and symptomatic endodontic infections. *Oral Microbiology and Immunology* **21**, 112–22.

281. Sakamoto M, Siqueira JF Jr, Rôças IN, Benno Y (2007) Bacterial reduction and persistence after endodontic treatment procedures. *Oral Microbiology and Immunology* **22**, 19–23.

282. Salyers AA, Whitt DD (1994) *Bacterial pathogenesis. A molecular approach*. Washington, DC: ASM Press.

283. Savarrio L, Mackenzie D, Riggio M, Saunders WP, Bagg J (2005) Detection of bacteraemias during non-surgical root canal treatment. *Journal of Dentistry* **33**, 293–303.

284. Scannapieco FA (1999) Role of oral bacteria in respiratory infection. *Journal of Periodontology* **70**, 793–802.

285. Schein B, Schilder H (1975) Endotoxin content in endodontically involved teeth. *Journal of Endodontics* **1**, 19–21.

286. Schonfeld SE, Greening AB, Glick DH, Frank AL, Simon JH, Herles BA (1982) Endotoxin activity in periapical lesions. *Oral Surgery, Oral Medicine, Oral Pathology* **53**, 82–7.

287. Schwandner R, Dziarski R, Wesche H, Rothe M, Kirschning CJ (1999) Peptidoglycan- and lipoteichoic acid-induced cell activation is mediated by toll-like receptor 2. *Journal of Biological Chemistry* **274**, 17406–9.

288. Sedgley C, Nagel A, Dahlén G, Reit C, Molander A (2006) Real-time quantitative polymerase chain reaction and culture analyses of *Enterococcus faecalis* in root canals. *Journal of Endodontics* **32**, 173–7.

289. Sedgley CM, Lennan SL, Appelbe OK (2005) Survival of *Enterococcus faecalis* in root canals ex vivo. *International Endodontic Journal* **38**, 735–42.

290. Sedgley CM, Molander A, Flannagan SE, Nagel AC, Appelbe OK, Clewell DB, *et al.* (2005) Virulence, phenotype and genotype characteristics of endodontic Enterococcus spp. *Oral Microbiology and Immunology* **20**, 10–19.

291. Sen BH, Piskin B, Demirci T (1995) Observation of bacteria and fungi in infected root canals and dentinal tubules by SEM. *Endodontics and Dental Traumatology* **11**, 6–9.

292. Sen BH, Safavi KE, Spångberg LS (1997) Growth patterns of *Candida albicans* in relation to radicular dentin. *Oral Surgery, Oral Medicine, Oral Pathology, Oral Radiology and Endodontics* **84**, 68–73.

293. Sen BH, Safavi KE, Spångberg LS (1997) Colonization of *Candida albicans* on cleaned human dental hard tissues. *Archives of Oral Biology* **42**, 513–20.

294. Seol JH, Cho BH, Chung CP, Bae KS (2006) Multiplex polymerase chain reaction detection of black-pigmented bacteria in infections of endodontic origin. *Journal of Endodontics* **32**, 110–14.

295. Shah HN, Collins DM (1988) Proposal for reclassification of *Bacteroides asaccharolyticus*, *Bacteroides gingivalis*, and *Bacteroides endodontalis* in a new genus, *Porphyromonas*. *International Journal of Systematic Bacteriology* **38**, 128–31.

296. Shah HN, Collins DM (1990) *Prevotella*, a new genus to include *Bacteroides melaninogenicus* and related species formerly classified in the genus *Bacteroides*. *International Journal of Systematic Bacteriology* **40**, 205–8.

297. Shalhav M, Fuss Z, Weiss EI (1997) In vitro antibacterial activity of a glass ionomer endodontic sealer. *Journal of Endodontics* **23**, 616–19.

298. Shapiro RA, Cunningham MD, Ratcliffe K, Seachord C, Blake J, Bajorath J, *et al.* (1997) Identification of CD14 residues involved in specific lipopolysaccharide recognition. *Infection and Immunity* **65**, 293–7.

299. Signoretto C, Lleo MM, Tafi MC, Boaretti M, Canepari P (2000) Cell wall chemical composition of *Enterococcus faecalis* in the viable but nonculturable state. *Applied and Environmental Microbiology* **66**, 1953–9.

300. Siqueira JF Jr, de Uzeda M (1996) Disinfection by calcium hydroxide pastes of dentinal tubules infected with two obligate and one facultative anaerobic bacteria. *Journal of Endodontics* **22**, 674–6.

301. Siqueira JF Jr, de Uzeda M, Fonseca ME (1996) A scanning electron microscopic evaluation of in vitro dentinal tubules penetration by selected anaerobic bacteria. *Journal of Endodontics* **22**, 308–10.

302. Siqueira JF Jr, Gonçalves RB (1996) Antibacterial activities of root canal sealers against selected anaerobic bacteria. *Journal of Endodontics* **22**, 89–90.

303. Siqueira JF Jr, Araujo MC, Garcia PF, Fraga RC, Dantas CJ (1997) Histological evaluation of the effectiveness of five instrumentation techniques for cleaning the apical third of root canals. *Journal of Endodontics* **23**, 499–502.

304. Siqueira JF Jr, Magalhaes FA, Lima KC, de Uzeda M (1998) Pathogenicity of facultative and obligate anaerobic bacteria in monoculture and combined with either *Prevotella intermedia* or *Prevotella nigrescens*. *Oral Microbiology and Immunology* **13**, 368–72.

305. Siqueira JF Jr, Favieri A, Gahyva SM, Moraes SR, Lima KC, Lopes HP (2000) Antimicrobial activity and flow rate of newer and established root canal sealers. *Journal of Endodontics* **26**, 274–77.

306. Siqueira JF Jr, Rôças IN, Favieri A, Santos KR (2000) Detection of *Treponema denticola* in endodontic infections by 16S rRNA gene-directed polymerase chain reaction. *Oral Microbiology and Immunology* **15**, 335–7.

307. Siqueira JF Jr, Rôças IN, Souto R, de Uzeda M, Colombo AP (2000) Checkerboard DNA–DNA hybridization analysis of endodontic infections. *Oral Surgery, Oral Medicine, Oral Pathology, Oral Radiology and Endodontics* **89**, 744–8.

308. Siqueira JF Jr (2001) Aetiology of root canal treatment failure: why well-treated teeth can fail. *International Endodontic Journal* **34**, 1–10.

309. Siqueira JF Jr, Lopes HP (2001) Bacteria on the apical root surfaces of untreated teeth with periradicular lesions: a scanning electron microscopy study. *International Endodontic Journal* **34**, 216–20.

310. Siqueira JF Jr, Rôças IN, Favieri A, Oliveira JC, Santos KR (2001) Polymerase chain reaction detection of *Treponema denticola* in endodontic infections within root canals. *International Endodontic Journal* **34**, 280–4.

311. Siqueira JF Jr, Rôças IN, Oliveira JC, Santos KR (2001) Detection of putative oral pathogens in acute periradicular abscesses by 16S rDNA-directed polymerase chain reaction. *Journal of Endodontics* **27**, 164–7.

312. Siqueira JF Jr, Rôças IN, Oliveira JC, Santos KR (2001) Molecular detection of black-pigmented

bacteria in infections of endodontic origin. *Journal of Endodontics* **27**, 563–6.

313. Siqueira JF Jr, Rôças IN, Souto R, Uzeda M, Colombo AP (2001) Microbiological evaluation of acute periradicular abscesses by DNA–DNA hybridization. *Oral Surgery, Oral Medicine, Oral Pathology, Oral Radiology and Endodontics* **92**, 451–7.

314. Siqueira JF Jr (2002) Endodontic infections: concepts, paradigms, and perspectives. *Oral Surgery, Oral Medicine, Oral Pathology, Oral Radiology and Endodontics* **94**, 281–93.

315. Siqueira JF Jr, Lima KC (2002) *Staphylococcus epidermidis* and *Staphylococcus xylosus* in a secondary root canal infection with persistent symptoms: a case report. *Australian Endodontic Journal* **28**, 61–3.

316. Siqueira JF Jr, Rôças IN (2002) *Dialister pneumosintes* can be a suspected endodontic pathogen. *Oral Surgery, Oral Medicine, Oral Pathology, Oral Radiology and Endodontics* **94**, 494–8.

317. Siqueira JF Jr, Rôças IN, de Uzeda M, Colombo AP, Santos KR (2002) Comparison of 16S rDNA-based PCR and checkerboard DNA–DNA hybridisation for detection of selected endodontic pathogens. *Journal of Medical Microbiology* **51**, 1090–96.

318. Siqueira JF Jr, Rôças IN, Lopes HP (2002) Patterns of microbial colonization in primary root canal infections. *Oral Surgery, Oral Medicine, Oral Pathology, Oral Radiology and Endodontics* **93**, 174–8.

319. Siqueira JF Jr, Rôças IN, Lopes HP, Elias CN, de Uzeda M (2002) Fungal infection of the radicular dentin. *Journal of Endodontics* **28**, 770–3.

320. Siqueira JF Jr, Rôças IN, Moraes SR, Santos KR (2002) Direct amplification of rRNA gene sequences for identification of selected oral pathogens in root canal infections. *International Endodontic Journal* **35**, 345–51.

321. Siqueira JF Jr, Rôças IN, Souto R, de Uzeda M, Colombo AP (2002) *Actinomyces* species, streptococci, and *Enterococcus faecalis* in primary root canal infections. *Journal of Endodontics* **28**, 168–72.

322. Siqueira JF Jr (2003) Periapical actinomycosis and infection with *Propionibacterium propionicum*. *Endodontic Topics* **6**, 78–95.

323. Siqueira JF Jr, Rôças IN (2003) *Bacteroides forsythus* in primary endodontic infections as detected by nested PCR. *Journal of Endodontics* **29**, 390–3.

324. Siqueira JF Jr, Rôças IN (2003) *Campylobacter gracilis* and *Campylobacter rectus* in primary endodontic infections. *International Endodontic Journal* **36**, 174–80.

325. Siqueira JF Jr, Rôças IN (2003) PCR-based identification of *Treponema maltophilum*, *T. amylovorum*, *T. medium*, and *T. lecithinolyticum* in primary root canal infections. *Archives of Oral Biology* **48**, 495–502.

326. Siqueira JF Jr, Rôças IN (2003) *Treponema socranskii* in primary endodontic infections as detected by nested PCR. *Journal of Endodontics* **29**, 244–7.

327. Siqueira JF Jr, Rôças IN (2003) *Pseudoramibacter alactolyticus* in primary endodontic infections. *Journal of Endodontics* **29**, 735–8.

328. Siqueira JF Jr, Rôças IN (2003) Detection of *Filifactor alocis* in endodontic infections associated with different forms of periradicular diseases. *Oral Microbiology and Immunology* **18**, 263–5.

329. Siqueira JF Jr, Rôças IN (2003) Positive and negative bacterial associations involving *Dialister pneumosintes* in primary endodontic infections. *Journal of Endodontics* **29**, 438–41.

330. Siqueira JF Jr, Rôças IN, Andrade AF, de Uzeda M (2003) *Peptostreptococcus micros* in primary endodontic infections as detected by 16S rDNA-based polymerase chain reaction. *Journal of Endodontics* **29**, 111–13.

331. Siqueira JF Jr, Barnett F (2004) Interappointment pain: mechanisms, diagnosis, and treatment. *Endodontic Topics* **7**, 93–109.

332. Siqueira JF Jr, Rôças IN (2004) Polymerase chain reaction-based analysis of microorganisms associated with failed endodontic treatment. *Oral Surgery, Oral Medicine, Oral Pathology, Oral Radiology and Endodontics* **97**, 85–94.

333. Siqueira JF Jr, Rôças IN (2004) *Treponema* species associated with abscesses of endodontic origin. *Oral Microbiology and Immunology* **19**, 336–9.

334. Siqueira JF Jr, Rôças IN (2004) Nested PCR detection of *Centipeda periodontii* in primary endodontic infections. *Journal of Endodontics* **30**, 135–7.

335. Siqueira JF Jr, Rôças IN, Alves FR, Santos KR (2004) Selected endodontic pathogens in the apical third of infected root canals: a molecular investigation. *Journal of Endodontics* **30**, 638–43.

336. Siqueira JF Jr, Rôças IN, Rosado AS (2004) Investigation of bacterial communities associated with asymptomatic and symptomatic endodontic infections by denaturing gradient gel electrophoresis fingerprinting approach. *Oral Microbiology and Immunology* **19**, 363–70.

337. Siqueira JF Jr, Sen BH (2004) Fungi in endodontic infections. *Oral Surgery, Oral Medicine, Oral Pathology, Oral Radiology and Endodontics* **97**, 632–41.

338. Siqueira JF Jr (2005) Reaction of periradicular tissues to root canal treatment: benefits and drawbacks. *Endodontic Topics* **10**, 123–47.

339. Siqueira JF Jr, Rôças IN (2005) Exploiting molecular methods to explore endodontic infections: Part 1 – current molecular technologies for microbiological diagnosis. *Journal of Endodontics* **31**, 411–23.

340. Siqueira JF Jr, Rôças IN (2005) Uncultivated phylotypes and newly named species associated with primary and persistent endodontic infections. *Journal of Clinical Microbiology* **43**, 3314–19.

341. Siqueira JF Jr, Rôças IN (2005) Exploiting molecular methods to explore endodontic infections: Part 2 – Redefining the endodontic microbiota. *Journal of Endodontics* **31**, 488–98.

342. Siqueira JF Jr, Rôças IN, Baumgartner JC, Xia T (2005) Searching for Archaea in infections of endodontic origin. *Journal of Endodontics* **31**, 719–22.

343. Siqueira JF Jr, Rôças IN, Cunha CD, Rosado AS (2005) Novel bacterial phylotypes in endodontic infections. *Journal of Dental Research* **84**, 565–9.

344. Siqueira JF Jr, Rôças IN (2003) Polymerase chain reaction detection of *Propionibacterium propionicus* and *Actinomyces radicidentis* in primary and persistent

endodontic infections. *Oral Surgery, Oral Medicine, Oral Pathology, Oral Radiology and Endodontics* **96**, 215–22.

345. Sirén EK, Haapasalo MP, Ranta K, Salmi P, Kerosuo EN (1997) Microbiological findings and clinical treatment procedures in endodontic cases selected for microbiological investigation. *International Endodontic Journal* **30**, 91–5.

346. Sjögren U, Happonen RP, Kahnberg KE, Sundqvist G (1988) Survival of *Arachnia propionica* in periapical tissue. *International Endodontic Journal* **21**, 277–82.

347. Sjögren U, Hagglund B, Sundqvist G, Wing K (1990) Factors affecting the long-term results of endodontic treatment. *Journal of Endodontics* **16**, 498–504.

348. Sjögren U, Hanstrom L, Happonen RP, Sundqvist G (1990) Extensive bone loss associated with periapical infection with *Bacteroides gingivalis*: a case report. *International Endodontic Journal* **23**, 254–62.

349. Sjögren U, Figdor D, Persson S, Sundqvist G (1997) Influence of infection at the time of root filling on the outcome of endodontic treatment of teeth with apical periodontitis. *International Endodontic Journal* **30**, 297–306.

350. Slots J (1998) Casual or causal relationship between periodontal infection and non-oral disease? *Journal of Dental Research* **77**, 1764–5.

351. Slots J (1999) *Actinobacillus actinomycetemcomitans* and *Porphyromonas gingivalis* in periodontal disease: introduction. *Periodontology 2000* **20**, 7–13.

352. Slots J, Sabeti M, Simon JH (2003) Herpesviruses in periapical pathosis: an etiopathogenic relationship? *Oral Surgery, Oral Medicine, Oral Pathology, Oral Radiology and Endodontics* **96**, 327–31.

353. Slots J (2005) Herpesviruses in periodontal diseases. *Periodontology 2000* **38**, 33–62.

354. Socransky SS (1979) Criteria for the infectious agents in dental caries and periodontal disease. *Journal of Clinical Periodontology* **6**, 16–21.

355. Socransky SS, Haffajee AD (1997) Microbiology of periodontal disease. In Lindhe J, Karring T, Lang NP, editors. *Clinical periodontology and implant dentistry*, pp. 138–188. Copenhagen: Munksgaard.

356. Socransky SS, Haffajee AD, Cugini MA, Smith C, Kent RL Jr (1998) Microbial complexes in subgingival plaque. *Journal of Clinical Periodontology* **25**, 134–44.

357. Socransky SS, Haffajee AD (2005) Periodontal microbial ecology. *Periodontology 2000* **38**, 135–87.

358. Spångberg LS, Barbosa SV, Lavigne GD (1993) AH 26 releases formaldehyde. *Journal of Endodontics* **19**, 596–8.

359. Spratt DA, Pratten J (2003) Biofilms and the oral cavity. *Reviews in Environmental Science and Biotechnology* **2**, 109–20.

360. Stashenko P, Yu SM (1989) T helper and T suppressor cell reversal during the development of induced rat periapical lesions. *Journal of Dental Research* **68**, 830–4.

361. Stashenko P (2002) Interrelationship of dental pulp and apical periodontitis. In Hargreaves KM, Goodis HE, editors. *Seltzer and Bender's dental pulp*, pp. 389–409. Chicago, IL: Quintessence.

362. Suau A, Bonnet R, Sutren M, Godon JJ, Gibson GR, Collins MD, Dore J (1999) Direct analysis of genes encoding 16S rRNA from complex communities reveals many novel molecular species within the human gut. *Applied and Environmental Microbiology* **65**, 4799–807.

363. Sunde PT, Tronstad L, Eribe ER, Lind PO, Olsen I (2000) Assessment of periradicular microbiota by DNA–DNA hybridization. *Endodontics and Dental Traumatology* **16**, 191–6.

364. Sunde PT, Olsen I, Debelian GJ, Tronstad L (2002) Microbiota of periapical lesions refractory to endodontic therapy. *Journal of Endodontics* **28**, 304–10.

365. Sunde PT, Olsen I, Gobel UB, Theegarten D, Winter S, Debelian GJ, et al. (2003) Fluorescence in situ hybridization (FISH) for direct visualization of bacteria in periapical lesions of asymptomatic root-filled teeth. *Microbiology* **149**, 1095–102.

366. Sundqvist G (1976) Bacteriological studies of necrotic dental pulps. Dissertation. Umea: University of Umea.

367. Sundqvist G, Carlsson J, Herrmann B, Tarnvik A (1985) Degradation of human immunoglobulins G and M and complement factors C3 and C5 by black-pigmented *Bacteroides*. *Journal of Medical Microbiology* **19**, 85–94.

368. Sundqvist G, Johansson E, Sjögren U (1989) Prevalence of black-pigmented bacteroides species in root canal infections. *Journal of Endodontics* **15**, 13–19.

369. Sundqvist G (1992) Associations between microbial species in dental root canal infections. *Oral Microbiology and Immunology* **7**, 257–62.

370. Sundqvist G (1992) Ecology of the root canal flora. *Journal of Endodontics* **18**, 427–30.

371. Sundqvist G (1993) Pathogenicity and virulence of black-pigmented gram-negative anaerobes. *FEMS Immunology and Medical Microbiology* **6**, 125–37.

372. Sundqvist G (1994) Taxonomy, ecology, and pathogenicity of the root canal flora. *Oral Surgery, Oral Medicine, Oral Pathology* **78**, 522–30.

373. Sundqvist G, Figdor D, Persson S, Sjögren U (1998) Microbiologic analysis of teeth with failed endodontic treatment and the outcome of conservative re-treatment. *Oral Surgery, Oral Medicine, Oral Pathology, Oral Radiology and Endodontics* **85**, 86–93.

374. Sundqvist G, Figdor D (2003) Life as an endodontic pathogen. Ecological differences between the untreated and root-filled root canals. *Endodontic Topics* **6**, 3–28.

375. Sundqvist GK, Eckerbom MI, Larsson AP, Sjögren UT (1979) Capacity of anaerobic bacteria from necrotic dental pulps to induce purulent infections. *Infection and Immunity* **25**, 685–93.

376. Sundqvist GK, Carlsson J, Herrmann BF, Hofling JF, Vaatainen A (1984) Degradation in vivo of the C3 protein of guinea-pig complement by a pathogenic strain of Bacteroides gingivalis. *Scandinavian Journal of Dental Research* **92**, 14–24.

377. Syrjänen J, Peltola J, Valtonen V, Livanainen M, Kaste M, Huttunen JK (1989) Dental infections in association with certain infarction in young and middle-aged men. *Journal of Internal Medicine* **225**, 179–84.

378. Tang G, Samaranayake LP, Yip HK, Chu FC, Tsang PC, Cheung BP (2003) Direct detection of *Actinomyces* spp. from infected root canals in a Chinese population: a study using PCR-based, oligonucleotide-DNA hybridization technique. *Journal of Dentistry* **31**, 559–68.

379. Tani-Ishii N, Wang CY, Tanner A, Stashenko P (1994) Changes in root canal microbiota during the development of rat periapical lesions. *Oral Microbiology and Immunology* **9**, 129–35.

380. Tendolkar PM, Baghdayan AS, Shankar N (2003) Pathogenic enterococci: new developments in the 21st century. *Cellular and Molecular Life Sciences* **60**, 2622–36.

381. ter Steeg PF, van der Hoeven JS (1989) Development of periodontal microflora on human serum. *Microbial Ecology in Health and Disease* **2**, 1–10.

382. ter Steeg PF, van der Hoeven JS (1990) Growth stimulation of *Treponema denticola* by periodontal microorganisms. *Antonie Van Leeuwenhoek* **57**, 63–70.

383. Tronstad L, Andreasen JO, Hasselgren G, Kristerson L, Riis I (1980) pH changes in dental tissues after root canal filling with calcium hydroxide. *Journal of Endodontics* **7**, 17–21.

384. Tronstad L, Barnett F, Riso K, Slots J (1987) Extraradicular endodontic infections. *Endodontics and Dental Traumatology* **3**, 86–90.

385. Tronstad L, Barnett F, Cervone F (1990) Periapical bacterial plaque in teeth refractory to endodontic treatment. *Endodontics and Dental Traumatology* **6**, 73–7.

386. Tronstad L, Sunde PT (2003) The evolving new understanding of endodontic infections. *Endodontic Topics* **6**, 57–77.

387. Trowbridge HO, Emling RC (1997) *Inflammation. A review of the process,* 5th edn. Chicago, IL: Quintessence.

388. van Amersfoort ES, van Berkel TJC, Kuiper J (2003) Receptors, mediators, and mechanisms involved in bacterial sepsis and septic shock. *Clinical Microbiology Reviews* **16**, 379–414.

389. van Steenbergen TJM, van der Mispel LMS, de Graaff J (1986) Effect of ammonia and volatile fatty acids produced by oral bacteria on tissue culture cells. *Journal of Dental Research* **65**, 909–12.

390. van Winkelhoff AJ, Carlee AW, de Graaff J (1985) *Bacteroides endodontalis* and others black-pigmented *Bacteroides* species in odontogenic abscesses. *Infection and Immunity* **49**, 494–8.

391. van Winkelhoff AJ, van Steenbergen TJ, de Graaff J (1992) *Porphyromonas (Bacteroides) endodontalis*: its role in endodontal infections. *Journal of Endodontics* **18**, 431–4.

392. van Winkelhoff AJ, Winkel EG, Barendregt D, Dellemijn-Kippuw N, Stijne A, van der Velden U (1997) beta-Lactamase producing bacteria in adult periodontitis. *Journal of Clinical Periodontology* **24**, 538–43.

393. van Winkelhoff AJ, Herrera D, Oteo A, Sanz M (2005) Antimicrobial profiles of periodontal pathogens isolated from periodontitis patients in The Netherlands and Spain. *Journal of Clinical Periodontology* **32**, 893–8.

394. Vianna ME, Horz HP, Gomes BP, Conrads G (2005) Microarrays complement culture methods for identification of bacteria in endodontic infections. *Oral Microbiology and Immunology* **20**, 253–8.

395. Vianna ME, Conrads G, Gomes BPF, Horz HP (2006) Identification and quantification of archaea involved in primary endodontic infections. *Journal of Clinical Microbiology* **44**, 1274–82.

396. Vianna ME, Horz HP, Gomes BP, Conrads G (2006) In vivo evaluation of microbial reduction after chemomechanical preparation of human root canals containing necrotic pulp tissue. *International Endodontic Journal* **39**, 484–92.

397. Waltimo T, Trope M, Haapasalo M, Ørstavik D (2005) Clinical efficacy of treatment procedures in endodontic infection control and one year follow-up of periapical healing. *Journal of Endodontics* **31**, 863–6.

398. Waltimo TM, Sirén EK, Torkko HL, Olsen I, Haapasalo MP (1997) Fungi in therapy-resistant apical periodontitis. *International Endodontic Journal* **30**, 96–101.

399. Waltimo TM, Ørstavik D, Sirén EK, Haapasalo MP (1999) In vitro susceptibility of *Candida albicans* to four disinfectants and their combinations. *International Endodontic Journal* **32**, 421–9.

400. Waltimo TM, Sirén EK, Ørstavik D, Haapasalo MP (1999) Susceptibility of oral *Candida* species to calcium hydroxide in vitro. *International Endodontic Journal* **32**, 94–8.

401. Waltimo TM, Ørstavik D, Sirén EK, Haapasalo MP (2000) In vitro yeast infection of human dentin. *Journal of Endodontics* **26**, 207–9.

402. Walton RE (1976) Histologic evaluation of different methods of enlarging the pulp canal space. *Journal of Endodontics* **2**, 304–11.

403. Wang JE, Dahle MK, McDonald M, Foster SJ, Aasen AO, Thiemermann C (2003) Peptidoglycan and lipoteichoic acid in Gram-positive bacterial sepsis: receptors, signal transduction, biological effects, and synergism. *Shock* **20**, 402–14.

404. Wara-Aswapati N, Boch JA, Auron PE (2003) Activation of interleukin 1beta gene transcription by human cytomegalovirus: molecular mechanisms and relevance to periodontitis. *Oral Microbiology and Immunology* **18**, 67–71.

405. Wasfy MO, McMahon KT, Minah GE, Falkler WA Jr (1992) Microbiological evaluation of periapical infections in Egypt. *Oral Microbiology and Immunology* **7**, 100–5.

406. Wayman BE, Murata SM, Almeida RJ, Fowler CB (1992) A bacteriological and histological evaluation of 58 periapical lesions. *Journal of Endodontics* **18**, 152–5.

407. Weiger R, Manncke B, Werner H, Lost C (1995) Microbial flora of sinus tracts and root canals of nonvital teeth. *Endodontics and Dental Traumatology* **11**, 15–19.

408. Weiger R, de Lucena J, Decker HE, Lost C (2002) Vitality status of microorganisms in infected human

root dentine. *International Endodontic Journal* **35**, 166–71.

409. Wen ZT, Burne RA (2004) LuxS-mediated signaling in *Streptococcus mutans* is involved in regulation of acid and oxidative stress tolerance and biofilm formation. *Journal of Bacteriology* **186**, 2682–91.

410. Whitney CG, Farley MM, Hadler J, Harrison LH, Lexau C, Reingold A, *et al.* (2000) Increasing prevalence of multidrug-resistant *Streptococcus pneumoniae* in the United States. *New England Journal of Medicine* **343**, 1917–24.

411. Williams JM, Trope M, Caplan DJ, Shugars DC (2006) Detection and quantitation of *Enterococcus faecalis* by real-time PCR (qPCR), reverse transcription-PCR (RT-PCR), and cultivation during endodontic treatment. *Journal of Endodontics* **32**, 715–21.

412. Wilson M, Reddi K, Henderson B (1996) Cytokine-inducing components of periodontopathogenic bacteria. *Journal of Periodontal Research* **31**, 393–407.

413. Withers H, Swift S, Williams P (2001) Quorum sensing as an integral component of gene regulatory networks in Gram-negative bacteria. *Current Opinion in Microbiology* **4**, 186–93.

414. Wu M-K, van der Sluis LWM, Wesselink PR (2003) The capability of two hand instrumentation techniques to remove the inner layer of dentine in oval canals. *International Endodontic Journal* **36**, 218–24.

415. Xia T, Baumgartner JC, David LL (2000) Isolation and identification of *Prevotella tannerae* from endodontic infections. *Oral Microbiology and Immunology* **15**, 273–5.

416. Xia T, Baumgartner JC (2003) Occurrence of *Actinomyces* in infections of endodontic origin. *Journal of Endodontics* **29**, 549–52.

417. Ying SC, Jiang H, Kim YB, Gewurz H (1993) C1q peptides bind endotoxin and inhibit endotoxin-initiated activation of the classical complement pathway. *Journal of Immunology* **150**, 304A.

418. Yoneda M, Hirofuji T, Anan H, Matsumoto A, Hamachi T, Nakayama K, *et al.* (2001) Mixed infection of *Porphyromonas gingivalis* and *Bacteroides forsythus* in a murine abscess model: involvement of gingipains in a synergistic effect. *Journal of Periodontal Research* **36**, 237–43.

419. Yoshida A, Ansai T, Takehara T, Kuramitsu HK (2005) LuxS-based signaling affects *Streptococcus mutans* biofilm formation. *Applied and Environmental Microbiology* **71**, 2372–80.

420. Yoshida M, Fukushima H, Yamamoto K, Ogawa K, Toda T, Sagawa H (1987) Correlation between clinical symptoms and microorganisms isolated from root canals of teeth with periapical pathosis. *Journal of Endodontics* **13**, 24–8.

421. Yuan L, Hillman JD, Progulske-Fox A (2005) Microarray analysis of quorum-sensing-regulated genes in *Porphyromonas gingivalis*. *Infection and Immunity* **73**, 4146–54.

422. Zhang Y, Wang T, Chen W, Yilmaz O, Park Y, Jung IY, Hackett M, Lamont RJ (2005) Differential protein expression by *Porphyromonas gingivalis* in response to secreted epithelial cell components. *Proteomics* **5**, 198–211.

423. Zoletti GO, Siqueira JF Jr, Santos KR (2006) Identification of *Enterococcus faecalis* in root-filled teeth with or without periradicular lesions by culture-dependent and -independent approaches. *Journal of Endodontics* **32**, 722–6.

424. Zou W, Bar-Shavit Z (2002) Dual modulation of osteoclast differentiation by lipopolysaccharide. *Journal of Bone and Mineral Research* **17**, 1211–18.

425. Zou W, Amcheslavsky A, Bar-Shavit Z (2003) CpG oligodeoxynucleotides modulate the osteoclastogenic activity of osteoblasts via Toll-like receptor 9. *Journal of Biological Chemistry* **278**, 16732–40.

426. Zuolo ML, Walton RE, Imura N (1992) Histologic evaluation of three endodontic instrument/preparation techniques. *Endodontics and Dental Traumatology* **8**, 125–9.

Chapter 6
Radiology of Apical Periodontitis

Dag Ørstavik and Tore A. Larheim

6.1 Introduction

Radiology is essential for all aspects of endodontic treatment: diagnosis, treatment planning, working length determination, control of obturation procedures, and follow-up controls. It is also indispensable for epidemiological surveys of apical periodontitis. The present chapter is concerned with radiology as a diagnostic aid [150] and as a tool for follow-up assessment and epidemiological studies, with limited discussion of the use of radiographs as technical aids during treatment.

Whereas acute inflammatory lesions usually are recognizable through their clinical signs and symptoms (Chapter 7), the more frequent, chronic apical periodontitis is detected mainly or exclusively by its radiological features.

The radiological diagnosis of apical periodontitis is often considered trivial and assigned low status and little emphasis in teaching programs as well as research. This is reflected by a scarcity of publications addressing the details of periapical radiography. However, the reliance on radiological interpretation for many treatment decisions makes it evident that extensive and factual-based knowledge of the radiological features of apical periodontitis is important both for the general practitioner and the specialist.

6.1.1 Principles of periapical radiography

The introduction of sophisticated radiographic techniques has provided an invaluable supplement to endodontic radiography. However, the intra-oral, periapical radiograph remains the standard for radiological diagnosis of apical periodontitis. Such radiographs therefore constitute the majority of the illustrations in this chapter. There are two principles of periapical radiography: the bisecting-angle and the paralleling technique. While the former technique may provide adequate information and in some instances be the only realistic approach, the paralleling technique has many practical and theoretical advantages and should be used whenever possible [51,52]. The use of film holders greatly facilitates reproducible exposure geometry, and parallel film/tooth placement reduces superimposition by neighboring structures.

6.2 Normal apical periodontium

The root apices vary in morphology, and they are embedded in bone of varying density and texture. This makes it difficult to define "normal periapical radiological features" [72]. But there are general features of the anatomy of the tooth apex, the periodontal ligament and the lamina dura of the alveolus which are of decisive importance for the interpretation of radiographic images of teeth in every tooth group. Superimposed on these common features, however, are site-specific and individual anatomical variations which may confound the diagnostic process.

The following are some key elements in the anatomy of the apical periodontium and surrounding structures which should be assessed on the radiograph.

6.2.1 Apex and pulp canal foramen

The tooth apex with the apical foramen and ramifications of the pulp is the most important structure in the development of apical periodontitis, since the pathologic processes most often occur in response to microbial infection of the pulp canal system. The tip of the root apex is usually at an angle to the long axis of the root, deviating in any direction (mesially, facially, distally, or lingually) depending on the tooth type and individual variations. Moreover, the apical foramen usually exits lateral to the anatomical tip of the apex, and the apparent apex on the radiograph seldom represents the true level of the foramen. While the apex is normally rounded and well defined, resorptive processes may occur or may have occurred which can lead to "blunting" of the root end on the radiograph. Apical root resorption may follow orthodontic movement of the teeth and other physical traumas [3,176], but it is also frequent during chronic apical periodontitis, where it may affect the apical foramen itself [25,109,191] (Fig. 6.1). Apical root resorption in apical periodontitis may stop spontaneously or following treatment, but it will leave a scar in the sense that the shape of the root tip is permanently altered despite recontouring and smoothening effects of new cementum deposition.

6.2.2 Cementum

The process of locating radiographically the apex and the foramen is further complicated by a variation in the amount of secondary cementum laid down at the tooth apex. This is done in response to attrition,

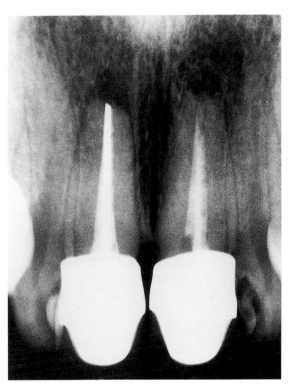

Fig. 6.1 Resorption of the apical parts of the roots of both maxillary central incisors associated with chronic apical periodontitis.

abrasion or other physiopathological processes of the clinical crown leading to extrusion of the tooth.

6.2.3 Periodontal ligament space

The precise, radiographic tracing of the tooth apex and its bony surroundings is made possible by the periodontal ligament (PDL). The PDL provides a radiolucent structure that gives contrast to the surrounding mineralized elements. While the PDL has a basic, minimal biological width that is assumed to prevent ankylosis of the tooth [205], it may be widened if the tooth has increased mobility [25]. Advanced marginal periodontitis often causes increased mobility of involved teeth, and the apical PDL in such cases may be widened substantially.

6.2.4 Lamina dura

The lamina dura is a radiological term applied to the cortical rim of bone immediately peripheral to the

PDL space. It is a continuation of the cortical plate. It may appear as an almost uninterrupted radiopaque wall around the root, but the blood, lymph and nerve supplies to the pulp and the PDL must cross the lamina dura through channels of varying sizes, and these channels sometimes appear to be reflected in radiographs as "perforations" in the lamina.

6.2.5 Cortical bone

Like other bones, the maxilla and the mandible are encased in cortical bone plates. The root tips are frequently located in close apposition to either the buccal/labial or the lingual cortical plates, with significant variation dependent primarily on tooth location (Fig. 6.2) [111]. Facial root apices and apices of single-rooted maxillary teeth usually touch the facial cortical plate; the lateral incisor is an exception in that its root apex frequently deviates palatally. In the maxilla, the facial cortical bone sometimes is discontinuous over the roots, leaving islands or strands of PDL suspended in soft tissue only [177]. This denudation may run from the apex to the marginal periodontium itself, but is hardly demonstrable in radiographs. Mandibular premolars may not infrequently be suspended in medullary bone; mandibular molar root tips tend to tilt towards the lingual cortical plate, whereas the incisors frequently are closer to the facial cortex.

6.2.6 Medullary bone

The organization of the medullary, central part of the mandible and maxilla varies in structure and density. The trabecular pattern which gives rise to the appearance of a texture on radiographs is typically fine granular in the maxilla and coarser with wider marrow spaces in the mandible. The organization of the trabeculae is determined by functional stress [18,56,64]; at times the functional suspension of teeth by the medullary bone organization may be visualized (Fig. 6.3) [166].

6.2.7 Neighboring anatomical structures

A number of anatomical bone structures may be superimposed on teeth in periapical radiographs [72]. The incisive canal is a channel-like structure between the upper central incisors. It may vary in size and shape from a thin line to a wedge- or heart-shaped, larger structure (Fig. 6.4), sometimes forming a cyst

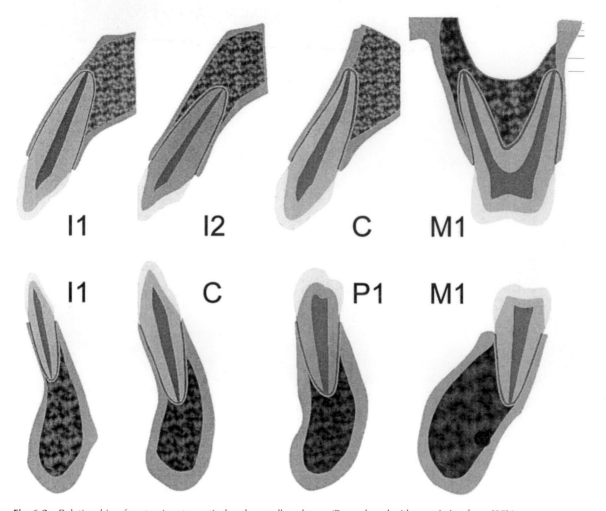

I1   I2   C   M1

I1   C   P1   M1

Fig. 6.2   Relationship of root apices to cortical and cancellous bone. (Reproduced with permission from [85].)

or cyst-like radiolucent area. The upper front part of the maxilla forms the floor of the front part of the nasal cavity. This floor appears as the radiopaque rim of two radiolucent areas and it is normally projected over the apices of the central incisors. Periapical radiographs of this region also frequently include the tip of the nose, which appears as a diffuse radiopacity over the apices. The canine fossa reduces the bone density over the maxillary lateral incisor sometimes to mimic apical periodontitis. The maxillary sinus has two extensions that typically appear over the premolars and the molars in the maxilla. Its border is a thin, radiopaque line, with one or several radiopaque lines inside the outer periphery. These septa are actually only folds of cortical bone projecting a few

millimeters into the sinus lumen. They are usually oriented vertically, although horizontal bony ridges also occur, and they vary in number, thickness and length. In the radiographs, maxillary sinus structures sometimes may mimic periapical pathosis. The variable morphology of the maxillary sinus makes it important that its outline is traced in periapical radiographs: the lower border of sinus lobes must be distinguished from outlines of apical cysts or granulomas and from slopes of the root apices and lamina dura projecting to the same area [169] (Fig. 6.5). The root apices of the first molar may have a distance of less than 0.5 mm to the sinus floor and at times there is no bony separation [85]. It then becomes impossible to trace the lamina dura around the roots. Three-rooted sec-

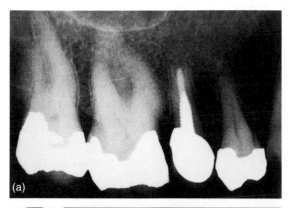

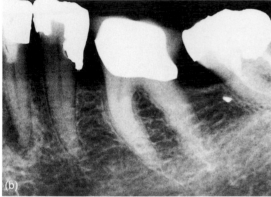

Fig. 6.3 The granular pattern of bone in maxilla (a) compared with the typical horizontal striations in the mandible (b) in the same patient.

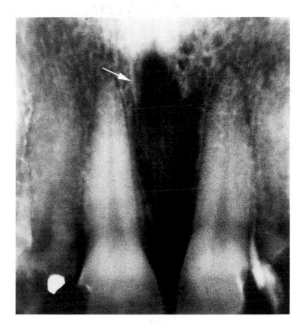

Fig. 6.4 The incisive canal.

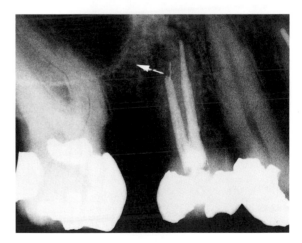

Fig. 6.5 The floor of the maxillary sinus uperimposed on the roots of the first maxillary molar. Tracing of an intact lamina dura on the radiograph and vitality testing of the first molar prevent a false diagnosis of apical peridontitis.

ond molars have apices located even closer to the maxillary sinus, and single-rooted molars may also be located in the immediate vicinity of the maxillary sinus [43]. The zygomatic arch supports the masseter muscle and may project over the apices of the maxillary molars. This can make distinction of periapical structures almost impossible (Fig. 6.6). Palatine tori may obscure details of the periapical structures.

In the mandible, the mental foramen is a well-known confounder for exact diagnosis of apical periodontitis of the canine or the first and, particularly, the second premolar. Usually located between the root apices of the premolars, the foramen is frequently, but not always, demonstrable on periapical radiographs. In some cases, it may mimic all the classical radiological signs of apical periodontitis (Fig. 6.7). Then tracing of the mandibular canal to the area of suspected pathology, or tracing of the lamina dura around the root apex would suggest the true nature

of the radiolucency. The mandibular canal runs in the mandible from the mandibular to the mental foramen, and may or may not show up on radiographs. Its proximity to the apices of the teeth in the area (Fig. 6.8) may affect the radiological appearance of the periapical region, and more importantly, lead to

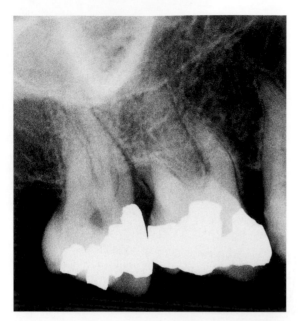

Fig. 6.6   The zygomatic arch is superimposed on the roots of the first and second molars.

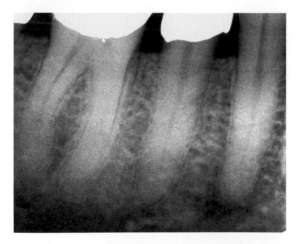

Fig. 6.7   The mental foramen superimposed on the periapical structures of the mandibular second premolar.

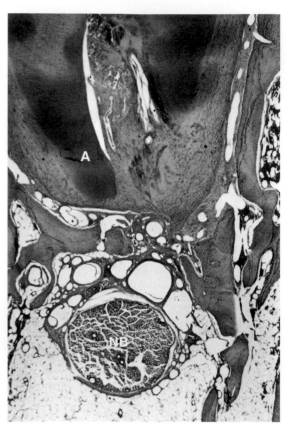

Fig. 6.8   Facio-lingual section of the first mandibular molar in the *Macaca fascicularis* monkey. The very close association between the tooth apex and the nerve bundle in the inferior alveolar canal is evident.

6.3 Established apical periodontitis

Established, chronic apical periodontitis (CAP) is a localized inflammatory response to pulpal infection developing from the periodontal ligament at the expense of bone, and appears radiographically as a reduction in mineral density of the affected area. Medullary and/or cortical bone has been replaced by soft tissue or liquid in the form of a granuloma or a cyst (Fig. 6.10).

6.3.1 Histological correlations

The histological description of a given disease process traditionally provides its defining characteristics. The validity and relevance of radiographic features are often considered to be mainly dependent on how

a risk of complications during conservative (Fig. 6.9) and surgical procedures in that region. Also in the mandible, tori and exostoses may obscure details of the periapical structures.

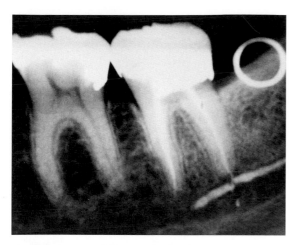

Fig. 6.9   Root canal filling material in the inferior alveolar canal associated with paresthesia of the inferior alveolar and mental nerves. (Reproduced from [139] with permission from *International Endodontic Journal*.)

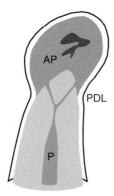

Fig. 6.10   The essential features of established, apical periodontitis. The apical lesion gives a droplet-shaped, radiolucent appearance; the PDL tapers off into the outer periphery of the lesion; the lamina dura is absent at the apex. The lesion itself is emanating from the necrotic/ infected contents of the root canal orifices at the root tip.

well they reflect the histological appearance of the disease. A number of studies have looked at the relationship between the histological and radiological characteristics of apical periodontitis [13,24,25,66, 96,161,182,204]. From these studies, a few generalizations may be made: (1) the radiographic appearance of CAP is always smaller than the histological extent of the lesion, (2) the absence of radiographic signs of CAP does not rule out its presence, whereas the presence of its key radiographic signs is virtually

pathognomonic, and (3) the radiograph cannot be used reliably to distinguish between a granuloma and a cyst.

By far the most extensive and penetrating study correlating the histology and the radiology of apical periodontitis was carried out by Brynolf [25]. The following is to a large degree based on her findings.

6.3.2 Stages in radiological features

A long-standing CAP of some extent is in most instances easily diagnosed in the radiograph. The problems arise when the radiographic signs are few and small, which typically occur when the lesion is young or of small size, and when other anatomical structures obscure the details of the periapical area. It is in these cases that the knowledge derived from the correlative studies has the greatest significance. A primary sign of apical periodontitis is bone structural changes: while the normal bone texture reflects the functional organization of bone, frequently with bone trabeculae radiating from the apical area, early stages of apical periodontitis are characterized by the disorganization of this pattern (Fig. 6.11). Sometimes the area of disorganization may be traced and separated from the surrounding, normal bone pattern; but it may also have a diffuse transition to normal bone. Widening of the PDL is traditionally taken as a sign of apical periodontitis (Fig. 6.12). However, it is a sign of limited significance, as this is also a feature of mobile teeth often associated with advanced marginal periodontitis, and the projection may favor its visualization. When a widened PDL reflects apical periodontitis, there is often a fairly sharp transition from the unaffected PDL coronally with a step up in size to the apical PDL affected by the inflammation. Another feature also frequently associated with apical periodontitis is disintegration of the lamina dura. While the breakdown of bone to accommodate the inflammatory response must include the lamina dura for expansion, in and by themselves the continuity and density of the lamina dura are weak signs of CAP [157]: the radiographic appearance of the structure is highly vulnerable to small individual variations in thickness; the number of normal canals perforating it may vary; and the exposure angle may affect its appearance. However, particularly when used in comparison with radiographs from a pre-diseased state of the same roots exposed from the same angle (parallel exposure technique), both the width of the PDL and the continuity of the lamina dura may help

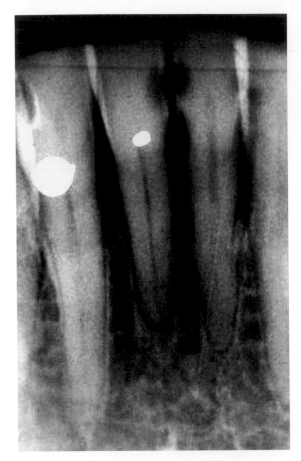

Fig. 6.11 Bone structural changes apically of the central incisor, associated with chronic, symptomatic pulpitis.

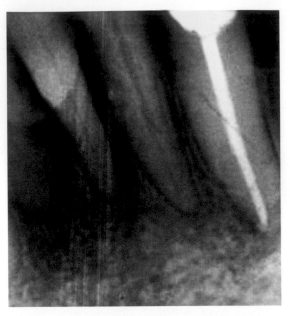

Fig. 6.12 Widened periodontal ligament of the central incisor associated with increased mobility.

in establishing the diagnosis. When net mineral loss of the periapical bone becomes evident, the diagnostic process is made much easier. Still, in the absence of a clear-cut 'radiolucency', true pathognomonic signs of CAP may be hard to identify. Following or accompanying the bone structural changes, one may see a change in appearance which may be described as a "shot-gun" effect: the basic fabric of the bone is intact, but the small marrow spaces have increased in size at the expense of the thickness of the bone spiculae (Fig. 6.13). These are also situations where it is important to judge whether the signs reflect a standing or healing CAP (see below).

A droplet-shaped radiolucency at an apex, with a PDL tapering into the normal areas at the lateral aspects of the root and the lamina dura absent, when combined with findings confirming a necrotic pulp, is pathognomonic of CAP (Fig. 6.10).

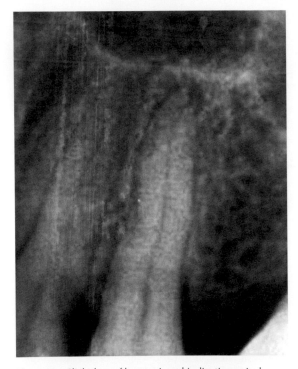

Fig. 6.13 Slight loss of bone mineral indicating apical periodontitis.

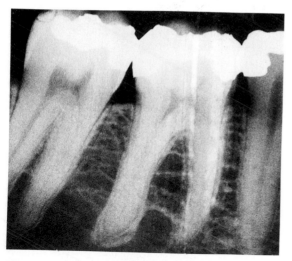

Fig. 6.14 Condensing apical periodontitis of the distal root of the mandibular first molar. Clinical inspection revealed a dentin fracture making endodontic treatment necessary.

Occasionally, however, CAP may develop adjacent to a partially necrotized and infected pulp with normal and vital pulp tissue apically. The extreme rarity of this situation makes it a minor, perhaps irrelevant clinical entity.

Acute or spreading features of initial as well as long-standing CAP may show texture changes around an intact lamina dura or beyond the borderline, enhanced or not, between the chronic lesion and the surrounding bone.

The reactive nature of bone sometimes produces denser bone in response particularly to low-grade irritants. Condensing apical periodontitis is a response typically to chronic pulpitis (Figs 6.14 and 6.15).

6.3.3 Cyst/granuloma formation

The expansion of the lesion is believed to continue until there is a balance between the protective function of the tissues and the virulence of the infecting organisms. The balance is promoted by the formation of a granuloma, which in turn may or may not develop into a cyst [17]. Expansion follows the path of least resistance, and the granuloma/cyst may be viewed as a soft tissue/fluid bag attached to the tooth at the site where the pulp canal exits. A cyst may also have separated completely from the root tip, forming a periapical "true" cyst [129,175]. The body of the lesion will

not necessarily project to the periapical area or a lateral or furcal portal of exit; it may be superimposed on structures coronal and lateral to the root itself. More often than not, the lesion will have a large part of it in these areas, which is one reason why the lesion in reality is larger than its radiographic appearance.

It is generally believed that the presence of a radiopaque rim surrounding a bone lesion indicates a more stable/slow-growing condition compared with diffusely demarcated lesions. This is supported by Brynolf's description of radiographs reflecting CAP with features of exacerbation: here, the bone peripheral to the central lesion shows an unclear border with radiations of radiolucent streaks into the surrounding areas [25]. On the other hand, we do not yet have data to associate particular radiographic features of CAP with the likelihood of imminent, acute clinical problems [157]. The recognition of some cystic lesions as being dissociated from the root apex [129,131] may reactivate the interest in radiographic differentiation of cysts and granulomas [172,193]. By conventional methods, however, differentiation between cysts and granulomas is hardly possible [206].

6.3.4 Regional variations in detectability

Generally, as endodontic treatment needs often arise from dental caries, CAP is frequent in teeth at high risk of caries. Moreover, since CAP is often associated with teeth which have had unsuccessful endodontic treatment, teeth with complex or difficult root canal anatomy, e.g., maxillary lateral incisors, first premolars and first molars, may be over-represented. It should be noted, however, that anatomical relationships may improve or impair the likelihood of detecting CAP. The relatively fewer superimposing structures in the mandible may make lesions in the lower jaw more easily detectable than in the maxilla. By contrast, lesions in maxillary molars may go undetected if the projection does not separate the zygomatic bone from the periapical area.

6.3.5 Lateral locations

The pulp canal system has exits to the periodontium in the apical delta, but also at other sites along the root. Infection of the pulp canal may therefore induce periodontitis at these sites. Apart from the localization to the area close to the pulpal exit, the radiographic appearance of such lesions is similar to apically located periodontitis; it is necessary, however

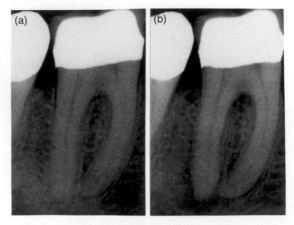

Fig. 6.15 Condensing apical periodontitis of the distal root of the lower first molar (a) developing in 6 months to chronic apical periodontitis (b).

to differentiate them from the lateral periodontal cyst and periodontitis of marginal origin. The localization of lateral canals may be difficult in conventional radiographs, and attempts to improve detectability with radiopaque agents and digital radiography have met with some limited success [167,171]. The root filling sometimes traces the lateral canal associated with the lesion (Fig. 6.16).

6.3.6 Furcal locations

Similarly, exits from the pulp canal system into the furcation area of multi-rooted teeth may give rise to inflammation in these locations. Such accessory canals in the furcation area of molars have been reported to occur in 76% of all molars [27]. The radiographic appearance is expectedly identical with similar lesions from marginal infection, and careful clinical investigation is necessary to identify the source of the infection to institute adequate treatment.

6.3.7 Impact of medullary vs cortical involvement

Generally speaking, as the cortices of the jaw bones contribute overwhelmingly to the total radiopacity of the periapical area, an inflammatory process which involves the medullary part of the bone only

or mainly, has less chance of becoming detectable on radiographs compared with lesions involving the cortex of the bone. Particularly in instances where the bone marrow is largely of soft tissue with few and thin bone trabeculae, the formation of a granuloma or cyst leaves little trace in mineralized tissue to become visible on the radiograph.

Based on extensive *in vitro* experimental studies, it was postulated that lesions could not be detected unless the cortical bone was involved, even perforated [14,107]. This was in striking contrast to the tradition of assigning great importance to the minuscule details of the integrity of the lamina dura or the width of the PDL. The correlative histological/radiological studies place the detectability somewhere in between: changes in bone texture and organization also reflecting medullary bone may be detectable, although with difficulty, on many radiographs [25,30,32]. Computed tomography (CT) scans have confirmed that it is possible to detect periapical lesion in conventional, periapical radiographs even when they do not impinge on the cortex [111].

6.4 Incipient apical periodontitis

6.4.1 Chronic inflammation of the pulp

Pulpal involvement from a carious lesion or a leaking restoration will not always result in the immediate infection and necrosis of the entire pulp canal system. A state of chronic pulpal inflammation may arise. In some cases a reactive bone tissue formation at the apex of the involved tooth can occur. This is termed condensing apical periodontitis [45,79]. Untreated, the condition may develop into rarefying apical periodontitis (Figs 6.15 and 6.17). Complete pulp extirpation and root filling may be necessary, but in selected cases, pulp healing and sometimes also apical bone restitution has been achieved by restorative treatment only. There does not appear to be any detailed description of the features of condensing apical periodontitis in the literature. It would appear that the lesion occupies a space around the apex that is similar in size and location to where a radiolucent lesion would be expected to occur, confirming a "region of interest" for the body's defenses of teeth predetermined for each root and location (see below). Hypermineralizaton has also been shown to occur following treatment of CAP [100] (Fig. 6.18).

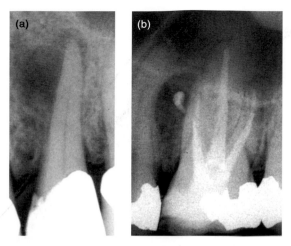

Fig. 6.16 Primary apical periodontitis (a) and root filling sealer extruding from a lateral canal associated with chronic apical periodontitis (b) in a lateral location.

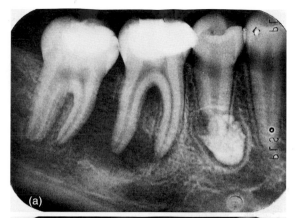

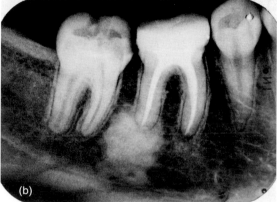

Fig. 6.18 Apical periodontitis (a) developing into condensing AP (b) after endodontic treatment of a lower right first molar. (The odontoma near the root of the premolar was extirpated and has no bearing on the issue.) (Reproduced from [94] with permission.)

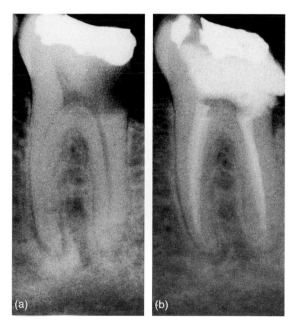

Fig. 6.17 Condensing apical periodontitis of the mesial root of the lower first molar (a) resolving in 6 months after endodontic treatment (b).

6.4.2 Transient apical breakdown; apical root resorption

This may occur following trauma, particularly luxation injuries, to anterior teeth. The trauma may result in loss of pulpal responsiveness, and radiographs may show resorptive processes of the apex and surrounding bone completely mimicking early stages of infectious apical periodontitis. However, if the pulp does not become infected, there is a potential for reversal of the process with repair of the root end surface and remodeling of the periapical bone structure including re-establishment of the lamina dura [5,21] (Fig. 6.19). Close monitoring of each case is however essential for detection of pulp necrosis and infection, which frequently occur [6].

6.5 Root-filled teeth with apical periodontitis

Spontaneous regression of apical periodontitis in untreated roots virtually never occurs. For root-filled

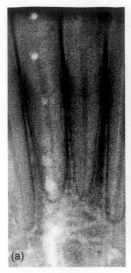
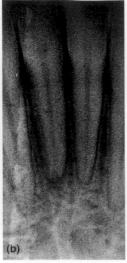
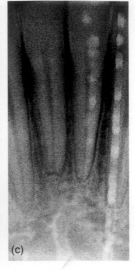

Fig. 6.19 Transient apical periodontitis. Immediately after a trauma to the lower right central incisor, there is no radiographic sign of disease (a). A lesion develops in the first few months (b) after trauma, but repair and resolution with intact pulp sensitivity is evident after 2 years (c). (Reproduced from [21] with permission.)

teeth, however, it may be hard to judge radiographically whether a lesion is in the process of healing, is stable, or expanding.

Histological studies of apical tissues of radiographically healed or healing apical periodontitis frequently show inflammation, often low-grade and limited in extent, but still signs of disease. The findings by Brynolf [25] that a majority of root-filled teeth had some, albeit small, signs of apical periodontitis also in radiographs, makes the diagnosis of apical periodontitis in root-filled teeth complex.

6.6 Characteristics of healing

6.6.1 Healing of apical periodontitis

Little is known about the radiographic characteristics of healing after root canal treatment of apical periodontitis. Repair of periradicular tissues consists of a complex regeneration involving bone, PDL and cementum. Immediately following instrumentation and filling of a root canal, there may actually be a transient increase in bone density for the first few weeks [137,140]. It has also been suggested that a periapical breakdown may persist for periods of years, but is ultimately resolved [55,180]. During healing, the area of mineral loss gradually fills with bone and the radiographic density increases. Whether bone is deposited concentrically from the periphery of the lesion or by spiculae projecting towards the

center, or both, is unknown. It appears, however, that healing of apical periodontitis is slow in comparison with the bone repair that takes place after surgical creation of a bone cavity [102,138,165]. If the cortical plate is perforated, bone deposition starts by reestablishment of the external cortical plate and then proceeds toward the center of the lesion [22,128]. The structure of the newly formed bone may differ from normal and may seem less organized. While it has been generally accepted that the PDL may remain widened mainly around excess filling material [180], it remains questionable whether complete healing has occurred in such cases [25]. A majority of root-filled teeth show some indication of bone structural change or minor rarefaction; this may be related to a protracted healing phase or reflect a limited residual infection [25,142].

6.6.2 Healing after surgery

The radiological appearance of the periapical tissues following apical surgery has some unique features [7]. The surgical procedure itself eliminates any residual mineralized mass over the lesion when it is excised or curetted, leaving a postoperative radiographic image of more pronounced radiolucency than preoperatively. When healing occurs, it is more variable in appearance and often irregular compared with the healing process following root canal treatment. The formation of apical scar tissue with bone trabeculae radiating from a center that may remain radiolucent

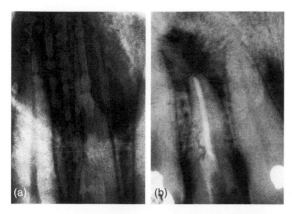

Fig. 6.20 A large lesion of chronic apical periodontitis (a) was treated conventionally with calcium hydroxide for 3 months and root filling. Five years afterwards, there is healing by scar tissue formation and no further growth of bone in the area (b).

indefinitely, is not uncommon (Fig. 6.20). Absence of apical periodontitis may still be diagnosed if the radiograph shows a continuous lamina dura and there are no clinical findings. Persistent radiolucencies may also be associated with healed lesions following root canal treatment, and are believed to occur when both cortical bone plates have been perforated by the inflammation itself or by the surgical procedures [124]. The presence of excess filling material is a possible source of persisting inflammation [130,211], but a limited foreign-body-type reaction to surplus material may not require retreatment.

6.7 Supplementary imaging to periapical radiography

In the majority of cases only one intraoral periapical radiograph is sufficient for the diagnostic assessment of apical periodontitis. However, more than one exposure may often be necessary [26], as in the evaluation of multi-rooted or traumatized teeth. Occclusal views may give valuable supplementary diagnostic information as well. In selected cases advanced imaging methods may add valuable diagnostic information. Cone-beam CT for jaw examinations demonstrates the tooth and the periapical area in both sagittal, coronal and axial planes (Fig. 6.21), and a destruction of for instance the buccal cortical plate may be clearly seen (Fig. 6.22). Advanced medical imaging, such as

multidetector CT, can add diagnostic information of therapeutic significance of the periapical area as well (Fig. 6.23) [103].

Chronic apical periodontitis may span in size from hardly detectable to involving a major part of the jaw bone (Fig. 6.24a). While panoramic radiography may not be as sensitive as periapical radiographs in the diagnosis of apical periodontitis [159], it is often valuable to get an impression of the size of large lesions. However, it will usually not be sufficient for evaluation of the association of such lesions with the maxillary sinus (Fig. 6.24b). CT can then be of great diagnostic value demonstrating the precise size and location as well as the integrity and displacement of the sinus walls (Fig. 6.24c). If there is a suspicion that the process involves the nasal cavity, CT is valuable to rule out the relationship, demonstrating for instance the lack of bony delineation between the pathological process and the anatomical structure (Fig. 6.25).

The apical lesion may also develop into maxillary sinusitis [47,168]. Conversely, the symptomatology of diseases originating in the maxillary sinuses may mimic apical periodontitis. These conditions may necessitate maxillary sinus imaging, which usually includes CT [103].

Apical surgery of lesions in the vicinity of the mandibular canal or mental foramen also dictates exact knowledge of the lesion's location in relation to these anatomical structures, representing another clinical situation where the use of advanced imaging methods has improved diagnostic and therapeutic performance [196].

The location and extent of a resorptive process within the tooth itself also poses special problems regarding treatment planning and surgical access. CT is a valuable adjunct also in these cases [82].

6.8 Differential diagnosis

The following is a listing of some relatively common lesions which may present difficulties in the differential diagnosis of apical periodontitis. In the differential diagnostic evaluation, particularly of larger jaw lesions, advanced imaging, predominantly CT, is increasingly used [103].

6.8.1 Marginal periodontitis

As the name periodontitis implies, inflammation originating from the tooth margin naturally shares

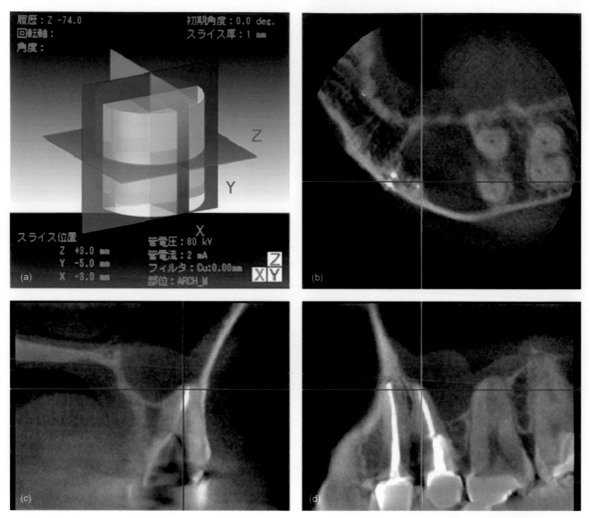

Fig. 6.21 Endodontically treated maxillary premolars with normal periapical structures. Some mucosal thickening in maxillary sinus. Cone beam CT with sections in axial (b), coronal (c) and sagittal (d) planes. The three image planes indicated by different colors (a). (Courtesy of Dr K. Honda, Nihon University School of Dentistry, Tokyo, Japan.)

some clinical and radiological features with periodontitis originating from pulpal infection. Apical responses to increased tooth mobility following marginal periodontitis have already been mentioned. Moreover, granulation tissue resulting from infection of the pocket may expand to the apical part of the root and mimic true apical periodontitis (Fig. 6.26). Sometimes a true pulpo-periodontal lesion is formed by pulpal and marginal infection reaching the apex. Such a condition can be reliably diagnosed with supplementary CT (Fig. 6.27). In this situation, infection control is virtually impossible and surgical intervention usually inevitable. This situation must be distinguished from a primary apical lesion with drainage through the periodontium; in this case, there may not necessarily be an established infection of the periodontium [190]. Resolution of both the apical process and the lateral involvement may be possible through endodontic treatment alone. Furcal responses to marginal infection may look indistinguishable on a radiograph from responses of the same area to infection of the pulp canal system. Pulp vitality testing and clinical assessment of marginal involvement is necessary for differential diagnosis.

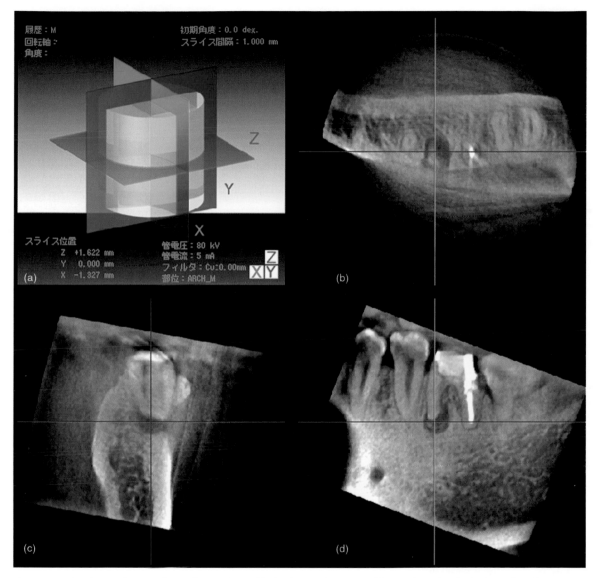

Fig. 6.22   Apical periodontitis of mesial root of mandibular first molar (no rootfilling in buccal or lingual canal) with destruction of the buccal cortex. Distal root with filling and normal periapical structures. Cone beam CT with sections in axial (b), coronal (c) and sagittal (d) planes. The three image planes indicated by different colors (a). (Courtesy of Dr K. Honda, Nihon University School of Dentistry, Tokyo, Japan.)

6.8.2 Root fracture

Root fractures, particularly vertical root fractures and cracked teeth, present particular problems of diagnosis [116,126,149,185] (Fig. 6.28). Initially, cracked teeth may not have infected pulps and the clinical situation may be resolved by conservative treatment without pulp extirpation (adhesive restorations, crown coverage). With time, infection is a certainty and lesion development follows, but with a more extended portal of exit which is reflected in the radiograph by the frequent occurrence of a radiolucency that runs along the greater part of the lateral

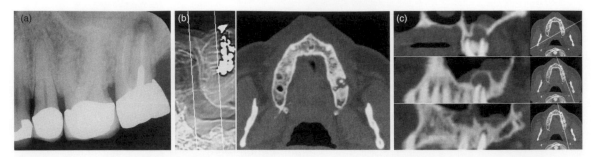

Fig. 6.23   Apical periodontitis of maxillary second molar, apparently rather small on intraoral radiograph (a). Axial CT scan with scout view indicating scanning area (left) demonstrates larger bone destruction around buccal roots than palatal root and destruction of buccal cortex (b). Different reformatted sections through the roots demonstrate corticated process particularly around buccal roots (c). (Reproduced from [103] with permission.)

aspect of the root [135]. Long-standing vertical root fractures may be viewed as a variant of apical periodontitis, in that there is indeed an infection of the pulp canal system that leads to the clinical or radiological manifestation of periodontitis. On the other hand, highly mobile teeth may show a radiographic image similar to vertical root fractures. Vertical root fractures have been associated with root-filled teeth where lateral forces during root filling condensation may have been excessive, or with stresses induced by post placement in root-filled teeth [136]. But it also occurs, although seldom, in intact or filled teeth with vital pulps [207]. The cracked tooth syndrome more frequently relates to fractured vital teeth where only a limited or no part of the periodontium is involved.

6.8.3 Osteomyelitis

Osteomyelitis may be a continuation of an apical periodontitis with spreading of the infection into the bone marrow [83,90] with a strong preference for the mandible. It is not dependent on an infected tooth as a reservoir of the causative organisms. The radiographic appearance is highly variable, but in the early phase the process is predominantly destructive (Fig. 6.29). CT is an excellent imaging method in the evaluation of osteomyelitis [103]. In addition to osteolytic areas also osteosclerotic areas may occur [68]. Occasionally, a periosteal reaction may be found [89,110] (Fig. 6.29), and all features may be seen in the same patient. Bone apposition is more commonly seen in younger patients and may lead to jaw asymmetry.

6.8.4 Cysts

Incisive canal cyst

The incisive canal may show a cystic development with clinical and radiographic features similar to apical periodontitis. It may project over one of the incisors, and the radiological tracing of the lamina dura of these teeth may not be easy [179] (Fig. 6.30). Tooth vitality responses are therefore particularly important in differential diagnosis.

Periodontal cyst

The periodontal cyst is a clinical entity that may be a source of diagnostic confusion. Typically, this cyst is located between roots in the mandibular canine/premolar area and is believed to originate from cellular or tissue remnants from the dental lamina in the periodontal ligament of the associated tooth. Tracing of a complete and intact lamina dura and the finding of vital pulps in neighboring teeth establishes the diagnosis. Treatment is by surgical excision.

Dentigerous cyst

Dentigerous (or follicular) cysts are associated with epithelium around the crowns of unerupted teeth. Usually, they do not present a major difficulty in differential diagnosis to apical periodontitis as the erupted teeth in the area will have uninterrupted lamina dura and vital pulps.

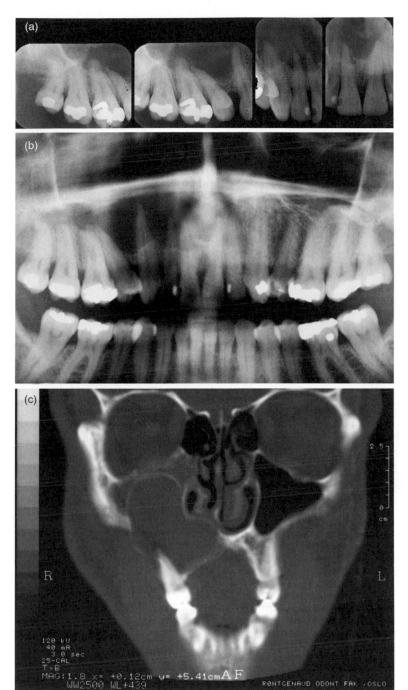

Fig. 6.24 Large maxillary radicular cyst. The process, associated with a nonvital lateral incisor cannot be distinguished from the maxillary sinus on intraoral radiographs (a). A panoramic view also cannot establish its size or its association with the maxillary sinus (b). Coronal CT scan demonstrates corticated process occupying most of maxillary sinus (almost to the orbit), expanding sinus walls and hard palate (c). (Reproduced from [103] with permission.)

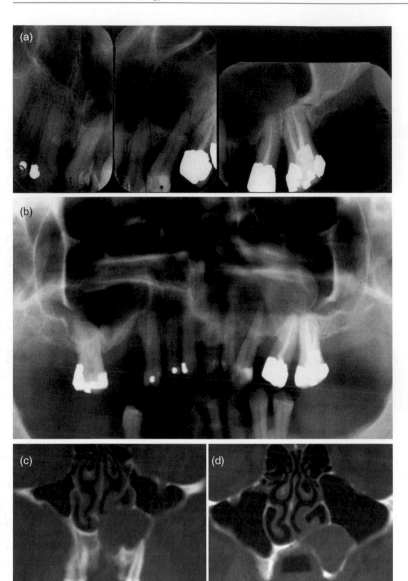

Fig. 6.25 Large maxillary radicular cyst. The periapical, corticated process associated with a nonvital lateral incisor cannot be distinguished from the nasal cavity on intraoral radiographs (a). A panoramic view also cannot establish an association with the nasal cavity (b). A coronal CT scan demonstrates a process involving nasal cavity without cortical delineation (c); however, a more posterior coronal CT scan demonstrates an intact, corticated outline (d). (Reproduced from [103] with permission.)

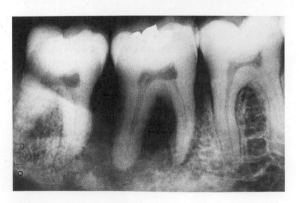

Fig. 6.26 Marginal periodontitis of the lower second molar extending to involve the apical area. All root canals were vital.

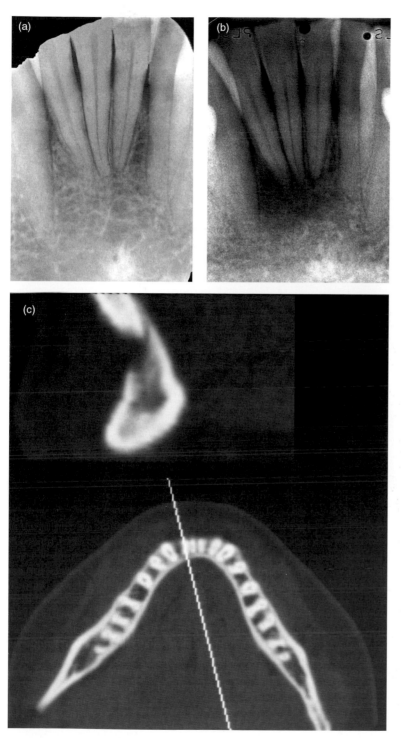

Fig. 6.27 Periodontal disease mimicking apical periodontitis. Normal periapical structures, but reduced marginal bone level in mandibular anterior region (a). Patient was under treatment for periodontal disease and had an abscess in this area. Three months later a new abscess developed and a periapical radiolucency was seen (b). Supplementary CT, reformatted perpendicular to the alveolar process, as seen by the cursor line on axial scan (lower), demonstrates destruction of buccal cortex and of the periapical area (c).

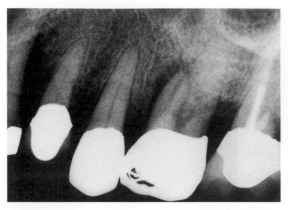

Fig. 6.28   Root fracture of the mesial root of the maxillary first molar.

6.8.5 Cystlike/non-neoplastic processes

Simple bone cyst (traumatic bone cyst)

This lesion is not a true cyst but simply a space without epithelial coverage. Its cause is unknown. Patients are usually young with most lesions occurring in the second decade of life. The mandible is more often affected than the maxilla, and the lesion is usually very well defined with extensions in between roots in the area, and may mimic apical periodontitis [160]. The traumatic bone cyst is known as an asymptomatic lesion often noted unintentionally during routine radiographic examinations. The lesion neither devitalizes the teeth within its borders, nor does it cause resorption of their roots. The well-demarcated traumatic bone cyst often projects into the intraradicular septa and hence has been described as having scalloped borders.

Giant cell granuloma

The giant cell granuloma usually presents as quite large (10–20 mm) radiolucencies with more or less well-defined borders, and with faint trabeculae often showing through the lesion [19,61,158,174,183]. Larger lesions frequently become multilocular [88]. A special case of foreign body giant cell granuloma at a root-filled tooth has been reported [130].

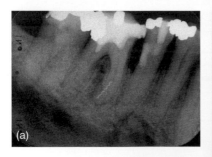

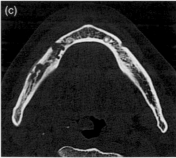

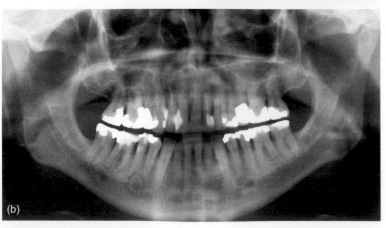

Fig. 6.29   Mandibular osteomyelitis. The patient had variable perimandibular swelling and variable pain. There is a fractured instrument in the mesial root of the first molar with a widened apical PDL, and a widened PDL of the second premolar with irregular bone destruction in the periapical area on intraoral radiograph (a). Panoramic view shows irregular bone structure in the periapical area of both molars and premolars, with a suspected sequester in the premolar region (b). Axial computed tomography scan demonstrates irregular bone destruction both in the premolar and molar areas with a widened mental foramen and some periosteal bone apposition buccally. No sequester formation could be confirmed (c). (Reproduced from [103] with permission.)

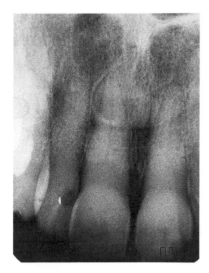

Fig. 6.30 Infected cyst of the incisive canal with minute fistula in the palate. The adjacent teeth responded normally to vitality tests.

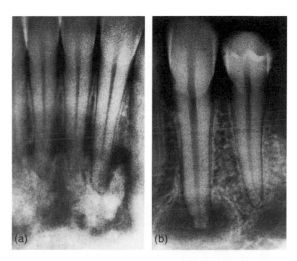

Fig. 6.31 Cemental dysplasia. The lesion in (a) shows a mixture of osteogenic and osteolytic features; in (b), the osteolytic reaction is deceptively similar to chronic apical periodontitis. [Figure (b) courtesy of Dr Agnar Halse.]

Osseous (cemental) dysplasia

This condition is also named periapical cemental dysplasia or periapical cementoma. Through its direct association with elements of the PDL, it may sometimes offer a challenge. However, the pulps of the affected teeth regularly test vital, and the correct diagnosis of the dysplasia should not be followed by any treatment. While idiopathic, it has been regarded as a reactive lesion, with no known source of irritation or stimulus. It shows a predilection for the anterior teeth of the mandible, and varies in expression from initially radiolucent to later more radiopaque structures (Fig. 6.31). The cementoblastoma is a related lesion characteristically associated with mandibular molars (Fig. 6.32).

6.8.6 Tumors

Keratocystic odontogenic tumor (odontogenic keratocyst)

This is a unicystic or multicystic tumor that was previously defined as a cyst, with a high recurrence rate after surgical excision. When multiple, lesions are usually part of the inherited naevoid basal cell carcinoma syndrome. It may mimic apical periodontitis when located close to the root apex (apices) and periapical area (Fig. 6.33). It is usually asymptomatic and may be large before detected, most frequently in

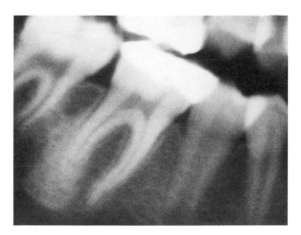

Fig. 6.32 Benign cementoblastoma with a mandibular lesion affecting the distal root of the first molar. The tooth is vital. (Courtesy of Dr Gunnar Thorseth.)

the mandible and in the second and third decades. Thus, a panoramic radiograph is frequently needed to observe the entire process (Fig. 6.33b). CT is usually necessary to demonstrate the occurrence of perforated cortical bones (Fig. 6.34) [103].

Ameloblastoma

Many jaw lesions occur as multilocular radiolucencies [91], and the ameloblastoma is probably the

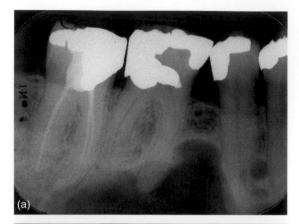

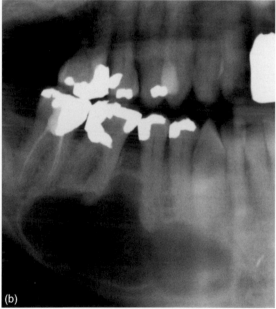

Fig. 6.33 Mandibular keratocystic odontogenic tumor (odontogenic keratocyst). Patient with hard perimandibular swelling and vital teeth. Corticated periapical radiolucency on intraoral radiograph (a). Panoramic view shows large corticated process occupying most of mandibular body, with caudal displacement of the mandibular canal in the periphery of the process (b). (Reproduced from [103] with permission.)

best known with bone trabeculae separating what appear to be lobes of the lesion in bone [58,152]. It typically occurs in the fourth or fifth decades of life, and the posterior parts of the mandible are most frequently affected. The ameloblastoma is characterized by frequently causing extensive resorption of

roots in the area, and the cortical bone plate may be expanded and perforated. Radiographic variants in some locations may present difficulties in differential diagnosis to apical periodontitis, in particular when it is unilocular (Fig. 6.35). The ameloblastoma is considered locally aggressive [134] and has definitive potential for malignant transformation [78,134].

Malignant tumors

Malignant tumors of the jaws are uncommon in most parts of the world, and seldom a differential diagnostic problem to apical peridontitis. Figure 6.36 is from a patient with some discomfort/pain and diffuse, slight swelling in the right upper jaw. Endodontical treatment was carried out for more than 6 months before the patient was referred for advanced imaging, and diffuse bone destruction suggestive of a tumor was detected. The tumour proved histologically to be a malignant lymphoma.

6.8.7 Other conditions

Primary hyperparathyroidism gives rise to a general radiolucent appearance of bone and may later give well-defined round or oval radiolucencies which may mimic apical periodontitis and which may also resemble ameloblastoma. Eosinophilic granuloma of bone may manifest itself in the bones and give radiologic signs not unlike apical periodontitis, sometimes also associated with pulpal necrosis of the involved teeth.

Bisphosphonate medication for osteoporosis may cause intrabony lesions that may look like apical periodontitis in radiographs [165].

6.9 Periapical radiology in clinical experiments and epidemiology

6.9.1 Success/failure analyses

The analysis of success and failure has a long tradition in endodontology and sets the discipline somewhat apart from, e.g., periodontics and cariology. The continuous onslaught by microbes in caries and marginal periodontitis makes any treatment temporary in nature; by contrast, the fact that it may be possible to eliminate infection from the root canal opens the way for definitive treatment with permanent "success".

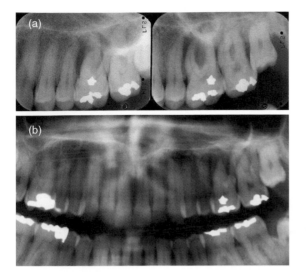
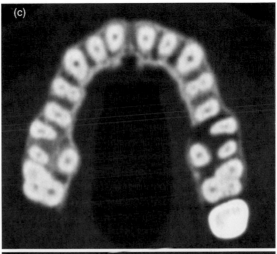
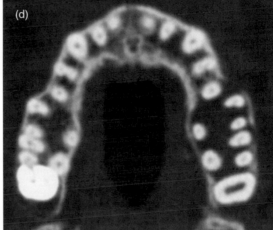

Fig. 6.34 Maxillary keratocystic odontogenic tumor (odontogenic keratocyst). Periapical radiolucency at first molar (which was vital) (a). Panoramic view suggests periapical radiolucency at second molar as well (b). Axial CT scan demonstrates expanded and thinned buccal and palatal cortex, the latter being perforated (c). A more cranial, axial CT scan demonstrates destruction of alveolar bone from the second premolar to the third molar and perforated buccal cortex (d).

Success/failure analyses are usually done by comparing the preoperative or immediate postoperative radiograph with subsequent radiographs taken at intervals after treatment (Fig. 6.37). Table 6.1 lists conventional criteria for success and failure derived from some of the most recognized studies [2,10,11,29,65,69,76,92,170,178,180].

The attractive feature of this type of analysis is the immediate subjective recognition, by clinicians, of its usefulness. Success or failure implies whether or not new treatment should be done [15,71,123], a key issue in diagnosis and treatment planning familiar to all practitioners. But the terms are compounds of a diagnosis, a description of treatment quality, and of

treatment need. This contributes to the difficulties in harmonizing what actually constitutes success or may require retreatment [44,153,155]. Furthermore, there are serious problems with the sensitivity and specificity of dental radiographic examination in general [40,59,60,62,63,105]. Therefore, results from such analyses carried out at different institutions and by different researchers are hardly comparable to each other. Moreover, the grouping of cases into only two categories gives low power to statistical methods applied to the results. It is also limiting for the applicability of the results that there is not a true measure of presence or absence of disease in the success/failure criteria.

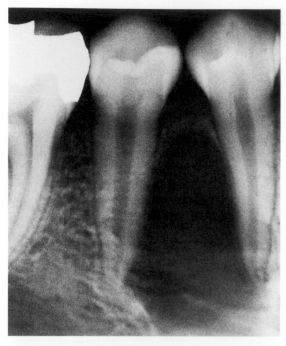

Fig. 6.35 Ameloblastoma located between the roots of the lower first and second premolar. (Courtesy of Dr Agnar Halse.)

6.9.2 Presence/absence of disease: probability assessments

The simple distinction between healthy and diseased roots in a single radiograph has some advantages: bias is reduced by reliance on radiological information from only one point in time and the information obtained may be used for several purposes. Combined with a scale to allow for uncertainties in the radiographic diagnosis, this concept has been applied to analyses of chronic apical periodontitis in

several clinical studies [100,154,156]. With different cut-off points for accepting a root as actually having disease, so called receiver operating characteristic (ROC) curves may be applied for more advanced statistical analyses of larger sets of data [154]. It has been shown that by applying strict criteria for the inclusion of a root as diseased, this system makes it possible to discern differences in the prevalence of apical periodontitis among groups of teeth [142]. One weakness of this scoring system is that it may be difficult to apply to clinical practice.

6.9.3 Index scoring systems: the periapical index

There is often strong bias in the selection of criteria for the definition of chronic apical periodontitis. A widened PDL and discontinuities in the lamina dura are frequently listed as such criteria [156], even though their actual association with the disease is not particularly strong. Little emphasis is placed on more subtle signs, such as structure disorganization and initial loss of mineral, although they may be more strongly associated with the disease. Based on a number of histology verified case radiographs from Brynolf's material [25], the periapical index (PAI) scoring system [142] offers a visual reference scale for assigning a health status to the periapex (Fig. 6.38). For radiographic assessment of the outcome of surgical endodontics, which has its own dynamics of healing, another strategy using stylized drawings of healing patterns has been presented [123].

Scoring systems with reference scales reduce bias, offer means of quantitative assessment of reproducibility, and have, by comparison with most other clinical/radiological systems, good statistical power [142] and a discriminatory ability comparable to automated densitometric analyses [38]. The PAI has found applications in studies comparing the clinical perfor-

Table 6.1 Conventional, radiographic criteria for the assessment of success and failure of endodontic treatment[a]

Treatment outcome	Radiographic criteria at time of follow-up
Success	The width and contour of the PDL is normal, or there is a slight radiolucent zone around excess filling material
Uncertain	The results are questionable [40]; there is an unsatisfactory control radiograph [84]; the tooth has been extracted for irrelevant causes [84]
Failure	There is a periradicular radiolucency [40]; decreased, unchanged, or new or increased rarefaction [84]

[a] From refs [40] and [84].

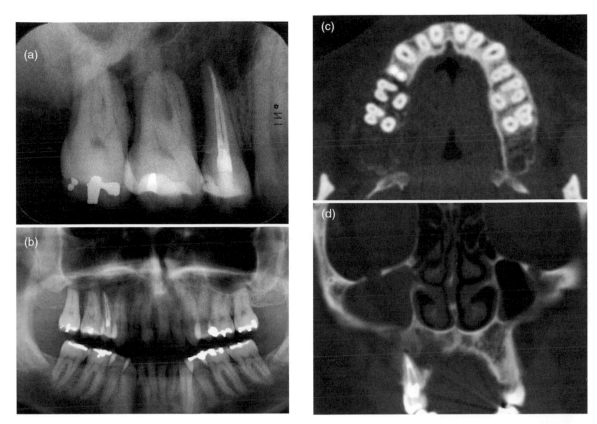

Fig. 6.36 Maxillary malignant lymphoma. Patient had had endodontic treatment for about 6 months and presented with some discomfort and a feeling of slight swelling of the right maxilla. Diffuse destruction of periapical bone, in particular around the root-filled tooth on intraoral radiograph (a). Panoramic view indicates destruction of alveolar bone in premolar and molar area including the tuber region (b). Axial computed tomography (CT) scan demonstrates irregular destruction of alveolar bone and entire tuber (c). Coronal CT scan demonstrates irregular destruction of hard palate and opacification of right maxillary sinus (d). (Reproduced from [103] with permission.)

mance of endodontic filling materials and techniques [50,141,143,192,198,199] and in epidemiologic studies [49] (Chapter 8). It is unfortunate, however, that there is an inadequate amount of reference material for mandibular and posterior teeth.

6.9.4 Surveys and epidemiology

Endodontics is an integral part of the health care aspect of dentistry. The effects of endodontic treatment efforts have a public health aspect as well as relating to the individual patient only. In epidemiological terms, it is of particular interest to see the effects on the prevalence of apical periodontitis.

Assessment of the incidence and prevalence of chronic apical periodontitis in different populations is important for many reasons. It may help to establish treatment needs and to relate treatment outcome to various technical and clinical factors of endodontic intervention (Chapter 8).

Only radiographic surveys are useful in the assessment of the occurrence of apical periodontitis. Both full-mouth-series of periapical radiographs and orthopantomograms have been used for this purpose. The PAI scoring system has been modified and applied to epidemiological and clinical comparative studies of treatment outcome. The possibility of comparisons among studies carried out with calibrated

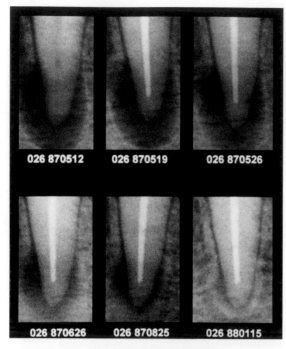

026 870512   026 870519   026 870526

026 870626   026 870825   026 880115

Fig. 6.37   Classical follow-up radiograph series. Preoperative and postoperative radiographs of the tooth apex mounted for assessment of success or failure. Final six digits show date of exposure.

observers makes this system attractive, and comparative data have been collected from all over the world [48,49,113,141,143,173] (Chapter 8).

6.9.5 Animal experiments

Experimental, animal studies with radiography of apical periodontitis are quite rare [156], and incursions into specific radiographic aspects even rarer. There are indications that pre-immunization of monkeys to infecting organisms may lead to more well-defined borders of the ensuing lesions [37]. Detection of radiographic lesions in bone of monkeys by conventional radiography has been reported after 2 months [86], but subtraction radiography was reported to allow identification of changes in the bone architecture as early as 7 days after infection of the pulp also in monkeys [144].

Initial signs of apical periodontitis in dogs may be visible on radiographs as early as 3 weeks after root canal infection. Lesions keep developing at 6 weeks, and become extensive at 11 and 14 weeks [54] (Fig. 6.39). The radiographic diagnosis may be more reliable at longer time intervals because the disease has become more extensive and there is naturally more time for changes in mineralization to occur [148]. Recent studies have however attempted to describe standardized ways of creating apical periodontitis in dogs, microbiologically and radiographically [186].

In rat molars periapical lesions develop rapidly after pulp exposure, with a maximum rate of bone loss and detectability in radiographs occurring within the first 2 weeks [108,187,210]. This reflects the most active phase of the pathogenic process, whereas later on, expansion occurs at a much slower rate if at all. The periapical lesion extends mesiodistally with resorption of medullary bone first, and then vertically with resorption of cortical bone and cementum [187].

6.10 Digital radiography

Conventional periapical radiography has its main strength in the large amount of information provided by each image. It is, however, essentially a tool for qualitative assessment of anatomical and pathological structures. Sensors for direct digitization are rapidly replacing physical films in dental practice. The use of charge-coupled device sensors or storage phosphor plates instead of radiographic film may reduce the amount of irradiation needed and can produce computer-displayed images that are instantly or through some seconds of scanning available for inspection and enhancement [203]. Speed and simplicity are important factors; the environmental problems associated with the chemicals used in development and fixation of radiographs and in the film itself are also eliminated. Originally, there was little if any gain in the information acquired; but while many systems still provide images of lower resolution than conventional radiographs, there is a steady development towards smaller pixel sizes that improves the resolution of the digitally acquired images. Long-term storage of digital images may also be seen as a problem, but this is easily solved by systematic software upgrades and proper copying of files. The sensors are also improved to replace the original bulky and stiff units of the first systems.

6.10.1 Diagnostic efficacy

Changes in radiographic density, or gray levels, are important visual features for the clinician to

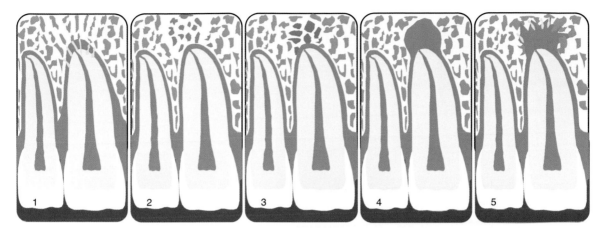

Fig. 6.38 The periapical index (PAI) scoring system is a visual reference scale for assigning a health status to the root. PAI score 1 shows little change in bone mineral content and any structural alterations reflect functional changes, usually increased mobility. PAI score 2 also shows little change in bone mineral content, but is characterized by a disorganization of the bone texture periapically. PAI score 3 has loss of mineral and may have a 'shot-gun' appearance. PAI score 4 has all the signs of classical, chronic apical periodontitis. PAI score 5 is similar, but with elements indicating expansion of the lesion: radiolucent streaks and structural disorganization peripheral to the body of the lesion may be characteristic. See also Fig. 8.2.

evaluate changes in bone pattern. The effects of enhancement on periapical lesion detection and/ or the application of measurement algorithms for dimensional assessment have been studied. *In vitro*, digital systems have been found to be at best as sensitive as conventional film, but more often than not, they show less detail [12,53,99,208]. Using ROC curves [75], the diagnostic efficacy with digital images is typically also comparable to or slightly inferior than that obtained with conventional radiographs [99,100,101,203].

Color-coding has been proposed as a means of detecting differences between sequential images to detect bone changes [189]. Assigning a color to a range of gray levels creates more visually striking images, but the image may lose some information in the process. For diagnostic purposes, retaining the original grayscale image seems preferable [115,168].

Texture analysis has been developed to identify the trabecular bone pattern and systemic or local changes caused by pathologic processes [28,120], but this method has not yet been applied to clinical work.

Contrasting with the diagnosis of caries and marginal periodontitis, image enhancement techniques seem to offer little to improve diagnostic performance in cases of apical periodontitis [100,101].

6.10.2 Quantitative assessments

Subtraction radiography and densitometric image analysis have been applied for monitoring bone density changes, also in apical periodontitis [145,209]. The principle of subtraction radiography is to eliminate, or even out all unchanging structures from a pair of radiographs, displaying only the area where changes in density have occurred. This makes the area of bone gain or loss contrast against a neutral grey background. In other densitometric image analysis techniques, the numeric density values are analyzed to quantify osseous changes in areas of interest.

Subtraction radiography requires that two radiographs be taken with similar contrast, density and angulation. Attention to detail is critical when exposing radiographs for the use in subtraction. Computer algorithms have been developed that can correct for variation in radiograph image density, contrast as well as geometry [163,164,201], and several attempts at applying subtraction radiography to apical periodontitis have been done, with variable success. However, some reports offer hope for improved efficacy [41,117]. This method can be used to monitor healing, respective development, of periapical and other bone lesions [97,98,137,140,195] (Fig. 6.40).

Digital subtraction in the diagnosis of periapical inflammatory changes has some problems [97,140].

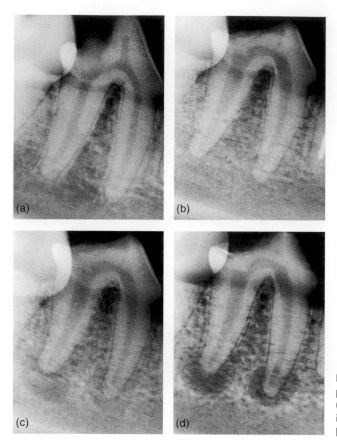

Fig. 6.39 Radiographs of a dog's mandibular premolar (a) before induction of apical periodontitis, (b), (c) and (d) 3, 11 and 14 weeks after pulpal inoculation with dental plaque. (Reproduced from [54] with permission.)

The background noise from variations in exposure geometry [9] and from normal bone structural changes over time reduces the sensitivity of this method for monitoring of periapical bone changes [140]. Moreover, early phases of chronic apical periodontitis may be characterized more by structural changes than by reductions in mineral density [25], which reduces the specificity of digital subtraction for this application [101,140].

Morphometric methods [23] were applied to conventional radiography for densitometric analyses of lesion size [43], and the same principle has been applied to digital images [80]. Good standardization of image geometry may be achieved with several methods. Customized film holders can stabilize the relationship between the teeth, film and X-ray source [162]; the X-ray source and the teeth may be stabilized using a cephalostat [87]; and the computer can be used to correct image distortion caused by film placement [201]. Reference points may be used to aid

in the superimposition of sequential radiographs in digital subtraction radiography [41,202]. It is possible to align serial images automatically as well as manually [165]. Other methods used in research include specialized computer software and a video camera to superimpose follow-up radiographs [38,93,140].

Contrast enhancement of the subtraction image may result in better visualization of some structures. Reddy *et al.* [151] used pseudocolor enhancement for the detection of small periodontal bone lesions, but they found that coloring did not add new information to the image. However, it may allow increased speed and efficiency for interpretation of subtraction images with greater confidence.

When densitometric analysis was performed together with histological evaluation of healing after surgical treatment of apical periodontitis in dogs [39], the average gray value of the surgical area on the subtraction images correlated with the histological evaluation of healing and the relative amount of

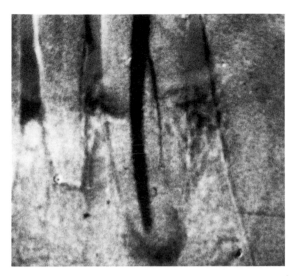

Fig. 6.40 Digital subtraction of radiographic images. The apical periodontitis of the mandibular canine was treated and controlled after 6 months. The numerical gray values in the control radiograph have been subtracted from their counterparts in the preoperative image, producing an image where areas of change stand out. The periapical change of the apical dark area may be analyzed quantitatively.

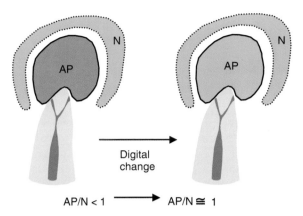

Fig. 6.41 Densitometric measurements of healing apical periodontitis. On the digitized radiograph taken at the time of root filling (left), an area is drawn (solid line) encircling the lesion and some of the structures peripheral to it. The area is stored in the computer. An area outside the lesion of presumed normal bone density (dotted line) is similarly delineated. These areas are automatically overlaid on the digitized radiographs taken at intervals later (right). The average gray value of the units (pixels) in each area is computed at the start (lower left) and later (lower right). The ratio of the average gray value of the lesion area (AP) to the average gray value of the normal area (N) (AP/N) increases with healing, usually approaching unity.

trabecular bone. Computer-based densitometric measurements have also been applied *in vivo* in humans in attempts to distinguish between radicular cysts and granulomas [172].

A more robust method for quantifying density changes over time has had considerable success [140]. By relating the density of the lesion area (region of interest) to a more peripheral and unaffected, normal bone area, a density ratio is obtained that may be monitored over time as a measure of development or healing of chronic apical periodontitis (Fig. 6.41) [140]. Under optimal conditions of exposure, film development and digitization or direct digital radiography, this method has been shown to give quantitative signs of healing within a month of initial treatment [93,140,147] (Fig. 6.42).

6.11 Advanced imaging methods

More information may be gained by the application of other, sophisticated medical imaging methods. In particular, magnetic resonance imaging (MRI) is

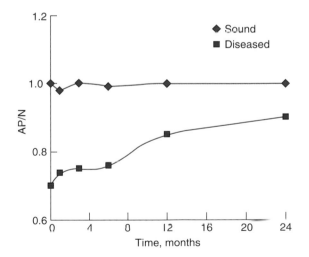

Fig. 6.42 Results of densitometric measurements with AP/N-ratios for a group of teeth treated for chronic apical periodontitis (diseased) and control teeth (sound) followed over 24 months. Note the sharp increase in AP/N ratio from 0 to 1 month and the continued, but less dramatic increase up to 12 and 24 months. (Modified from [41] with permission.)

increasingly used for advanced maxillofacial diagnostic imaging [67,84,103,132,193,196].

6.11.1 MRI

Changes in hydrogen content, also in soft tissues, alter the strength of the MRI signal. In this way inflammation, for instance, may become visible. The imaging method has been used to show edema at the apex of teeth with inflamed pulps, and to demonstrate dentigerous cysts and their relation to surrounding tissues [57]. It has been applied to studies of periapical lesions including osteomyelitis [114]. MRI has also been analyzed for differential diagnosis of odontogenic tumours and cysts [119] and to follow longitudinally a myxoma [81]. MRI can reveal septa chiefly made of soft tissue with few or thin bone structures, and it may have particular advantages in demonstrating multilocularity in some cases [118]. MRI may be particularly valuable in the evaluation of larger cystic processes of the jaws as a supplement to CT aiming to determine the nature of the process. The method is also indicated in selected cases of osteomyelitis supplementing CT [103].

6.11.2 Medical (multidetector) CT

CT may be helpful in the detection and diagnosis of a variety of jaw lesions; cysts [1,35,95], giant cell granulomas [19] and other conditions [20,31], as reviewed extensively by Larheim and Westesson [103]. Particularly, software designed for dental applications has been found useful [1,19,20,95]. Its use for routine diagnosis is still hampered by the relatively high radiation exposure and moderate resolution. CT scans are, however, particularly important for the overall orientation in the operative field, e.g., for detection and localization of adjoining structures (maxillary sinus; nasal cavity, mandibular canal, mental foramen) and for detailing complex root anatomy that may be blurred from surrounding structures in periapical films [35,132].

6.11.3 Cone-beam CT

A high-resolution CT that uses a small conical beam and reconstructs images in any direction by means of a software program that runs on a personal computer has been developed for dental applications [8]. This imaging technique, exclusively applied for jaw examinations, may be useful also for depicting periapical lesions [8,197].

6.11.4 Micro CT

As the thickness of the plane visualized in CT scans is still quite high, attempts at developing microsystems continue. Currently the use of microcomputer tomography technology in humans is restricted to samples of no larger than a few millimeters, e.g., biopsies from the iliac crest [46], or as an *in vitro* non-invasive method for three-dimensional reconstruction of root canals [146]. Systems are improving, and fairly high resolution may be obtained with current systems [104,106].

6.11.5 Conventional tomography

Conventional tomography provides sharp imaging of a section or plane through the tissues, whereas those outside it may be blurred. The blurred structures appear in tomograms as homogenous, low contrast shadows allowing the detection of lesions in the object layer. Dental radiography units that include a tomographic imaging mode are available; these visualize dentoalveolar structures in detail, and the sensitivity in visualizing periapical bone lesions is higher for premolar and molar regions compared with periapical films [184].

6.11.6 Tuned-aperture computed tomography (TACT)

The system uses a set of digital radiographic images and the software forms a layering of images that can be viewed in "slices" [128,194,200]. The system may have advantages over conventional film in the visualization of root resorptions [133], and root fractures [126,127]. It may also help in evaluations of dental caries and has been applied to simulated osseous defects [75,77,128,194,200].

6.11.7 Ultrasound

Ultrasound is a real-time technique that has also been applied to the diagnosis of apical periodontitis [33,34,70]. Since sound waves do not pass through bone, only lesions that are not covered by bone can be examined, but with that provisio, it is possible to discriminate fluid, soft tissue and small mineral particles and to study blood flow. For particular applications, ultrasound would be safe and may be easy to use, if suitable sensors were available.

6.11.8 Nuclear techniques

Scintigraphic images may be obtained after introducing a radionuclide to the patient. The uptake of radionuclides in different parts of body may be registered by gamma camera counts of the amount of radiation emitted from tissues. The uptake of the radionuclide is generally greater in tissues with high metabolic activity and is increased in inflamed areas. This makes early detection of lesion in bones possible.

Many dental diseases such as pulpitis and apical periodontitis may cause abnormal uptake on skeletal images, where they may appear before clinical evidence of the inflammatory disease [181]. Scintigraphy also aided the localization of an active root canal infection that could not be clinically localized [188].

6.12 Concluding remarks

The radiographic diagnosis of chronic apical periodontitis is complex, and is confounded by several anatomical and biological variables. While diagnosis is easy when well-defined, pathognomonic radiolucencies are present, the detection and grading of weak radiographic signs of chronic apical periodontitis may be extremely difficult. Systems for training and calibration of observers have improved diagnostic performance and the methods for clinical and epidemiological research on apical periodontitis, and digital manipulations show great potential for the detection of subtle changes indicating disease. Advanced imaging, in particular CT, has become an essential tool in many clinical situations; with increased availability and reduced radiation dosage, this technique offers the spatial resolution that has been lacking in most other radiographic methods.

6.13 References

1. Abrahams JJ, Oliverio PJ (1993) Odontogenic cysts: improved imaging with a dental CT software program. *American Journal of Neuroradiology* **14**, 367–74.
2. Adenubi JO, Rule DC (1976) Success rate for root fillings in young patients. A retrospective analysis of treated cases. *British Dental Journal* **141**, 237–41.
3. Ahlgren J (1993) A 10-year evaluation of the quality of orthodontic treatment *Swedish Dental Journal* **17**, 201–9.
4. Ahlqwist JR, Halling A, Hollender L (1986) Rotational panoramic radiography in epidemiological studies on dental health. *Swedish Dental Journal* **10**, 79–84.
5. Andreasen FM (1986) Transient apical breakdown and its relation to color and sensibility changes after luxation injuries to teeth. *Endodontics and Dental Traumatology* **2**, 2–19.
6. Andreasen FM, Pedersen BV (1985) Prognosis of luxated permanent teeth – the development of pulp necrosis. *Endodontics and Dental Traumatology* **1**, 207–20.
7. Andreasen JO, Rud J (1972) Correlation between histology and radiography in the assessment of healing after endodontic surgery. *International Journal of Oral Surgery* **1**, 161–73.
8. Arai Y, Tammisalo E, Iwai K, Hashimoto K, Shinoda K (1999) Development of a compact computed tomographic apparatus for dental use. *Dentomaxillofacial Radiology* **28**, 245–8.
9. Araki K, Kitamori H, Yoshiura K, Okuda H, Ohki M (1992) Standardized lateral oblique projection of the mandible for digital subtraction radiography. *Dentomaxillofacial Radiology* **21**, 88–92.
10. Barbakow FH, Cleaton-Jones P, Friedman D (1980) An evaluation of 566 cases of root canal therapy in general dental practice. 2. Postoperative observations. *Journal of Endodontics* **6**, 485–9.
11. Barbakow FH, Cleaton-Jones PE, Friedman D (1981) Endodontic treatment of teeth with periapical radiolucent areas in a general dental practice. *Oral Surgery, Oral Medicine, Oral Pathology* **51**, 552–9.
12. Barbat J, Messer HH (1998) Detectability of artificial periapical lesions using direct digital and conventional radiography. *Journal of Endodontics* **24**, 837–42.
13. Barthel CR, Zimmer S, Trope M (2004) Relationship of radiologic and histologic signs of inflammation in human root-filled teeth. *Journal of Endodontics* **30**, 75–9.
14. Bender IB, Seltzer S (1961) Roentgenographic and direct observation of experimental lesions of bone. *Journal of the American Dental Association* **62**, 157–62.
15. Bender IB, Seltzer S, Soltanoff W (1966) Endodontic success – a reappraisal of criteria. *Oral Surgery, Oral Medicine, Oral Pathology* **22**, 780–802.
16. Bender IB (1982) Factors influencing the radiographic appearance of bone lesions *Journal of Endodontics* **8**, 161–70.
17. Bhaskar SN (1966) Periapical lesions – types, incidence and clinical features. *Oral Surgery, Oral Medicine, Oral Pathology* **21**, 657–71.
18. Biewener AA, Fazzalari NL, Konieczynski DD, Baudinette RV (1996) Adaptive changes in trabecular architecture in relation to functional strain patterns and disuse. *Bone* **19**, 1–8.
19. Bodner L, Bar-Ziv J (1996) Radiographic features of central giant cell granuloma of the jaws in children. *Pediatric Radiology* **26**, 148–51.

20. Bodner L, Sarnat H, Bar-Ziv J, Kaffe I (1996) Computed tomography in pediatric oral and maxillofacial surgery. *Journal of Dentistry for Children* **63**, 32–8.

21. Boyd KS (1995) Transient apical breakdown following subluxation injury: a case report. *Endodontics and Dental Traumatology* **11**, 37–40.

22. Boyne PH, Harvey WL (1961) The effects of osseus implant material on regeneration of alveolar cortex. *Oral Surgery, Oral Medicine, Oral Pathology* **14**, 369–73.

23. Boysen H, Giörtz-Carlsen E, Ånerud Å (1972) Root canal therapy. A radiographic control. *Danish Tandlaegebladet* **76**, 425–37.

24. Briseno-Marroquin B, Willershausen-Zonchen B, Pistorius A, Goller M (1995) The reliability of apical x-ray pictures in the diagnosis of mandibular bone lesions. A review of the literature and in-vitro study. *Schweizerische Monatsschrift für Zahnmedizin* **105**, 1142–8.

25. Brynolf I (1967) Histological and roentgenological study of periapical region of human upper incisors. *Odontologisk Revy* **18**, suppl.11.

26. Brynolf I (1970) Roentgenologic periapical diagnosis. One, two or more roentgenograms? *Swedish Dental Journal* **63**, 345–50.

27. Burch JG, Hulen S (1974) A study of the presence of accessory foramina and the topography of molar furcations. *Oral Surgery, Oral Medicine, Oral Pathology* **38**, 451–5.

28. Caputo B, Gigante GE (2000) Analysis of periapical lesion using statistical textural features. *Studies in Health Technology and Informatics* **77**, 1231–4.

29. Castagnola L (1950) 1000 Fälle von Gangränbehandlung nach der Walkhoffschen Methode aus dem statistischen Material der Konservierenden Abteilung. *Schweizerische Monatsschrift für Zahnmedizin* **11**, 1033.

30. Cavalcanti MG, Ruprecht A, Johnson WT, Southard TE, Jakobsen J (2002) The contribution of trabecular bone to the visibility of the lamina dura: an in vitro radiographic study. *Oral Surgery, Oral Medicine, Oral Pathology, Oral Radiology and Endodontics* **93**, 118–22.

31. Cholia SS, Wilson PH, Makdissi J (2005) Multiple idiopathic external apical root resorption: report of four cases. *Dentomaxillofacial Radiology* **34**, 240–6.

32. Colosi D, Potluri A, Islam S, Geha H, Lurie A (2003) Bone trabeculae are visible on periapical images. *Oral Surgery, Oral Medicine, Oral Pathology, Oral Radiology and Endodontics* **96**, 772–3.

33. Cotti E, Campisi G, Ambu R, Dettori C (2003) Ultrasound real-time imaging in the differential diagnosis of periapical lesions. *International Endodontic Journal* **36**, 556–63.

34. Cotti E, Campisi G, Garau V, Puddu G (2002) A new technique for the study of periapical bone lesions: ultrasound real time imaging. *International Endodontic Journal* **35**, 148–52.

35. Cotti E, Vargiu P, Dettori C, Mallarini G (1999) Computerized tomography in the management and follow-up of extensive periapical lesion. *Endodontics and Dental Traumatology* **15**, 186–9.

36. Czajka J, Rushton VE, Shearer AC, Horner K (1996) Sensitometric and image quality performance of "rapid" intraoral film processing techniques. *British Journal of Radiology* **69**, 49–58.

37. Dahlén G, Fabricius L, Heyden G, Holm SE, Möller ÅJR (1982) Apical periodontitis induced by selected bacterial strains in root canals of immunized and non-immunized monkeys. *Scandinavian Journal of Dental Research* **90**, 207–16.

38. Delano EO, Ludlow JB, Ørstavik D, Tyndall D, Trope M (2001) Comparison between PAI and quantitative digital radiographic assessment of apical healing after endodontic treatment *Oral Surgery, Oral Medicine, Oral Pathology, Oral Radiology and Endodontics* **92**, 108–15.

39. Delano EO, Tyndall D, Ludlow JB, Trope M, Lost C (1998) Quantitative radiographic follow-up of apical surgery: a radiometric and histologic correlation. *Journal of Endodontics* **24**, 420–6.

40. Douglass CW, Valachovic RW, Wijesinha A, Chauncey HH, Kapur KK (1986) Clinical efficacy of dental radiography in the detection of dental caries and periodontal diseases. *Oral Surgery, Oral Medicine, Oral Pathology* **62**, 330–9.

41. Dove SB, McDavid WD, Hamilton KE (2000) Analysis of sensitivity and specifity of a new digital subtraction system. An in vitro study. *Oral Surgery, Oral Medicine, Oral Pathology Oral Radiology and Endodontics* **89**, 771–6.

42. Duinkerke AS, van de Poel AC, Doesburg WH, Lemmens WA (1977) Densitometric analysis of experimentally produced periapical radiolucencies. *Oral Surgery, Oral Medicine, Oral Pathology* **43**, 782–97.

43. Eberhardt JA, Torabinejad M, Christiansen EL (1992) A computed tomographic study of the distances between the maxillary sinus floor and the apices of the maxillary posterior teeth. *Oral Surgery, Oral Medicine, Oral Pathology* **73**, 345–6.

44. Eckerbom M, Andersson J-E, Magnusson T (1986) Interobserver variation in radiographic examination of endodontic variables. *Endodontics and Dental Traumatology* **2**, 243–6.

45. Eliasson S, Halvarsson C, Ljungheimer C (1984) Periapical condensing osteitis and endodontic treatment. *Oral Surgery, Oral Medicine, Oral Pathology* **57**, 195–9.

46. Engelke K, Graeff W, Meiss L, Hahn M, Delling G (1993) High spatial resolution imaging of bone mineral using computed microtomography. Comparison with microradiography and uncalcified histologic sections. *Investigative Radiology* **28**, 341–9.

47. Ericson S, Welander U (1966) Local hyperplasia of the maxillary sinus mucosa after elimination of adjacent periapical osteitis. *Odontology Revy* **17**, 153–9.

48. Eriksen HM, Berset GP, Hansen BF, Bjertness E (1995) Changes in endodontic status 1973–1993 among 35-year-olds in Oslo, Norway. *International Endodontic Journal* **28**, 129–32.

49. Eriksen HM, Bjertness E, Ørstavik D (1988) Prevalence and quality of endodontic treatment in an urban adult population in Norway. *Endodontics and Dental Traumatology* **4**, 122–6.

50. Eriksen HM, Ørstavik D, Kerekes K (1988) Healing of apical periodontitis after endodontic treatment using three different root canal sealers. *Endodontics and Dental Traumatology* **4**, 114–17.

51. Forsberg J, Halse A (1994) Radiographic simulation of a periapical lesion comparing the paralleling and the bisecting-angle techniques. *International Endodontic Journal* **27**, 133–8.

52. Forsberg J, Halse A (1997) Periapical radiolucencies as evaluated by bisecting angle and paralleling radiographic techniques. *International Endodontic Journal* **30**, 115–23.

53. Friedlander LT, Love RM, Chandler NP (2002) A comparison of phosphor-plate digital images with conventional radiographs for the perceived clarity of fine endodontic files and periapical lesions. *Oral Surgery, Oral Medicine, Oral Pathology, Oral Radiology and Endodontics* **93**, 321–7.

54. Friedman S, Torneck CD, Komorowski R, Ouzounian Z, Syrtash P, Kaufman A (1997) In vivo model for assessing the functional efficacy of endodontic filling materials and techniques. *Journal of Endodontics* **23**, 557–61.

55. Fristad I, Molven O, Halse A (2004) Nonsurgically retreated root filled teeth – radiographic findings after 20–27 years. *International Endodontic Journal* **37**, 12–18.

56. Frost HM (1994) Wolff law and bone's structural adaptations to mechanical usage – an overview for clinicians. *Angle Orthodontist* **64**, 175–88.

57. Gahleitner A, Solar P, Nasel C, Homolka P, Youssefzadeh S, Ertl L, *et al.* (1999) Magnetic resonance tomography and dental radiology (Dental-MRT). *Radiologe* **39**, 1044–50.

58. Gardner DG (1996) Some current concepts on the pathology of ameloblastomas. *Oral Surgery, Oral Medicine, Oral Pathology* **82**, 660–9.

59. Gelfand DW, Ott DJ (1985) Methodological considerations in comparing imaging methods. *American Journal of Roentgenology* **144**, 1117–21.

60. Gelfand M, Sunderman E, Goldman JM (1983) Reliability of radiographic interpretations. *Journal of Endodontics* **9**, 71–5.

61. Giusto TJ, Baer PN (1996) A peripheral giant cell granuloma mimicking a combined endodontic-periodontic lesion. *Periodontal Clinical Investigation* **18**, 17–19.

62. Goldman M, Pearson AH, Darzenta N (1972) Endodontic success – who's reading the radiograph? *Oral Surgery, Oral Medicine, Oral Pathology* **33**, 432–7.

63. Goldman M, Pearson AH, Darzenta N (1974) Reliability of radiographic interpretations. *Oral Surgery, Oral Medicine, Oral Pathology* **38**, 287–93.

64. Goldstein SA, Matthews LS, Kuhn JL, Hollister SJ (1991) Trabecular bone remodeling – an experimental model. *Journal of Biomechanics* **24**, 135.

65. Grahnén H, Hansson L (1961) The prognosis of pulp and root canal therapy. A clinical and radiographic follow-up examination. *Odontologisk Revy* **12**, 146–65.

66. Green TL, Walton RE, Taylor JK, Merrell P (1997) Radiographic and histologic periapical findings of root canal treated teeth in cadaver. *Oral Surgery, Oral Medicine, Oral Pathology, Oral Radiology and Endodontics* **83**, 707–11.

67. Grimm WD, Wentz K, Boedecker T, Eberhard J, Jackowski J, Kamann W (1995) Use of ultrafast computed tomography in dental surgery: A case report. *Endodontics and Dental Traumatology* **11**, 297–300.

68. Groot RH, van Merkesteyn JP, Bras J (1996) Diffuse sclerosing osteomyelitis and florid osseous dysplasia. *Oral Surgery, Oral Medicine, Oral Pathology* **81**, 333–42.

69. Grung B, Molven O, Halse A (1990) Periapical surgery in a Norwegian county hospital: follow-up findings of 477 teeth. *Journal of Endodontics* **16**, 411–17.

70. Gundappa M, Ng S, Whaites E (2006) Comparison of ultrasound, digital and conventional radiography in differentiating periapical lesions. *Dentomaxillofacial Radiology* **35**, 326–33.

71. Halse A, Molven O, Grung B (1991) Follow-up after periapical surgery: the value of the one-year control. *Endodontics and Dental Traumatology* **7**, 246–50.

72. Halstead CL, Hoard BC (1991) Dental radiology and oral pathology. *Current Problems in Diagnostic Radiology* **20**, 187–235.

73. Hanley JA, McNeil BJ (1982) The meaning and use of the area under a receiver operating characteristic (ROC) curve. *Radiology* **143**, 29–36.

74. Hannig C, Dullin C, Hulsmann M, Heidrich G (2005) Three-dimensional, non-destructive visualization of vertical root fractures using flat panel volume detector computer tomography: an ex vivo in vitro case report. *International Endodontic Journal* **38**, 904–13.

75. Harase Y, Araki K, Okano T (2006) Accuracy of extraoral tuned aperture computed tomography (TACT) for proximal caries detection. *Oral Surgery, Oral Medicine, Oral Pathology, Oral Radiology and Endodontics* **101**, 791–6.

76. Harty FJ, Parkins BJ, Wengraf AM (1970) Success rate in root canal therapy. A retrospective study on conventional cases. *British Dental Journal* **128**, 65–70.

77. Hayakawa Y, Yamamoto K, Kousuge Y, Kobayashi N, Wakoh M, Sekiguchi H, *et al.* (2003) Clinical validity of the interactive and low-dose three-dimensional dento-alveolar imaging system, tuned-aperture computed tomography. *Bulletin of Tokyo Dental College* **44**, 159–67.

78. Hayashi N, Iwata J, Masaoka N, Ueno H, Ohtsuki Y, Moriki T (1997) Ameloblastoma of the mandible metastasizing to the orbit with malignant transformation. A histopathological and immunohistochemical study. *Virchows Archives* **430**, 501–7.

79. Hedin M, Polhagen L (1971) Follow-up study of periradicular bone condensation. *Scandinavian Journal of Dental Research* **79**, 436–40.

80. Heling I, Bialla-Shenkman S, Turetzky A, Horwitz J, Sela J (2001) The outcome of teeth with periapical periodontitis treated with nonsurgical endodontic treatment: a computerized morphometric study. *Quintessence International* **32**, 397–400.

81. Hisatomi M, Asaumi J, Konouchi H, Yanagi Y, Matsuzaki H, Kishi K (2003) Comparison of radiographic and MRI features of a root-diverging odontogenic myxoma, with discussion of the differential diagnosis of lesions likely to move roots. *Oral Diseases* **9**, 152–7.

82. Holberg C, Steinhauser S, Geis P, Rudzki-Janson I (2005) Cone-beam computed tomography in orthodontics: benefits and limitations. *Journal of Orofacial Orthopedics* **66**, 434–44.

83. Hovi L, Saarinen UM, Donner U, Lindqvist C (1996) Opportunistic osteomyelitis in the jaws of children on immunosuppressive chemotherapy. *Journal of Pediatric Hematology and Oncology* **18**, 90–4.

84. Huang CH, Brunsvold MA (2006) Maxillary sinusitis and periapical abscess following periodontal therapy: a case report using three-dimensional evaluation. *Journal of Periodontology* **77**, 129–34.

85. Huumonen S, Ørstavik D (2002) Radiological aspects of apical periodontitis *Endodontic Topics* **1**, 3–25.

86. Jansson L, Ehnevid H, Lindskog S, Blomlof L (1993) Development of periapical lesions. *Swedish Dental Journal* **17**, 85–93.

87. Jeffcoat MK, Reddy MS, Webber RC, Ruttimann UE (1987) Extraoral control of geometry for digital subtraction radiography. *Journal of Periodontal Research* **22**, 396–402.

88. Kaffe I, Ardekian L, Taicher S, Littner MM, Buchner A (1996) Radiologic features of central giant cell granuloma of the jaws. *Oral Surgery, Oral Medicine, Oral Pathology* **81**, 720–6.

89. Kannan SK, Sandhya G, Selvarani R (2006) Periostitis ossificans (Garre's osteomyelitis) radiographic study of two cases. *International Journal of Paediatric Dentistry* **16**, 59–64.

90. Kashima I, Tajima K, Nishimura K, Yamane R, Saraya M, Sasakura Y, *et al.* (1990) Diagnostic imaging of diseases affecting the mandible with the use of computed panoramic radiography. *Oral Surgery, Oral Medicine, Oral Pathology* **70**, 110–16.

91. Katz JO, Underhill TE (1994) Multilocular radiolucencies. *Dental Clinics of North America* **38**, 63–81.

92. Kerekes K, Tronstad L (1979) Long-term results of endodontic treatment performed with a standardized technique. *Journal of Endodontics* **5**, 83–90.

93. Kerosuo E, Ørstavik D (1997) Application of computerised image analysis to monitoring endodontic therapy: reproducibility and comparison with visual assessment. *Dentomaxillofacial Radiology* **26**, 79–84.

94. Kosti E, Lambrianidis T, Chatzisavvas P, Molyvdas I (2004) Healing of a radiolucent periradicular lesion with periradicular radiopacity. *Journal of Endodontics* **30**, 548–50.

95. Krennmair G, Lenglinger F (1995) Imaging of mandibular cysts with a dental computed tomography software program. *International Journal of Oral and Maxillofacial Surgery* **24**, 48–52.

96. Kronfeld R (1940) Correlation between clinical and pathological diagnosis in chronic apical periodontitis. In *Proceedings Dental Centenary Celebration*. Baltimorem, MD: Waverly Press, pp. 409–24.

97. Kullendorff B, Gröndahl K, Rohlin M, Henrikson CO (1988) Subtraction radiography for the detection of periapical bone lesions. *Endodontics and Dental Traumatology* **4**, 253–9.

98. Kullendorff B, Gröndahl K, Rohlin M, Nilsson M (1992) Subtraction radiography of interradicular bone lesions. *Acta Odontologica Scandinavica* **50**, 259–67.

99. Kullendorff B, Nilsson M (1996) Diagnostic accuracy of direct digital dental radiography for the detection of periapical bone lesions. II. Effects on diagnostic accuracy after application of image processing. *Oral Surgery, Oral Medicine, Oral Pathology* **82**, 585–9.

100. Kullendorff B, Nilsson M, Rohlin M (1996) Diagnostic accuracy of direct digital dental radiography for the detection of periapical bone lesions. I. Overall comparison between conventional and direct digital radiography. *Oral Surgery, Oral Medicine, Oral Pathology* **82**, 344–50.

101. Kullendorff B, Petersson K, Rohlin M (1997) Direct digital radiography for the detection of periapical bone lesions. A clinical study. *Endodontics and Dental Traumatology* **13**, 183–9.

102. Kvist T, Reit C (1999) Results of endodontic retreatment: a randomized clinical study comparing surgical and nonsurgical procedures. *Journal of Endodontics* **12**, 814–17.

103. Larheim TA, Westesson PL (2006) *Maxillofacial imaging*. Berlin: Springer.

104. Laib A, Ruegsegger P (1999) Calibration of trabecular bone structure measurements of in vivo three-dimensional peripheral quantitative computed tomography with 28-microm-resolution microcomputed tomography. *Bone* **24**, 35–9.

105. Lambrianidis T (1985) Observer variations in radiographic evaluation of endodontic therapy. *Endodontics and Dental Traumatology* **1**, 235–41.

106. Lee SJ, Jang KH, Spångberg LS, Kim E, Jung IY, Lee CY, *et al.* (2006) Three-dimensional visualization of a mandibular first molar with three distal roots using computer-aided rapid prototyping. *Oral Surgery, Oral Medicine, Oral Pathology, Oral Radiology and Endodontics* **101**, 668–74.

107. Lee SJ, Messer HH (1986) Radiographic appearance of artificially prepared periapical lesions confined to cancellous bone. *International Endodontic Journal* **19**, 64–72.

108. Lin SK, Hong CY, Chang HH, Chiang CP, Chen CS, Jeng JH, *et al.* (2000) Immunolocalization of macrophages and transforming growth factor beta 1 in induced rat periapical lesions. *Journal of Endodontics* **26**, 335–40.

109. Lomcali G, Sen BH, Cankaya H (1996) Scanning electron microscopic observations of apical root surfaces of teeth with apical periodontitis *Endodontics and Dental Traumatology* **12**, 70–6.

110. Marks JM, Dunkelberger FB (1980) Paget's disease. *Journal of the American Dental Association* **101**, 49–52.

111. Marmary Y, Koter T, Heling I (1999) The effect of periapical rarefying osteitis on cortical and cancellous bone. A study comparing conventional radiographs with computed tomography. *Dentomaxillofacial Radiology* **28**, 267–71.

112. Marmary Y, Kutiner G (1986) A radiographic survey of periapical jawbone lesions. *Oral Surgery, Oral Medicine, Oral Pathology* **61**, 405–8.

113. Marques MD, Moreira B, Eriksen HM (1998) Prevalence of apical periodontitis and results of endodontic treatment in an adult, Portuguese population. *International Endodontic Journal* **31**, 161–5.

114. Matteson SR, Deahl ST, Alder ME, Nummikoski PV (1996) Advanced imaging methods. *Critical Reviews in Oral Biology and Medicine* **7**, 346–95.

115. Meier AW, Brown CE, Miles DA, Analoui M (1996) Interpretation of chemically created periapical lesions using direct digital imaging. *Journal of Endodontics* **22**, 516–20.

116. Meister F, Lommel TJ, Gerstein H (1980) Diagnosis and possible causes of vertical root fractures. *Oral Surgery, Oral Medicine, Oral Pathology* **49**, 243–53.

117. Mikrogeorgis G, Lyroudia K, Molyvdas I, Nikolaidis N, Pitas I (2004) Digital radiograph registration and subtraction: a useful tool for the evaluation of the progress of chronic apical periodontitis. *Journal of Endodontics* **30**, 513–17.

118. Minami M, Kaneda T, Yamamoto H, Ozawa K, Itai Y, Ozawa M, *et al.* (1992) Ameloblastoma in the maxillomandibular region – MR imaging. *Radiology* **184**, 389–93.

119. Minami M, Kaneda T, Ozawa K, Yamamoto H, Itai Y, Ozawa M, *et al.* (1996) Cystic lesions of the maxillomandibular region: MR imaging distinction of odontogenic keratocysts and ameloblastomas from other cysts. *American Journal of Roentgenology* **166**, 943–9.

120. Mol A, Dunn SM, van der Stelt PF (1992) Diagnosing of periapical bone lesions on radiographs by means of texture analysis. *Oral Surgery, Oral Medicine, Oral Pathology* **73**, 746–50.

121. Molander B, Ahlqwist M, Gröndahl HG, Hollender L (1992) Comparison of panoramic and intraoral radiography for the diagnosis of caries and periapical pathology. *Dentomaxillofacial Radiology* **22**, 28–32.

122. Molander B, Ahlqwist M, Gröndal H-G (1995) Panoramic and restrictive intraoral radiography in comprehensive oral radiographic diagnosis. *European Journal of Oral Sciences* **103**, 191–8.

123. Molven O, Halse A, Grung B (1987) Observer strategy and the radiographic classification of healing after endodontic surgery. *International Journal of Oral and Maxillofacial Surgery* **16**, 432–9.

124. Molven O, Halse A, Grung B (1996) Incomplete healing (scar tissue) after periapical surgery – radiographic findings 8 to 12 years after treatment. *Journal of Endodontics* **22**, 264–8.

125. Morfis AS (1990) Vertical root fractures. *Oral Surgery, Oral Medicine, Oral Pathology* **69**, 631–5.

126. Nair MK, Gröndahl HG, Webber RL, Nair UP, Wallace JA (2003) Effect of iterative restoration on the detection of artificially induced vertical radicular fractures by Tuned Aperture Computed Tomography. *Oral Surgery, Oral Medicine, Oral Pathology, Oral Radiology and Endodontics* **96**, 118–25.

127. Nair MK, Nair UDP, Gröndahl HG, Webber RL, Wallace JA (2001) Detection of artificially induced vertical radicular fractures using tuned aperture computed tomography. *European Journal of Oral Sciences* **109**, 375–9.

128. Nair MK, Tyndall DA, Ludlow JB, May K (1998) Tuned aperture computer tomography and detection of recurrent caries. *Dentomafillofacial Radiology* **32**, 23–30.

129. Nair PNR, Pajarola G, Schroeder HE (1996) Types and incidence of human periapical lesions obtained with extracted teeth. *Oral Surgery, Oral Medicine, Oral Pathology* **81**, 93–102.

130. Nair PNR, Sjögren U, Krey G, Sundqvist G (1990) Therapy-resistant foreign body giant cell granuloma at the periapex of a root-filled human tooth. *Journal of Endodontics* **16**, 589–95.

131. Nair R (1998) New perspectives on radicular cysts: do they heal? *International Endodontic Journal* **31**, 155–60.

132. Nakata K, Naitoh M, Izumi M, Inamoto K, Ariji E, Nakamura H (2006) Effectiveness of dental computed tomography in diagnostic imaging of periradicular lesion of each root of a multirooted tooth: a case report. *Journal of Endodontics* **32**, 583–7.

133. Nance R, Tyndall D, Levin LG, Trope M (2000) Diagnosis of external root resorption using TACT (tuned-aperture computed tomography). *Endodontics and Dental Traumatology* **16**, 24–8.

134. Nastri AL, Wiesenfeld D, Radden BG, Eveson J, Scully C (1995) Maxillary ameloblastoma: a retrospective study of 13 cases. *British Journal of Oral and Maxillofacial Surgery* **33**, 28–32.

135. Nicopoulou-Karayianni K, Bragger U, Lang NP (1997) Patterns of periodontal destruction associated with incomplete root fractures. *Dentomaxillofacial Radiology* **26**, 321–6.

136. Obermayr G, Walton RE, Leary JM, Krell KV (1991) Vertical root fracture and relative deformation during obturation and post cementation. *Journal of Prosthetic Dentistry* **66**, 181–7.

137. Ørstavik D (1991) Radiographic evaluation of apical periodontitis and endodontic treatment results: a computer approach. *International Dental Journal* **41**, 89–98.

138. Ørstavik D (1996) Time-course and risk analyses of the development and healing of chronic apical periodontitis in man. *International Endodontic Journal* **29**, 150–5.

139. Ørstavik D, Brodin P, Aas E (1983) Paraesthesia following endodontic treatment. survey of the literature and report of a case. *International Endodontic Journal* **16**, 167–72.

140. Ørstavik D, Farrants G, Wahl T, Kerekes K (1990) Image analysis of endodontic radiographs: digital subtraction and quantitative densitometry. *Endodontics and Dental Traumatology* **6**, 6–11.

141. Ørstavik D, Hørsted-Bindslev P (1993) A comparison of endodontic treatment results at two dental schools. *International Endodontic Journal* **26**, 348–54.

142. Ørstavik D, Kerekes K, Eriksen HM (1986) The periapical index: A scoring system for radiographic assessment of apical periodontitis. *Endodontics and Dental Traumatology* **2**, 20–34.

143. Ørstavik D, Kerekes K, Eriksen HM (1987) Clinical performance of three endodontic sealers. *Endodontics and Dental Traumatology* **3**, 178–86.

144. Ørstavik D, Mjör IA (1992) Usage test of four endodontic sealers in *Macaca fascicularis* monkeys. *Oral Surgery, Oral Medicine, Oral Pathology* **73**, 337–44.

145. Pascon EA, Introcaso JH, Langeland K (1987) Development of predictable periapical lesion monitored by subtraction radiography. *Endodontics and Dental Traumatology* **3**, 192–208.

146. Peters OA, Laib A, Rüesegger P, Barbakov F (2000) Three-dimensional analysis of root canal geometry by high-resolution computed tomography. *Journal of Dental Research* **79**, 1405–9.

147. Pettiette MT, Delano EO, Trope M (2001) Evaluation of success rate of endodontic treatment performed by students with stainless-steel K-files and nickel-titanium hand files. *Journal of Endodontics* **27**, 124–7.

148. Pitt Ford TR (1984) The radiographic detection of periapical lesions in dogs. *Oral Surgery, Oral Medicine, Oral Pathology* **57**, 662–7.

149. Polson AM (1977) Periodontal destruction associated with vertical root fracture. *Journal of Periodontology* **18**, 53–9.

150. Priebe WA, Lazonsky JP, Wuehrman AH (1954) Value of the roentgenographic film in the differential diagnosis of periapical lesions. *Oral Surgery, Oral Medicine, Oral Pathology* **7**, 979–83.

151. Reddy MS, Bruch JM, Jeffcoat MK, Williams RC (1991) Contrast enhancement as an aid to interpretation in digital subtraction radiography. *Oral Surgery, Oral Medicine, Oral Pathology* **71**, 763–9.

152. Reichart PA, Philipsen HP, Sonner S (1995) Ameloblastoma: biological profile of 3677 cases. *European Journal of Cancer Research and Clinical Oncology* **31B**, 86–99.

153. Reit C (1987) Decision strategies in endodontics: on the design of a recall program. *Endodontics and Dental Traumatology* **3**, 233–9.

154. Reit C, Gröndahl HG (1983) Application of statistical decision theory to radiographic diagnosis of endodontically treated teeth. *Scandinavian Journal of Dental Research* **91**, 213–18.

155. Reit C, Gröndahl HG (1984) Management of periapical lesions in endodontically treated teeth. A study on clinical decision making. *Swedish Dental Journal* **8**, 1–7.

156. Reit C, Hollander L (1983) Radiographic evaluation of endodontic therapy and the influence of observer variation. *Scandinavian Journal of Dental Research* **91**, 205–12.

157. Ricucci D, Mannocci F, Ford TR (2006) A study of periapical lesions correlating the presence of a radiopaque lamina with histological findings. *Oral Surgery, Oral Medicine, Oral Pathology, Oral Radiology and Endodontics* **101**, 389–94.

158. Roberson JB, Crocker DJ, Schiller T (1997) The diagnosis and treatment of central giant cell granuloma. *Journal of the American Dental Association* **128**, 81–4.

159. Rohlin M, Kullendorff B, Ahlqwist M, Henrikson CO, Hollender L, Stenström B (1989) Comparison between panoramic and periapical radiography in the diagnosis of periapical bone lesions. *Dentomaxillofacial Radiology* **18**, 151–5.

160. Rosen DJ, Ardekian L, Machtei EE, Peled M, Manor R, Laufer D (1997) Traumatic bone cyst resembling apical periodontitis. *Journal of Periodontology* **68**, 1019–21.

161. Rowe AHR, Binnie WH (1974) Correlation between radiological and histological changes following root canal treatment. *Journal of the British Endodontic Society* **7**, 57–63.

162. Rudolph DJ, White SC (1988) Film-holding instruments for intraoral subtraction radiography. *Oral Surgery, Oral Medicine, Oral Pathology* **65**, 767–72.

163. Ruttimann UE, Webber RL, Schmidt E (1986) A robust digital method for film contrast correction in subtraction radiography. *Journal of Periodontal Research* **21**, 486–95.

164. Samarabandu J, Allen KM, Hausmann E, Acharya R (1994) Algorithm for the automated alignment of radiographs for image subtraction. *Oral Surgery, Oral Medicine, Oral Pathology* **77**, 75–9.

165. Sarathy AP, Bourgeois SL Jr, Goodell GG (2005) Bisphosphonate-associated osteonecrosis of the jaws and endodontic treatment: two case reports. *Journal of Endodontics* **31**, 759–63. Erratum in: *Journal of Endodontics* **31**, 835–6.

166. Sato H, Kawamura A, Yamaguchi M, Kasai K (2005) Relationship between masticatory function and internal structure of the mandible based on computed tomography findings. *American Journal of Orthodontics and Dentofacial Orthopedics* **128**, 766–73.

167. Scarfe WC, Czerniejewski VJ, Farman AG, Avant SL, Molteni R (1999) In vivo accuracy and reliability of color-coded image enhancements for the assessment of periradicular lesion dimensions. *Oral Surgery, Oral Medicine, Oral Pathology, Oral Radiology and Endodontics* **88**, 603–11.

168. Scarfe WC, Fana CR Jr, Farman AG (1995) Radiographic detection of accessory/lateral canals: use of RadioVisioGraphy and Hypaque. *Journal of Endodontics* **21**, 185–90.

169. Selden H (1974) The interrelationship between the maxillary sinus and endodontics. *Oral Surgery, Oral Medicine, Oral Pathology* **4**, 623–9.

170. Seltzer S, Bender IB, Turkenkopf S (1963) Factors affecting successful repair after root canal therapy. *Journal of the American Dental Association* **52**, 651–62.

171. Shearer AC, Wasti F, Wilson NH (1996) The use of a radiopaque contrast medium in endodontic radiography. *International Endodontic Journal* **29**, 95–8.

172. Shrout MK, Hall JM, Hildebolt CE (1993) Differentiation of periapical granulomas and radicular cysts by digital radiometric analysis. *Oral Surgery, Oral Medicine, Oral Pathology,* **76**, 356–61.

173. Sidaravicius B, Aleksejuniene J, Eriksen HM (1999) Endodontic treatment and prevalence of apical periodontitis in an adult population of Vilnius, Lithuania. *Endodontics and Dental Traumatology* **15**, 210–15.

174. Sidhu MS, Parkash H, Sidhu SS (1995) Central giant cell granuloma of jaws – review of 19 cases. *British Journal of Oral and Maxillofacial Surgery* **33**, 43–6.

175. Simon JH. (1980) Incidence of periapical cysts in relation to the root canal. *Journal of Endodontics* **6**, 845–8.

176. Sismanidou C, Lindskog S (1995) Spatial and temporal repair patterns of orthodontically induced surface resorption patches *European Journal of Oral Science* **103**, 292–8.

177. Skoglund A, Persson G (1985) A follow-up study of apicoectomized teeth with total loss of the buccal bone plate. *Oral Surgery, Oral Medicine, Oral Pathology* **59**, 78–81.

178. Smith CS, Setchell DJ, Harty FJ (1993) Factors influencing the success of conventional root canal therapy – a five-year retrospective study. *International Endodontic Journal* **26**, 321–33.

179. Staretz LR, Brada BJ, Schott TR (1990) Well-defined radiolucent lesion in the maxillary anterior region. *Journal of the American Dental Association* **120**, 335–6.

180. Strindberg LZ (1956) The dependence of the results of pulp therapy on certain factors. An analytical study based on radiographic and clinical follow-up examinations. Dissertation. *Acta Odontologica Scandinavia* **14** (suppl 21), 1–174.

181. Strittmatter EJ, Keller DL, LaBounty GL, Lewis DM, Graham GD (1989) The relationship between radionuclide bone scans and dental examinations. *Oral Surgery, Oral Medicine, Oral Pathology* **68**, 576–81.

182. Syrjänen S, Tammisalo E, Lilja R, Syrjänen K (1982) Radiological interpretation of the periapical cysts and granulomas. *Dentomaxillofacial Radiology* **11**, 89–92.

183. Tallan EM, Olsen KD, McCaffrey TV, Unni KK, Lund BA (1994) Advanced giant cell granuloma: a twenty-year study. *Otolaryngology – Head and Neck Surgery* **110**, 413–18.

184. Tammisalo T, Luostarinen T, Vähätalo K, Neva M (1996) Detailed tomography of periapical and periodontal lesions. Diagnostic accuracy compared with periapical radiography. *Dentomaxillofacial Radiology* **25**, 89–96.

185. Tamse A, Fuss Z, Lustig J, Ganor Y, Kaffe I (1999) Radiographic features of vertically fractured, endodontically treated maxillary premolars. *Oral Surgery, Oral Medicine, Oral Pathology, Oral Radiology and Endodontics* **88**, 348–52.

186. Tanomaru-Filho M, Poliseli-Neto A, Leonardo MR, Silva LA, Tanomaru JM, Ito IY. (2005) Methods of experimental induction of periapical inflammation. Microbiological and radiographic evaluation. *International Endodontic Journal* **38**, 477–82.

187. Teixeira FB, Gomes BPFA, Ferraz CCR, Souza-Filho J, Zaia AA (2000) Radiographic analysis of the development of periapical lesions in normal rats, sialoadenectomized and sialoadenenectomized-immunosuppressed rats. *Endodontics and Dental Traumatology* **16**, 154–7.

188. Telfer N, Abelson SH, Witmer RR (1980) Role of bone imaging in the diagnosis of active root canal infections: case report. *Journal of Endodontics* **6**, 570–2.

189. Thorell LG, Smith WJ (1991) *Using computer color effectively.* Upper Saddle River, NJ: Prentice Hall.

190. Torabinejad M, Trope M (1996) Endodontic and periodontal interrelationships. In Walton RE, Torabinejad M, editors. *Principles and practice of endodontics.* Philadelphia, PA: WB Saunders.

191. Tronstad L (1988) Root resorption – etiology, terminology and clinical manifestations. *Endodontics and Dental Traumatology* **4**, 241–52.

192. Trope M, Delano EO, Ørstavik D (1999) Endodontic treatment of teeth with apical periodontitis: Single vs. multivisit treatment. *Journal of Endodontics* **25**, 345–50.

193. Trope M, Pettigrew J, Petras J, Barnett F, Tronstad L (1989) Differentiation of radicular cyst and granulomas using computerized tomography. *Endodontics and Dental Traumatology* **5**, 69–72.

194. Tyndall DA, Clifton TL, Webber RL, Ludlow JB, Horton RA (1997) TACT imaging of primary caries. *Oral Surgery, Oral Medicine, Oral Pathology* **84**, 214–25.

195. Tyndall DA, Kapa SF, Bagnell CP (1990) Digital subtraction radiography for detecting cortical and cancellous bone changes in the periapical region. *Journal of Endodontics* **16**, 173–8.

196. Velvart P, Hecker H, Tillinger G (2001) Detection of the apical lesion and the mandibular canal in conventional radiography and computed tomography. *Oral Surgery, Oral Medicine, Oral Pathology, Oral Radiology and Endodontics* **92**, 682–8.

197. von Stechow D, Balto K, Stashenko P, Muller R (2003) Three-dimensional quantitation of periradicular bone destruction by micro-computed tomography. *Journal of Endodontics* **29**, 252–6.

198. Waltimo T, Boiesen J, Eriksen HM, Ørstavik D (2001) Clinical performance of 3 endodontic sealers. *Oral Surgery, Oral Medicine, Oral Pathology, Oral Radiology and Endodontics* **92**, 89–92.

199. Wang X, Wang J, Zhang G (1999) [Analysis on curative effects of teeth with chronic apical periodontitis in elderly people] [In Chinese]. *Zhonghua Kou Qiang Yi Xue Za Zhi* **34**, 16–18.

200. Webber RL, Horton RA, Underhill TE, Ludlow JB, Tyndall DA (1996) Comparison of film, direct digital, and tuned aperture computed tomography images to identify the location of crestal defects around endosseous implants. *Oral Surgery, Oral Medicine, Oral Pathology, Oral Radiology and Endodontics* **81**, 480–90.

201. Webber RL, Ruttimann UE, Groenhuis AJ (1984) Computer correction of projective distortions in dental radiography. *Journal of Dental Research* **63**, 1032–6.

202. Wenzel A (1989). Effect of manual compared with reference point superimposition on image quality in digital subtraction radiography. *Dentomaxillofacial Radiology* **18**, 145–50.

203. Wenzel A, Gröndahl HG (1995) Direct digital radiography in the dental office. *International Dental Journal* **119**, 27–34.

204. Weski O (1914) Röntgenologisch-mikroskopische Studien aus dem Gebiete der Kieferpathologie. *Korrespondanze-Blätter für Zahnärzte* **42**, 244–69.

205. Wesselink PR, Beertsen W (1994) Repair processes in the periodontium following dentoalveolar ankylosis – the effect of masticatory function. *Journal of Clinical Periodontology* **21**, 472–8.

206. White SC, Sapp JP, Seto BG, Mankovich NJ (1994) Absence of radiometric differentiation between periapical cyst and granulomas. *Oral Surgery, Oral Medicine, Oral Pathology* **78**, 650–4.

207. Yang SF, Rivera EM, Walton RE (1995) Vertical root fracture in nonendodontically treated teeth. *Journal of Endodontics* **21**, 337–9.

208. Yokota ET, Miles DA, Newton CW, Brown CE Jr (1994) Interpretation of periapical lesions using RadioVisioGraphy. *Journal of Endodontics* **20**, 490–4.

209. Yoshioka T, Kobayashi C, Suda H, Sasaki T (2002) An observation of the healing process of periapical lesions by digital subtraction radiography. *Journal of Endodontics* **28**, 589–91.

210. Yu SM, Stashenko P (1987) Identification of inflammatory cells in developing rat periapical lesions. *Journal of Endodontics* **13**, 535–40.

211. Yusuf H (1982) The significance of the presence of foreign material periapically as a cause of failure of root treatment. *Oral Surgery, Oral Medicine, Oral Pathology* **54**, 566–74.

Chapter 7
Clinical Manifestations and Diagnosis

Asgeir Sigurdsson

7.1 Introduction

Correct pulpal diagnosis is the key to all endodontic treatments. It is paramount to have established a clinical diagnosis of the pulp and the periapical tissue before cutting access into the pulp chamber or doing any other treatment to a tooth or a patient. This clinical diagnosis should be based on history of symptoms, presenting symptoms, diagnostic tests, and clinical findings. If it is not possible to establish the diagnosis or a differential diagnosis cannot be ruled out, therapy should not be initiated until further evaluation has been done or second opinion gained.

Unfortunately, there is a poor correlation between clinical symptomatology and pulpal histopathology [5,32,34,45,67,116]. Previous attempts made to diagnose accurately the condition of the pulp based only on clinical signs and symptoms, on electric pulp and/or thermal tests and radiography have not been very successful [24,34,87].

Since symptoms or test results have such a limited predictor of pulpal and periapical status, as much information as possible should be collected about the presentation and history of symptoms and as many tests that are practical should be conducted prior to a formulation of final diagnosis. Thus, clinical signs and symptoms, diagnostic tests in addition to a comprehensive knowledge of the reaction of the pulp to caries, operative manipulations, trauma, and periodontal disease, enable us to establish an empirical pulp diagnosis only.

In the past there has been a variety of different pulpal diagnostic terms introduced in the literature [5,113]. Many of these have been very elaborate and almost all classifications have been very descriptive of the assumed histological appearance of the pulp. However, due to obvious reasons, the assessment of the histology is impossible with current technology without removing the pulp. In more recent times the trend has been to move away from these elaborate classifications and to use a somewhat modified version that Morse *et al.* suggested in 1977 [85]. Even though this classification refers to some degree to histological status of the pulp, it helps the clinician to decide on treatment because there is no crossover between categories in terms of treatment needs.

7.2 Pulpal diagnostic terms

7.2.1 Healthy pulp

According to the definition, a healthy pulp is vital, asymptomatic, and without any inflammation. This diagnostic term is only used if the pulp needs to be removed and the tooth root-filled for restorative reasons, e.g., need for a post space or when shortening an extruded tooth. Additionally, this term is used in case of dental trauma when a crown of a tooth breaks off, exposing the pulp, but then is treated within the first 30–48 hours [54].

7.2.2 Reversible pulpitis

This term implies that the pulp is vital, but inflamed to some degree. Symptoms can be very misleading, ranging from none at all to very sharp sensation asso-

ciated with a thermal stimuli. Through information gathered during testing (see below), it is predicted that the inflammation should heal once the irritant, like deep caries, is removed, or when an exposed dentin surface is sealed again. The mild trauma with subsequent inflammation can cause small regions of neurogenic inflammation and sufficient mechanical damage to stimulate nerve sprouting reaction [19] and thereby possibly cause exaggerated response to vitality tests, indicating more severe inflammation than actually there is. As already stated, clinical signs or symptoms or diagnostic test do not, in many cases, correlate with the histopathologic status of the pulp [5,34,45,69,113,116]. There is, however, quite a high risk of diagnosing a pulp with mild symptoms as being reversibly, inflamed, when actually the pulp is irreversibly inflamed (see below). It is therefore very important to recall all patients with a diagnosis of reversible pulpitis a few weeks after treatment and reevaluate all appropriate symptoms and vitality tests. A telephone consultation is not enough in these cases, because the pulp may have become necrotic and thereby give the false impression to the patient that the problem has been resolved. The history of symptoms will mainly reveal provoked pain or sensation, and the tooth will only bother the patient when the tooth is exposed to a hot and/or cold stimulus.

7.2.3 Irreversible pulpitis

This term implies that the pulp is still vital, but so inflamed that it will not be able to heal again. Therefore, it needs to be removed and root canal therapy done. In almost all cases, if this condition is left alone the pulp will eventually become necrotic, and then bacteria will have an easy access to the apex and periapical structures. Symptoms can be rather misleading. It has been well documented that in many cases an apparent irreversible pulpitis is asymptomatic. Studies have reported that dental pulps can progress to necrosis without pain in 26–60% of all cases [3,12]. It is of interest to note that according to a recent study neither gender nor tooth type seems to matter in such cases of asymptomatic pulpitis [81], or "painless pulpitis" [53].

7.2.4 Necrotic pulp

When the pulp necroses, the necrotic part of the pulpal space is filled with sterile debris at best, but no vital structures. The distinction between partial and total necrosis can be very important in cases of immature teeth, where the presence of intact pulp tissue apically may ensure continued root development. The only way to confirm vitality in those cases is to enter the pulp chamber and remove the necrotic debris down to a vital pulp stub.

7.2.5 Infected pulp/infected pulpal space

Infection of the pulp may affect only part of the pulp canal, such as in a recent pulpal exposure by trauma or caries, or when just one or two roots in multirooted teeth are involved. The space that is left once the pulp has become completely necrotic can be sterile in the case of trauma where the blood supply to the tooth was cut off, but where there is no ingrowth of bacteria from the coronal part of the tooth. In most cases though, the pulp has become necrotic secondary to bacterial invasion through caries or fracture in the crown and therefore the space is infected. It has been shown that all teeth with periapical lesions have infected pulp spaces [10]. Teeth that do not have a periapical lesion may or may not be infected, as it is well known that there has to be a significant loss of bone structure before it becomes radiographically apparent [8].

7.3 Symptomatology of pulpal disease

Dental training focuses on diagnosing a problem by visual means, such as assessing restorations, clinical signs of oral health or disease, and radiographs. However, when diagnosing origins of pain, most of the diagnosis is done by collecting anamnestic information, i.e., what we hear, and not what we can see [96]. In fact, visual clues may throw us off the track and lead to an incorrect diagnosis. Therefore, it is important to listen carefully to patients and to systematically review all their present symptoms as well as the history of the symptoms prior to coming to a conclusion about the cause.

7.3.1 Presenting symptoms

Presenting symptoms are, by definition, symptoms that are recognizable during the consultation. The presenting symptoms, while suggestive, cannot be used alone to make the final diagnosis.

Pain free

It is well established that pulpitis is, as a rule, painless [3,9,34,54,81]. Lack of pain is therefore not a good indicator of the presence, severity, or reversibility of pulpitis. The reasons, however, for the variability of pain symptoms in pulpitis are not well known. At least in some cases the progression of the inflammation may either be so rapid that there is no pain, or so slow that the classical inflammatory mediators participating in the pain process never reach a critical level [81]. A more likely explanation would be that there is effective modification by local as well as centrally mediated systems. There are several local regulatory factors and systems in the pulp. Endogenous opioid, adrenergic sympathetic and nitric oxide systems exist in the pulp [20,57,98], and there is a good indication that, for example, somatostatin may inhibit pulpal pain activation under certain conditions [22,57,125].

Sharp pain

If the pain is short and only associated with a stimulus, like cold air or fluid, it is likely to be mediated only by the A-delta neurofibers that are normally active throughout the dentin–pulp complex [9,122]. Therefore, complaints of only provoked pain may possibly indicate only mild inflammation. Vital pulp therapy may be sufficient to treat the condition, e.g., by removing a shallow caries lesion, replacing a leaky restoration, or covering up exposed root surfaces.

Severe pain that lingers

There is building evidence that the classical inflammatory mediators that cause pain are released in the pulp in direct proportion to the insult. Serotonin (5-TH) can sensitize intradental A-fibers resulting in increased responsiveness [97], and bradykinin has been shown to be in significant higher concentration in irreversibly inflamed human pulps [69]. It is not only the inflammatory mediators that are associated with pulpal pain. Recent studies have also demonstrated that neuropetides from the nociceptive nerve fibers present in the pulp [calcitonin gene-related peptide (CGRP), neurokinin A (NKA) and substance P] are in significantly higher concentrations in symptomatic compared to asymptomatic pulps [15,89]. Initially, these mediators and peptides will affect primarily the more peripheral A-delta fibers, but when the inflammation reaches deeper structures, the C-fibers will be affected as well. This will cause their firing threshold to be lower and make the receptive field larger [92]. Therefore, it is important when the patient is questioned about lingering pain after the stimulus has been removed to ask not only about the time it took the pain to go away, but also about the quality of the lingering sensation. A dull, throbbing, pain component of the lingering pain indicates that more C-fibers are involved and that there is an increased likelihood of severe inflammation. This can be used, with caution, to predict if the pulp is likely to be irreversibly inflamed or not.

Pain on heat, relieved by cold

It is interesting and generally accepted that there are not nearly as many complaints about heat in normal pulp compared to cold sensitivity. However, when there is severe inflammation in the pulp there seems to be a strong tendency for heat sensitivity, especially in latter stages of the disease. Studies on this are scarce, but clinical experience indicates that when a patient complains about severe heat sensitivity it is almost certain that the pulp is irreversibly inflamed. In the past it was theorized that this was due to increased intrapulpal pressure when heat was applied to the tooth and the increased pressure caused increased neural activity [12]. The same activity was not seen by a similar degree of cooling [12] and hence it was thought that this was related to a pressure increase. Recently, it has become clear that this is an incomplete explanation at best. It is more likely that clinical heat sensitivity is due to a reaction of the heat-sensitive pulpal nerves. Heat-sensitive C-fibers are not easily stimulated under normal circumstances, but they become more active with more extensive inflammation [20]. When the pulp becomes inflamed, the nerves respond due to the influx of inflammatory mediators into the inflamed area as well as due to secretion of neuropetides. This response will cause the nerves to undergo both local and centrally mediated changes, changes which are likely to explain the alterations in pulpal sensitivity seen in pulpitis. An example, symptoms of throbbing pain associated with pulpitis [20], could be allodynia in pressure-sensitive fibers. The same would hold for a tooth with heat sensitivity alleviated by cold. The firing threshold of heat-sensitive fibers may be lowered so much by the inflammatory mediators that in extreme cases the normal body temperature would activate those nerves and cause pain. The only relief

to the pain is then to cool the tooth to below ambient temperature [65].

Pain on biting, when the pulp has been confirmed to be vital

This may be indicative of a severe inflammation involving the pulp and periodontium, and differential diagnosis to nonpulp-related conditions must be carefully considered. If the pulp is involved, the clinical finding suggests at least some necrosis within the pulp and an irreversible pulpitis of the vital tissue [115,116].

Referred pain

As the inflammation progresses in the pulp there is an increased tendency for the pain to be referred to a site remote from the tooth. It has been shown that pain from one tooth can be referred to another adjacent tooth or even to the opposite arch as well as to remote areas like the ear, clavicle and temple. In a classic study on referral patterns from teeth with pulpitis, Glick [48] showed that there were certain tendencies in referral patterns. Upper teeth tended to refer the pain to the zygomatic or temporal areas. Mandibular molars were more likely to refer the pain back to the ear or even to the occipital area. Pain from a tooth may be referred between the arches, but never across the midline of the face. The mechanisms for referred pain are not fully understood, but it is clear that both peripheral and central mechanisms are responsible [119,124]. It is interesting to note that soft tissue structures, such as temporal and masseter muscles, can refer pain in similar fashion from the tissue to the teeth [127]. Therefore, it is important to palpate any pain in the head and neck area that the patient reports away from the teeth. If the palpation increases the pain report then there is a strong possibility that the patient is suffering from muscular pain rather than dental pain (see Section 7.10).

7.3.2 History of the presenting symptoms

A number of factors related to a history of the patient's chief complaint are important to predicting irreversibility of pulpal inflammation. These include the following.

Character of the pain: dental versus pulpal pain

In dentinal pain, the sharp rapid pain in response to external stimuli is a reaction of the fast conducting A-delta fibers. They extend $150\,\mu m$ into the dentin and are normally active throughout the dentin–pulp complex [50,72,76]. The deeper seated, slower and unmyelinated C-fiber are for the most part unresponsive to all but very intense stimulus in normal, noninflamed pulp [20,89]. When a long and intense enough stimulus is placed on a healthy pulp, there is first sharp pain, mediated by the A-delta fibers, followed by second, poorly localized, dull pain sensation [62]. Complaints of only provoked pain indicate therefore possibly only mild inflammation that a vital pulp therapy would be sufficient to treat, such as removing a shallow caries lesion, replacing a leaky restoration or covering up exposed root surfaces. However, when bacteria or bacterial products start to affect the pulp, inflammatory mediators will affect nerve fibers resulting in a lower threshold to firing especially the C-fibers [68]. The history of the pain can be very revealing if it follows the pattern of starting as primarily temperature sensitivity, with sharp defined pain episodes, and then changing to a more dull, throbbing ache that is increasing in severity. This is important for two reasons: first, it indicates a shift in pain consistent with more activation of the C-fibers that would then indicate increased inflammation; secondly, it has been shown that self-reports of intensity and quality of dental pain are a valid predictor of whether or not the pulpal inflammation is reversible or not [49,118].

Severe pain

Self-reports on the intensity and quality of toothache pain seem to be valid predictors of whether the pulpal inflammation is reversible or not [49]. It has also been shown that the more severe the pain is, and the longer it has been symptomatic, the more likely it is that irreversible inflammation is present [9]. However, the reported severity of pain can be misleading due to the subjectivity of the sensation. Fear of dentists, for example, has been shown to result in an exaggerated perception of pain and response to diagnostic stimuli [66].

Spontaneous (unprovoked) pulpal pain

Probably the clearest sign of an irreversibly inflamed pulp is the history of spontaneous pain, which will inflict the patient without any thermal stimulation to the teeth, and may even wake the patient up from a sound sleep [116]. Inflammation can cause spontaneous pain sensations in the affected area, and may at times prolong sensitivity to innocuous stimuli, which in the absence of inflammation would not cause any pain sensation (allodynia). This spontaneous activity is thought to be, at least in part, caused by the effects of inflammatory mediators on peripheral nociceptive nerve endings, primarily C-fibers [91]. These effects on the nerve endings will activate and/or sensitize them and cause local as well as central release of substance P and CGRP [33,51,134]. These neuropeptides can then further increase the release of inflammatory mediators, creating a positive feedback loop or a vicious cycle. This vicious cycle is sometimes referred to as neurogenic inflammation [52].

7.4 Clinical findings

The findings of the clinical examination, in addition to an extensive knowledge of the pulpal reaction to external irritants, is important for arriving at a correct diagnosis. A clinical examination is critical since pulpitis is frequently painless [81] and also because of the lack of correlation between symptomatology, diagnostic tests and the histopathologic state of the pulp [5,34,45,69,113,116].

7.4.1 Carious pulpal exposure

Scientific evidence indicates that when the pulp is exposed directly to caries, bacteria have already penetrated the pulp ahead of the caries lesion and formed micro-abscesses [67,78,108,115]. Therefore, the pulp should always be considered irreversibly inflamed if it has a carious exposure. Only in cases where root development is incomplete should an attempt be made to estimate the level at which the pulp is inflamed or infected and apexogenesis attempted [115].

7.4.2 Age related changes

With age, the pulp is reduced in size and volume due to continued dentin formation. Its content of cellular components decreases relative to the number and thickness of collagen fibers [30]. There is also a decrease in the number of blood vessels and nerves, and an increased incidence of calcification and pulp stones [56]. Although it has not been shown experimentally, these changes have been assumed to result in a pulp which is less likely to reverse an inflammatory response compared to a young pulp. On the other hand, the pulp may remain vital for indefinite time periods following extensive degenerative changes.

7.4.3 Periodontal disease

It has been reported that a moderate-to-severe periodontal disease will result in a pulp which is "prematurely" aged [11,109,116] (Fig. 7.1). Thus, a pulp in a periodontally involved tooth is also thought to be less resistant to inflammation than that in a tooth with a healthy pulp. However, this view is not universally accepted since Mazur and Massler [74] found no difference in the pulp status of teeth with or without periodontal disease.

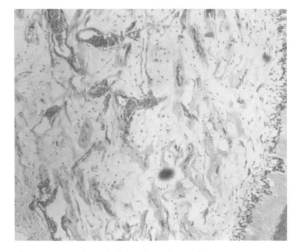

Fig. 7.1   Histological slide of a pulp, mid-root section, that was diagnosed with a vital pulp, but extracted due to extensive periodontal disease.

7.4.4 Previous pulpal insults

Previous pulpal insults such as caries, caries removal, and restorative procedures can all result in tubule sclerosis, reparative dentin formation, and fibrosis of the pulp. It has been hypothesized that this "premature" aging of the pulp may render it less likely to heal than an unstressed pulp [116].

7.5 Diagnostic testing

Unfortunately many clinicians rely solely on diagnostic tests for their diagnosis. It is important to remember that most commonly used test systems do not actually assess the vitality (blood circulation) of the pulp and they do not give much, if any, indication about presence or severity of inflammation in the pulp. The main reasons for doing a pulp test are to reproduce and, primarily, to localize the symptoms and to assess the severity of the symptoms. With every test it has to be remembered that the responses are subjective and some patients will have the tendency to exaggerate, while others understate the pain felt [37,66].

7.5.1 Sensitivity tests

Sensitivity tests include the electric pulp test (EPT) and thermal tests. The primary function of these tests it to differentiate a vital from a nonvital pulp. By the use of these tests the nerve fibers in the pulp are activated, eliciting a reaction from the patient. The patient response is subjective, so that care must be taken to differentiate a "fearful" positive response from a true one [37,66,86]. This is usually accomplished by comparing the patient's response with that of a contralateral or neighboring tooth and revisiting the tested teeth to ensure consistency. Care must also be taken to clean and dry the teeth so that conduction of the stimulus to the periodontal ligament or to adjacent teeth is minimized.

As stated above, the main disadvantage of these tests, apart from their subjectivity, is the fact that an assumption has to be made that the presence of nerve fibers in the pulp correlates to a vital blood supply. While this assumption is valid most of the time, in a number of cases the blood supply in the pulp will be lost before the degeneration of nerves in the pulp, resulting in an incorrect diagnosis of pulpal vitality [103]. Conversely, it is known that, especially after luxation injury, vital pulps sometimes do not respond to sensitivity tests shortly after the trauma, but at a follow-up appointment a few weeks to few months later, normal responses are observed [80,121].

Electric pulp test

The electric pulp testers activate the nerve bundle in the pulp, probably mainly the A-delta fibers. The unmyelinated C-fibers of the pulp may [86] or may not respond [88]. The main problem with this type of test is the many variables that need to be taken into account, some of which cannot be controlled. Key issues are location of the probe on the tooth (as far away as possible from the gingival), conductivity between the instrument and the tooth, rate of stimulus intensity increase, isolation of the tooth tested from adjacent teeth, and prevention of shunting to the gingiva by drying the crown. It is not possible to control for the thickness and electric resistance of the enamel and dentin, the presence of restorations and caries, and the functionality of the nerve complex in the pulp.

The two stimulating modes available are so-called bipolar and monopolar. The bipolar mode presumably is more accurate because the current is confined to the coronal pulp [73,87,107]. However, most electric pulp testers are still monopolar [88].

Procedure. The tooth and surrounding teeth are dried. The pulp test probe is placed on the incisal edge or cusp tip corresponding to the pulp horn of the tooth [7,43,83] (Fig. 7.2). Contact between the probe and tooth is facilitated by the use of a conducting medium such as toothpaste or fluoride gel [27]. The circuit must be completed with a lip contact or the patient holding the handle of the electric pulp tester. The amount of current is increased slowly with the patient instructed to indicate (e.g. by raising the hand) if a tingling or other sensation is felt.

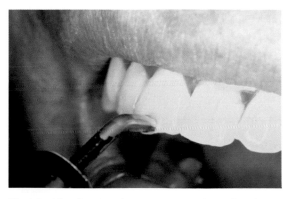

Fig. 7.2 The electric pulp tester (EPT) probe is placed on the incisal edge of a maxillary anterior tooth. The tooth is thoroughly dried and contact between the probe and surface of the crown is facilitated by a conduction medium like toothpaste or fluoride gel.

Diagnostic information. A response, within reasonable intensity, to a stimulus is an indication of a vital pulp tissue. The response level however does not indicate the health of the pulp or reversibility of inflammation that might be present in the pulp, because no correlation has been shown between the electric pain threshold in a pulp and histological condition [69,87,116]. However, no response is a strong indicator of a necrotic pulp in most teeth [103,116]. Seltzer *et al*. found complete necrosis in 72% and localized necrosis of the pulp in 25.7% of those teeth that did not respond to EPT [116]. Thus, if it is accepted that even localized necrosis is an indication for the need of pulpectomy in a mature tooth, 97.7% of cases with no response to EPT will require a pulpectomy or the debridement of a necrotic pulp.

It is also important to remember that responses to EPT are unreliable shortly after dental trauma [121. Also, in teeth with incomplete root formation, EPT may be very unreliable [43,44]. This is possibly due to the fact that the nerve plexus of Raschkow does not fully develop until the very late stages of root formation [41]. Thus, the pulpal nerves do not reach the odontoblasts, predentin, or dentin, as in fully developed teeth that have reached normal occlusion. In young teeth the cold test, especially with carbon dioxode ice, is more reliable than EPT [43].

Thermal tests: cold test

Probably the most commonly used test in dental offices is some form of cold test. It is important to realize that this testing method, like EPT and heat, only gives an indication of functional nerve fibers, rather than information about the vitality status (blood flow) of the pulp.

The initial response to any cold stimulus is generated by cold-sensitive A-delta fibers [62] activated by hydrodynamic forces. The temperature change causes a rapid movement of fluids in the dental tubules, a movement that then activates the intratubular nerves [15,17]. Moreover, in animal models, the cold-sensitive A-delta fibers respond uniformly to rapid lowering of the tooth temperature [62], while the initial high-frequency discharge rate falls off as the rate of temperature change decreases, and stops completely when the temperature reaches a steady level. This is a good indication that the sharp initial sensation when a cold stimulus is applied to the tooth is caused by the A-delta fibers and subsides when those fibers stop firing once the movement of the intratubular fluid stops.

The C-fibers also show a quite uniform, but very different, reaction. The C-fibers start to discharge after a short latency and then the discharge rate is low [62]. In an experimental study in humans [79], the subjects reported sensations that could be interpreted as being comparable to a phasic type of activation of the A- and C-fibers in an animal study. There was a distinct, sharp and with short latency (1.6 s) pain felt when the tooth was rapidly cooled. The latter pain was described as dull, burning pain, which was difficult to localize. These findings support the assumption that the response behavior of the human pulp nerves is comparable to those of an animal model: the first sharp pain is evoked by intradental A-delta fibers and then later, once the interdental temperature is changed sufficiently, the C-fibers are activated and are responsible for the dull, throbbing and aching sensation. Subsequently, other research groups have come to similar or the same conclusions, although with somewhat different research approaches. It is important to note, however, that the studies providing the data for these mechanisms were done on relatively normal, healthy pulps [1].

Very few studies have been done to investigate pain sensation in inflamed human pulps. There appears to be only a poor correlation between estimates of pain magnitude and the total A-delta nerve activity in patients that were clinically diagnosed with pulpitis [2]. However, abnormal, but positive, responses are equally distributed among the pulps of teeth with varying degrees of inflammation [34,116]. Therefore, a positive cold test response only indicates vitality, but not if the pulp is reversibly or irreversibly inflamed; no response is very indicative of a necrotic pulp [34,116].

Historically ice and ethyl chloride spray have been used for cold testing, but both have several problems that have led to new approaches. Both are not very cold: ethyl chloride is only about −4°C and ice is at or just above 0°C. An additional problem with water is that once it melts, very cold water can drip on adjacent teeth and thereby give false positive responses. Carbon dioxide ice pencils have now been available for over 20 years. They are safe to use on vital pulps and will not cause damage to enamel or pulpal tissue *in vivo* [59,101,102]. The carbon dioxide ice may also be more dependable than ethyl chloride and water ice in producing a positive response, and in young patients with incomplete root formation, carbon dioxide ice seems to be more reliable than EPT [42]. Additionally the carbon dioxide ice appears more reliable than

EPT in patients undergoing orthodontic movement of teeth [23].

More recently a refrigerant spray, dichlorodifluoromethane, has been introduced. It has the advantage of being supplied in spray cans; it can be stored at the chairside; and it has a lower start-up cost compared to carbon dioxide ice. It is, however, not as cold as carbon dioxide ice (boiling point close to −50°C). It appears that there is no difference between tetrafluoroethane and carbon dioxide ice in producing a pulp response regardless of tooth type or presence of restoration [61].

If several vitality tests are planned on a patient, it seems that the sequence and interval between EPT and cold vitality testing with dichlorodifluoromethane do not affect the reliability of pulpal diagnostic testing [99].

Procedure. As with the EPT, care needs to be taken to dry the tooth and surrounding teeth. The cold object should be placed on the incisal edge or close to a pulp horn for optimum results. The cold test should be administered gently, as a placement of the very cold ice or object could cause rapid and severe pain, especially in the anterior teeth (Fig. 7.3).

Diagnostic information. Abnormal, but positive, responses are equally distributed among the pulps of teeth in all diagnostic categories [34,116]. Therefore a positive response is an indication that the pulp is at least partially vital, but it does not indicate if inflammation is reversible if present. Despite the lack of an apparent clear correlation between cold response and histological appearance of the pulp, clinical experience indicates that an exaggerated response, which quickly turns into a dull aching pain, coupled with other signs, such as a history of pain and spontaneous pain, strongly indicates a pulpal inflammation that is most likely irreversible.

Thermal tests: heat test

Less common, but probably a more clinically informative temperature test, is some form of heat test. The main problem with this approach is that many commonly used tests can cause excessive heat that may damage the pulp or adjacent tissue, and others are cumbersome to apply. Therefore, the clinical use of heat tests is somewhat limited.

The normal pulp reaction and sensation to heat is similar to cold. It is in most cases biphasic, where ini-

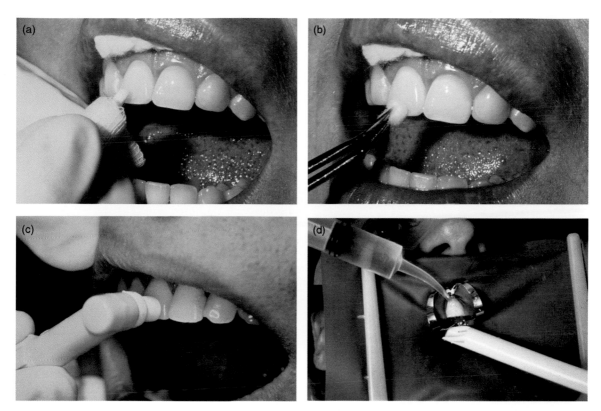

Fig. 7.3   Thermal sensitivity test with (a) CO_2 frozen stick ($-70°C$), (b) cotton pellet sprayed with dichlorodifluoromethane (DDM) ($-50°C$), (c) prophy rubber cup without any lubrication used to heat the tooth surface, (d) single tooth rubber dam isolation and irrigation with hot water.

tially the A-delta fibers are activated and then later, if the stimulus is maintained, a dull, radiating pain follows [17,89,90]. It has been shown in *in vivo* human studies that hot gutta percha induced a more complex neural response pattern than ethyl chloride. The hot gutta percha evoked a response in three phases, where the third phase was a slow spontaneous emerging activity in the absence of physical stimulus, and this activity was not felt by the healthy and pain-free test subjects [2].

Procedure. Several heat tests have been advocated. One is to heat gutta percha over a flame and then place it on a lubricated surface of the crown towards the incisal edge [86]. The problem with this approach is that there is little control over the heat and the gutta percha tends to stick on the tooth and thereby cause continued heating of the tooth after the bulk material is removed. Using a prophy cup or a rubber wheel without lubrication has also been advocated,

but again there is no control over the heat generated. A better, but cumbersome, approach is to put the patient in a supine position, isolate a single tooth with a rubber dam and then bathe the exposed tooth in hot water. Once a response has been noted the rubber dam is moved mesially by one tooth and the procedure repeated. One starts distal to the suspected tooth so that if there is a leakage through the dam, the hot water will not drip on the suspected tooth and thereby give a false positive response.

Diagnostic information. No correlation has been found between an abnormal response to heat and histological diagnosis. [34,116]. It is, however, generally accepted that when there is severe inflammation in the pulp there seems to be a tendency for extreme heat sensitivity. Studies on this are scarce, but clinical experience indicates that when a patient complains about severe heat sensitivity the pulp is usually irreversibly inflamed. This is confirmed to some degree in animal studies where it has been shown that the nerves stimulated by heat are located in similar areas as markers for pain responses in symptomatic pulpitis [26,27].

7.5.2 Mechanical tests

Percussion and palpation tests technically are not vitality tests, but rather give an indication about periodontal and/or periapical inflammation. It has been stated that pain is more likely to be elicited on percussion when there is a partial or total necrosis present in the pulp [114] and, as such, an indirect assessment of the status of the pulp. Other causes for percussion sensitivity, such as recent traumatic occlusion, high filling, etc., obviously need to be ruled out. The same seems to be the case when the periapical area is sensitive to palpation, but the pulp is still vital [114]. Presence of percussion and/or palpation sensitivity in conjunction with a vital pulp with hypersensitivity to thermal stimulation is indicative of a pulp that is severely, and thus most likely irreversibly, inflamed [114]. However, if the tooth is not sensitive to percussion and/or palpation, inflammation is not necessarily absent [116].

Percussion

This test is properly performed with the handle of a mouth mirror. The aim is to determine the presence/absence of inflammation in the apical periodontium.

Procedure. The mouth mirror handle is used to percuss not only the occlusal, but also facial and lingual surfaces of the teeth. The teeth should be percussed in a random order so that the patient does not respond to "anticipates" rather than real pain.

Diagnostic information. As stated before, a positive percussion test indicates inflammation of the periradicular tissues. Care must be taken, when interpreting the results of the percussion tests, to rule out a positive response due to periodontal diseases or cuspal fracture. This is particularly difficult in cases where the pulp vitality tests indicate a vital pulp. The results of other diagnostic tests and presenting symptoms need to be used to differentiate periodontitis of marginal or endodontic origin.

Palpation

This test is used to detect inflammation in the mucoperiosteum around the root of the tooth. It may be possible to detect tenderness, fluctuation, hardness or crepitius before extensive swelling is present.

Procedure. The index finger is pressed against the bone through the mucosa. When pressure is felt, the finger is rolled causing sensitivity if inflammation is present. As with percussion, the test should be performed in a random fashion and the results obtained should be compared to a contralateral tooth or neighboring teeth.

Diagnostic information. Similar to the percussion test, a positive response when palpating over the root tip is a reliable indicator of periapical inflammation. However, if a positive response is not elicited, inflammation is not necessarily absent [116].

7.5.3 Radiographic examination

The radiographic examination is one of many tests, and the findings should always be evaluated together with those of presenting symptoms and clinical examination as well as with those of the other tests. All radiographs should be taken using holders which allow parallelism and standardization. If comparative radiographs will be required on follow-up it is useful to fabricate a rubber bite-block so that the angulation of the follow-up radiographs will be as similar as possible (Fig. 7.4).

Diagnostic information. The radiograph cannot detect pulpal inflammation directly. However, caries or defective restorations seen on the radiograph will indicate pulp inflammation [71]. Condensing apical periodontitis is a near pathognomonic sign of pulpitis (Fig. 7.5). Signs of obliteration and calcification (diffuse or as pulp stones) may be considered, but are not directly correlated with inflammatory reactions in the pulp. Also, the presence of an apical radiolucency of endodontic origin may be a good indication that necrosis or a necrotic zone is present in the pulp space.

7.5.4 Experimental testing methods

Sensitivity tests of pulp vitality require functional nerves to respond to a stimulus. Pulp with effective

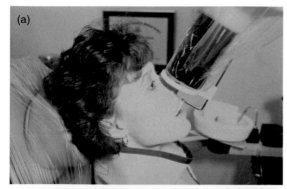

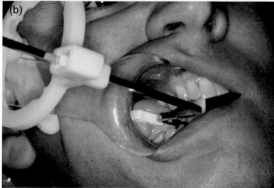

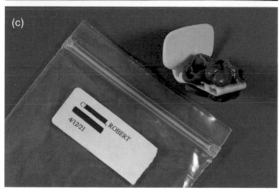

Fig. 7.4 (a) All radiographs should be taken using holders which allow parallelism and standardization. (b) If comparative radiographs will be required on follow-up, it is useful to fabricate a customized rubber bite-block using putty impression material. (c) The bite registration is then stored along with the film holder.

circulation and vital cells, but with severed or compromised nerves, may be misdiagnosed as being necrotic or nonvital by these tests. Therefore, attempts have been made to demonstrate pulpal vitality based on blood circulation. Several experimental methods

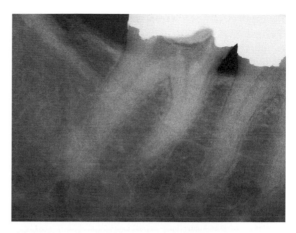

Fig. 7.5 A radiograph showing condensing apical periodontitis associated with the distal root of a lower molar. The tooth had been restored some years earlier, with what appears to be direct pulp capping. The patient reported hypersensitivity to cold for some weeks prior to seeking help.

have been proposed, such as crown surface temperature measurements [38–40], Xenon-133 radioisotope injection [63,64], photoplethymography [16], pulse oximetry [111], dual wavelength spectrophotomerty [25,83,94,133], and laser Doppler flowmetry (LDF) [47,80]. Unfortunately most of these approaches, despite experimental demonstration of very accurate and reliable findings, have never been made available commercially for pulp vitality assessment.

Laser Doppler flowmetry

Presently, the only commercially available pulpal blood flow assessment method is LDF. This technique was developed initially in order to assess blood flow in microvasculature systems, e.g., retina, mesentery, renal cortex, and skin [58]. More recently it was shown to be able to detect blood circulation in teeth, first in animals [46,47] and later in humans [47,80]. The first machines on the market had a light beam generated with a helium/neon lamp at 632.8 nm. This wavelength was chosen because it was shown to be scattered by moving erythrocytes [132]. More recently, a light beam closer to the infrared wavelength (700–810 nm) has been shown to be better suited for dental applications [95]. These machines emit a light from the end of a fiber cable that is placed on the tooth of interest. The light beam will undergo a frequency shift if it hits moving erythrocytes in the pulp. The backscattered light is picked up by photodetectors that are embedded in the fiber. The wavelength shift is then calculated by the machine and it produces an arbitrary number often referred to as perfusion units (PU) or flux, which in most machines is calculated as number of cells multiplied by the average velocity. No current laser Doppler instrument can present absolute perfusion values (e.g. ml/min/100 g tissue), therefore, comparison between different individuals, or even within the same individual or tooth, is difficult, and a very careful calibration of the laser Doppler machine is essential when monitoring a tooth or teeth over time. Moreover, laser Doppler technology does not allow for assessment of the degree of inflammatory changes in the pulpal tissue.

The main issue with LDF is, like all other vitality tests, the risks of false positive and false negative results. For LDF these can be both from movement artifacts associated with the probe placement on the tooth as well as scattering of the light beam from surrounding tissue, e.g., gingiva. It has been shown that if a tooth is tested without masking the adjacent gingiva, the blood flow in the gingiva may significantly affect the reading, so therefore each tooth assessed with the laser Doppler should be carefully isolated with opaque rubber dam [122].

The laser Doppler technique has many desirable qualities. It has been shown to be objective, noninvasive, and accurate in detecting revascularization of the pulp in young traumatized teeth [47,82].

In recent animal studies where revascularization was monitored by LDF and then later confirmed by histological observation, it was shown that LDF readings correctly predicted the pulp status (vital vs nonvital) in 83.7% of the readings and were able to confirm the vitality or necrosis in those teeth as early as 2–3 weeks after the trauma [105,135]. This is a vast improvement compared to more traditional testing methods of EPT or cold, where it may take up to 10 weeks to confirm revascularization, during which time significant damage could occur on a root surface of a tooth that did not undergo revascularization, because the root canal space became infected.

7.6 Formulation of a pulpal diagnosis

The diagnosis is made using the information obtained above (see Table 7.1).

7.6.1 Key factors

Necrotic versus vital

Using the patient's presenting symptomatology and the results of as many diagnostic tests as possible, it should be possible to determine accurately if the pulp is necrotic or vital. If the pulp is necrotic, the choice of treatment is root canal therapy, if the tooth is to be maintained for an extended period.

Table 7.1 The formulation of a pulpal diagnosis

		Vital pulp	
Symptom, test, supporting information	Necrotic pulp	Irreversibly inflamed	Reversibly inflamed
Pulp test	Negative	Positive	Positive
Key factors			
Pulpal exposure		Present	Absent
Pain to percussion		Present	Absent
Related factors			
Severe pain		Present	Absent
Spontaneous pain		Present	Absent
Past history of pain		Present	Absent
Pain that lingers		Present	Absent
Pain to hot, relieved by cold		Present	Absent
Factors related to treatment plan			
Age, periodontal disease, previous pulpal insults		Questionable (complex treatment plan)	Questionable (simple treatment plan)

It is a much greater challenge to differentiate a reversible from an irreversible pulpitis. For this determination, the presenting symptomatology and its history (subjective) and clinical findings are used.

Pulp exposure

As already discussed, if on excavation the pulp is found to be exposed to bacteria, an irreversible pulpitis can confidently be diagnosed. Treatment is then extirpation of the whole pulp and root canal filling as a preventive measure. An exception would be a case of a very young tooth with incomplete root formation. In these cases a temporary (few months to a year) partial pulpotomy would be indicated in an attempt to allow the apex to fully form prior to initiation of complete root canal therapy.

7.6.2 Related factors

A history of severe pain, spontaneous pain, a past history of pain in the same tooth, or referred pain, are all indications of an irreversible pulpitis.

All other related factors, such as age, periodontal status, and previous pulpal and treatment history, must be taken into account, but are less suggestive.

7.6.3 Treatment planning

It has been stressed continuously that with methods of diagnosis available today, the diagnosis of an irreversible pulpitis is at best an "educated guess" and mistakes are inevitable. Because of this fact, the overall treatment plan for the patient should play a role in the choice of pulpectomy or conservative therapy.

For example, if a tooth is the only tooth in the arch needing treatment and the long-term restoration is to be a simple amalgam or resin (Fig. 7.6) a conservative approach can be attempted without pulpectomy, even though some of the related factors suggest a moderate inflammation is present. With the same presenting signs and symptoms, a tooth planned as an abutment for a bridge which would be difficult to treat endodontically subsequent to possible failure of conservative treatment, might preferentially be subjected to immediate pulpectomy without an attempt at conservative treatment.

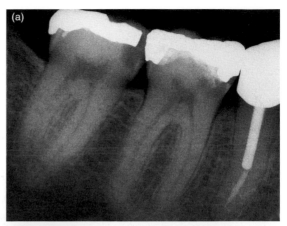

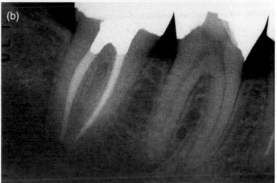

Fig. 7.6   Radiograph (a) showing two lower molars both with extensive and deep carious lesions. Patient complained about severe pain of few days' duration, but was unable to determine which tooth was causing the pain. Pulpal test were inconclusive on which tooth had more severe pulpal inflammation. After caries excavation a caries perforation was found in the second molar, but not the first. The second molar was treated with root canal therapy, the first with vital pulp therapy and restoration. (b) At 1-year recall the first molar responded normally to pulpal tests and both teeth were normal to percussion and palpation.

7.7 Periapical diagnostic terms

The term apical periodontitis implies that there is an inflammation in the periodontal ligament caused by infection of the pulp or of the necrotic pulp space. The noxious material and bacterial byproducts have passed to the periodontium through the apical foramina. If communication between the pulp space and surrounding periodontium is present through furcation or accessory canals, periodontal inflammation can result in these locations as well (Fig. 7.7).

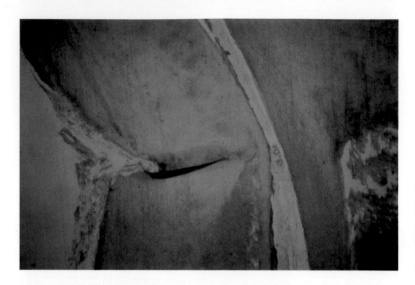

Fig. 7.7   Histological section of root pulp in accessory canal of a tooth with moderated periodontal disease. A localized area of inflammation (arrow) corresponds to the plaque at the opening of the accessory canal. (Courtesy of Dr Samuel Seltzer.)

Histologically, the lesion is predominated by chronic inflammatory cells with the overall appearance of a granuloma or cyst [13].

As with pulpal inflammation, the periapical inflammation can be symptom free and then only diagnosed in a chronic phase on a periapical radiograph. However, if there is a periapical lesion detectable on a radiograph it is almost certainly caused by an infection in the root canal system, irrespective of the tooth's history or the occurrence of symptoms [10]. As always, if the patient is symptomatic it is important to be able to diagnose the source prior to treatment. Treatment is always to remove the irritant that causes the symptoms or lesion. This could be accomplished by simple occlusal adjustment in cases of occlusal trauma, but as the cause is usually bacteria in the root canal system, the only predictable treatment is to completely disinfect the canal space followed by obturation and a good coronal seal. Antibiotic therapy alone is not effective [42].

7.7.1 Acute apical periodontitis

Acute apical periodontitis (AAP) usually implies that the apical inflammation started in the acute phase. By definition there are minimal or no radiographic changes associated with this diagnostic term. There can be several causes for this inflammation. Most benign would be occlusal trauma. If that is the case, the pulp should be vital and unaffected. However, in the case of bacterial infection the pulp is either severely and irreversibly inflamed and usually partly or totally necrotic.

An AAP can also be superimposed on a previously chronic lesion (see Phoenix abscess below).

7.7.2 Chronic apical periodontitis

Chronic apical periodontitis (CAP) implies that the apical periodontitis is of some duration without or with minor symptoms. The condition may be suspected when the pulp is necrotic with radiographic signs of apical periodontitis (radiolucency or rarely a radiopacity) (Fig. 7.8).

7.7.3 Apical periodontitis with abscess (APA, Phoenix abscess)

Here the periapical inflammation has caused a purulent breakdown of periapical tissues with accumulation of pus in the periodontium, subperiosteally, submucosally, and/or subcutaneously. Commonly, this acute inflammation is superimposed on a previous CAP and has been termed a Phoenix abscess. Treatment is aimed primarily at eliminating the source of the abscess, the infection of the pulpal space, and antibiotics are only used as a supplemental treatment if the patient is showing systemic effects of the infection.

7.7.4 Apical periodontitis with sinus tract

This diagnostic term implies that periapical exudate discharges on a body surface, establishing a traceable sinus tract with periapical drainage (Fig. 7.9).

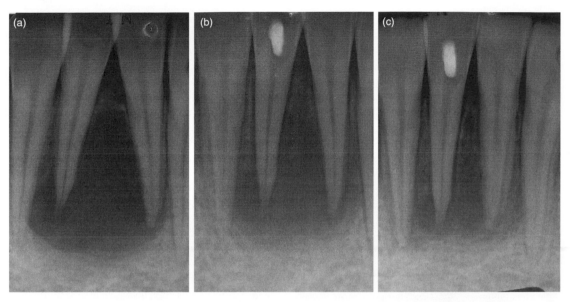

Fig. 7.8 A 13-year-old patient asymptomatic, apart from noticing some firm enlargement facial to his lower anterior teeth. Radiographic evaluation revealed large periapical radiolucency with the roots of the central incisors pushed distally (a). The right central incisor did not respond to cold, but the left one did. Diagnosis of necrotic pulp with chronic apical periodontitis (CAP) was made. Six weeks after placing calcium hydroxide in the root canal system there was significant improvement of the periapical lesion (b). After 3 months of calcium hydroxide treatment there was almost complete resolution of the lesion (c).

7.8 Symptomatology of periapical disease

The same diagnostic steps should take place for the diagnosis of periodontal pathosis as described above for the pulp. The patient's presenting symptoms are carefully evaluated, diagnostic tests are performed, clinical findings recorded, and the information is compiled to make the tentative diagnosis.

7.8.1 Acute apical periodontitis

Traumatic occlusion

Presenting symptoms. Patients complain of pain on biting, eating or "when the teeth come into contact".

History. Commonly the patient has recently had a dental procedure performed which has resulted in a restoration where the occlusion is not balanced, leaving high contact.

Clinical findings. There is often evidence of a new restoration(s) in the area.

Diagnostic tests. Response to thermal and electrical sensitivity testing is normal. Pain is elicited to percussion, and on rare occasions to palpation as well. Radiographic findings are usually nonspecific.

Treatment. The occlusion should be adjusted so that premature contacts are removed. The patient should return for a follow-up visit to ensure that the acute apical inflammation has subsided and the pulp has remained vital.

AAP with acute pulpitis

This condition has already been discussed in pulpal diagnosis. AAP in conjunction with an acute pulpitis indicates an irreversible pulpitis [115].

Treatment. Pulpectomy (see Chapter 10). Recall is at 1–4 weeks for reevaluation of the original diagnosis and confirmation that the apical inflammation has subsided so that root canal therapy can be completed. A permanent restoration is placed as soon as possible after obturation of the root canal(s) to prevent coronal leakage with subsequent CAP [70,129].

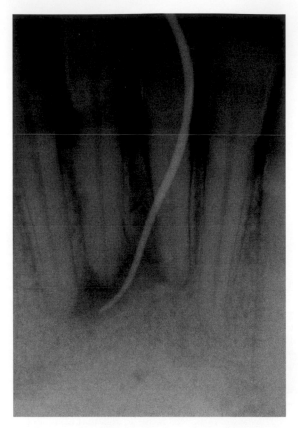

Fig. 7.9 A radiograph of a sinus tract that has been traced with size 40 gutta percha. Note that the exit of the tract was distal to the left central incisor but traced to the right central incisor.

Acute exacerbation of CAP

Presenting symptoms. Patient complains of pain on biting, eating, or "when the teeth come into contact". There may also be episodes of spontaneous and intense pain, as well as swelling and malaise.

History. The history in these cases is varied. In some cases the patient reports episodes of previous pain or there is a recent restoration placed in the tooth. In other cases the patient may tell a previous history of pulpal pain which later subsided. Sometimes root canal therapy has been performed on the tooth previously.

Clinical findings. These are consistent with a tooth with a necrotic pulp or a previous root filling. Examples would be a deep carious lesion, a previous pulp capping, a large restoration, or full coverage crown (Fig. 7.10).

Diagnostic tests. There is no response to thermal and electrical sensitivity tests. There will be pain to percussion and/or palpation. An apical radiolucency is present on radiographic examination, indicating the presence of CAP in addition to the acute exacerbation.

Treatment. The treatment involves complete root canal instrumentation and disinfection with antibacterial irrigation and intracanal medication of the root canal system [21] (see Chapter 11). Since abscess

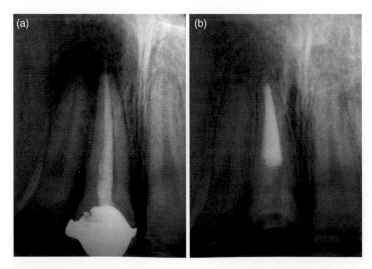

Fig. 7.10 (a) A radiograph of a patient that became symptomatic and presented with facial swelling to right central and lateral incisors. The radiographic image indicated a chronic apical periodontitis associated with the lateral incisor. However, it responded normally to vitality tests. It was therefore decided to retreat the central incisor with removal of the obturation material and calcium hydroxide application. (b) One-year recall radiograph showing complete resolution of periapical lesion. (Courtesy of Dr Cecilia Bourguignon.)

formation has not yet occurred, drainage is not possible. For the same reason antibiotic therapy is not required. Pain medication is prescribed as needed. Recall is at 1–4 weeks for reevaluation of the original diagnosis and for confirmation that the apical inflammation has subsided, after which the canal is obturated. A permanent restoration is placed as soon as possible for prevention of coronal leakage.

7.8.2 Chronic apical periodontitis

Presenting symptoms. Typically the patient is asymptomatic. The condition may be diagnosed on a routine recall radiograph, or a restoration may have been required on a tooth which when tested for vitality shows no response.

History and clinical findings. These are as in acute exacerbation of CAP. Pain may have been completely absent.

Diagnostic tests. There is no response to thermal and EPT tests. Percussion and/or palpation tests are usually negative, although slight sensitivity may be present.

Radiographic findings. Since these cases are largely asymptomatic, the diagnosis of CAP is made primarily on radiographic evidence of the presence of radiolucency (or rarely on opacity) (see Chapter 6) (Fig. 7.8). It is possible for an apical periodontitis to go undetected radiographically [8]), so that pulp necrosis and infection is evident only after initiation of endodontic therapy. A revised diagnosis of probable CAP should then be made and the tooth treated accordingly (Chapter 11).

Treatment. Effective disinfection of the root canal system will result in reversal of the CAP.

7.8.3 Apical periodontitis with abscess

During acute phases of apical periodontitis (primary acute or an exacerbation of chronic lesion), the infection may develop to produce an accumulation of pus and formation of an abscess. From this point, the inflammation may become chronic, but in some cases continues with the formation of a clinical abscess. There is an increase in tissue pressure, bone resorption is initiated by inflammatory mediators, and the pus escapes first through the bone and underneath the periosteum and then, if the periosteum is penetrated, into the tissue spaces.

The exact location of the accumulation of fluids is dependent on the anatomical location of the root apex relative to the facial muscles [84]. Most commonly the drainage is buccal into the oral vestibule. A rare complication is spread from maxillary and mandibular third molars via the pterhygoid plexus causing a cavernous sinus thombophlebitis and impairment of cerebral vascular drainage [55]. In the mandibular teeth the most serious spread would be from the premolar or molar teeth lingually under the mylohyoid muscle and into the retropharyngeal space. Ludwig's angina is a bilateral retropharyngeal spread which may become serious through a blockage of the airway [123]. In most cases the pus will break through the intraoral mucosa to a surface. Occasionally, the abscess will drain extraorally on or under the chin or below the mandible.

Presenting symptoms. Symptoms will vary according to the stage of progression of the inflammatory process. Initially, the symptoms may be minor with pain on biting, eating or occlusal contact. As pus builds under the periosteum, the pain increases in intensity and can in time be excruciating. When the periosteum is penetrated by the pus, diffuse swelling may develop (Fig. 7.11). The penetration of the periosteum by the pus is usually accompanied by a release of pressure and a considerable reduction in the pain.

History and clinical findings. These are the same as in CAP.

Diagnostic tests. There is no response to thermal or electrical sensitivity tests. Pain on percussion and/or palpation is elicited which can sometimes be severe, depending on the stage of the process.

Radiographic findings. The stage of development of the abscess determines the radiographic picture. At the early states of abscess formation radiographic signs of inflammation may be minimal if any. As the abscess spreads and more bone is destroyed the radiographic signs of apical periodontitis will be more obvious. In the case of an acute excacerbation of a chronic lesion, the signs of apical periodontitis are present throughout.

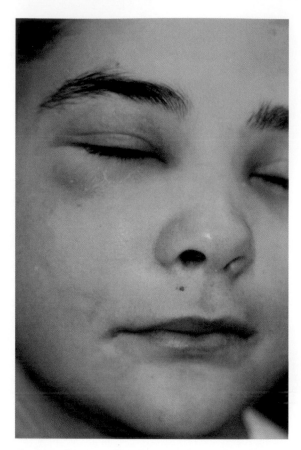

Fig. 7.11   Severe swelling due to an abscessed maxillary first premolar tooth. Pus has broken through the periosteum and caused severe and very serious swelling around the orbit.

Treatment. Treatment principles are the same as for all teeth with apical periodontitis, i.e., the disinfection of the root canal (see Chapter 11). Additionally, in the case of an acute abscess, concerns of spread of the infection in the tissue spaces (cellulitis) and pain control must be addressed in the treatment protocol.

7.8.4 Apical periodontitis with sinus tract

This occurs when apical inflammatory exudate drains to a body surface, as a sinus tract has developed. The formation of a sinus tract may be the mechanism with which the body controls the infection, or it may indicate a specific infection of some, as yet unknown, bacterial combination. It may develop as a result of an abscess as described above or be without preceding symptoms, and the diagnosis may be made without the patient even being aware of its existence. When long standing, the tract can become completely epithelialized [6]. With adequate disinfection of the root canal and resolution of the periapical inflammation, the epithelium, if present, will in most cases disintegrate. Commonly, the sinus tract will drain on the mucosa adjacent to the offending tooth. However, the opening may be at some distance from the involved tooth (Fig. 7.9) or drain through the periodontal ligament mimicking a periodontal pocket (Fig. 7.12). For this reason, it is important to perform a thorough diagnostic examination and not rely on the presence and location of the sinus tract opening.

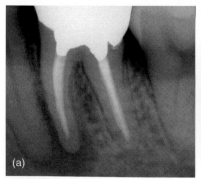
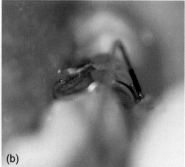
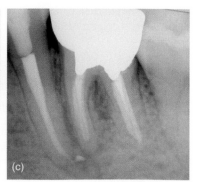

Fig. 7.12   A sinus tract of endodontic origin can be misdiagnosed as periodontal disease or as clinical sings of root fracture. (a) A root canal therapy was done on a first lower left molar with necrotic pulp and chronic apical periodontitis. (b) The root canal therapy did not eliminate a narrow deep pocket that was located on the facial aspect of the mesial root of the molar. (c) Further investigation revealed the premolar having necrotic pulp and once treated the sinus tract in the sulcus healed and a 1-year recall radiograph revealed almost complete periapical healing. (Courtesy of Dr George Shuping.)

Presenting symptoms. Generally, when a sinus tract is present in conjunction with the apical periodontitis, pain is absent or very mild and swelling is minimal. This is due to the lack of pressure build-up under the periosteum or adjacent tissues.

History and clinical findings. A history consistent with that described for CAP or APA is possible.

Diagnostic tests. The tooth is nonresponsive to thermal or EPT tests. There is no or only light pain to percussion and/or palpation.

Radiographic findings. Radiographic evidence of chronic apical periodontitis is usually present, but the location of the sinus tract on the mucosa does not always correspond to the offending tooth. Therefore, it is important to race the sinus tract with an opaque objcct, for instance a size 35 or 40 gutta perha cone, to determine the origin of the tract. Care must be taken not to force the cone and thereby create a false tract, which could lead to an incorrect diagnosis.

Treatment. Disinfection of the root canal system should result in reversal of the CAP and the sinus tract will disappear within days or a few weeks. In rare cases, the sinus tract will not heal because the infection is primarily located extraradicularly [128] and antibiotic therapy and/or surgical treatment may become necessary.

Differential diagnosis of a sinus tract and periodontal disease

A sinus tract of endodontic origin can be misdiagnosed as periodontal disease, particularly when it drains through the sulcular area (Fig. 7.12). Table 7.2 outlines important differences between the two diseases [126,129]. If doubt exists as to the origin of the tract/pocket, curettage of the periodontal ligament should be delayed so as not to damage the cemental layer which may be intact. A sinus tract of endodontic origin can heal completely if the cemental layer has not been damaged by curetting. Treatment of periodontal diseases should be delayed until healing is assessed after endodontic treatment.

7.9 Formulation of a periapical diagnosis

The diagnosis is made using the information obtained above (see Table 7.3)

Table 7.2   Differential diagnosis of an endodontic sinus tract versus a periodontal pocket

Test applied	Periodontal pocket	Endodontic sinus tract
Vitality testing	Within normal limits	No response
Perio probing	Wide pockets	Narrow tract
Clinical status of the tooth	Minimal caries/restorations	Evidence of caries/restorations
General periodontal condition	Poor	Within normal limits
Dark field spirochete count	>30%	<10%

Table 7.3   The formulation of periapical diagnosis

Diagnosis	Presenting symptoms		Radiographic signs	Other findings
	Pain	Swelling		
Acute apical periodontitis	Yes	No	Normal PDL	
Chronic apical periodontitis	No	No	Periapical radiolucency	
Apical periodontitis with abscess	Yes/no	Yes	Initially normal PDL. In late stage some widening	
Apical periodontitis with sinus tract	No	No	Usually periapical radiolucency	Draining sinustract

7.9.1 Key factors

Periapical diseases associated with the root canal system are always caused by bacteria and/or bacterial byproducts. Elimination of those should ensure resolution of the disease and healing.

7.9.2 Related factors

Diagnosis of periodontal versus endodontic causes for periapical diseases is crucial for correct and proper treatment of the disease.

7.10 Differential diagnosis

Prior to any invasive treatment of teeth, including endodontic or extraction, all possible differential diagnoses have to be ruled out. Careful history of the chief complaint should be taken, and all changes in the pattern of the pain should be explored as well as the current status of the pain. If any pain in the head and neck, away from the oral region, is reported that should be noted and those areas palpated with a firm finger pressure prior to the intraoral examination.

The following is a brief summary of many common nondental diseases that can cause pain in the oral region. It is important to note that this list is not meant to be all inclusive so vigilance should be kept at all times.

7.10.1 Temporomandibular disorder

By definition temporomandibular disorder (TMD) is a chronic self-reported pain (over 6 months' duation) in the face, temporomandibular joint (TMJ), and/or neck [35]. This diagnostic term includes both myalgia of the facial and neck muscles, arthralgia of the TMJ, and a combination of the two. The etiology of this disease is unknown. In the past it was thought that environmental factors combined with hyperactivity of the muscles were the main reasons for this disease [75]. More recently indications have emerged that at least some of the reasons are genetically based [30].

Differential diagnosis. TMD pain is usually reported to be felt as deep, annoying pain that does not have a very clear location, but is felt rather diffusely over the affected area. Palpation of the affected muscle or joint will cause an increase in the pain. This increased pain sensation can also be felt in referred locations of the pain, such as the teeth. Teeth in the affected area should respond normally to vitality testing and percussion/palpation.

7.10.2 Sinusitis

Inflammation in the maxillary sinus due to infection or reaction (allergy) can cause pressure on the maxillary branch of the trigeminal nerve. The pain is usually felt as diffuse pressure pain in the maxilla. If the trigeminal nerve is pressured, multiple teeth are affected.

Differential diagnosis. There is in most cases history of nasal congestion or a cold. The pain in the teeth usually gets worse with sudden movements, such as when running up and down steps. The percussion test is unreliable because the test itself can cause sudden movement of the fluid in the sinus and thereby give a false positive response. This may be turned to a diagnostic advantage in that if many teeth are sensitive to percussion, it is a sign of possible sinusitis. Also, it is possible that teeth in the affected area have lower cold sensitive threshold. Again most teeth in the area will be affected rather than just one.

7.10.3 Angina pectoris

It has been stated that up to 18% of patients with angina report pain in the mandible only (unilaterally on the left or bilateral) rather than in the more traditional areas of the left shoulder blade and/or arm [93]. The pain is usually associated with some physical exercises and/or emotional stress, and it is not localized to a specific tooth, but rather to the body of the mandible.

Differential diagnosis. Careful evaluation of medial history should reveal risk factors for cardiac disease, such as smoking, obesity, lack of exercise, etc. Teeth in the area should respond normally to vitality tests. If there is any suspicion that the patient is suffering from angina, immediate referral to emergency services in a hospital is necessary.

7.10.4 Trigeminal neuralgia

Patients suffering from trigeminal neuralgia, or tic douloureux, usually complain of a severe, electric, stabbing pain that comes in a burst. It seems to affect mainly women of 50 years or older. The etiology of it is unknown; there are two main competing theories. One calls for anatomical lesions locally in the affected area [104,106] and the other that the trigeminal root is compressed in the area of the pons, usually by an artery, vein or in rare cases a small neoplasm [60].

Differential diagnosis. There are few very distinctive characteristics of the trigeminal neuralgia pain that differentiate it from pulpitis. By definition there is a trigger point that when touched will cause pain. It can be hard to find the trigger in some cases, but carefully asking the patient to show what he or she is doing when the pain starts may give an indication. The second is that the pain episodes are very short: a maximum of a few seconds. The third indication is that most often this kind of pain does not affect the patient's sleeping patterns because the patient seems to subconsciously learn to stay away from the trigger during sleeping. Teeth on the affected area should respond normally to vitality tests.

7.10.5 Atypical odontalgia, neuropathic pain

This neurological disease can start in a similar way to trigeminal neuralgia, but then progresses to being a more dull, radiating, diffuse pain that only seems to get worse with treatment such as endodontic therapy or extraction. Again the etiology is unknown, but there is now building evidence that this is deafferentation pain or more commonly referred to as phantom pain [77]. There have been some suggestions that obsessive–compulsive or perfectionist psychological traits are common in patients suffering from atypical odontalgia [77]. However, it is not clear if this is a byproduct of the disease or if it is a true predisposing factor. An important aspect is that if this is a deafferentation pain then any invasive procedure carries a high risk of further exacerbating the condition.

Differential diagnosis. The pain is usually continuous, dull, throbbing, radiating, and/or burning, and it is not affected by temperature. It can be felt by the patient originating from a specific tooth or teeth. Treatment of those teeth does not relieve the pain, but may enhance it further. Local or even regional anesthesia is often inconclusive, but teeth in the area usually respond normally to vitality tests if they have not already been subjected to root canal therapy.

7.10.6 Herpes zoster

In 1892 the association between varicella and herpes zoster was first made [131]. It is now well established that a herpes zoster infection (shingles) requires preexposure to the varicella-zoster virus. The primary varicella virus infection causes an acute, generally mild, infection (chicken pox). Then the virus establishes latency somewhere within sensory ganglia. The virus is then later reactivated to cause a herpes zoster outbreak. The most important etiologic factors

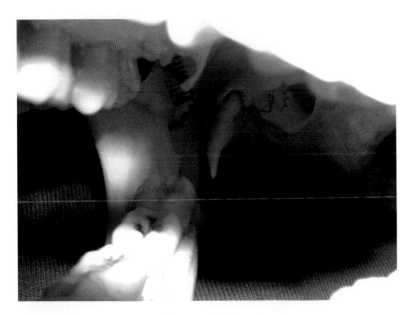

Fig. 7.13 A clinical slide of a dried skull that has part of the tendon from the stylo process to the hyoid bone calcified. The close proximity to the ramus of mandible causes pain with movements of the head as well as with opening and closing the mouth, causing symptoms associated with Eagle's syndrome.

for these outbreaks are increased age, compromised immune system, and emotional stress. Recent events perceived as stressful seem to be an important factor [110]. During the prodromal stage, prior to vesicular skin eruptions usually there is very severe pain from the affected nerve segment which can be confused with odontogenic pain if the virus has affected the second or third branch of the trigeminal nerve [120].

Differential diagnosis. During the first few days after activation of the virus there are no skin lesions, but the pain is severe and closely mimics dental pain. Therefore, it can be difficult to diagnose the shingles at this stage. And to compound the problem, vitality tests are not always reliable. In cases of unusually severe pain, frequently in two or more teeth. This combined with the patient having some of the risk factors listed above, one should be suspicious of herpes zoster infection and refer for evaluation immediately. After the vesicles have formed on the affected skin, diagnosis is simple (Fig. 7.14).

7.10.7 Cluster headache

Presenting symptoms are usually pain in the suborbital or retro-orbital area of the face, which can be confused with odontogenic pain on upper canine or premolar. It is usually associated with several teeth. The condition seems to affect males six times more often than females, and the most common age range is 35–50 years. It has been hypothesized that the cause is similar to migraine and related to episodic vasodilatation. The pain attack usually lasts for 30–90 min and is often triggered by a stimulus such as smoke, light, smell, etc. Recently a case report was published where the use of cocaine caused cluster-like pain [100]. Of note is that the onset of the pain was not immediate after the cocaine use, but some time after (30 min to 2 h later) and a new administration of cocaine for the most part relieved the pain.

Differential diagnosis. Usually the pain is not felt in a tooth, but rather in several teeth; it is not initiated by temperature changes in the oral cavity and it may be associated with nasal congestion and lacrimation of the eye on the affected side. If cluster headache is suspected and the patient is having an attack when he or she is in the dental office, administering oxygen for a few minutes (up to 15 min) will in most cases completely eliminate the pain. All teeth in the affected area should respond normally to vitality tests.

7.10.8 Salivary glands

The chief complaint is moderate to severe pain in the affected area usually associated with eating. Patients could have swelling that mimics apical periodontitis with abscess. This is caused by submandibular/parotid gland infection or blockage.

Differential diagnosis. Even though the patient may report the pain as being most severe when he or she is chewing food, most often the pain actually starts

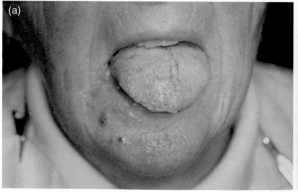
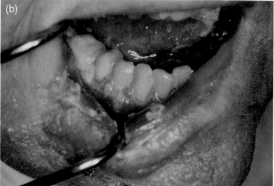

Fig. 7.14   This patient that had sought treatment for severe toothache in the lower right premolar area presented 2 days later with fluid-filled vesicles on the right side of the chin and mucosal changes on the tongue (a). Note the sharp midline changes, where the lesions abruptly stop and where the innervations end at midline both on the chin and tongue. (b) After a further 2 days the oral lesions became severe [120].

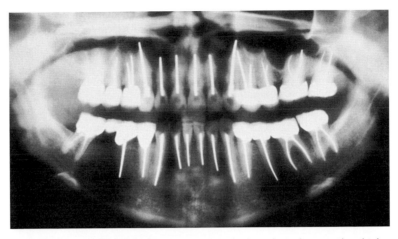

Fig. 7.15   An orthopantograph of a patient who had sought and received multiple endodontic therapies followed by crowns and other restorations over a period of 18 months. The patient was referred to a specialty clinic for evaluation and possible need for apicoectomy of lower right second molar. No treatment was rendered at that time, but the previous need for all the endodontic therapies, as well as multiple other medical treatments, was questioned. After consultation with a psychiatrist the patient was diagnosed with Munchausen syndrome and received psychological treatment recommended for that diagnosis.

prior to eating, when the saliva flow has increased due to the smell or stimulus of food. The area where the gland is affected shows decreased or absent salivary flow. Teeth on the affected area should respond normally to vitality tests.

7.10.9 Eagle's syndrome

Here the chief complaint is moderate to severe pain when swallowing, turning the head, and/or when opening the mouth wide. This has been reported to be associated with dysphagia, otalgia, and headache with dizziness [28]. The cause of this syndrome is that the tendon from the stylo process to the hyoid bone calcifies such that it starts to impede on the structures lateral between the process and the ramus of the mandible (Fig. 7.13).

Differential diagnosis. Digital palpation of the tonsillar fossa on the affected side is likely to cause the typical pain. On occasion, the process can be visualized on an orthophantogram, but currently specific computed tomography scans are indicated to confirm the diagnosis. Teeth on the affected side should respond normally to vitality tests.

7.10.10 Munchausen syndrome

There are patients who suffer from psychological disorders that manifest in looking for unnecessary medical help. This may be at least in part because of drug-seeking tendencies, but in rare cases it has a true psychological reason where the patients are only interested in receiving as much medical care as possible. This is irrespective of whether they are offered pain relievers or other drugs associated with the treatment [14]. This disease has been called Munchausen syndrome for those who are seeking medical treatment for various illnesses, and somatoform pain disorder for those who apparently suffer from cognitive perception of pain that does not seem to have any physical reasons [112].

Differential diagnosis. Patients suffering from these psychological disorders are often well-read people who have even studied medical and dental textbooks in detail. Therefore, it can initially be difficult to differentiate what is a true problem versus a disease that the patient has heard or read about. A careful medical history usually reveals multiple and often convoluted medical treatments that do fit the appearance of the patient. Vitality testing can be unreliable because these patients try to deceive the clinician (Fig. 7.15).

7.11 References

1. Ahlquist ML, Frazen OG (1994) Encoding of the subjective intensity or sharp dental pain. *Endodontics and Dental Traumatology* **10**, 153–66.
2. Ahlquist ML, Frazen OG (1994) Inflammation and dental pain in man. *Endodontics and Dental Traumatology* **10**, 201–9.
3. Barbakow F, Cleaton-Jones P, Friedman D (1981) Endodontic treatment of teeth with periapical radiolucent areas in a general practice. *Oral Surgery, Oral Medicine, Oral Pathology* **51**, 552–9.
4. Barthel CR, Rosenkranz B, Leuenberg A, Roulet JF (200) Pulp capping of carious exposures: treatment outcome after 5 and 10 years: a retrospective study. *Journal of Endodontics* **26**, 525–8.
5. Baume LJ (1970) Diagnosis of diseases of the pulp. *Oral Surgery, Oral Medicine, Oral Pathology* **29**, 102–16.
6. Baumgartner JC, Pickett AB, Muller JT (1984) Microscopic examination of oral sinus tracts and their associated periapical lesions. *Journal of Endodontics* **10**, 146–52.
7. Bender IB, Landau MA, Fonsecca S, Trowbridge HO (1989) The optimal placement site of the electrode in electric pulp testing of the 12 anterior teeth. *Journal of the American Dental Association* **118**, 305–10.
8. Bender IB, Seltzer S (1961) Roentgenographic and direct observation of experimental lesions in bone. *Journal of the American Dental Association* **62**, 157–62.
9. Bender IB (2000) Reversible and irreversible painful pulpitides: diagnosis and treatment. *Australian Endodontic Journal* **26**, 10–14.
10. Bergenholtz G. (1974) Microorganisms from necrotic pulp of traumatized teeth. *Odontologisk Revy* **25**, 347–58.
11. Bergenholtz G, Lindhe J (1978) Effects of experimentally induced marginal periodontitis an periodontal scaling on the dental pulp. *Journal of Clinical Periocontology* **5**, 59–65.
12. Beveridge EE, Brown AC (1965) The measurement of human dental intrapulpal pressure and its response to clinical variables. *Oral Surgery, Oral Medicine, Oral Pathology* **19**, 655–72.
13. Bhaskar SN (1966) Periapical lesions – types, incidence, and clinical features. *Oral Surgery, Oral Medicine, Oral Pathology* **21**, 657–71.
14. Bjil P (1995) Psychogenic pain in dentistry. *Compendium* **16**, 45–54.
15. Bowles WR, Withrow JC, Lepinski AM, Hargreaves KM (2003) Tissue levels of immunoreactive substance P are increased in patients with irreversible pulpitis. *Journal of Endodontics* **29**, 265–7.
16. Brannstrom M, Linden LA, Astrom A (1967) The hydrodynamics of the dental tubule and of pulp fluid. A discussion of its significance in relation to dentinal sensitivity. *Caries Research* **1**, 310–17.
17. Brannstrom M, Johnson G (1970) Movement of the dentin and pulp liquids on application of thermal stimuli. An in vitro study. *Acta Odontologica Scandinavica* **28**, 59–70.
18. Brannstrom M, Astrom A (1972) The hydrodynamics of the dentine: its possible relationship to dental pain. *International Dental Journal* **22**, 219–27.
19. Byers MR, Narhi MV, Mecifi KB (1988) Acute and chronic reactions of dental sensory nerve fibers to hydrodynamic stimulation or injury. *Anatomical Records* **221**, 872–83.
20. Byers MR, Narhi MVO (1999) Dental injury models: Experimental tools for understanding neuroinflammatory interactions and polymodal nocicpetor functions. *Critical Review in Oral Biology and Medicine* **10**, 4–39.
21. Bysröm A, Claesson R, Sundquist G (1985) The antibacterial effect of camphorated paramonochlorophenol, camphorated phenol and calcium hydroxid in the treatment of infected root canals. *Endodontics and Dental Traumatology* **1**, 170–5.
22. Casasco A, Calligaro A, Casasco M (1990) Peptidergic nerves in human dental pulp. An immunocytochemical study. *Histochemistry* **95**, 115–21.
23. Cave SG, Freer TJ, Podlich HM (2002) Pulp-test responses in orthodontic patients. *Australian Orthodontic Journal* **18**, 27–34.
24. Chambers IG (1982) The role and methods of pulp testing in oral diagnosis. *International Endodontic Journal* **15**, 1–5.
25. Chance B (1951) Rapid and sensitive spectrophotometry: III. A double beam apparatus. *Review of Scientific Instruments* **22**, 634–8.
26. Chattipakorn SC, Light AR, Narhi M, Maixner W (2001) The effects of noxious dental heating on the jaw-opening reflex and trigeminal Fos expression in the ferret. *Journal of Pain* **2**, 345–53.
27. Chattipakorn SC, Sigurdsson A, Light AR, Narhi M, Maixner W (2002) Trigeminal c-Fos expression and behavioral responses to pulpal inflammation in ferrets. *Pain* **99**, 61–9.
28. Cooley RL, Robinson SF (1980) Variables associated with electric pulp testing. *Oral Surgery, Oral Medicine, Oral Pathology* **50**, 66–73.
29. Correll RW, Wescott WB (1982) Eagle's syndrome diagnosed after history of headache, dysphagia, otalgia, and limited neck movement. *Journal of the American Dental Association* **104**, 491–2.
30. Diatchenko L, Slade GD, Nackley AG, Bhalang K, Sigurdsson A, *et al.* (2005) Genetic basis for individual variations in pain perception and the development of a chronic pain condition. *Human Molecular Genetics* **14**, 135–43.
31. Domine L, Holz J (1991) The aging of the human pulp–dentin organ. *Schweizer Monatsschrift für Zahnmedizin* **101**, 725–33.
32. Dowden WE, Langeland K (1969) A correlation of pulpal histopathology with clinical symptoms. *Journal of Dental Research* **48**, 183 (abstract No. 569).
33. Dubner R, Ruda MA (1992) Activity-dependent neuronal plasticity following tissue injury and inflammation. *Trends in Neuroscience* **15**, 96–103.
34. Dummer PMH, Hicks R, Huws D (1980) Clinical signs and symptoms in pulp disease. *International Endodontic Journal* **13**, 27–35.

35. Dworkin S, LaResche L. (1992) Research diagnostic criteria for temporomandibular disorder: Review, criteria, examinations and specifications. *Journal of Craniomandibular Disorder* **6**, 301–55.

36. Garfunkel A, Sela J, Almansky M (1987) Dental pulp pathosis: Clinicopathologic correlation based on 109 cases. *Oral Surgery, Oral Medicine, Oral Pathology* **35**, 110–17.

37. Eli I (1993) Dental anxiety: a cause for possible misdiagnosis of tooth vitality. *International Endodontic Journal* **26**, 251–3.

38. Fanibunda KB (1985) A laboratory study to investigate the differentiation of pulp vitality in human teeth by temperature measurement. *Journal of Dentistry* **13**, 295–303.

39. Fanibunda KB (1986) The feasibility of temperature measurement as a diagnostic procedure in human teeth. *Journal of Dentistry* **14**, 126–8.

40. Fanibunda KB (1986) Diagnosis of tooth vitality by crown surface temperature measurement: A clinical evaluation. *Journal of Dentistry* **14**, 160–4.

41. Fearnhead RW (1963) The histologic demonstration of nerve fibers in dentin. In Andersen DJ, editor. *Sensory mechanisms in dentine*, p. 15. New York: Pergamon Press.

42. Fouad AF, Rivera EM, Walton RE (1996) Penicillin as a supplement in resolving the localized acute apical abscess. *Oral Surgery, Oral Medicine, Oral Pathology* **81**, 590–5.

43. Fulling HJ, Andereasen JO (1976) Influence of maturation status and tooth type of permanent teeth upon electrometric and thermal pulp testing procedures. *Scandinavian Journal of Dental Research* **84**, 291–6.

44. Fuss Z, Trowbridge H, Bender IB, Rickoff B, Sorin S. Assessment of reliability of electrical and thermal pulp testing. *Journal of Endodontics* **12**, 301–5.

45. Garfunkel A, Sela J, Almansky M (1973) Dental pulp pathosis: Clinicopathologic correlation based on 109 cases. *Oral Surgery, Oral Medicine, Oral Pathology* **35**, 110–17.

46. Gazelius B, Edwall B, Olgart L, Lundberg JM, Hokfelt T, Fisher JA (1987) Vasodilatory effects and coexistence of calcitonin gene related peptide (CGRP) and substance P in sensory nerves of cat dental pulp. *Acta Physiologica Scandinavica* **130**, 33–40.

47. Gazelius B, Olgart L, Edwall B, Edwall L (1986) Non-invasive recording of blood flow in human dental pulp. *Endodontics and Dental Traumatology* **2**, 219–21.

48. Glick DH (1962) Locating referred pulpal pains. *Oral Surgery, Oral Medicine, Oral Pathology* **15**, 613–23.

49. Grushka M, Sessle BJ. (1984) Application of the McGill pain questionnaire to the differentiation of toothache pain. *Pain* **19**, 49–57.

50. Hagerstram G (1976) The origin of impulses recorded from dentinal cavities in the tooth of the cat. *Acta Physiologica Scandinavica* **97**, 121–8.

51. Hargreaves KM Roszkowski MT, Jackson DL, Swift JQ (1995) Orofacial pain; peripheral mechanisms. In Fricton JR, Dubner R, editors. *Advances in pain research and therapy*, pp. 33–42, Vol. 21. New York: Raven Press.

52. Hargreaves KM (2002) Pain mechanism of the pulpo-dentin complex. In Hargreaves KM, Goodis HE, editors. *Dental pulp*, p. 183. Chicago, IL: Quintessence.

53. Hasler JE, Mitchell DF (1970) Painless pulpitis. *Journal of the American Dental Association* **81**, 671–7.

54. Heide S, Mjör IA (1983) Pulp reaction to experimental exposures in young permanent monkey teeth. *International Endodontic Journal* **16**, 11–19.

55. Henig EF, Derschowitx T, Shalit M, Toledo E, Tikva P, Aviv T (1978) Brain abscess following dental infection. *Oral Surgery, Oral Medicine, Oral Pathology* **45**, 955–8.

56. Hillmann G, Geurtsen W (1997) Light-microscopical investigation of the distribution of extracellular matrix molecules and calcifications in human dental pulps of various ages. *Cell, Tissue Research* **289**, 145–54.

57. Hirvonen T, Hippi P, Narhi M (1998) The effect of an opioid antagonist and a somatostatin antagonist on the nerve function in normal and inflamed pulp. *Journal of Dental Research* **77**, 1329.

58. Holloway GA (1983) Laser Doppler measurement of cutaneous blood flow. In Rolfe P, editor. *Non-invasive physiological measurements*, p. 11. London: Academic Press.

59. Ingram TA, Peters DD (1983) Evaluation of the effects of carbon dioxide used as a pulpal test. 2. In vivo effect on canine enamel and pulpal tissue. *Journal of Endodontics* **9**, 296–303.

60. Jannetta PJ (1967) Arterial compression of the trigeminal nerve at the pons in patients with trigeminal neuralgia. *Journal of Neurosurgery* **26**(Suppl), 159–62.

61. Jones VR, Rivera EM, Walton RE (2002) Comparison of carbon dioxide versus refrigerant spray to determine pulpal responsiveness. *Journal of Endodontics* **28**, 531–3.

62. Jyvasjarvi E, Kniffki DK (1987) Cold stimulation of teeth: a comparison between the responses of cat intradental A- and C-fibers and human sensations. *Journal of Physiology* **391**, 193–207.

63. Kim S, Dorscher-Kim J, Liu MT, Trowbridge H (1988) Biphasic pulp blood flow response to substance P in the dog as measured with radiolabeld, microsphere injection method. *Archives of Oral Biology* **33**, 305–9.

64. Kim S, Schuessler G, Chien S (1983) Measurement of blood flow in the dental pulp of dogs with Xe-133 washout method. *Archives of Oral Biology* **28**, 501–5.

65. Klausen B, Helbo M, Dabelsteen E (1985) A differential diagnostic approach to the symptomatology of acute dental pain. *Oral Surgery, Oral Medicine, Oral Pathology* **59**, 297–301.

66. Klepac RK, Dowling J, Hauge G, McDonald M (1980) Reports of pain after dental treatment, electrical tooth pulp stimulation and cutaneous shock. *Journal of the American Dental Association* **100**, 692–5.

67. Langeland, K (1981) Management of the inflamed pulp associated with deep carious lesion. *Journal of Endodontics* **7**, 169–81.

68. Lepinski M, Hargreaves KM, Goodis HE, Bowles WR (2000) Bradykinin levels in dental pulp by microdialysis. *Journal of Endodontics* **26**, 744–7.

69. Lundy T, Stanley HR (1969) Correlation of pulpal histopathology and clinical symptoms in human teeth

subjected to experimental irritation. *Oral Surgery, Oral Medicine, Oral Pathology* 27, 187–201.

70. Madison S, Wilcox LR (1988) An evaluation of coronal microleakage in endodontically treated teeth. III. In vivo study. *Journal of Endodontics* 14, 455–8.

71. Massler M (1967) Pulpal reaction to dental caries. *International Dental Journal* 17, 441–60.

72. Matthews B (1977) Responses of intradental nerves to electrical and thermal stimulation of teeth in dogs. *Journal of Physiology* 264, 641–64.

73. Matthews B, Searle BN (1976) Electrical stimulation of teeth. *Pain* 2, 245–51.

74. Mazur B, Massler M (1964) Influence of periodontal disease on the dental pulp. *Oral Surgery, Oral Medicine, Oral Pathology* 17, 592–603.

75. MacGregor A, Griffiths G, Baker J, Spector T (1997) Determinants of pressure pain threshold in adult twins: Evidence that shared environmental influences predominate. *Pain* 73, 253–7.

76. McGrath PA Gracely RH Dubner R, Heft MW (1983) Non-pain and pain sensations evoked by tooth pulp stimulation. *Pain* 15, 377–88.

77. Marbach J (1996) Orofacial phantom pain: Theory and phenomenology. *Journal of the American Dental Association* 127, 221–9.

78. Martin FE (2003) Carious pulpitis: microbiological and histopathological considerations. *Australian Endodontic Journal* 29, 134–7.

79. Mengel MK, Stiefenhofer AE, Jyvasjarvi E, Kniffki KD (1993) Pain sensation during cold stimulation of the teeth: differential reflection of A delta and C fibre activity? *Pain* 55, 159–69.

80. Mesaros SV, Trope M (1997) Revascularization of trumatized teeth assessed by laser Doppler flowmetry: Case Report. *Endodontics and Dental Traumatology* 13, 24–30.

81. Michaelson PL, Holland GR (2002) Is pulpitis painful? *Intentional Endodontic Journal* 35, 829–32.

82. Millard HD (1973) Electric pulp testers. *Journal of the American Dental Association* 86, 872–3.

83. Milikan GA (1942) The oxymeter, an instrument for measuring continuously the oxygen saturation of arterial blood in man. *Review of Scientific Instruments* 13, 434–7.

84. Morse DR (1972) Oral pathways of infection: with special reference to endodontics. *Journal of the British Endodontic Society* 6, 13–16.

85. Morse DR, Seltzer S, Sinai I, Biron G (1977) Endodontic classification. *Journal of the American Dental Association* 94, 685–9.

86. Mumford JM (1964) Evaluation of gutta percha and ethyl chloride in pulp testing. *British Dental Journal* 116, 338–32.87. Mumford JM (1967) Thermal and electrical stimulation of teeth in the diagnosis of pulpal and periapical disease. *Proceedings of the Royal Society of Medicine* 60, 197–202.

88. Narhi M, Virtanen A, Kuhta J, Huopaniemi T (1979) Electrical stimulation of teeth with pulp tester in the cat. *Scandinavian Journal of Dental Resarch* 87, 32–8.

89. Narhi M, Jyvasjarvi E, Hirvonen T, Huopaniemi T. (1982) Activation of heat sensitive nerve fibers in the dental pulp of the cat. *Pain* 14, 317–26.

90. Narhi MVO, Hirvonen T, Hakamaki MOK (1982) Activation of intradental nerves in the dog to some stimuli applied to the dentin. *Archives of Oral Biology* 27, 1053–8.

91. Narhi M, Jyvasjarvi E, Virtanen A, Huopaniemi T, Ngassapa D, Hirvonen T (1992) Role of intradental A and C type nerve fibers in dental pain mechanisms. *Proceedings of the Finnish Dental Society* 88 (suppl 1), 507–16.

92. Narhi MVO, Yamamoto H, Ngassapa D, Hirvonen T (1998) Function of interadental nociceptors in normal and inflamed teeth. In Shjimono M, Maeda T, Suda H, Takahash K, editors. *Dentin/pulp complex*, pp, 136–40. Tokyo: Quintessence.

93. Natkin E (1974) Treatment of endodontic emergencies. *Dental Clinics of North America.* 18, 243–55.

94. Nissan R, Trope M, Zheng C-D, Chance B (1992) Dual wavelength spectrophotometry as a diagnostic test of the pulpchamber contents. *Oral Surgery, Oral Medicine, Oral Pathology* 74, 508–14.

95. Odor TM, Pitt Ford TR, McDonald F (1996) Effect of wavelength and bandwidth on the clinical reliability of laser Doppler recordings. *Endodontics and Dental Traumatology* 12, 9–15.

96. Okeson JP (1996) *Orofacial pain.* Philadelphia, PA: Quintessence.

97. Olgart LM (1985) The role of local factors in dentin and pulp intradental pain mechanisms. *Journal of Dental Research* 64, 572–8.

98. Olgart LM (1996) Neural control of pulpal blood flow. *Critical Reviews in Oral Biology and Medicine* 7, 159–71.

99. Pantera EA, Anderson RW, Pantera CT (1993) Reliability of electric pulp testing after pulpal testing with dichlorodifluoromethane. *Journal of Endodontics* 19, 312–14.

100. Penarrocha M, Bagan J, Penarrocha M, Silverstre F (2000) Cluster headache and cocaine use. *Oral Surgery, Oral Medicine, Oral Pathology* 90, 271–4.

101. Peters DD, Lorton L, Mader CL, Augsburger RA, Ingram TA (1983) Evaluation of the effects of carbon dioxide used as a pulpal test. 1. In vitro effect on human enamel. *Journal of Endodontics* 9, 219–27.

102. Peters DD, Mader CL, Connelly JC (1986) Evaluation of the effects of carbon dioxide used as a pulpal test. 3. In vivo effect on human enamel. *Journal of Endodontics* 12, 13–20.

103. Petersson K, Soderstrom C, Kiani-Anaraki M, Levy G (1999) Evaluation of the ability of thermal and electrical tests to register pulp vitality. *Endodontics and Dental Traumatology* 15, 127–31.

104. Ratner EJ, Person P, Kleinman DJ, Shklar G, Socranksy SS (1979) Jawbone cavities and trigeminal and atypical facial neuralgias. *Oral Surgery, Oral Medicine, Oral Pathology* 48, 3–20.

105. Ritter AL, Ritter AV, Murrah V, Sigurdsson A, Trope M (2004) Pulp revascularization of replanted immature dog teeth after treatment with minocycline and doxycycline assessed by laser Doppler flowmetry, radiography, and histology. *Dental Traumatology* 20, 75–84.

106. Roberts AM, Person P (1979) Etiology and treatment of idiopathic trigeminal and atypical facial neuralgias. *Oral Surgery, Oral Medicine, Oral Pathology* **48**, 298–308.

107. Robinson PP (1987) A comparison of monopolar and bipolar electrical stimuli and thermal stimuli in determining the vitality of autotransplanted human teeth. *Archives of Oral Biology* **32**, 191–4.

108. Rodd HD, Boissonade FM (2005) Vascular status in human primary and permanent teeth in health and disease. *European Journal of Oral Science* **113**, 128–34.

109. Rubach WC, Mitchell DF (1965) Periodontal disease, accessory canals and pulp pathosis. *Journal of Periodontology* **36**, 34–9.

110. Schmader K, Studenski S, MacMillan J, Grufferman S, Cohen HJ (1990) Are stressful life events risk factors for herpes zoster? *Journal of the American Geriatric Society* **38**, 1188–94.

111. Schnettler JM, Wallance JA (1991) Pulse oximetry as a diagnostic tool of pulpal vitality. *Journal of Endodontics* **17**, 488–90.

112. Scully C, Eveson JW, Porter SR (1995) Munchausen's syndrome: oral presentations. *British Dental Journal* **178**, 65–7.

113. Seltzer S (1972) Classification of pulpal pathosis. *Oral Surgery, Oral Medicine, Oral Pathology* **34**, 269–80.

114. Seltzer S (1990) *Odontalgia (tooth pain) diagnostic and therapeutic considerations.* Philadelphia, PA: Temple University.

115. Seltzer S, Bender IB (1985) *The dental pulp*, 3rd edn. Philadelphia, PA: Lippincott.

116. Seltzer S, Bender IB, Zionitz M (1963) The dynamics of pulp inflammation: correlation between diagnostic data and actual histologic finding in the pulp. *Oral Surgery, Oral Medicine, Oral Pathology* **16**, 846–71.

117. Seltzer S, Bender IB, Zionitz M (1963) The interrelationship of pulp and periodontal disease. *Oral Surgery, Oral Medicine, Oral Pathology* **16**, 1474–90.

118. Sessle B (1987) Neurophysiology of orofacial pain. *Dental Clinics of North America* **31**, 595–614.

119. Sigurdsson, A, Maixner W (1994) Effects of experimental and clinical noxious counterirritants on pain perception. *Pain* **57**, 2 65–75.

120. Sigurdsson A, Jackway JR (1995) Herpes zoster infection presenting as an acute pulpitis. *Oral Surgery, Oral Medicine, Oral Pathology* **80**, 92–5.

121. Skiller V (1960) The prognosis for young teeth loosened after mechanical injuries. *Acta Odontologica Scandinavica* **18**, 171–7.

122. Soo-ampon S, Vongsavan N, Soo-ampon M, Chuckpaiwong S, Matthews B (2003) The sources of laser Doppler blood-flow signals recorded from human teeth. *Archives of Oral Biology* **48**, 353–60.

123. Stone A, Stratigos GT (1979) Mandibular odontogenic infection with serious complications. *Oral Surgery, Oral Medicine, Oral Pathology* **47**, 395–400.

124. Suda H, Sunakawa M, Yamamoto H (1995) Orofacial referred pain; its physiological bases and case report. In Shimono M, Maeda T, Suda H, Takahashi K, editors. *Dentin/pulp complex.* Tokyo: Quintessence,

125. Taddese A, Nah S-Y, McClesky EW (1995) Selective opioid inhibition of small nociceptive neurons. *Science* **270**, 1366–69.

126. Torabinejad M, Trope M (1996) Endodontic and periodontal interrelationships. In Walton RE, Torabinejad M, editors. *Principles and practice of endodontics*, pp. 442–56. Philadelphia, PA: WB Saunders.

127. Travell G, Simons D (1983) *Myofacial pain and dysfunction.* Baltimore, MD: Williams & Wilkins.

128. Tronstad L, Mjör IA (1972) Capping the inflamed pulp. *Oral Surgery, Oral Medicine, Oral Pathology* **34**, 477–85.

129. Trope M, Tronstad L, Rosenbert E, Listgarten M (1988) Darkfield microscopy as a diagnostic aid in differentiating exudates from endodontic and periodontal abscess. *Journal of Endodontics* **12**, 35–8.

130. Trope M, Chow E, Nissan R (1995) In vitro endotoxin penetration of coronally unsealed endodontically treated teeth. *Endodontics and Dental Traumatology* **11**, 90–4.

131. Von Bokay I (1909) Ueber den aetiologischen Zusammenhang der Varicellen mit gewissen Faellen von Herpes Zoster. *Wien Klinsher Wochenschriftung* **39** (suppl), 1323–37.

132. Wilder-Smith PE (1988) A new method for the non invasive recording of blood flow in human dental pulp. *International Endodontic Journal* **21**, 307–12.

133. Wood EH, Geraci JE (1949) Photoelectric determination of arterial oxygen saturation in man. *International Endodontic Journal* **21**, 307–12.

134. Woolf C (1999) Transcriptional and posttranslational plasticity and the generation of inflammatory pain. *Proceedings of the National Academia of Science* **96**, 7723–30.

135. Yanpiset K, Vongsavan N, Sigurdsson A, Trope M. (2001) Efficacy of laser Doppler flowmetry for the diagnosis of revascularization of reimplanted immature dog teeth. *Dental Traumatology* **17**, 63–70.

Chapter 8
Epidemiology of Apical Periodontitis

Harald M. Eriksen

8.1 Introduction

Apical periodontitis is an acute or chronic inflammatory lesion around the apex of a tooth caused by bacterial infection of the pulp and root canal system. The aim of endodontic treatment is either to prevent the development of apical periodontitis or to establish conditions for healing. This implies that the principle of endodontic treatment should be based on infection control and elimination of bacteria from the root canal [10,70,81].

Evaluation of endodontic treatment is primarily based on radiographic recording of the periapical structures [59,73,74], while clinical signs and symptoms may contribute additional information regarding clinical function and patient satisfaction. There are two essential questions related to the occurrence of apical periodontitis and its treatment:

- Is it possible, with present knowledge and modern principles of endodontic treatment, to control and eliminate apical periodontitis?
- To what extent are we, as a dental profession, succeeding in achieving that goal?

The first question may be answered by using information from experimental and clinical research (see Chapters 3–7, 11, and 12). An appropriate answer to the last question can only be assessed using an epidemiologic approach.

8.2 Epidemiology: general aspects

8.2.1 Definitions and aims

In health care, the basic difference between an experimental, a clinical, and an epidemiological approach is that experimental research is primarily concerned with disease mechanisms under strictly controlled laboratory conditions, usually far from "real-life" conditions. Clinical research focuses on the individual and their health problems while epidemiology discloses diseases as they appear in defined groups (cohorts) or populations. Epidemiologic investigations may in addition include estimates on disease determinants and thereby contribute to risk prediction, prevention, and health care strategies.

Traditionally, dentistry focuses on treatment of individuals. Epidemiology is considered to belong to public health policy and health planners and with limited relevance to dental practice and individual patients. However, epidemiologic research has more to offer dental practice than results from health surveys. Epidemiologic knowledge can answer questions such as:

- Is the manifestation and nature of a disease as it appears in an individual similar to most other cases or is it unusual?
- What are the major causes and contributing factors for a specific condition or disease in society, and are these factors considered in individual treatment strategies?
- Are there certain social and other characteristics about the group(s) from where the majority of cases appear?
- What is the probability that the disease will respond to a specific treatment?

- What are the reasons for differences in treatment outcome between specialists and general practitioners?

To be answered properly, these questions depend on epidemiologic data in addition to information from experimental and clinical research. However, to comprehend the information from these different fields of research, the difference in criteria and methods applied must be acknowledged. In addition, translational research and principles based on complexity theory have recently been developed in order to assure relevance of knowledge from different levels of organization [24,69].

8.2.2 Epidemiologic research

There are at least five basic reasons for performing an epidemiologic investigation:

- to describe health status in a defined population
- to explain the etiology and contributing factors of a specific disease
- to control or eradicate a disease
- to predict the occurrence of a disease
- to collect data in order to test hypotheses about the appearance of a disease.

Depending on the purpose of the investigation, an appropriate design of the study should be determined (Fig. 8.1).

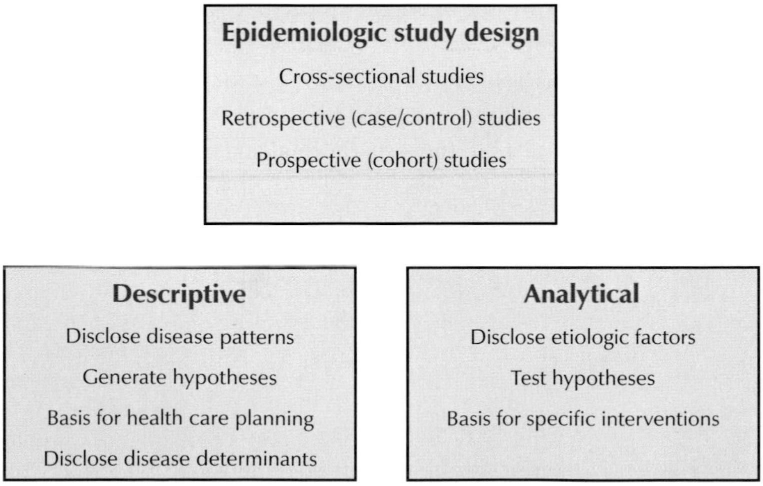

Epidemiologic study design

Cross-sectional studies

Retrospective (case/control) studies

Prospective (cohort) studies

Descriptive

Disclose disease patterns

Generate hypotheses

Basis for health care planning

Disclose disease determinants

Analytical

Disclose etiologic factors

Test hypotheses

Basis for specific interventions

Fig. 8.1 Design of epidemiologic studies and utilization of epidemiologic data.

Descriptive epidemiology

With descriptive epidemiology, the occurrence of a disease is described with respect to time, location and characteristics of the population studied. A study can be cross-sectional (recording the prevalence at a certain time), retrospective (using historical data), or prospective (recording incidence and prevalence of a disease by following a population over time using a longitudinal design). Descriptive epidemiology does not disclose etiologic factors but may initiate hypotheses about possible cause/effect associations. Such hypotheses may be tested by analytical epidemiology or in experimental or controlled clinical studies.

Analytical epidemiology

Analytical epidemiology includes at least three different study designs:

• Observational studies where exposure to a known set of agents differs between groups or individuals.
• Detection of possible differences related to healthy and unhealthy individuals, or groups with different prevalence of a disease.
• Case/control studies where "cases" have been exposed to a certain agent as the "controls" have not.

The case/control study design is close to a controlled clinical study and represents a borderline between epidemiologic and clinical research. In this presentation a distinction between epidemiologic and controlled clinical studies will be made. Clinical studies are usually conducted on highly selected groups of individuals (students, referrals, university or specialty clinic patients). In addition, treatment is often performed by highly motivated and skilled personnel under optimal conditions (no time constraints, no payment involved, etc.) which indicates what might be obtained rather what is usually achieved by a specific procedure. Again, epidemiology will give the probability of a certain outcome of a specific procedure, while a clinical study indicates what might be achieved under optimal conditions. This difference is highly relevant for endodontic treatment of apical periodontitis. The results from abundant clinical studies in endodontics should therefore not be erroneously interpreted as valid for what is usually achieved in general practice and being representative for the population in general [20].

8.2.3 Elements of an epidemiologic study

The study population

In epidemiologic studies, it is of crucial importance to define the population of interest. The defined population constitutes the denominator for the results obtained. Even if results may have general validity, generalization is only directly relevant for this population. To avoid unnecessary work without losing too much precision, a defined sampling procedure is performed in epidemiologic research.

Sampling

To secure a representative sample drawn from a defined population, certain principles have to be followed:

• Randomness (each individual in the defined population has an equal chance to be drawn).
• A sufficient number of individuals included (the fewer included, the lower is the power of the final result).

Measurements

In epidemiologic research, characteristics are recorded according to defined criteria, usually presented as index systems. The criteria applied should be:

• measurable (operationalized)
• mutually exclusive
• meaningful regarding the condition under investigation
• reproducible
• communicable.

The periapical index (PAI) system (Fig. 8.2) for registration of apical periodontitis is an example of a criterion that complies with the requirements listed above [59]. Reproducibility should be secured by calibration of investigator(s). A κ-value is usually given in order to indicate the level of precision (reproducibility).

There has been, and still is, a debate about the advantages of using objectively defined criteria instead of just a success/failure judgment of endodontic treatment based on the presence or absence of apical periodontitis. With a defined index system, results from different studies can be compared. It is therefore recommended that a defined index system is used in epidemiologic research [20].

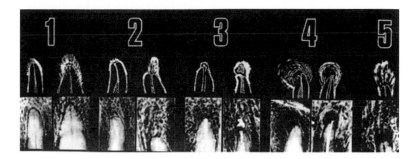

Fig. 8.2 The periapical index (PAI) is based on a combination of radiographic and histologic characteristics. (Reproduced from [59] with permission from Munksgaard.)

Reliability and validity

Even when applying well-defined criteria, by well-trained and calibrated investigators, misjudgments will always occur. These errors may be of two kinds:

- overlooking a pathological process (a false negative registration)
- erroneously interpreting a normal condition as pathological (a false positive registration).

There are consequences linked to both over- and under-registration of pathological conditions. It is impossible to eliminate false registrations entirely, and the challenge is to acknowledge them and take into consideration possible consequences. This becomes even more important in treatment results from individual dentists in case or clinical reports. The wide diversity in recording apical periodontitis and suggested treatment of choice documented by Reit and Hollender [74] is thought provoking in this context and will be considered in more detail at the end of the chapter.

Evaluation of epidemiologic data

Statistical evaluation is essential in epidemiology. Statistical evaluations focus on probabilities, and an appreciation of epidemiologic data thereby represents a contrast to the need and demand for certainty, a feature intimately linked to clinical decision-making. The quality of the collected data determines the choice of appropriate statistical methods. Nonparametric methods should be used for nominal and ordinal data, while interval data are usually analyzed by parametric statistical methods. Multivariate statistical methods, i.e., methods calculating the combined effect of different variables acting together and estimating their relative importance for the final outcome, have become more common in connection with extensive use of computerized data [1].

8.3 Epidemiology in endodontic research

Endodontology represents a field where, until recently, epidemiologic data have been scarce. Based on a survey of scientific endodontic journals, this has, however, gradually changed over the past few years [25]. Major textbooks in cariology and periodontology have for many years presented extensive epidemiologic documentation on prevalence of disease. This is not the case for endodontic textbooks. An exception may be Ingle and Bakland's "Washington study" which contains some epidemiologic characteristics [40,41]. In general, systematic description of symptoms, technical details and clinical procedures seem to be of major concern in the endodontic literature. There is also a lack of epidemiologic data on apical periodontitis in textbooks of oral pathology, oral radiology, and oral diagnosis thereby demonstrating the lack of a population-based approach to endodontic conditions.

There is a need to assess critically teaching practices and research approaches in endodontics. In a survey among US dental schools regarding possible areas for endodontic research, epidemiology was not mentioned among a total of 35 different topics [16]. Furthermore, guidelines for endodontic teaching programs do not regularly include endodontic epidemiology [26]. In an extensive survey of the state of the art and science of endodontics published in 2005 [76] the focus is mainly on technical details and endodontic epidemiology is not mentioned. Major oral health surveys either exclude radiographic documentation or apply only bitewing radiographs for caries/periodontal documentation, excluding the opportunities for endodontic evaluation [20].

8.3.1 Prevalence of apical periodontitis

Epidemiologic data about prevalence of apical periodontitis were primarily found from Scandinavian investigations, but during the past 15 years a number of international epidemiologic studies have been published contributing to a broader documentation of prevalence of apical periodontitis and endodontic treatment outcome in different societies [25,30,38,82]. A survey of available documentation including frequencies of subjects affected is given in Table 8.1. A mean of approximately one tooth per individual with apical periodontitis was detected. However, this was unevenly distributed in the populations studied. In Fig. 8.3 an overview of prevalence

of apical periodontitis and remaining teeth in various Swedish populations is presented. There is an age profile whereby older age increases the risk of apical periodontitis. There is also an uneven distribution among individuals, as half the individuals had no apical periodontitis (Table 8.1). Even when considering the skewness in distribution, apical periodontitis is widespread and constitutes both a diagnostic and a treatment challenge of large proportions. It is also both relevant and interesting to compare the prevalence of apical periodontitis with the prevalence of severe marginal periodontitis (inflamed periodontal pockets >5.5 mm, CPITN score 4) in different populations. Apical periodontitis appears to be more

Table 8.1 Prevalence of apical periodontitis in percentage of remaining teeth and percentage of individuals affected according to age

Reference	Age group (years)				
	20–30	30–40	40–50	50–60	60+
Apical periodontitis in % of remaining teeth					
Bergenholtz *et al.* 1973 [6] (Sweden)	2.9	5.2	7.3	8.4	7.7
Axelsson *et al.* 1977 [3] (Sweden)	2.0	4.1	5.5	6.5	8.7
Hugoson *et al.* 1986 [37] (Sweden)	1.2	3.6	5.5	8.0	9.0
Ödesjö *et al.* 1990 [58] (Sweden)	1.0	2.4	3.0	4.3	7.6
Eriksen and Bjertness 1991 [22] (Norway)		1.5	4.8		
Eriksen *et al.* 1995 [21] (Norway)		0.6			
Marques *et al.* 1998 [56] (Portugal)		2.0			
Sidaravicius *et al.* 1999 [77] (Lithuania)		7.2			
Kirkevang *et al.* 2001 [47] (Denmark)	0.6	1.8	3.1	6.6	9.2
Jimenez-Pinzon *et al.* 2004 [42] (Spain)	3.9	4.1	3.8	5.4	5.5
Loftus *et al.* 2005 [55] (Ireland)	1.2	2.3	2.2	2.7	2.5
Mean value	1.8	3.2	4.5	6.0	7.2
Apical periodontitis in % of individuals					
Lavstedt 1978 [54] (Sweden)	42	48	46	55	69
Laurell *et al.* 1983 [53] (Sweden)	12	39	51	56	68
Ödesjö *et al.* 1990 [58] (Sweden)	22	42	46	61	48
Eriksen *et al.* 1988 [23] (Norway)		30	49		
Eriksen *et al.* 1995 [21] (Norway)		14			
Marques *et al.* 1998 [56] (Portugal)		27			
Sidaravicius *et al.* 1999 [77] (Lithuania)		70			
Jimenez-Pinzon *et al.* 2004 [42] (Spain)	64	80	38	60	85
Kabak and Abbott 2005 [44] (Belarus)	45	85	85	82	85
Mean value	37	48	53	63	71

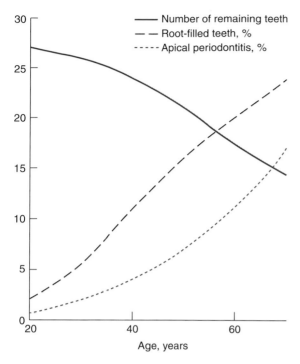

Fig. 8.3 Root-filled teeth and teeth with apical periodontitis given as percentage of remaining teeth of various Swedish populations [3,37,53,54]. (Reproduced from [20] with permission from Munksgaard.)

prevalent [22,23,37,53,54,58] than severe forms of marginal periodontitis [35,67,68] in selected European populations [25].

8.3.2 Intraoral distribution of apical periodontitis

Data both from epidemiologic and clinical research indicate that lateral maxillary incisors, first maxillary premolars, and first mandibular molars are the most prevalent teeth presenting with apical periodontitis [54]. This is usually explained by anatomical characteristics (apical deviations, accessory canals) resulting in unsuccessful endodontic treatment.

8.3.3 Acute and chronic apical periodontitis

To estimate the frequency of exacerbations of chronic apical periodontitis, longitudinal prospective epidemiologic investigations would offer the best opportunities. However, such investigations do not exist, in part due to ethical considerations. However, repetitive cross-sectional studies of the same sample also offer opportunities for proper estimates. Petersson *et al.* in Malmö, Sweden [62,64,66] and Eriksen *et al.* in Oslo, Norway [21] have both performed such investigations by reevaluating the endodontic status in the same individuals after 11 and 15 years, respectively. Both studies demonstrated that about half of the teeth with chronic apical periodontitis at the first investigation had been treated/retreated or extracted during the observation period. These data may indicate an incidence of exacerbations of less than 5% annually for chronic apical periodontitis. For the individual practitioner dealing with recall patients, less than one in 20 teeth with apical periodontitis will be in need of acute treatment between yearly recall appointments. However, within a 10-year period half of them may, and this represents the calculated risk of consciously leaving a tooth with apical periodontitis untreated.

8.3.4 Apical periodontitis and reasons for extractions

Dental caries and its sequelae, including apical periodontitis, seem to represent the most prevalent reasons for extraction of teeth. There is, however, an age profile where some investigations report periodontal problems to be a more prevalent reason than caries in higher age groups [51]. As apical periodontitis is usually not defined as a specific case for extraction, it is difficult to estimate its relative importance for extraction of teeth in society. It has been suggested that 10% of extractions performed among adult Swedes were due to apical periodontitis [18]. In a survey of 31 investigations dealing with reasons for extraction of permanent teeth [52], in only three [8,18,43] was apical periodontitis mentioned explicitly as the reason for extraction. One of them was an investigation performed by Brekhus as early as 1929 [8]. An interesting observation was that some additional investigations mentioned "failed endodontic treatment" and "pain" as reasons for extraction without explicitly defining pulpitis or apical periodontitis [4,12,72,83]. It can therefore be concluded that apical periodontitis has not been appreciated as a "disease" compared to, for instance, marginal periodontitis, but rather considered as a sequel to dental caries.

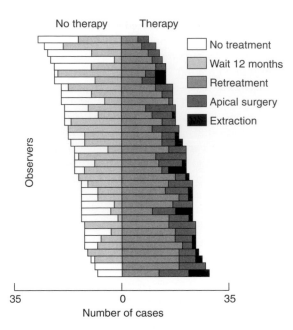

Fig. 8.4 Decisions made by 35 dentists on 33 cases. Each bar represents one observer. (Reproduced from [73] with permission from Swedish Dental Journal.)

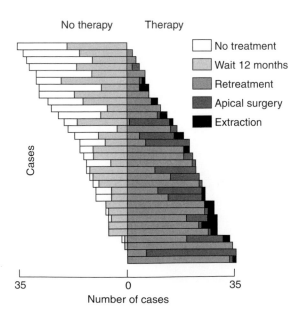

Fig. 8.5 Distribution of decisions made by 35 dentists on 33 cases. Each bar represents one case. (Reproduced from [73] with permission from *Swedish Dental Journal*.)

8.3.5 Radiographic diagnosis

The diagnosis of apical periodontitis based on radiographs is an uncertain process with wide variations among dentists [59,73,74]. This is linked both to the perception of the observed lesions per se and the perceived need for appropriate treatment (Figs 8.4 and 8.5). It has also been demonstrated that treatment suggestions are influenced both by the previous treatment performed and the planned restorative treatment for the tooth in question [63]. This makes the success/failure evaluation, commonly applied both in clinical and epidemiological endodontic investigations, a very uncertain procedure. It further indicates a lack of concern for the disease, i.e., apical periodontitis, underlying all endodontic treatment.

8.3.6 Epidemiologic versus clinical studies

There is a substantial discrepancy between the results of endodontic treatment recorded in epidemiological studies and in controlled clinical studies (Table 8.2). Based on evaluation of radiographs success rates of 77–94% are indicated from well-controlled clinical studies compared to 35–78% indicated from epidemiological studies. The former represent treatment performed by specialists or students under well-controlled and supervised conditions while the latter represent general practice. This discrepancy does not create problems of interpretation in relation to clinical endodontics if clinicians and researchers are both aware of the difference between clinical and epidemiological studies. If, however, results from well-controlled clinical studies are used uncritically as guidelines and standards for endodontic treatment in society, frustration and communication problems might result. The discrepancy between these two types of investigations should initiate analyses of major factors, explaining this difference and pragmatic solutions based on the possibilities and limitations related to general practice. Then what is ideally obtainable may serve as an inspiration instead of creating ignorance and the feeling of inferiority versus "the experts". It is interesting to observe that two recently published epidemiological investigations from the USA conclude with success rates similar to Scandinavian studies, and a close correlation between quality of the root canal filling and apical periodontitis [9,71]. In one of the studies [71], the quality and sealing ability of the coronal restoration

Table 8.2　Results of endodontic treatment based on the presence of apical periodontitis evaluated from radiographs. Comparison between clinical and epidemiological studies

Reference	Age Mean	(range)	Success	Uncertain	Failure
Clinical studies					
Strindberg 1956 [80] (Sweden)			87	3	10
Grahnén and Hansson 1961 [32] (Sweden)			83	5	12
Grossman et al. 1964 [33] (USA)			90	1	9
Engström et al. 1965 [19] (Sweden)			77	6	17
Harty et al. 1970 [36] (UK)	29	(15–45)	90	0	10
Molven 1974 [57] (Norway)	42	(15–65)	87	13	
Kerekes and Tronstad 1979 [46] (Norway)	48	(10–80)	91	4	5
Barbakow et al. 1980 [5] (South Africa)			87		13
Ingle 1985 [40] (USA)			94		6
Ørstavik et al. 1987 [60] (Norway)	46	(20–80)	93		7
Friedman et al. 1995 [28] (Canada)			81		19
Caliskan et al. 1996 [11] (USA)			81	8	11
Sjögren et al. 1990 [78] (Sweden)			91		9
Peters et al. 2002 [61] (The Netherlands)			76	21	3
Mean value			86	6	9
Epidemiological studies					
Bergenholtz et al. 1973 [6] (Sweden)	45	(20–70)	69		31
Kerekes and Bervell 1976 [45] (Norway)	33	(20–60)	75		25
Axelsson et al. 1977 [3] (Sweden)	45	(20–70)	75		25
Laurell et al. 1983 [53] (Sweden)	45	(20–70)	75		25
Hugoson et al. 1986 [37] (Sweden)	50	(20–80)	70		30
Allard and Palmquist 1986 [2] (Sweden)	73	(65–80)	73		27
Petersson et al. 1986 [65] (Sweden)		(20–60)	69		31
Bergström et al. 1987 [7] (Sweden)	41	(21–60)	71		29
Eriksen et al. 1988 [23] (Norway)	35		66		34
Eckerbom et al. 1989 [17] (Sweden)	45	(20–60+)	77		23
Eriksen and Bjertness [22] 1991 (Norway)	50		64		36
Ödesjö et al. 1990 [58] (Sweden)	45	(20–80)	75		25
Imfeld 1991 [39] (Switzerland)	66		69		31
De Cleen et al. 1993 [13] (Belgium)	38	(20–59+)	61		39
Buckley and Spångberg 1995 [9] (USA)	45		69		31
Ray and Trope 1995 [71] (USA)			61		39
Saunders et al. 1997 [75] (Scotland)		(20–60+)	42		58
Weiger et al. 1997 [84] (Germany)	39		61		
Marques et al. 1998 [56] (Portugal)	35	(30–39)	78		22
Sidaravicius et al. 1999 [77] (Lithuania)	40	(35–44)	65		35
De Moor et al. 2000 [14] (Belgium)	>18		60		40
Kirkevang et al. 2001 [47] (Denmark)		(20–60)	48		52
Dugas et al. 2003 [15] (Canada)		(25–40)	56		44
Dugas et al. 2003 [15] (Canada)		(25–40)	49		51
Jimenez-Pinzon et al. 2004 [42] (Spain)	37	(18–60+)	35		65
Kabak and Abbott 2005 [44] (Belarus)	46	(15–65+)	55		45
Loftus et al. 2005 [55] (Ireland)			75		25
Georgopoulou et al. 2005 [31] (Greece)	48	(16–77)	40		60
Mean value	45		63		37

was also found to correlate with the final outcome of endodontic treatment.

There is no doubt that the quality of endodontic treatment in society should be improved. Lack of epidemiological data, both descriptive and analytical, has so far represented a limitation in exchange of ideas between epidemiologists and clinicians. This situation is, however, about to change.

Information published within clinical science can be divided into three categories: case reports, well-controlled clinical studies, and epidemiology. This is of relevance to clinical endodontology. Case reports usually represent extremes in cost–benefit and not what might usually be expected from endodontic treatment. The unusual is the issue and even when summed up, the results represent averages of extremes and can be misleading as guidelines for clinical practice.

8.3.7 Cost–benefit considerations

The interplay between health outcomes and resources invested in general versus specialist practice is illustrated in Fig. 8.6. Simple cases may be treated more effectively in general practice, while for complicated cases specialists may provide treatment at a lower cost–benefit ratio. An interplay between clinical and epidemiological data and knowledge is necessary in order to define the breakpoint where the two lines are crossing, indicating a proper balance between specialists and general practice. Results from selected case reports are frequently used in such discussions, but are of little relevance and can even be misleading when used uncritically.

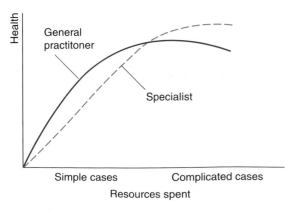

Fig. 8.6 Hypothetical cost–benefit calculation of general/specialist treatment according to severity of the case.

8.3.8 Reasons for treatment failure

While the prevalence of apical periodontitis related to endodontically treated teeth under well-controlled conditions is markedly lower [27,28] than what is reported from epidemiologic studies [25] (Table 8.2), there is general agreement about the most common reasons for treatment failures [27,78]. From epidemiologic studies, the technical quality of the treatment performed (complete/incomplete and optimal length/over- or under-extended root filling) strongly influences the final outcome. This is also documented from clinical studies [27]. There are, however, obvious limitations linked to the analysis of reasons for failures in both these types of studies.

In epidemiologic studies, only the quality of the root filling and the periapical conditions as they appear in radiographs constitute the basis for evaluation. The treatment conditions, e.g., asepsis, materials used, age of the filling and accessibility, are unknown. Thereby, the evaluation of reasons for failure is limited to what can be observed at the time of investigation. Some factors having an indirect impact on the treatment result cannot be evaluated. With a few exceptions [1,22] a consistent lack of multivariate approaches, disclosing the relative importance of various factors acting together also represents a problem. This is a challenge for epidemiologists dealing with endodontic problems, particularly because such analyses will be of direct relevance to general practice.

A series of epidemiologic dental health studies on 35-year-old people in Oslo, Norway, has included information on endodontic conditions [22,79]. By introducing the presence of apical periodontitis as the dependent variable and dental health, social and behavioral variables as independent variables in a multiple regression analysis, previous endodontic treatment, oral hygiene, and caries experience appeared as the strongest determinants. The total set of variables explained 27% of the total distribution of apical periodontitis studied [22]. Details regarding endodontic treatment, e.g., asepsis, materials used, quality of treatment, were unavailable and therefore not included in the analyses. Even with this limitation, 27% explained variance must be considered satisfactory as a meaningful evaluation of the results. Previous endodontic treatment as the strongest determinant for the presence of apical periodontitis indicates that the present treatment procedures, as they are applied in general practice in the population studied, do not solve the problem. This finding is supported by many clinical and epidemiologic studies [27,48,49,50].

8.3.9 Apicectomy and apical periodontitis

Nonsurgical endodontic treatment is the method of choice in most instances. It has repeatedly been shown that when root canal treatment is properly performed, surgical intervention can usually be avoided. However, when apical periodontitis persists either due to an inaccessible root canal, persistent extra-radicular infection, foreign bodies in the periapical tissues, or for other unknown reasons, apical surgery may be indicated. Index systems based on the pattern of apical structures after surgical removal are established and success rates of up to 90% are reported from specialist practices [34] while epidemiologic data are lacking.

8.3.10 General epidemiologic considerations

Too frequently, epidemiologic data on the distribution of apical periodontitis are presented as average values. The reduction of data to calculated means may hide valuable information related to the following questions:

- Who is suffering from apical periodontitis and who may require special attention?
- Who will benefit from eventual interventions, e.g., changing diagnostic routines and recommended changes of treatment?
- How many cases of apical periodontitis need to be retreated and what characterizes these cases?

Study designs carefully considering such questions should be implemented in future studies.

8.4 Conclusions

Two questions were raised initially in this chapter:

- Is it possible with present-day knowledge and modern principles of endodontic treatment to control and eliminate apical periodontitis?
- To what extent are we as a dental profession succeeding in eradicating apical periodontitis?

The following answers may be given based on epidemiologic information about apical periodontitis:

- Experimental and clinical research has demonstrated that over 90% success may be achieved by applying modern principles of endodontic treatment based on infection control.
- Epidemiologic research has clearly demonstrated that the potential for this knowledge is not fully utilized in general practice.

The challenges for the future must be to implement the principles documented by experimental and clinical research within the framework of general practice and, in addition, develop relevant procedures for using specialty competence when necessary.

8.4.1 Technical quality

Epidemiologic studies have clearly documented a strong association between technical quality of root fillings and prevalence of apical periodontitis. However, what is unclear is whether this quality problem is due to lack of knowledge, use of inappropriate materials, lack of clinical skills, economic considerations, or attitude/quality consciousness. Epidemiologic research should try to focus on these questions in a multifactorial perspective.

8.4.2 Infection control

Apical periodontitis is an infectious disease and epidemiologic research indirectly confirms that anti-infective measures such as the use of rubber dam and proper antiseptic irrigation during treatment are essential for success.

8.4.3 Biological considerations

The prevalence of apical periodontitis has been intimately linked to endodontic treatment. It should be acknowledged that apical periodontitis frequently is a sequel to inadequate management of dental caries and inferior prosthetic treatment. Ultimately, caries prevention may therefore be the ideal way of solving the major part of apical periodontitis in society, rather than exclusively concentrating on improved endodontic techniques and procedures.

8.5 References

1. Aleksejuniene J, Eriksen HM, Sidaravicius B, Haapasalo M (2000) Apical periodontitis and related factors in an adult Lithuanian population. *Oral Surgery,*

Oral Medicine, Oral Pathology, Oral Radiology and Endodontics **90**, 95–101.

2. Allard U, Palmquist S (1986) A radiographic survey of periapical conditions in elderly people in a Swedish county population. *Endodontics and Dental Traumatology* **2**, 103–8.

3. Axelsson P, Hugoson A, Koch G, Ludvigsson H-G, Paulander J, Pettersson S, *et al.* (1977) Tandhälsotillståndet hos 1000 peroner I åldrarna 3 till 70 år inom Jönköping Kommun. III. Röntgendiagnostisk undersökning av tänder och käker. *Tandläkartidningen* **69**, 1006–17.

4. Bailit HL, Braun R, Maryniuk GA, Camp P (1987) Is periodontal disease the primary cause of tooth extraction in adults? *Journal of the American Dental Association* **114**, 40–5.

5. Barbakow FH, Cleaton-Jones P, Friedman D (1980) An evaluation of 566 cases of root canal therapy in general dental practice. 2. Postoperative observations. *Journal of Endodontics* **6**, 485–9.

6. Bergenholtz G, Malmcrona E, Milton R (1973) Endodontisk behandling och periapikalstatus. I. Röntgenologisk undersökningav frekvensen av endodontiskt behandlade tänder och frekvensen apikala destruktioner. *Tandläkartidningen* **65**, 64–73.

7. Bergström J, Eliasson S, Ahlberg KF (1987) Periapical status in subjects with regular dental care habits. *Community Dentistry and Oral Epidemiology* **15**, 236–9.

8. Brekhus PJ (1929) Dental disease and its relation to the loss of human teeth. *Journal of the American Dental Association* **16**, 2237–47.

9. Buckley M, Spångberg LSW (1995) The prevalence and technical quality of endodontic treatment in an American subpopulation. *Oral Surgery, Oral Medicine, Oral Pathology* **79**, 92–100.

10. Byström A (1986) Evaluation of endodontic treatment of teeth with apical periodontitis. Thesis. Umeå: University of Umeå.

11. Caliskan MK, Sen BH (1996) Endodontic treatment of teeth with apical periodontitis using calcium hydroxide: a long-term study. *Endodontics and Dental Traumatology* **12**, 215–21.

12. Corbet EF, Davies WIR (1990) Reasons given for tooth extraction in Hong Kong. *Community Dental Health* **8**, 121–30.

13. De Cleen MJH, Schuurs AHB, Wesselink PR, Wu MK (1993) Periapical status and prevalence of endodontic treatment in adult Dutch population. *International Endodontic Journal* **26**, 112–19.

14. De Moor RGJ, Hommez GMG, DeBoever JG, Delme KIM, Martens GEI (2000) Periapical health related to the quality of root canal treatment in a Belgian population. *International Endodontic Journal* **33**, 113–20.

15. Dugas NN, Lawrence HP, Teplitsky PE, Pharoah MJ, Friedman S (2003) Periapical health and treatment quality assessment of root-filled teeth in two Canadian populations. *International Endodontic Journal* **36**, 181–92.

16. Dumsha TC, Gutmann JL (1986) The status and direction of endodontic research for the 1980s. *Journal of Endodontics* **12**, 174–6.

17. Eckerbom M, Andersson JE, Magnusson T (1989) A longitudinal study of changes in frequency and technical standard of endodontic treatment in a Swedish population. *Endodontics and Dental Traumatology* **5**, 27–31.

18. Eckerbom M, Magnusson T, Martinsson T (1992) Reasons for and incidence of tooth mortality in a Swedish population. *Endodontics and Dental Traumatology* **8**, 230–4.

19. Engström B, Lundberg M (1965) The correlation between positive culture and the prognosis of root canal therapy after pulpectomy. *Odontologisk Revy* **16**, 193–203.

20. Eriksen HM (1991) Endodontology – epidemiologic considerations. *Endodontics and Dental Traumatology* **7**, 189–95.

21. Eriksen HM, Berset GP, Hansen BF, Bjertness E (1995) Changes in endodontic status 1973–1993 among 35-year-olds in Oslo, Norway. *International Endodontic Journal* **28**, 129–32.

22. Eriksen HM, Bjertness E (1991) Prevalence of apical periodontitis and results of endodontic treatment in middle-aged adults in Norway. *Endodontics and Dental Traumatology* **7**, 1–4.

23. Eriksen HM, Bjertness E, Ørstavik D (1988) Prevalence and quality of endodontic treatment in an adult, urban population in Norway. *Endodontics and Dental Traumatology* **4**, 122–6.

24. Eriksen HM, Dimitrov V (2003) Ecology of oral health: a complexity perspective. *European Journal of Oral Sciences* **111**, 285–90.

25. Eriksen HM, Kirkevang L-L, Petersson K (2002) Endodontic epidemiology and treatment outcome: general considerations. *Endodontic Topics* **2**, 1–9.

26. European Society for Endodontology (1992) Undergraduate curriculum guidelines for endodontology. *International Endodontic Journal* **25**, 169–72.

27. Friedman S (2002) Prognosis of initial endodontic therapy. *Endodontic Topics* **2**, 59–88.

28. Friedman S, Abitbol S, Lawrence HP (2003) Treatment outcome in endodontics: The Toronto study. Phase 1: Initial treatment. *Journal of Endodontics* **29**, 787–93.

29. Friedman S, Lost C, Zarrabian M, Trope M (1995) Evaluation of success and failure after endodontic therapy using a glass ionomer cement. *Journal of Endodontics* **21**, 384–90.

30. Frisk F, Hakeberg M (2006) Socio-economic risk indicators for apical periodontitis. *Acta Odontologica Scandinavica* **64**, 123–8.

31. Georgoupoulou MK, Spanaki-Voreadi AP, Pantazis N, Kontakiotis EG (2005) Frequency and distribution of root filled teeth and apical periodontitis in a Greek population. *International Endodontic Journal* **38**, 105–11.

32. Grahnén H, Hansson L (1961) The prognosis of pulp and root canal therapy. A clinical and radiographic follow-up examination. *Odontologisk Revy* **12**, 146–65.

33. Grossman LI, Shephard LI, Pearson LA (1964) Roentgenologic and clinical evaluation of endodontically treated teeth. *Oral Surgery, Oral Medicine, Oral Pathology* **17**, 368–74.

34. Grung B, Molven O, Halse A (1990) Periapical surgery in a Norwegian county hospital: follow-up findings in 477 teeth. *Journal of Endodontics* **16**, 411–17.

35. Grytten J, Holst D, Gjermo P (1989) Validity of CPITN's hierarchial scoring method for describing prevalence of periodontal conditions. *Community Dentistry and Oral Epidemiology* **17**, 300–3.

36. Harty FJ, Parkins BJ, Wengraf AM (1970) Success rate in root canal therapy. A retrospective study on conventional cases. *British Dental Journal* **128**, 65–70.

37. Hugoson A, Koch G, Bergendahl T, Hallonsten AL, Laurell L, Lundgren D, *et al.* (1986) Oral health of individuals aged 3–80 years in Jönköping, Sweden, in 1973 and 1983. II. A review of clinical and radiographic findings. *Swedish Dental Journal* **10**, 175–94.

38. Hülsmann M (1995) Epidemiologische Daten zur Endodontie (I). *Endodontie* **3**, 193–203.

39. Imfeld TN (1991) Prevalence and quality of endodontic treatment in an elderly, urban population in Switzerland. *Journal of Endodontics* **17**, 604–7.

40. Ingle JI, Bakland LK (1985) Modern endodontic therapy. In Ingle JI, Bakland LK, editors. *Endodontics*, 3rd edn, p. 34. Philadelphia, PA: Lea & Febiger.

41. Ingle JI, Bakland LK, editors (1994) *Endodontics,* 4th edn. Baltimore, MD: Williams & Wilkins.

42. Jimenez-Pinzon A, Segura-Egea JJ, Poyato-Ferrera M, Velasco-Ortega E, Rios-Santos JV (2004) prevalence of apical periodontitis and frequency of root-filled teeth in an adult Spanish population. *International Endodontic Journal* **37**, 167–73.

43. Johansen SB, Johansen JR (1977) A survey of causes of permanent tooth extractions in South Australia. *Australian Dental Journal* **22**, 238–42.

44. Kabak Y, Abbott PV (2005) Prevalence of apical periodontitis and the quality of endodontic treatment in an adult Belarusian population. *International Endodontic Journal* **38**, 238–45.

45. Kerekes K, Bervell SFA (1976) En røntgenologisk vurdering av endodontisk behandlingsbehov. *Den Norske Tannlaegeforenings Tidende* **86**, 248–54.

46. Kerekes K, Tronstad L (1979) Long term results of endodontic treatment performed with a standardized technique. *Journal of Endodontics* **5**, 83–90.

47. Kirkevang L-L, Hörsted-Bindslev P, Ørstavik D, Wenzel A (2001) Frequency and distribution of endodontically treated teeth and apical periodontitis in an urban Danish population. *International Endodontic Journal* **34**, 198–205.

48. Kirkevang LL, Vaeth M, Horsted-Bindslev P, Wenzel A (2006) Longitudinal study of periapical and endodontic status in a Danish population. *International Endodontic Journal.* **39**, 100–7.

49. Kirkevang LL, Vaeth M, Wenzel A (2004) Tooth-specific risk indicators for apical periodontitis. *Oral Surgery, Oral Medicine, Oral Pathology, Oral Radiology and Endodontics* **97**, 739–44.

50. Kirkevang LL, Wenzel A (2003) Risk indicators for apical periodontitis. *Community Dentistry and Oral Epidemiology.* **31**, 59–67.

51. Klock KS, Haugejorden O (1991) Primary reasons for extractions of permanent teeth in Norway: Changes from 1968 to 1988. *Community Dentistry and Oral Epidemiology* **19**, 336–41.

52. Klock KS (1995) A multidimensional study of aspects relating to extractions of permanent teeth in Norway. Thesis. Bergen: University of Bergen.

53. Laurell L, Holm G, Hedin M (1983) Tandhälsan hos vuksna i Gävleborgs län. *Tandläkartidningen* **75**, 759–77.

54. Lavstedt S (1978) Behovet av tandhälsovård och tandsjukvård hos en normalpopulation. rebusundersökningen II. *Tandläkartidningen* **70**, 971–91.

55. Loftus JJ, Keating AP, McCartan BE (2005) Periapical status and quality of endodontic treatment in an adult Irish population. *International Endodontic Journal* **38**, 81–6.

56. Marques MD, Moreira B, Eriksen HM (1998) Prevalence of apical periodontitis and results of endodontic treatment in an adult, Portuguese population. *International Endodontic Journal* **31**, 161–5.

57. Molven O (1974) The frequency, technical standard and results of endodontic therapy. Thesis. Bergen: University of Bergen.

58. Ödesjö B, Hellden L, Salonen L, Langeland K (1990) Prevalence of previous endodontic treatment, technical standard and occurrence of periapical lesions in a randomly selected adult general population. *Endodontics and Dental Traumatology* **6**, 265–72.

59. Ørstavik D, Kerekes K, Eriksen HM (1986) The periapical index: a scoring system for radiographic assessment of apical periodontitis. *Endodontics and Dental Traumatology* **2**, 20–34.

60. Ørstavik D, Kerekes K, Eriksen HM (1987) Clinical performance of three endodontic sealers. *Endodontics and Dental Traumatology* **3**, 178–86.

61. Peters LB, Wesselink PR (2002) Periapical healing of endodontically treated teeth in one and two visits obturated in the presence or absence of detectable microorganisms. *International Endodontic Journal* **35**, 660–67.

62. Petersson K, Håkansson R, Håkansson J, Olsson B, Wennberg A (1991) Follow-up study of endodontic status in an adult Swedish population. *Endodontics and Dental Traumatology* **7**, 221–5.

63. Petersson K, Lewin B, Håkansson J, Olsson B, Wennberg A (1989) Endodontic status and suggested treatment in a population requiring substantial dental care. *Endodontics and Dental Traumatology* **5**, 153–8.

64. Petersson K, Pamenius M, Eliasson A, Narby B, Holender F, Palmqvist S, Hakansson J (2006) 20-year follow-up of patients receiving high-cost dental care within the Swedish Dental Insurance System: 1977–1978 to 1998–2000. *Swedish Dental Journal* **30**, 77–86.

65. Petersson K, Petersson A, Olsson B, Håkansson J, Wennberg A (1986) Technical quality of root fillings in an adult Swedish population. *Endodontics and Dental Traumatology* **2**, 99–102.

66. Petersson K (1993) Endodontic status of mandibular premolars and molars in an adult Swedish population. A longitudinal study 1974–1985. *Endodontics and Dental Traumatology* **9**, 13–18.

67. Pilot T, Miyazaki H, Leclercq MH, Barmes DE (1992) Profiles of periodontal conditions in older age cohorts

measured by CPITN. *International Dental Journal* **42**, 23–30.

68. Pilot T, Miyazaki H (1991) Periodontal conditions in Europe. *Journal of Clinical Periodontology* **18**, 353–7.

69. Pober JS, Neuhauser CS, Pober JM (2001) Obstacles facing translational research in academic medical centers. *FASEB Journal* **15**, 2303–13.

70. Portenier I (2005) Factors confounding the *in vitro* activity of root canal disinfectants against *Enterococcus faecalis*. Thesis. Oslo: University of Oslo.

71. Ray HA, Trope M (1995) Periapical status endodontically treated teeth in relation to the root filling and the coronal restoration. *International Endodontic Journal* **28**, 12–18.

72. Reich E, Hiller KA (1993) Reasons for tooth extractions in the western states of Germany. *Community Dentistry and Oral Epidemiology* **21**, 379–83.

73. Reit C, Gröndahl H-G (1984) Management of periapical lesions in endodontically treated teeth. A study on clinical decision making. *Swedish Dental Journal* **8**, 1–7.

74. Reit C, Hollender L (1983) Radiographic evaluation of endodontic therapy and the influence of observer variation. *Scandinavian Journal of Dental Research* **91**, 205–12.

75. Saunders WP, Saunders EM, Sadiq J, Cruickshank E (1997) Technical standard of root canal treatment in an adult Scottish sub-population. *British Dental Journal* **182**, 382–6.

76. Sharbahang S (2005) State of the art and science of endodontics. *Journal of the American Dental Association* **136**, 40–52.

77. Sidaravicius B, Aleksejuniene J, Eriksen HM (1999) Endodontic treatment and prevalence of apical periodontitis in an adult population of Vilnius, Lithuania. *Endodontics and Dental Traumatology* **15**, 210–15.

78. Sjögren U, Hägglund B, Sundqvist G, Wing K (1990) Factors affecting the long-term results of endodontic treatment. *Journal of Endodontics* **16**, 498–504.

79. Skudutyte-Rysstad R, Eriksen HM (2006) Endodontic status amongst 35-year-old Oslo citizens and changes over a 30-year period. *International Endodontic Journal*. **39**, 637–42.

80. Strindberg LZ (1956) The dependence of the results of pulp therapy on certain factors. An analytic study based on clinical, radiographic and clinical follow-up examinations. *Acta Odontologica Scandinavica* Suppl. 21.

81. Sundqvist G, Figdor D, Persson S, Sjögren U (1998) Microbiologic analysis of teeth with failed endodontic treatment and the outcome of conservative retreatment. *Oral Surgery, Oral Medicine, Oral Pathology, Oral Radiology and Endodontics* **85**, 86–93.

82. Tsuneishi M, Yamamoto T, Yamanaka R, Tamaki N, Sakamoto T, Tsuji K, Watanabe T (2005) Radiographic evaluation of periapical status and prevalence of endodontic treatment in an adult Japanese population. *Oral Surgery, Oral Medicine, Oral Pathology, Oral Radiology and Endodontics* **100**, 631–5.

83. Vignarajah S (1993) Various reasons for permanent tooth extractions in a Carribean population – Antigua. *International Dental Journal* **43**, 207–12.

84. Weiger R, Hitzler S, Hemle G, Lost C (1997) Periapical status of root canal fillings and estimated endodontic treatment needs in an urban German population. *Endodontics and Dental Traumatology* **13**, 69–74.

Chapter 9

Prevention and Management of Apical Periodontitis in Primary Teeth

Heather Pitt Ford

9.1 Introduction

In spite of the great advances in prevention of dental caries by water fluoridation, better control of oral hygiene, and use of pit and fissure sealants, primary teeth are still lost prematurely due to caries and its sequelae. The reasons for retaining primary teeth include prevention of pain, maintenance of aesthetics, speech and mastication, preservation of arch length and the avoidance of drifting of permanent teeth, and subsequent malocclusion [97]. Preventive endodontics in primary teeth should aim first to prevent pulp exposure, inflammation or death of the pulp, or second to preserve the vitality of the remaining pulp if part has become irreversibly diseased, thus allowing normal exfoliation and preventing damage to the successional tooth. It has been shown that untreated inflammation and infection of a primary tooth can damage the tooth germ of the permanent successor and surrounding structures [26]. Retention of a non-vital primary tooth may lead to deflection of the permanent successor [25]. If root canal treatment does become necessary care must be taken not to damage the underlying permanent tooth.

Two questions concerning pulp conservation that confront the dentist are how to protect the pulp, and how to encourage healing of a damaged pulp. What is the treatment of choice to minimize the risk of death of the pulp, thus preventing damage to the developing permanent tooth germ, or to avoid the need to extract the tooth? An analysis of these factors can be better understood after reviewing the physiology and pathology of the pulp–dentin complex [61,62].

9.2 Pulp–dentin complex

The dentin and the pulp must be studied together because, in spite of their great physical dissimilarities, these tissues are interdependent and react as a single physiological unit. The coronal part of the pulp is covered by dentin and enamel and the radicular part by dentin and cementum. As long as their continuity is maintained, the pulp is protected and remains healthy. Occasionally, a great force applied on the apical blood supply, such as trauma, may produce changes in the pulp leading to its degeneration or death. However, most pathologic pulp conditions begin with a breach of one of the outer protective barriers, e.g., by dental caries, fractures, attrition, or operative procedures [18]. As a result, a communication is established between the pulp and the oral cavity, via the dentinal tubules or directly. Under these conditions, bacteria and their toxins may permeate the tubules causing stimulation of the odontoblasts, to lay down reactionary dentin. However, if the infection is more severe, inflammation and possibly death of the pulp ensues. Because primary teeth have a thinner layer of enamel and dentin than permanent teeth and wider dentin tubules this process tends to take place very rapidly, and is especially evident in the case of nursing bottle caries in very young children.

9.2.1 Dentin and dentin permeability

Dentin of primary teeth is a calcified tissue traversed by millions of tubules so that it is quite porous. Its structure is similar to that of permanent teeth. The tubules contain a fluid similar to extracellular fluid. If, as a result of dental caries, bacterial toxins penetrate the fluid space, they become a source of injurious agents to the pulp. The surface area occupied by tubules at different levels is a function of tubule density and diameter. At the dentino-enamel junction only a small area is occupied by tubules but this figure increases substantially at the periphery of the pulp chamber. The clinical implications of this configuration are important because, if dentin becomes exposed and some of the tissue is removed, the greater the depth, the greater the permeability [77]; in a deep cavity the pulp is more susceptible to bacterial irritation, although this is modulated by the lessened permeability of carious dentin [120].

9.2.2 Pulp

The pulp is in intimate contact with dentin, which is protected by enamel and cementum. The pulp contains cells, intercellular substance, fibers and other elements, such as vessels and nerves. Histological studies on the pulps of primary teeth have shown their similarity to those of permanent teeth [45,162]. The odontoblasts line the periphery of the pulp space and extend their cytoplasmic processes into the dentinal tubules. The pattern of the odontoblast layer is: columnar odontoblasts in the coronal pulp, cuboidal cells in the middle region and flat ones in the apical region. Beneath the odontoblast layer is the cell-free zone that contains a plexus of unmyelinated nerves and blood capillaries. The principal roles of the pulp are formation of the dentin and participation in the defense process. The pulp contains large blood vessels that are orientated coronally and exhibit increased branching as they approach the subodontoblast layer [125]. Numerous capillaries are evenly distributed around the peripheral regions and small arterioles are located more centrally. Small arterioles also run parallel to the subodontoblastic nerve plexus. Primary teeth appear more vascular in the mid-coronal region than permanent teeth [134]. Mature primary teeth contain pulp that is well innervated and has many nerve endings terminating in or near the odontoblast layer, with a number penetrating into dentin [35].

It has been shown that there are quantitative differences in coronal nerve distribution between the dentitions, with permanent teeth demonstrating a greater innervation density in all regions investigated [132]; however, the authors caution against speculation that this may have functional significance in terms of nociceptive potential.

There appear to be no significant differences in overall innervation (or peptide-related innervation) of blood vessels between primary and permanent teeth, indicating that pulpal blood flow is likely to be subject to similar neurological control mechanisms in both dentitions [133]. Collagenous fibers appear coarse, densely packed and coronally orientated in the apical third of the pulp, whereas in the middle and coronal thirds, the fibers are thin, loosely packed and randomly orientated. This distribution of collagen fibers is similar to that in permanent teeth. Immune cells have been shown to extend their cytoplasmic processes into the dentinal tubules [71]. It has been suggested that immune cells in the coronal pulp of human primary teeth play an inductive role in the differentiation, migration and/or activation of the osteoclasts and cementoblast-like cells during the stages of tooth resorption [71]; however, other work suggests that their role in resorption is unclear [5].

9.2.3 Morphology of the root canal system

Root canal treatment presupposes a thorough knowledge of the anatomy of the teeth and their root canal systems. Some characteristics are common to all primary teeth. The root to crown ratio is greater than that of permanent teeth. The roots of primary teeth are more slender, and in the molars, they diverge more widely to allow room for the permanent tooth germs. The roots of the primary teeth do not complete their formation until several years after tooth eruption, and their physiological resorption begins soon thereafter. This process usually starts on the surface closest to the permanent tooth germs. The developing permanent teeth lie lingual and apical to the primary anterior teeth. Because of this relationship, resorption of the primary incisors is initiated on the lingual surface in the apical third of the root. In molars, it starts on the inner surfaces of the roots. This has implications for the shifting location of the apical foramen.

In the newly completed roots of primary teeth, the apical foramina are located near the anatomical apices of the roots. However, as resorption progresses, the root is shortened and the foramen moves coronally. From the radiograph it may not be possible to discern the exact site of the foramen because resorption may not be symmetrical, and it may erode one of the walls to the point of opening a communication with the periodontium at a site coronal to the apical-most extent of the root observed on the radiograph. Many primary teeth have accessory canals in the furcation region (Fig. 9.1) [175]. For these reasons the inflammatory lesion associated with a primary tooth is better termed periradicular rather than periapical. In some cases resorption even separates part of the roots of a molar.

Understanding the morphogenesis of the teeth permits a better comprehension of the common variations that occur in the form and number of root canals. During root formation, the apical foramen of each root has a wide opening limited by Hertwig's root sheath, but deposition of additional dentin and cementum creates multiple apical ramifications of the canal as it exits the root [63], just as in permanent teeth.

The form and shape of the root canals of anterior primary teeth resemble the form and shape of the exterior of the teeth. In the maxilla, the canals of the primary central and lateral incisors are almost round but slightly compressed in the bucco-lingual

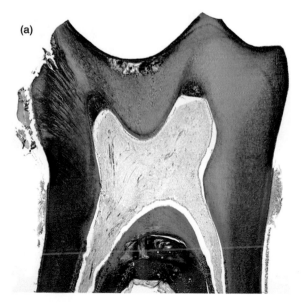
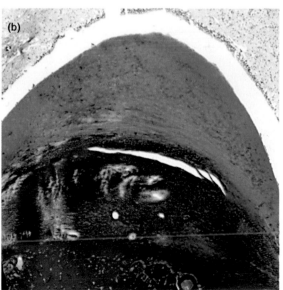

Fig. 9.1 (a) Histological section of a primary molar showing dental caries (left) normal pulp, and canals in the furcation (original magnification ×10). (b) Higher magnification of furcation showing canals and secondary dentin laid over the furcation. Masson's trichrome stain (original magnification ×50).

direction. These teeth have one canal. Apical rami-fications or accessory and lateral canals are rare but do exist. The pulp chamber in the maxillary incisors is situated in a facial position. In the mandible, the root canals of the primary incisors are flattened on the mesial and distal aspects. These root surfaces are sometimes grooved, leading to a narrowing down of the root canal and possible division into two canals, yet the incidence of two canals is low. Occasionally lateral and accessory canals are observed. The pulp chamber of mandibular primary incisors is in a lingual position.

The morphology of the root canal system of primary molar teeth has been well documented and studied by injection–corrosion methods [63,181] and is considered briefly here.

At the beginning of root formation each molar root had only one root canal. Following continued root formation, the morphology of the root canals changed, producing variations in the number and size of canals. The deposition of irritation dentin was responsible for the variation. In addition to variation in the number of root canals, there are lateral branches, communication between canals, apical ramifications, and fusion of roots.

Average lengths of individual root canals have been reviewed [140]; the complexity of the root canal system has also been demonstrated using newer methods, such as computerized tomography [180]. In a clinical study buccal roots of mandibular molars were shown to be longer than lingual roots; this has been attributed to resorption following development of the germ of the permanent successor [128].

9.3 Pulp and periradicular disease

9.3.1 Etiology

Dental caries is the most common cause of pulp injury in primary teeth (Fig. 9.2). Injury is also caused by dental trauma [4]. Pulp changes resulting from caries range from early formation of reactionary dentin under initial caries, to accumulation of chronic inflammatory exudate under deep carious lesions [162]. If carious dentin or biofilm is sealed in a deep cavity, pulp inflammation begins within hours, but following removal of the irritant and sealing the cavity, the pulp can recover. Healing in experimentally inflamed pulps was noted after 7–8 days [100]. Moderate to severe inflammation of the pulp may heal if the irritating agents are removed from the dentin [10]. The close correlation between dentin and pulp has also been investigated [152]. However, in the usual process of dental caries, invasion of dentin occurs gradually and it can be slowed by the pulp–dentin reaction of tubular sclerosis [120,159].

9.3.2 Pulp reactions

Primary teeth are capable of a defense reaction similar to that of permanent teeth, even where the pulp is inflamed as a result of dental caries [159]. With mild-to-moderate stimuli, dentin with a relatively normal structure has been formed (Fig. 9.3) [74]. Areas devoid of tubules had a similar appearance to regular intertubular dentin, and occluded tubules had a higher mineral content than intertubular dentin [74].

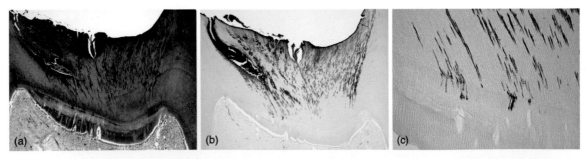

Fig. 9.2 (a) Histological section of a primary molar with occlusal caries and new regular dentin formed under affected tubules; the odontoblast layer is intact, Masson's trichrome stain (original magnification ×20). (b) Adjacent section stained for bacteria with a large cleft (left) filled with bacterial biofilm, Brown and Brenn stain (original magnification ×20). (c) Higher magnification of caries showing bacteria in original dentinal tubules and entering tubules of newly formed dentin, Brown and Brenn stain (original magnification ×100).

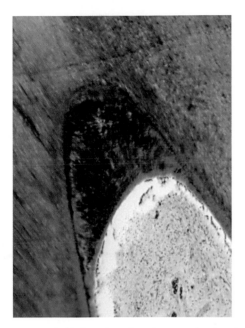

Fig. 9.3 Histological section of a primary molar showing new dentin laid down in the pulp horn, Masson's trichrome stain (original magnification ×50); this is a higher magnification of part of Figure 9.1.

Reparative dentin in human primary teeth is secreted by a new generation of odontoblast-like cells that have been subject to strong stimuli, e.g., trauma or deep active caries associated with pulpal inflammation [75]. In response to strong stimuli the morphology of the tissue is varied, indicating that different stimuli lead to induction of hard-tissue-forming cells that produce different types of hard tissue (Fig. 9.4) [75]. In the pulp chamber and especially in the root canals, resorption had often occurred, indicating that signals giving rise to odontoclasts were also present. Resorption was often followed by deposition of various amounts of cementum-like repair tissue [75]. Primary tooth pulp has been shown to maintain its healing and defense capacity against the advancing carious lesion and progressive root resorption [151], suggesting that vital pulp therapy is appropriate if the status of the pulp is accurately diagnosed.

The severity of the pulp reaction to dental caries and to operative procedures is inversely related to the remaining dentin thickness and degree of calcification of the remaining dentin over the pulp. The primary pulp is surrounded by a relatively thin layer of calcified tissues and the small dimensions of these tissues together with wide dentin tubules facilitate rapid spread of bacterial toxins to the pulp. In

(a)

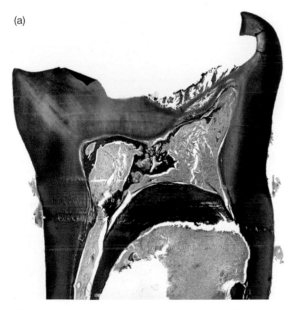

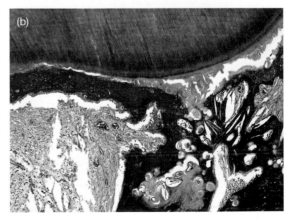

Fig. 9.4 (a) Histological section of a primary molar showing severe responses to caries: irregular calcification and severe inflammation (original magnification ×10). (b) At higher magnification the calcification appears more like bone than dentin, and odontoblasts are not visible, Masson's trichrome stain (original magnification ×50).

primary teeth with inflammation of the pulp the average thickness of remaining dentin between the most deeply penetrating bacteria and the pulp was shown to be 0.6 mm, and the maximal width of dentin between the pulp and the most deeply penetrating bacteria associated with pulpitis was 1.8 mm, suggesting that the primary pulp responds to more superficial dentin caries than does that of permanent teeth [126]. In a study of primary incisors extracted from very young children with advanced rampant caries some pulps were shown to be healthy histologically under <0.5 mm remaining dentin [38]. In primary teeth with proximal caries the majority of teeth showed inflammation involving the pulp horn, well before the pulp was clinically exposed [34]. Few of these teeth, however, showed inflammation in the radicular pulp [34]. In a study of cariously exposed primary teeth with no clinical symptoms or radiological signs of total chronic pulpitis, healthy pulp in the roots was shown in 30 of 37 teeth by histological examination [144].

A poor correlation has been found between the clinical and histological findings in the pulps of primary teeth in two studies [37,38], but better correlation was found in another [144]. Increased neural density and leukocyte concentration have been shown within the pulp horns in both dentitions as caries progressed [132,135]. Healing of a damaged pulp requires the inflammatory changes to be reversed, so it is important to treat the tooth in the early stages of inflammation. When the carious lesion reaches the pulp, the inflammatory process may become irreversible (Fig. 9.5), and in time involve the entire coronal part. Thus, carious primary teeth judged clinically free of inflammation may have profound undetected pulpal changes [34]. Immune cells have been shown to increase in number in the areas affected by dental caries, attrition or restorative procedures, implicating their role in immunosurveillance [71]. There has recently been interest in natural methods of tissue repair, which have been shown to mimic dentinogenic events during tooth development [163]. Dentin has been shown to be capable of producing bioactive molecules in appropriate conditions. Traditional clinical strategies are potentially capable of exploiting endogenous signaling molecules in the tissues to develop more effective treatment methods. Application of exogenous signaling molecules offers opportunities for development of new therapies [163]. It has been shown that transforming growth factor (TGF)-β may be solubilized from dentin by some conditioning agents, and it has been suggested that these may be involved in the repair process [153]. A more abundant blood supply may possibly explain the finding of hyperplastic pulpitis (pulp polyp) in primary and young permanent teeth, in comparison with its rarity in older individuals (Fig. 9.6).

(a)

(b)

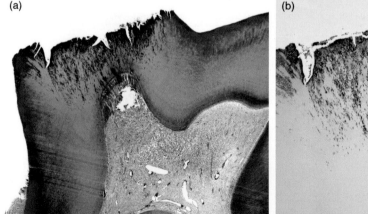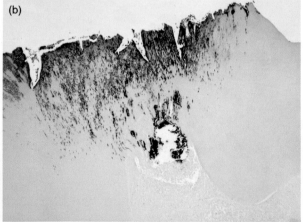

Fig. 9.5   (a) Histological section of a primary molar showing a pulp horn abscess under caries, Masson's trichrome stain (original magnification ×10). (b) Adjacent section stained for bacteria present in the dentin and in the pulp abscess, Brown and Brenn stain (original magnification ×50).

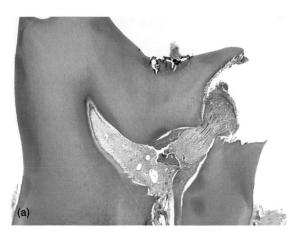
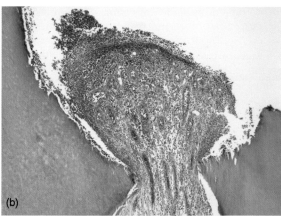

Fig. 9.6   (a) Histological section of a primary molar with a pulp polyp extending into an approximal cavity, and partial pulp calcification, Masson's trichrome stain (original magnification ×10). (b) Higher magnification of pulp polyp showing inflammatory cells and blood vessels (original magnification ×50).

9.3.3 Periradicular disease

Severe inflammation and infection of the pulp result in the formation of inflammatory lesions in the periodontal ligament and alveolar bone, where there is communication with the inflamed or infected canal. The flora of the infected primary molar has seldom been investigated in regard to obligate anaerobes but one study confirmed its similarity to that of infected permanent teeth [141]. The main site of apical periodontitis in permanent teeth is around the root apex, while in primary molars the lesions can be found anywhere along the root but it is much more common to find a lesion in the furcation (Fig. 9.7). The furcation area of molars, which encompasses the region around the division of the roots, is of special significance in the primary dentition due to its close anatomical relationship with the follicle of the developing premolar and its implication in periradicular disease. Carious exposure of the pulp in primary molars frequently results in pulp necrosis and a radiolucency in the furcation. Extraction of such teeth shows granulation tissue attached to the external root surfaces and this is viewed as a sequel of pulp infection. The search for an explanation for furcation lesions has led to examination of alternative pathways of extension of infection: e.g., pulp–periodontal canals (from the pulp chamber to the furcation periodontal ligament), porosity of the floor of the chamber, and lateral canals. Inflammation may spread from the pulp to the periodontal ligament via lateral canals. Periradicular lesions may be explained by the establish-

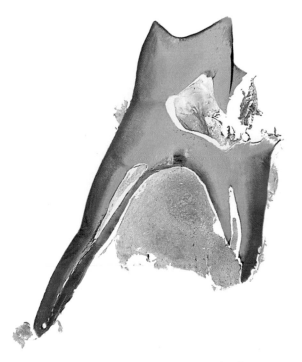

Fig. 9.7   Histological section of a primary molar showing an inflammatory lesion in the furcation connecting with the root end of the resorbed root (right), Masson's trichrome stain (original magnification ×10).

ment of pulpo-periodontal communications caused by resorption of the canal wall [105,106] or furcation area [128] (Figs 9.4 and 9.8).

Large furcation canals are present at the floor of the pulp chamber in some nonhuman species animals, [158,174], but these have been found less commonly in human teeth. The presence of accessory canals in abscessed primary molars has been studied to ascertain whether they were the reason for the interradicular site of the abscess [9,29,78, 101,104,117,118,129,173,175]. One recent study, in which teeth were examined using scanning electron microscopy, reported that the incidence of accessory foramina was significantly larger in primary than in permanent molars and some of those in primary teeth had larger diameters [29]. In a study of primary molars 78% were shown to have accessory canals in the furcation area [175]. However it is suggested that since accessory canals were not found in the pulp floors of all infected primary molars, these may not be the sole reason for interradicular radiolucency [175]. Various prevalences have been found, but not all of these studies could confirm the continuity or patency of these canals. It is therefore considered that these may be the cause of abscess formation in the furcation but should not necessarily be considered the sole reason. A histological study of infected primary molars showed structural alterations in the dentin and cementum of their pulpal floors [104]. The tubules were distorted or not observable, the

matrix was amorphous and deeply stained, suggesting hypocalcification and an increase in organic matrix. In the cementum there was evidence of thinning or breakdown, and often complete loss of the cementum lining the furcation of the roots. These changes generally appeared in the regions adjacent to disrupted dentin [104]. During tooth formation the development of separate mineralization centers for interradicular dentin of primary molars may be a factor [114]. Periradicular inflammation and infection have been shown to affect the development of the underlying permanent tooth [26,99].

Apical periodontitis of endodontic origin

The most common lesion of inflammatory origin is chronic apical periodontitis, sometimes called a "granuloma". The cell composition is similar to that in the permanent dentition and epithelial proliferation may also be seen [87]. Exacerbation of the process results in its transformation into a periradicular abscess that may be clinically acute or chronic.

Radicular cysts on primary teeth have also been reported; in some cases the permanent tooth bud was displaced [87]. The formation of cysts has been correlated with endodontic therapy in primary teeth [143]; however one study [93] confirmed that 36 out of 49 lesions suspected to be cysts associated with primary teeth, were indeed cysts but only four teeth had had previous treatment. Stimulation of the dentigerous epithelium of the permanent successor by the inflammatory lesion has also been reported [99,164].

9.3.4 Classification of pulp disease in primary teeth

Acute pulpitis may follow trauma, or may follow chronic pulpitis in a carious tooth. The classification of chronic pulpitis is based on the distinction between coronal partial pulpitis and total pulpitis [90]. In the case of pulp exposure due to dental caries, if there is no history of pain or only of momentary induced pain, the diagnosis is chronic coronal pulpitis. There should be lack of tenderness to palpation and to percussion, and it is important to confirm that the radiograph indicates no disease. This diagnosis may be confirmed at the time of intervention by the following signs: the exposed pulp tissue is light red and it bleeds moderately. The diagnosis of chronic total pulpitis is related to a history of spontaneous, shooting or persistent pain, and tenderness to palpa-

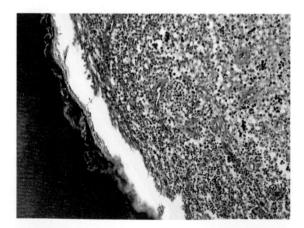

Fig. 9.8 Histological section of a primary molar showing external root resorption through to the pulp space, Masson's trichrome stain (original magnification ×100); this is a higher magnification of the coronal part of the root in Fig. 9.4.

tion, to percussion or even to touch. In these cases the exposed pulp tissue will bleed continuously and the radiograph may present pathologic findings such as resorption or furcation involvement [90].

9.3.5 Clinical diagnosis

Before taking any decision about dental treatment, it is important to make a comprehensive clinical examination in order to reach a diagnosis.

Medical history

An accurate medical history is important because a child with a systemic condition or disease may require a different approach from that for a healthy child.

Case history

The case history in a child may be difficult to obtain and may sometimes contain misleading information. The child may answer in a way that he or she thinks is best or the parents will point to the tooth with the largest cavity or darkest color. An important part of the history is usually that concerning the history of pain and its quality. Spontaneous, throbbing, or continuous pain that may keep the child awake at night is considered of pulpal origin, indicating advanced and irreversible pulp damage [144]. An important consideration in differential diagnosis is spontaneous throbbing pain caused by food impaction: it is associated with an inflamed dental papilla and bone destruction and not related to the state of the pulp.

Clinical visual examination

Clinical examination should include extraoral and intraoral examination. The teeth should be examined for evidence of caries as well as for sequels of trauma; changes in color should be noted [64,67]. The soft tissues are checked for any sign of redness, swelling, sinus tract, or fluctuation, related to pulp disease. Mobility may also be related to the pulp condition, but it must be distinguished from that accompanying normal exfoliation of the tooth.

Clinical tests

These include vitality (sensitivity) tests or percussion and are less reliable in a child [6]. Changes in eye contact may reveal more than the spoken word [90]. Furthermore, children may have severe pulp disease without any symptoms. Nerve endings degenerate and their number diminishes with physiological root resorption [13]. The diagnostic problems of primary teeth have been demonstrated in comparisons of clinical and histological findings [37,144]. Since sensitivity testing is not normally useful in primary teeth [6,95], necrosis of the pulp is diagnosed by a combination of other signs and symptoms: visually by color or the presence of swelling or a sinus tract, by tenderness to pressure or mobility beyond what would be expected physiologically, and by radiological examination.

Radiological examination

The clinical examination cannot be completed without radiological evaluation. Bitewing films best show the proximity of dental caries to the pulp, the depth of restorations and their relationship to pulp horns and vertical bitewings are particularly useful to show the furcation area. The pulp space should be examined for calcifications [79] and internal resorption. It is important to check the interradicular space for furcation involvement and the apical region for radiolucency. If the tip of the root cannot be seen in the bitewing radiograph, a periapical radiograph should be taken when pulp disease is suspected. The integrity of the lamina dura, presence of internal or external resorption of the roots, and the state of physiological root resorption should be checked. Information about the stage of resorption is important for planning the most appropriate treatment and may warrant having a radiograph of the contralateral teeth for comparison. If a sinus tract is present clinically, its origin should be correlated with the radiological findings. Whenever a decision must be made whether the treatment will be root canal treatment or extraction, a radiograph is mandatory to ascertain the extent of root resorption and also the presence and position of the developing permanent tooth.

9.4 Endodontic therapy of primary teeth

The objective of endodontic treatment of a tooth with an affected pulp is first to maintain the integrity of the dental arch, the oral tissues and the patient's general health, and second to prevent or treat pain of dental origin. Because immune cells in the dental pulp are reported to be involved in physiological root resorption, it is important where possible to maintain the vitality of the radicular pulp [151]. The different types of treatment have been categorized [3]. Because different research methods have been used in different studies it has not been possible to compare directly the various methods of pulp treatment.

9.5 Prevention of periradicular disease

9.5.1 Protective base

This is a material placed on the pulpal or axial walls of a cavity preparation between the restorative material and the pulp. The dentin of primary teeth is thin and permeable. It is important to prevent infection of the pulp through microleakage and microbial colonization of the space between the filling material and the dentinal wall [17]. Reinforced zinc oxide/eugenol or glass ionomer cement may be placed over the pulpal floor. Alternatively, hybridization of the surface between the dentin floor and a restorative resin is recommended [27].

9.5.2 Stepwise excavation and indirect pulp capping

The pediatric dentistry literature has not always distinguished between these terms. Currently, the practice of leaving softened caries, i.e., infected material, in the tooth, is not condoned by endodontists (see Chapter 10). Stepwise excavation implies the removal of soft caries short of pulp exposure and sealing the cavity to allow reactionary dentine to form. The cavity is then reentered, at least 2 months later, more than once if necessary, and further caries removed, until no softened caries remains over the pulp. One study of primary teeth compared excavation of all caries without consideration of exposure of the pulp, with removing the caries in two or more visits until all carious dentine had been removed [91]. This technique, which was termed stepwise excavation, significantly reduced the number of carious exposures in primary molars; it may therefore avoid a considerable number of pulp treatments [91].

Indirect pulp capping has been described as the removal of gross caries and sealing the cavity for a time with a biocompatible material [95]. Caries is removed just short of pulp exposure and the pulp protected so that the caries becomes arrested and the pulp can repair itself by laying down reactionary dentin [95]. In this way, pulp exposure with the concomitant danger of infection is avoided. The decision to apply this treatment must be made after meticulous examination. This treatment is recommended for patients when a preoperative diagnosis suggests no signs of pulp degeneration [46]. The tooth must present only deep caries without detectable exposure of the pulp, and must be symptomless or only show signs of reversible pulpitis. The remaining dentin has been presumed to be "affected", but "uninfected" [94]. Prior to permanent restoration, a protective base must be placed. Both zinc oxide/eugenol and calcium hydroxide cements as sub-bases stimulate reactionary dentin [72] or allow it to form [27]. In the first of these two studies, the teeth were reentered and residual caries removed. Important considerations for the success of this type of treatment are a healthy pulp and an efficient seal to prevent leakage and infection, or reinfection, of the dentin. It has been suggested that cavity conditioners may release TGF-β from the tissues promoting a reactionary response from the odontoblasts [46,153,163].

The success rate of indirect pulp capping has been shown to be higher than that of formocresol pulpotomy in the treatment of deep dentinal caries in primary teeth [41]. In another study [2] the success of indirect pulp capping in posterior primary teeth was 95%. Failure was associated with primary first molars, which are more difficult to restore with amalgam restorations as opposed to preformed metal crowns, and second with calcium hydroxide used alone as a liner with no base over it. Bases used were resin modified glass ionomer cement, zinc oxide/eugenol, or a luting agent when a preformed metal crown was used [2]. A higher success rate was achieved with indirect pulp therapy compared to formocresol pulpotomy in primary teeth with deep carious lesions approaching the pulp, especially those with reversible pulpitis [167]. A higher success rate was found for indirect pulp capping following caries control procedures [167].

There has been controversy as to whether it is safe to leave softened dentin in the base of the cavity. It has been shown that bonded and sealed composite restorations over cavitated lesions stopped clinical progress of these lesions for 10 years [98]. If the residual caries cannot be completely removed the sealing capacities of the filling material seem to be more important than its cariostatic properties [169].

9.5.3 Direct pulp capping

Direct pulp capping of primary teeth has had limited success in the past and there is controversy over its use. This is the placement of a protective dressing over an exposed pulp to preserve its vitality. Success in permanent teeth has been linked with the expectation that the pulp will respond by apposition of a reparative dentin bridge, thus closing again the exposed pulp cavity [27]. This procedure has been recommended in permanent teeth for pinpoint exposures that occur during operative work on a tooth with an otherwise healthy pulp. The dressing of choice used over the exposed site has traditionally been calcium hydroxide to stimulate dentin formation. Nevertheless, in primary teeth, direct pulp capping has been considered inadvisable because its application to carious teeth has been linked with internal resorption [166]. There is a concern that calcium hydroxide will promote internal resorption, but there does not appear to be evidence that pulp capping will cause a similar response [122]; failure may be amplified by existing inflammation and pulp capping should be limited to mechanical exposures.

Although there is reluctance to advocate the practice of direct pulp capping in cariously exposed primary molars, it has been shown that there are no marked differences in caries-induced vascular changes between the two dentitions, and therefore the subject should be reappraised [134]. Direct pulp capping in primary teeth has been suggested using dentin bonding agents, which are stated to achieve a hermetic seal [76]. This is reported to overcome the disadvantages of calcium hydroxide such as moisture susceptibility, failure to bond to dentin and contribution to imperfect reparative dentin that may ultimately lead to bacterial invasion. Other authors are reluctant to advocate dental adhesives for direct pulp capping until more successful human studies have been reported [122]. This technique has been reported to be successful in permanent teeth in the absence of bacterial leakage [27]. The use of hard set calcium hydroxide cements such as Dycal (Dentsply) has been suggested [76]. Mineral trioxide aggregate (MTA) has been used successfully for pulp capping in permanent teeth [161]. It has been used successfully in a case report of a primary tooth [16], but there is

no controlled study. Although dentists will normally perform a pulpotomy to treat a small exposure in a primary tooth, it has been suggested that this may be unnecessary [122].

A recent review has suggested that direct pulp capping of a carious pulp exposure in a primary tooth is not to be recommended except in older children, 1–2 years prior to normal exfoliation [46].

9.5.4 Pulpotomy

Partial pulpotomy

Partial (or Cvek) pulpotomy is now the treatment of choice for vital exposure in permanent teeth [28]. This has traditionally been done with calcium hydroxide. As yet there is little literature on the use of the technique in primary teeth. It has been shown to give an 83% success rate in primary molars with chronic coronal pulpitis [148] and has been suggested for fractured primary incisors [80].

Full coronal pulpotomy

Two types of full coronal pulpotomy have traditionally been used for the treatment of primary teeth: first, so-called "vital" pulpotomy, in which part or all of the radicular pulp remains vital, and secondly "nonvital" pulpotomy where the pulp tissue in the roots is irreversibly damaged and treatment aims simply at disinfection of the radicular pulp tissue. The latter technique is not now recommended [33], and where indicated root canal treatment of primary teeth is the treatment of choice.

Vital pulpotomy

"Vital" full coronal pulpotomy has traditionally been the most widely accepted treatment for primary teeth with a traumatic or carious exposure or even when caries has not reached the pulp, where there is believed to be no inflammation of the radicular pulp [7,31,95,145,156,176,177]. Full coronal pulpotomy is the surgical amputation of the entire coronal pulp. When a carious lesion approaches the pulp, the reaction may involve a large volume of the pulp chamber. As it is believed that healing of a pulp wound can only take place in tissue with no more than reversible inflammatory changes, it is very important to evaluate the state of the pulp at the time of intervention, by taking a careful history and examining the teeth and relevant radiographs. After amputation the radicular pulp stumps should be covered with a protective dressing and the cavity effectively sealed. The ideal dressing material after pulpotomy must be bactericidal, promote healing of the radicular pulp, be biocompatible, and not interfere with the physiological process of root resorption. An ideal pulp-dressing material has for many years been sought and numerous dressing procedures have been suggested.

Indications and contraindications

Indications for vital pulpotomy include teeth with carious, mechanical or traumatic exposure of the pulp, free of spontaneous pain or pathological radiological findings. Some dentists favor this approach when caries is approaching the pulp, especially if the patient is being treated under a general anesthetic and therefore retreatment is particularly undesirable. Contraindications for vital pulpotomy in primary teeth are: an unrestorable tooth, physiological root resorption of more than one third of the root, a history of spontaneous or persistent pain, presence of a sinus tract, increased tooth mobility or any pathological finding on the radiographs, such as presence of extensive calcifications, internal resorption in the pulp cavity, or interradicular bone loss. Pulpotomy in primary teeth is contraindicated in patients at risk of infective endocarditis or with a compromised immune system because it cannot be guaranteed that all infected material has been removed. During the procedure, light red blood and vital tissue should be visible at the root canal orifices and hemorrhage should be readily controlled; this latter observation implies that the remaining tissue is free from inflammation [95].

More recently there has been a move towards more conservative methods of treatment where damage to the coronal pulp is believed to be limited, with the use of indirect pulp capping [95], stepwise excavation [91], or partial pulpotomy [148]. Because of the difficulty in determining the state of the pulp of primary teeth clinically, and because many children with grossly carious teeth are of necessity treated under general anesthesia, dentists choose to perform the more radical treatment in order to avoid the risk involved in repeated anesthesia. Treatment planning may also be influenced by the large treatment load which may be required in very young children with rampant caries. It is important to correct diet and oral hygiene if pulp treatment is to be successful. It has also been shown that both indirect pulp treatment and formocresol pulpotomy were more successful after caries control by removing gross caries and sealing the cavities that reduced the bacterial load prior to treatment [167].

Formocresol

For many years the material of choice for pulpotomy in primary teeth has been formocresol [96]. However there has been much concern over its toxicity, and it has greatly lost favor since the International Agency for Research on Cancer classified formaldehyde as a carcinogen in humans [70]; many other materials and methods have been investigated.

Formocresol was introduced at the beginning of the twentieth century, and is a combination of formaldehyde and cresol [19]. Formaldehyde can form methylol derivatives with various amino acids and nucleic acids; then, a slow secondary reaction can lead to intermolecular and/or intramolecular methylene cross-links. These reactions denature and fix protein and nucleic acids; they also deactivate autolytic lysosomes and bacterial toxins. There has long been concern about the potential carcinogenic and mutagenic effects of formocresol reacting with nucleic acids [14,82,83,107,108,112,119,179]. Cresol is capable of dissolving membranes and probably contributes to the observed loss of cellular detail in the area beneath the medicament [54]. Formocresol is very cytotoxic and the immune response in the pulp tissue caused by formaldehyde may probably preclude healing [15]. Concern has long been voiced about the diffusion of formaldehyde into the systemic circulation; labeled carbon introduced into the formaldehyde component of formocresol [14,109,171] or tritiated formalin [72] has been found in numerous organs shortly after the material was used in pulpotomy.

The results of clinical and histological studies carried out on formocresol pulpotomy vary widely and are somewhat controversial. A clinical 3-year follow-up study of formocresol pulpotomy in primary teeth reported a progressively decreasing survival rate of 91% at 3 months, 83% at 12 months and only 70% after 36 months [137]. In a histological study involving 110 roots [90], it was concluded that formocresol did not produce healing in even one root, confirming a previous hypothesis [15]. The treatment resulted in chronic inflammation in the residual tissue, and there was no evidence of ingrowth of new tissue. These observations agree with previously reported findings [136]. The rationale for its use seemed to be the exchange of an acute inflammatory or infected state for subclinical chronic inflammation [90]. The fact that internal resorptive defects remain small and sometimes cannot be detected on a radiograph is attributed to the severe damage to the residual tissue that also destroys its capacity to resorb [90].

To reduce the exposure of the child to formaldehyde, it was suggested to dilute Buckley's formocresol. Animal research demonstrated that a 1:5 dilution was just as effective in inhibiting enzymes *in vivo* as was a full strength preparation [86]; clinical studies with this dilution also yielded good results [47,48,102,155]. Formocresol has enjoyed popularity because it can give clinical success even when the radicular pulp is nonvital. Diagnosis of a healthy radicular pulp is therefore not necessary for clinical success [131].

Alternatives to formocresol

The shortcomings of formocresol and the debate about the safety of formaldehyde have led to the search for alternative pulpotomy dressings. Currently ferric sulfate has enjoyed widespread success [43], acting as a hemostatic agent, calcium hydroxide is being further investigated and MTA has shown good results, but is expensive. Other materials suggested have included glutaraldehyde, bone morphogenic protein [110,111], and collagen gel [53]. Electrosurgery [115,138] and lasers [150] involve the application of another form of energy to eliminate residual infectious processes and coagulate the surface without the use of pharmacotherapeutic agents. Those methods that do not involve fixing the tissues are dependent on correct diagnosis of healthy radicular pulp. The move away from formocresol has led to more root canal treatment and, in less favorable circumstances, more extractions.

Glutaraldehyde

Glutaraldehyde, proposed as an alternative to formocresol, is an aliphatic dialdehyde [121]. It is considered a mild fixative [50] and reported as less toxic than formaldehyde [36,123,124]. It is a good antibacterial agent. However, little difference has been found between formocresol and glutaraldehyde as regards toxicity, mutagenicity, and systemic distribution [44]. A further study found a relatively high failure rate with 2% buffered glutaraldehyde and concluded that this did not justify its recommendation as a substitute for formocresol [49]. It has been used in spite of a

mediocre clinical success rate and controversial histological findings [11,137].

Calcium hydroxide

Calcium hydroxide has been used successfully for vital pulp therapy in permanent teeth [146]. The dressing used is a calcium hydroxide preparation with a high alkaline potential that produces surface necrosis. The pulp is expected to respond with the typical repair process described in direct pulp capping [146] and a dentin bridge over the coronal parts of the canals [178]; the radicular pulp tissue is expected to remain healthy in order to allow normal exfoliation to occur. If this process fails due to the presence of inflammatory cells in the radicular tissue at the time of dressing, massive internal resorption can follow and premature loss of the tooth can occur [145,146]. Calcium hydroxide has shown less favorable results clinically than formocresol [168].

The use of calcium hydroxide in the primary dentition has long been contraindicated for either direct pulp capping or pulpotomy following unfavorable reports and an association with internal resorption [46,89,146]. In these investigations the failures were attributed to chronic pulp inflammation and internal resorption. It was considered that internal resorption may have been due to overstimulation of the primary pulp by the highly alkaline calcium hydroxide that caused metaplasia in the pulp tissue leading to formation of odontoclasts [147]; however these studies did not consider the possible role of infection between the restoration and dentin. It would be hoped that adhesive restorations or preformed metal crowns could overcome this problem. In a study of calcium hydroxide pulpotomies [12], it was considered that the dominating factor for success was not the calcium hydroxide dressing but the state of the pulp. The difficulty of obtaining hemostasis has been considered as contributing to failure [145]. These teeth were treated using an aseptic technique, but in those that failed it is unclear whether subsequent infection contributed.

Coronal seal has been shown to be important in the success of endodontic treatment in permanent teeth [142]. Correct diagnosis and better control of bleeding have been considered to contribute to the success of partial pulpotomy with calcium hydroxide in primary teeth [148]. A study of full coronal pulpotomies in 106 extensively carious primary molars using calcium hydroxide followed by a light cured cavity sealing material showed an 80% success rate after 2 years. The success rate has been higher in teeth restored with a stainless steel crown rather than amalgam [57], suggesting that coronal seal is important. Because this technique relies on a healthy radicular pulp correct diagnosis is essential.

Ferric sulfate

This material has recently found favor as a pulpotomy dressing following the move away from formocresol (Fig. 9.9). Ferric sulfate is a hemostatic agent, used at a 15.5% dilution, and it is applied to the pulp stumps using a rubbing action for 15 s. Because the material has only limited antibacterial action it is very important to have a correct diagnosis. There should be no inflammation of the radicular pulp. A study that used

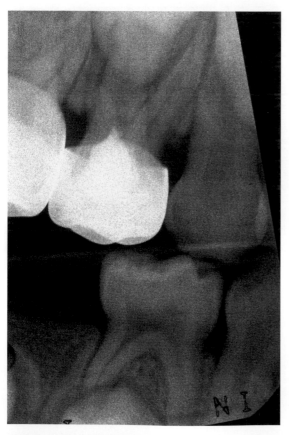

Fig. 9.9   Radiograph of a primary maxillary first molar treated by pulpotomy using ferric sulfate 1 year previously. (Courtesy of Dr Evelyn Sheehy.)

histological examination to compare ferric sulfate with a 20% dilution of formocresol found a similar outcome [51]. A further histological study came to a similar conclusion, but also noted that pulpotomies may be clinically successful in the presence of adverse histological reactions [23]. Clinical studies found comparable results [52,69,92] or slightly less favorable radiological results [154]. Both methods can lead to early exfoliation [165].

An evidence-based assessment of ferric sulfate versus formocresol primary molar pulpotomy concluded that in human carious primary molars with reversible coronal pulpitis, pulpotomies performed with either formocresol or ferric sulfate were likely to have a similar outcome [85]. Another review recommended the use of ferric sulfate, and noted that although internal resorption was seen it was small and unchanged over time or repaired with hard tissue [116]. The outcome of ferric sulfate pulpotomy has been compared with that of root canal treatment, one with incisors and the other with molars, in carious primary teeth where removal of caries was likely to produce a vital exposure [21,22]. The incisors were restored with acid-etched composite resin, and the molars with stainless-steel crowns. Both studies concluded that root canal treatment was more successful [21,22].

MTA

This material has recently been developed for use in endodontics. It has been shown to prevent microleakage, be biocompatible, and to promote regeneration of the original tissues when placed in contact with the dental pulp or periradicular tissues [161]. It has a pH of approx 11.0 and a setting time of 3 h. The constituents include calcium and silicate; a product of the setting reaction is calcium hydroxide [20]. It has been shown to be successful in pulpotomy in primary teeth and to compare favorably with formocresol (Fig. 9.10) [1,36,42,60,65,139]. In one study internal resorption was found in both groups and it was suggested that this was not necessarily an indication of failure, but could be followed up, with the expectation of arrest of the process and calcific metamorphosis [65]. One study compared MTA with bioactive glass, ferric sulfate, and formocresol [139]. MTA performed very well causing dentin bridge formation while simultaneously maintaining normal pulp structure. Bioactive glass induced an inflammatory response at 2 weeks with resolution at 4 weeks. Ferric

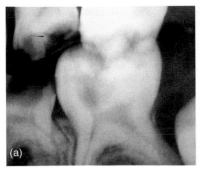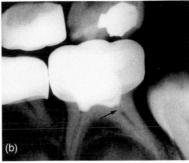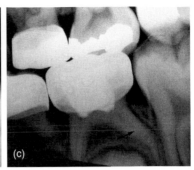

Fig. 9.10 Radiographs of a primary mandibular second molar treated by pulpotomy using mineral trioxide aggregate. (a) Carious mandibular second molar. (b) Nine months after pulpotomy: a calcific bridge (arrowed) has formed in the distal root. (c) Twenty-two months after pulpotomy the distal canal appears almost completely calcified (arrowed). (Reproduced by permission from Eidelman *et al.* [36].)

sulfate showed moderate inflammation of the pulp at 2 and 4 weeks [139]. Gray MTA, which contains some iron, was found to be superior to the white variety [1]. There is at present limited clinical evidence, but this material promises to be successful.

Laser

Lasers (argon, Nd:YAG, and carbon dioxide) have been used on amputated pulps in pulpotomies in primary molars, and success has been reported, although this technique is not widely used [40,84,150,172].

Electrosurgery

Electrosurgery has been used for pulpotomy. Two clinical studies comparing it with formocresol showed no significant difference [32,130]; however a histological study showed less pulpal inflammation in teeth treated with electrosurgical coronal pulp removal than in teeth treated with formocresol [39].

9.6 Root canal treatment in primary teeth

Root canal treatment is now considered the treatment of choice for primary teeth with irreversible inflammation extending into the radicular pulp where extraction is not indicated [33]. As long ago as 1972 it was suggested that it was desirable to retain nonvital primary teeth and that root canal treatment could be successfully carried out on these teeth, but

that this treatment had been neglected [12]. It was suggested that this may have been due to a number of factors: lack of familiarity with the morphology, time involved, the temporary nature of the teeth, the need for absorbable materials, and difficulty in their handling, problems with taking radiographs and behavior management [12]. Little research has been done into root canal treatment of primary teeth compared to permanent teeth.

The endodontic anatomy of primary molars is difficult to predict because of the balance of resorption and hard tissue deposition [128]. These authors suggested that root length was the most reliable predictor of the integrity of the root, with the borderline of being able to treat at 4 mm. Resorptive areas that appeared at furcation level when root length was between 7 and 10 mm became perforating when root length was less than 4 mm. A study examining success of pulpectomy found no adverse effect on the succedaneous tooth if the treatment was correctly done, but there was a 20% chance of altering its path of eruption [25]. This study showed an overall success rate of 78%, the most important preoperative predictor of failure being excess resorption of the primary tooth due to infection; when excess root resorption was >1 mm the success rate was only 23%; this was statistically significant.

A study of filling techniques found a lentulo-spiral filler to be the most effective method of filling curved canals [8]. A further study of endodontic techniques on extracted primary incisors examined three filling techniques using an incremental technique, a lentulo-spiral filler and a pressure syringe; no statistically significant difference was found when these were evaluated radiologically in two planes [30].

A filling material used in primary teeth should be absorbable and should not set into a hard mass which could deflect the erupting permanent tooth; it should induce vital periapical tissue to seal the canal with calcified or connective tissue, and be harmless to the adjacent tooth germ [66]. A study comparing zinc oxide/eugenol with Kri paste (Farmachemie AG, Zurich, Switzerland), a mixture of 80% iodoform, camphorated monochlorophenol, and menthol, found Kri paste significantly more successful in primary first molars compared with second molars, and in maxillary rather than mandibular teeth [66]. The authors suggested that this may have been due to the relative difficulty of filling with a thicker paste. Teeth which were overfilled with Kri paste did better than those overfilled with zinc oxide/eugenol. Kri paste has been considered to contain too much iodoform and to be absorbed too quickly from the canal [127]. Another study found Kri paste to be a successful root-filling material in primary teeth [55]. This author suggested that iodoform paste is less likely to deflect the underlying permanent tooth than the harder zinc oxide/eugenol. Other authors state that if pure zinc oxide/eugenol is extruded from the roots it is entirely absorbable and that this, inserted as a paste, is the filling material of choice as it is absorbed at the same rate as the root [33]. These authors recommended filling to within 1 mm of the apex. They cautioned against using zinc oxide/eugenol with additives that might retard absorption. A histological study comparing zinc oxide/eugenol and calcium hydroxide pulpectomies in primary molars found zinc oxide/eugenol to be more successful [24].

Vitapex (Neo Dental Chemical Products Co., Tokyo, Japan) is a mixture of calcium hydroxide and iodoform that gave good clinical and histological results [88,103,113]. Maisto's paste has been used [157]; the basic components are similar to those of Kri paste but the additives are considered important: zinc oxide controls the speed of absorption so that it is at the same rate as the root [81]; thymol is a disinfectant; and lanolin improves the handling of the paste. The effects of various materials on the root canal flora have been investigated [160].

Disinfection of the canals is important as primary teeth have narrow ribbon-like canals with many ramifications. It is also very important to avoid damage to the successional tooth and it is therefore important not to instrument beyond the apex [33]. However, if infection persists the disease will remain. The use of an electronic apex locator has been found to be effective in primary teeth [73].

9.7 Restoration

Much early work does not state how teeth were restored following treatment of the primary tooth dental pulp. In permanent teeth this has been shown to be of vital importance for the success of endodontic treatment as it is essential to prevent bacterial leakage around the crown and thence to the pulp or root canal [142]. Primary teeth restored with a preformed metal crown following pulpotomy did better than those restored with amalgam [57]. It has been suggested that pulpotomized primary teeth could be restored with a single surface amalgam rather than a stainless-steel crown if the tooth was within a short period of exfoliation [68]. A study investigating cements for use with stainless-steel crowns concluded that adhesive cements significantly reduced microleakage, but suggested that further long-term results were required [149]. A later study found that bonding agents and resin-based restorations were able to provide the best total margin protection; stainless-steel crowns cemented with glass ionomer cement were unable to seal teeth, and amalgam, glass ionomer cement, and intermediate restorative material (IRM) restorations did not appear to be leakage-resistant materials for pulpotomies of primary molars [58]. A radiological assessment of primary molar pulpotomies found resin-based materials for restorations were inferior to stainless-steel crowns for a successful outcome of intraradicular radiolucencies [59].

9.8 Trauma to primary teeth

Trauma is a frequent cause of loss of vitality of anterior primary teeth. The pulp may be affected by luxation injuries, or by fractures of the crown or root. In luxation injuries, the pulp may be damaged by crushing or severance of the apical vessels. The tooth may become nonvital and discolored, but unless infection intervenes there may be no need for pulp treatment [64]. Not infrequently the pulp may calcify as a repair mechanism, when the crown will acquire a yellowish hue; intervention is not indicated. Recent fractures of the crown involving the pulp may be treated by minimal pulpotomy, or pulp capping if cooperation does not allow pulpotomy. If the pulp does become nonvital root canal treatment may be indicated if cooperation allows. Root fractures do not normally require intervention. If the coronal fragment becomes necrotic it can be removed [4]. The apical fragment will almost always remain vital and should be left *in situ* to resorb or exfoliate naturally. Replantation of primary teeth is not indicated because of the risk of damage to the permanent tooth germ [4].

Clinicians should always be aware in the case of trauma to children's teeth of the possibility of nonaccidental injury [170].

9.9 References

1. Agamy HA, Bakry NS, Mounir MMF, Avery D (2004) Comparison of mineral trioxide aggregate and formocresol as pulp-capping agents in pulpotomized primary teeth. *Pediatric Dentistry* **26**, 302–9.
2. Al-Zayer MA, Staffron LH, Feigal RJ, Welch KB (2003) Indirect pulp treatment of primary posterior teeth: a retrospective study. *Pediatric Dentistry* **25**, 29–36.
3. American Academy of Pediatric Dentistry (2004) Guideline on pulp therapy for primary and young permanent teeth. *Pediatric Dentistry* **26**, 115–19.
4. Andreasen J, Andreasen FM, Bakland LK, Flores MT (2003) Injuries to the primary dentition. In *Traumatic dental injuries. A manual*, pp. 52–55, 2nd edn. Copenhagen: Blackwell Munksgaard.
5. Angelova A, Takagi Y, Okiji T, Kaneko T, Yamashita Y (2004) Immunocompetent cells in the pulp of human deciduous teeth. *Archives of Oral Biology* **49**, 29–36.
6. Asfour MA, Millar BJ, Smith PB (1996) An assessment of the reliability of pulp testing deciduous teeth. *International Journal of Paediatric Dentistry* **6**, 163–6.
7. Avram DC, Pulver F (1989) Pulpotomy medicaments for vital primary teeth. Surveys to determine use and attitudes in pediatric dental practice and in dental schools throughout the world. *ASDC Journal of Dentistry for Children* **56**, 426–34.
8. Aylard SR, Johnson R (1987) Assessment of filling techniques for primary teeth. *Pediatric Dentistry* **9**, 195–8.
9. Bendek S, Correa C, Donado J (1993) Estudio en microscopia electronica de barrido del piso de la camera pulpar en molares deciduos. Bogota, Colombia: *Universidad Odontologica* **12**, 33–7.
10. Bergenholtz G (1981) Inflammatory response of the dental pulp to bacterial irritation. *Journal of Endodontics* **7**, 100–4.
11. Berger JE (1965) Pulp tissue reaction to formocresol and zinc oxide-eugenol. *Journal of Dentistry for Children* **32**, 13–28.
12. Berk H, Krakow AA (1972) A comparison of the management of pulpal pathosis in deciduous and permanent teeth. *Oral Surgery, Oral Medicine, Oral Pathology* **34**, 944–55.
13. Bernick S (1959) Innervation of the teeth and periodontium. *Dental Clinics of North America* **3**, 503–14.
14. Block RM, Lewis RD, Hirsch J, Coffey J, Langeland K (1983) Systemic distribution of [^{14}C]-labeled paraformaldehyde incorporated within formocresol following pulpotomies in dogs. *Journal of Endodontics* **9**, 176–89.
15. Block RM, Lewis RD, Sheats JB, Fawley J (1977) Cell-mediated immune response to dog pulp tissue altered by formocresol within the root canal. *Journal of Endodontics* **3**, 424–30.
16. Bodem O, Blumenshine S, Zeh D, Koch MJ (2004) Direct pulp capping with mineral trioxide aggregate in a primary molar: a case report. *International Journal of Paediatric Dentistry* **14**, 376–9.
17. Brännström M (1984) Communication between the oral cavity and the dental pulp associated with restorative treatment. *Operative Dentistry* **9**, 57–68.
18. Brännström M, Lind PO (1965) Pulpal response to early dental caries. *Journal of Dental Research* **44**, 1045–50.
19. Buckley JP (1904) A rational treatment for putrescent pulps. *Dental Review* **18**, 1193–7.
20. Camilleri J, Montesin FE, Brady K, Sweeny R, Curtis RV, Pitt Ford TR (2005) The constitution of mineral trioxide aggregate. *Dental Materials* **21**, 297–303.
21. Casas MJ, Kenny DJ, Johnston DH, Judd PL, Layug MA (2004) Outcomes of vital primary incisor ferric sulphate pulpotomy and root canal therapy. *Journal of Canadian Dental Association* **70**, 34–8.
22. Casas MJ, Layug MA, Kenny DJ, Johnston DH, Judd PL (2003) Two-year outcomes of primary molar ferric sulphate pulpotomy and root canal therapy. *Pediatric Dentistry* **25**, 97–102.
23. Cleaton-Jones P, Duggal M, Parak R, Williams S, Setzer S (2002) Ferric sulphate and formocresol pulpotomies in baboon primary molars: histological responses. *European Journal of Paediatric Dentistry* **3**, 121–5.
24. Cleaton-Jones P, Duggal M, Parak R, Williams S, Setzer S (2004) Zinc oxide-eugenol and calcium hydroxide pulpotomies in baboon primary molars: histological responses. *European Journal of Paediatric Dentistry* **5**, 131–5.
25. Coll J, Sadrian R (1996) Predicting pulpectomy success and its relationship to exfoliation and succedaneous dentition. *Pediatric Dentistry* **18**, 57–63.
26. Cordeiro MM, Roch MJ (2005) The effects of periradicular inflammation and infection on a primary tooth and permanent successor. *Journal of Clinical Paediatric Dentistry* **29**, 193–200.
27. Cox CF, Suzuki S (1994) Re-evaluating pulp protection: calcium hydroxide liners vs. cohesive hybridization. *Journal of the American Dental Association* **125**, 823–31.
28. Cvek M (1978) A clinical report on partial pulpotomy and capping with calcium hydroxide in permanent incisors with complicated crown fracture. *Journal of Endodontics* **4**, 232–7.

29. Dammaschke T, Witt M, Ott K, Schafer E (2004) Scanning electron microscope investigation of incidence, location, and size of accessory foramina in primary and permanent molars. *Quintessence International* **35**, 699–705.

30. Dandashi MB, Nazif MM, Zullo T, Elliott MA, Schneider LG, Czonstkowsky M (1993) An in vitro comparison of three endodontic techniques for primary incisors. *Pediatric Dentistry* **15**, 254–6.

31. Davis MJ, Myers R, Switkes MD (1982) Glutaraldehyde: an alternative to formocresol for vital pulp therapy. *ASDC Journal of Dentistry for Children* **49**, 176–80.

32. Dean JA, Mack RB, Fulkerson BT, Sanders BJ (2002) Comparison of electrosurgical and formocresol pulpotomy procedures in children. *International Journal of Paediatric Dentistry* **12**, 177–82.

33. Duggal MS, Curzon MEJ, Fayle SA, Toumba KJ, Robertson AJ (2002) *Restorative techniques in paediatric dentistry*, 2nd edn. London: Martin Dunitz.

34. Duggal MS, Nooh A, High A (2002) Response of the primary pulp to inflammation: a review of the Leeds studies and challenges for the future. *European Journal of Paediatric Dentistry* **14**, 111–14.

35. Egan CA, Hector MP, Bishop MA (1999) On the pulpal nerve supply in primary human teeth: evidence for the innervation of primary dentine. *International Journal of Paediatric Dentistry* **9**, 57–66.

36. Eidelman E, Holan G, Fuks A (2001) Mineral trioxide aggregate vs formocresol in pulpotomized primary molars: a preliminary report. *Pediatric Dentistry* **23**, 15–18.

37. Eidelman E, Touma B, Ulmansky M (1968) Pulp pathology in deciduous teeth. Clinical and histological correlations. *Israel Journal of Medical Sciences* **4**, 1244–8.

38. Eidelman E, Ulmansky M, Michaeli Y (1992) Histopathology of the pulp in primary incisors with deep dentinal caries. *Pediatric Dentistry* **14**, 372–5.

39. El-Meligy O, Abdalla M, El-Baraway S, El-Tekya M, Dean JA (2001) Histological evaluation of electrosurgery and formocresol pulpotomy techniques in primary teeth in dogs. *Journal of Clinical Pediatric Dentistry* **26**, 81–5.

40. Elliott RD, Roberts MW, Burkes J, Phillips C (1999) Evaluation of the carbon dioxide laser on vital human primary pulp tissue. *Pediatric Dentistry* **21**, 327–31.

41. Farooq NS, Coll JA, Kuwabara A, Shelton P (2000) Success rate of formrcresol pulpotomy and indirect pulp therapy in the treatment of deep dentinal caries in primary teeth. *Pediatric Dentistry* **22**, 278–86.

42. Farsi N, Alamoudi N, Balto K, Mushayt A (2005) Success of mineral trioxide aggregate in pulpotomized primary molars. *Journal of Clinical Pediatric Dentistry* **29**, 307–11.

43. Fei AL, Udin RD, Johnson R (1991) A clinical study of ferric sulfate as a pulpotomy agent in primary teeth. *Pediatric Dentistry* **13**, 327–32.

44. Feigal RJ, Messer HH (1990) A critical look at glutaraldehyde. *Pediatric Dentistry* **12**, 69–71.

45. Fox AG, Heeley JD (1980) Histological study of pulps of human primary teeth. *Archives of Oral Biology* **25**, 103–10.

46. Fuks AB (2002) Current concepts in vital primary pulp therapy. *Pediatric Dentistry* **3**, 115–20.

47. Fuks AB, Bimstein E (1981) Clinical evaluation of diluted formocresol pulpotomies in primary teeth of school children. *Pediatric Dentistry* **3**, 321–4.

48. Fuks AB, Bimstein E, Bruchim A (1983) Radiographic and histologic evaluation of the effect of two concentrations of formocresol on pulpotomized primary and young permanent teeth in monkeys. *Pediatric Dentistry* **5**, 9–13.

49. Fuks AB, Bimstein E, Guelmann M, Klein H (1990) Assessment of a 2 percent buffered glutaraldehyde solution in pulpotomized primary teeth of schoolchildren. *ASDC Journal of Dentistry for Children* **57**, 371–5.

50. Fuks AB, Bimstein E, Michaeli Y (1986) Glutaraldehyde as a pulp dressing after pulpotomy in primary teeth of baboon monkeys. *Pediatric Dentistry* **8**, 32–6.

51. Fuks A, Eidelman E. Cleaton-Jones P, Michaeli Y (1997) Pulp response to ferric sulphate, diluted formocresol and IRM in pulpotomised baboon teeth. *Journal of Dentistry for Children* **64**, 254–9.

52. Fuks AB, Holan G, Davis JM, Eidelman E (1997) Ferric sulphate versus dilute formocresol in pulpotomized primary molars: long term follow-up. *Pediatric Dentistry* **19**, 327–30.

53. Fuks AB, Michaeli Y, Sofer-Saks B, Shoshan S (1984) Enriched collagen solution as a pulp dressing in pulpotomized teeth in monkeys. *Pediatric Dentistry* **6**, 243–7.

54. Fulton R, Ranly DM (1979) An autoradiographic study of formocresol pulpotomies in rat molars using ^{3}H-formaldehyde. *Journal of Endodontics* **5**, 71–8.

55. Garcia-Godoy F (1987) Evaluation of an iodoform paste in root canal therapy for infected primary teeth. *ASDC Journal of Dentistry for Children* **54**, 30–4.

56. Garcia-Godoy F, Ranly DM (1987) Clinical evaluation of pulpotomies with ZOE as the vehicle for glutaraldehyde. *Pediatric Dentistry* **9**, 144–6.

57. Gruythuysen R, Weerheijm K (1997) Calcium hydroxide pulpotomy with a light-cured cavity-sealing material after two years. *Journal of Dentistry for Children* **64**, 251–3.

58. Guelmann M, Bookmyer KL, Villalta P, Garcia-Godoy F (2004) Microleakage of restorative techniques for pulpotomised primary molars. *Journal of Dentistry for Children* **71**, 209–11.

59. Guelmann M, McIlwain MF, Primosch RE (2005) Radiographic assessment of primary molar pulpotomies restored with resin-based materials *Pediatric Dentistry* **27**, 24–7.

60. Hegde N, Amitha M (2005) Mineral trioxide aggregate as a pulpotomy agent in primary molars: an in vivo study. *Indian Society of Pedodontics and Preventive Dentistry* **23**, 13–16.

61. Heyeraas K (1980) Blood flow and vascular pressure in the dental pulp. *Acta Odontologica Scandinavica* **38**, 135–44.

62. Heyeraas KJ, Kvinnsland I (1992) Tissue pressure and blood flow in pulpal inflammation. *Proceedings of the Finnish Dental Society* **88**, Supplement 1, 393–401.
63. Hibbard ED, Ireland RL (1957) Morphology of the root canals of the primary molar teeth. *Journal of Dentistry for Children* **24**, 250–7.
64. Holan G (2006) Long-term effect of different treatment modalities for traumatized primary incisors presenting dark coronal discoloration with no other signs of injury. *Dental Traumatology* **22**, 14–17.
65. Holan F, Eidelman E, Fuks A (2005) Long-term evaluation of pulpotomy in primary molars using mineral trioxide aggregate or formocresol. *Pediatric Dentistry* **27**, 129–36.
66. Holan G, Fuks AB (1993) A comparison of pulpectomies using ZnOE and Kri paste in primary molars: a retrospective study. *Pediatric Dentistry* **15**, 403–7.
67. Holan G, Fuks AB (1996) The diagnostic value of coronal dark-gray discoloration in primary teeth following traumatic injuries. *Pediatric Dentistry* **18**, 224–7.
68. Holan G, Fuks AB, Keltz N (2002) Success rate of formocresol pulpotomy in primary molars restored with stainless steel crown vs amalgam. *Pediatric Dentistry* **24**, 212–16.
69. Ibricevic H, al-Jame Q (2000) Ferric sulphate as pulpotomy agent in primary teeth: twenty month clinical follow-up. *Journal of Clinical Pediatric Dentistry* **24**, 269–72.
70. International Agency for Research on Cancer (2004) Press Release no 153. http://www.iarc.fr/ENG/Press_Releases/archives/pr153a.html
71. Kannari N, Ohshima H, Maeda T, Noda T, Takano Y (1998) Class II MHC antigen-expressing cells in the pulp tissue of human deciduous teeth prior to shedding. *Archives of Histology and Cytology* **61**, 1–15.
72. Kerkhove BC, Herman SC, Klein AI, McDonald RE (1967) A clinical and television densitometric evaluation of the indirect pulp capping technique. *Journal of Dentistry for Children* **34**, 192–201.
73. Kielbassa A, Muller U, Monting J (2003) Clinical evaluation of measuring accuracy of Root ZX in primary teeth. *Oral Surgery, Oral Medicine, Oral Pathology, Oral Radiology and Endodontics* **95**, 94–100.
74. Klinge RF (1999) A microradiographic and electron microscope study of tertiary dentine in human deciduous teeth. *Acta Odontologica Scandinavica* **57**, 87–92.
75. Klinge RF (2001) Further observations on tertiary dentine in human deciduous teeth. *Advances in Dental Research* **15**, 76–9.
76. Kopel HM (1997) The pulp capping procedure in primary teeth 'revisited'. *Journal of Dentistry for Children* **64**, 327–33.
77. Koutsi V, Noonan RG, Horner JA, Simpson MD, Matthews WG, Pashley DH (1994) The effect of dentin depth on the permeability and ultrastructure of primary molars. *Pediatric Dentistry* **16**, 29–35.
78. Kramer PF, Faraco Junior IM, Meira R (2003) A SEM investigation of accessory foramina in the furcation area of primary molars. *Journal of Clinical Pediatric Dentistry* **27**, 157–61.

79. Kumar S, Chandra S, Jaiswal JN (1990) Pulp calcifications in primary teeth. *Journal of Endodontics* **16**, 218–20.
80. Kupietzky A, Holan, G (2003) Treatment of crown fractures with pulp exposure in primary incisors. *Pediatric Dentistry* **25**, 241–7.
81. Leonardo MR, Canzani GH, Berbert A, Fernandez EG, Lia RC (1982) Reaccion a la pasta lentamente reabsorbible en el tejido periapical de perros. *Revista de la Asociacion Odontologica Argentina* **70**, 217–21.
82. Lewis BB, Chestner SB (1981) Formaldehyde in dentistry: a review of mutagenic and carcinogenic potential. *Journal of the American Dental Association* **103**, 429–34.
83. Lewis B (1998) Formaldehyde in dentistry: a review for the millennium. *Journal of Clinical Pediatric Dentistry* **22**, 167–77.
84. Liu J, Chen L, Chao S (1999) Laser pulpotomy of primary teeth. *Pediatric Dentistry* **21**, 128–9.
85. Loh A, O'Hoy P, Tran X, Charles R, Hughes A, Kubo K, Messer LB (2004) Evidence-based assessment: evaluation of the formocresol versus ferric sulphate primary molar pulpotomy. *Pediatric Dentistry* **26**, 401–9.
86. Loos PJ, Han SS (1971) An enzyme histochemical study of the effect of various concentrations of formocresol on connective tissues. *Oral Surgery, Oral Medicine, Oral Pathology* **31**, 571–85.
87. Lustmann J, Shear M (1985) Radicular cysts arising from deciduous teeth. Review of the literature and report of 23 cases. *International Journal of Oral Surgery* **14**, 153–61.
88. Machida Y (1982) Root canal therapy in deciduous teeth. *Journal of the Tokyo Dental Association* **36**, 796–802.
89. Magnusson B (1970) Therapeutic pulpotomy in primary molars – clinical and histological follow-up. *Odontologisk Revy* **21**, 415–31.
90. Magnusson BO (1980) Pulpotomy in primary molars: long-term clinical and histological evaluation. *International Endodontic Journal* **13**, 143–55.
91. Magnusson BO, Sundell SO (1977) Stepwise excavation of deep carious lesions in primary molars. *Journal of the International Association of Dentistry for Children* **8**, 36–40.
92. Markovic D, Zivojinovic M, Vucctic M (2005) Evaluation of three pulpotomy medicaments in primary teeth. *European Journal of Paediatric Dentistry* **3**, 133–8.
93. Mass E, Kaplan I, Hirshberg A (1995) A clinical and histological study of radicular cysts associated with primary molars. *Journal of Oral Pathology and Medicine* **24**, 458–61.
94. Massler M (1967) Preventive endodontics: vital pulp therapy. *Dental Clinics of North America* **11**, 663–73.
95. McDonald RE, Avery DR, Dean J (2004) Treatment of deep caries, vital pulp exposure, and pulpless teeth. In McDonald RE, Avery DR, Dean J, editors. *Dentistry for the child and adolescent*, pp. 388–412, 8th edn. St Louis, MO: Mosby,

96. Mejare I (1979) Pulpotomy of primary molars with coronal or total pulpitis using formocresol technique. *Scandinavian Journal of Dental Research* **57**, 208–16.

97. Melsen B, Terp S (1982) The influence of extractions caries cause on the development of malocclusion and need for orthodontic treatment. *Swedish Dental Journal* Supplement **15**, 163–9.

98. Mertz-Fairhurst EJ, Curtis JW, Ergle JW, Rueggeberg FA, Adair SM (1998) Ultraconservative and cariostatic sealed restorations. *Journal of the American Dental Association* **129**, 55–66.

99. Messer LB, Cline JT, Korf NW (1980) Long term effects of primary molar pulpotomies on succedaneous bicuspids. *Journal of Dental Research* **59**, 116–23.

100. Mjör IA, Tronstad L (1972) Experimentally induced pulpitis. *Oral Surgery, Oral Medicine, Oral Pathology* **34**, 102–8.

101. Morabito A, Defabianis P (1992) A SEM investigation on pulpal-periodontal connections in primary teeth. *Journal of Dentistry for Children* **59**, 53–7.

102. Morawa AP, Straffon LH, Han SS, Corpron RE (1975) Clinical evaluation of pulpotomies using dilute formocresol. *ASDC Journal of Dentistry for Children* **42**, 360–3.

103. Mortazavi M, Mesbahi M (2004) Comparison of zinc oxide and eugenol, and Vitapex for root canal treatment of necrotic primary teeth. *International Journal of Paediatric Dentistry* **14**, 417–24.

104. Moss SJ, Addelston H, Goldsmith ED (1965) Histologic study of pulpal floor of deciduous molars. *Journal of the American Dental Association* **70**, 372–9.

105. Myers DR, Battenhouse MR, Barenie JT, McKinney RV (1987) Histopathology of furcation lesions associated with pulp degeneration in primary molars. *Paediatric Dentistry* **9**, 289–92.

106. Myers DR, Durham LC, Hanes CM, Barenie JT, McKinney RV (1988) Histopathology of radiolucent furcation lesions associated with pulpotomy-treated primary molars. *Pediatric Dentistry* **10**, 291–4.

107. Myers DR, Pashley DH, Whitford GM, McKinney RV (1981) The acute toxicity of high doses of systemically administered formocresol in dogs. *Pediatric Dentistry* **3**, 37–41.

108. Myers DR, Pashley DH, Whitford GM, McKinney RV (1983) Tissue changes induced by the absorption of formocresol from pulpotomy sites in dogs. *Pediatric Dentistry* **5**, 6–8.

109. Myers DR, Shoaf HK, Dirksen TR, Pashley DH, Whitford GM, Reynolds KE (1978) Distribution of ^{14}C-formaldehyde after pulpotomy with formocresol. *Journal of the American Dental Association* **96**, 805–13.

110. Nakashima M (1994) Induction of dentine formation on canine amputated pulp by recombinant human bone morphogenic proteins BMP-2 and -4. *Journal of Dental Research* **73**, 1515–22.

111. Nakashima M (2005) Bone morphogenic proteins in dentin regeneration for potential use in endodontic therapy. *Cytokine Growth Factor Review* **16**, 369–76.

112. Nunn JH, Smeaton I, Gilroy J (1996) The development of formocresol as a medicament for primary molar pulpotomy procedures. *ASDC Journal of Dentistry for Children* **63**, 51–3.

113. Nurko C, Ranly DR, Garcia-Godoy F, Lakshmyya K (2000) Resorption of calcium hydroxide/iodoform paste (Vitapex) in root canal therapy for primary teeth: a case report. *Pediatric Dentistry* **22**, 517–20.

114. Ooë T, Gohdo S (1984) The development of the human interradicular dentine as revealed by tetracycline-labelling. *Archives of Oral Biology* **29**, 257–62.

115. Oztas N, Ulusu T, Oygur T, Cokpefin F (1994) Comparison of electrosurgery and formocresol as pulpotomy techniques in dog primary teeth. *Journal of Clinical Pediatric Dentistry* **18**, 285–9.

116. Papagiannoulis L (2002) Clinical studies on ferric sulphate as a pulpotomy medicament in primary teeth. *European Journal of Paediatric Dentistry* **3**, 126–32.

117. Paras LG, Rapp R, Piesco NP, Zeichner SJ, Zullo TG (1993) An investigation of accessory canals in furcation areas of human primary molars. Part 2. Latex perfusion studies of the internal and external furcation areas to demonstrate accessory canals. *Journal of Clinical Pediatric Dentistry* **17**, 71–7.

118. Paras LG, Rapp R, Piesco NP, Zeichner SJ, Zullo TG (1993) An investigation of accessory foramina in human primary molars. Part 1. SEM observations of frequency, size and location of accessory foramina in the internal and external furcation areas. *Journal of Clinical Pediatric Dentistry* **17**, 65–9.

119. Pashley EL, Myers DR, Pashley DH, Whitford GM (1980) Systemic distribution of ^{14}C-formaldehyde from formocresol treated pulpotomy sites. *Journal of Dental Research* **59**, 602–8.

120. Pashley EL, Talman R, Horner JA, Pashley DH (1991) Permeability of normal versus carious dentin. *Endodontics and Dental Traumatology* **7**, 207–11.

121. Pearse AGE (1980) The chemistry of fixation. In *Histochemistry, theoretical and applied*, pp 101–2. Edinburgh: Churchill Livingstone.

122. Ranly DM, Garcia-Godoy (2000) Current and potential pulp therapies for primary and young permanent teeth. *Journal of Dentistry* **28**, 153–61.

123. Ranly DM, Horn D (1990) Distribution, metabolism, and excretion of [^{14}C] glutaraldehyde. *Journal of Endodontics* **16**, 135–9.

124. Ranly DM, Lazzari EP (1983) A biochemical study of two bifunctional reagents as alternatives to formocresol. *Journal of Dental Research* **62**, 1054–7.

125. Rapp R (1992) Vascular pathways within pulpal tissue of human primary teeth. *Journal of Clinical Pediatric Dentistry* **16**, 183–201.

126. Rayner JA, Southam JC (1979) Pulp changes in deciduous teeth associated with deep carious dentine. *Journal of Dentistry* **7**, 39–42.

127. Rifkin A (1980) A simple effective, safe technique for the root canal treatment of abscessed primary teeth. *ASDC Journal of Dentistry for Children* **47**, 435–41.

128. Rimondini L, Baroni C (1995) Morphologic criteria for root canal treatment of primary molars undergoing resorption. *Endodontics and Dental Traumatology* **11**, 136–41.

129. Ringelstein D, Seow WK (1989) The prevalence of furcation foramina in primary molars. *Pediatric Dentistry* **11**, 198–202.

130. Rivera N, Reyes E, Mazzaoui S, Moron A (2003) Pulpal therapy for primary teeth: formocresol vs electrosurgery: a clinical study. *Journal of Dentistry for Children* **70**, 71–3.

131. Roberts JF (1996) Treatment of vital and non-vital primary molar teeth by one-stage formocresol pulpotomy: clinical success and effect on age at exfoliation. *British Dental Journal* **6**, 111–15.

132. Rodd HD, Boissonade FM (2001) Innervation of human tooth pulp in relation to caries and dentition type. *Journal of Dental Research* **80**, 389–93.

133. Rodd HD, Boissonade FM (2003) Immunocytochemical investigation of neurovascular relationships in human tooth pulp. *Journal of Anatomy* **202**, 195–203.

134. Rodd HD, Boissonade FM (2005) Vascular status in human primary and permanent teeth in health and disease. *European Journal of Oral Science* **113**, 128–34.

135. Rodd HD, Boissonade FM (2006) Immunocytochemical investigation of immune cells within human primary and permanent tooth pulp. *International Journal of Paediatric Dentistry* **16**, 2–9.

136. Rolling I, Hasselgren G, Tronstad L (1976) Morphologic and enzyme histochemical observations on the pulp of human primary molars 3 to 5 years after formocresol treatment. *Oral Surgery, Oral Medicine, Oral Pathology* **42**, 518–28.

137. Rolling I, Thylstrup A (1975) A 3-year clinical follow-up study of pulpotomized primary molars treated with the formocresol technique. *Scandinavian Journal of Dental Research* **83**, 47–53.

138. Ruemping DR, Morton TH, Anderson MW (1983) Electrosurgical pulpotomy in primates – a comparison with formocresol pulpotomy. *Pediatric Dentistry* **5**, 14–18.

139. Salako N, Joseph B, Ritwik P, Salonen J, John P, Junaid TA (2003) Comparison of bioactive glass, mineral trioxide aggregate, ferric sulphate, and formocresol as pulpotomy agents in rat molar. *Dental Traumatology* **19**, 314–20.

140. Salama FS, Anderson RW, McKnight-Haynes C, Barenie JT, Myers DR (1992) Anatomy of primary incisor and molar root canals. *Pediatric Dentistry* **14**, 117–18.

141. Sato T, Hoshino E, Uematsu H, Noda T (1993) Predominant obligate anaerobes in necrotic pulps of human deciduous teeth. *Microbial Ecology in Health and Disease* **6**, 269–75.

142. Saunders WP, Saunders E (1997) Coronal leakage as a cause of failure in root canal therapy. *Endodontics and Dental Traumatology* **10**, 105–8.

143. Savage NW, Adkins KF, Weir AV, Grundy GE (1986) An histological study of cystic lesions following pulp therapy in deciduous teeth. *Journal of Oral Pathology* **15**, 209–12.

144. Schroder U (1977) Agreement between clinical and histologic findings in chronic coronal pulpitis in primary teeth. *Scandinavian Journal of Dental Research* **85**, 583–7.

145. Schroder U (1978) A 2-year follow-up of primary molars, pulpotomized with a gentle technique and capped with calcium hydroxide. *Scandinavian Journal of Dental Research* **86**, 273–8.

146. Schroder U, Granath LE (1971) Early reaction of intact human teeth to calcium hydroxide following experimental pulpotomy and its significance to the development of hard tissue barrier. *Odontologisk Revy* **22**, 379–95.

147. Schroder U, Granath LE (1971) On internal dentine resorption in deciduous molars treated by pulpotomy and capped with calcium hydroxide. *Odontologisk Revy* **22**, 179–88.

148. Schroder U, Szpringer-Nodzak M, Janicha J, Wacinska M, Budny J, Mlosek K (1987) A one-year follow-up of partial pulpotomy and calcium hydroxide capping in primary molars. *Endodontics and Dental Traumatology* **6**, 304–6.

149. Shiflett K, White SN (1997) Microleakage of cements for stainless steel crowns. *Pediatric Dentistry* **19**, 262–6.

150. Shoji S, Nakamura M, Horiuchi H (1985) Histopathological changes in dental pulps irradiated by CO_2 laser: a preliminary report on laser pulpotomy. *Journal of Endodontics* **11**, 379–84.

151. Simsek S, Durutürk L (2005) A flow cytometric analysis of the biodefensive response of deciduous tooth pulp to carious stimuli during physiological root resorption. *Archives of Oral Biology* **50**, 461–8.

152. Skogedal O, Tronstad L (1977) An attempt to correlate dentin, and pulp changes in human carious teeth. *Oral Surgery, Oral Medicine, Oral Pathology* **43**, 135–40.

153. Smith AJ, Smith G (1998) Solubilization of TGFβ1 by dentine conditioning agents. *Journal of Dental Research* **77**, 1034 (abstract 3224).

154. Smith NL, Seale NS, Nunn ME (2000) Ferric sulphate pulpotomy in primary molars: a retrospective study. *Pediatric Dentistry* **22**, 192–9.

155. Straffon LH, Han SS (1970) Effects of varying concentrations of formocresol on RNA synthesis of connective tissues in sponge implants. *Oral Surgery, Oral Medicine, Oral Pathology* **29**, 915–25.

156. Sweet CA (1955) Treatment of vital primary teeth with pulpal involvement. Therapeutic pulpotomy. *Journal of the Colorado Dental Association* **33**, 10–14.

157. Tagger E, Sarnat H (1984) Root canal therapy of infected primary teeth. *Acta de Odontologica Pediatrica* **5**, 63–6.

158. Tagger M, Massler M (1975) Periapical tissue reactions after pulp exposure in rat molars. *Oral Surgery, Oral Medicine, Oral Pathology* **39**, 304–17.

159. Taylor BR, Berman DS, Johnson NW (1971) The response of pulp and dentine to dental caries in primary molars. *Journal of the International Association of Dentistry for Children* **2**, 3–9.

160. Tchaou WS, Turng BF, Minah GE, Coll JA (1995) In vitro inhibition of bacteria from root canals of primary teeth by various dental materials. *Pediatric Dentistry* **17**, 351–5.

161. Torabinejad M, Chivian N (1999) Clinical applications of mineral trioxide aggregate. *Journal of Endodontics* **25**, 197–205.

162. Trowbridge HO (2002) Histology of pulpal inflammation. In Hargreaves KM, Goodis HE, editors. *Seltzer & Bender's dental pulp*, pp. 227–45. Chicago, IL: Quintessence.

163. Tziafas D, Smith AJ, Lesot H (2000) Designing new treatment strategies in vital pulp therapies. *Journal of Dentistry* **28**, 77–92.

164. Valderhaug J (1974) Periapical inflammation in primary teeth and its effect on the permanent successors. *International Journal of Oral Surgery* **3**, 171–82.

165. Vargas KG, Packham B (2005) Radiographic success of ferric sulphate and formocresol pulpotomies in relation to early exfoliation. *Pediatric Dentistry* **27**, 233–7.

166. Via WF (1955) Evaluation of deciduous molars treated by pulpotomy and calcium hydroxide. *Journal of the American Dental Association* **50**, 34–43.

167. Vij R, Col JA, Shelton P, Farooq NS (2004) Caries control and other variables associated with success of primary molar vital pulp therapy. *Paediatric Dentistry* **26**, 214–19.

168. Waterhouse PJ, Nunn JH, Whitworth JM (2000) An investigation of the relative efficacy of Buckley's formocresol and calcium hydroxide in primary molar vital pulp therapy. *British Dental Journal* **188**, 32–6.

169. Weerheijm KL, Groen HJ (1999) The residual caries dilemma. *Community Dentistry and Oral Epidemiology* **27**, 436–41.

170. Wellbury RR, Murphy JM (1998) The dental practitioner's role in protecting children from abuse. *British Dental Journal* **24**, 61–5.

171. Wemes JC, Purdell-Lewis D, Jongebloed W, Vaalburg W (1982) Diffusion of carbon-14-labeled formocresol and glutaraldehyde in tooth structures. *Oral Surgery, Oral Medicine, Oral Pathology* **54**, 341–6.

172. Wilkerson MK, Hill SD, Arcoria CJ (1996) Effects of the argon laser on primary tooth pulpotomies in swine. *Journal of Clinical Laser Medicine and Surgery* **14**, 37–42.

173. Winter GB (1962) Abscess formation in connexion with deciduous molar teeth. *Archives of Oral Biology* **7**, 373–9.

174. Winter GB, Kramer IRH (1965) Changes in periodontal membrane and bone following experimental pulpal injury in deciduous molar teeth in kittens. *Archives of Oral Biology* **10**, 279–89.

175. Wrbas K, Kielbassa AM, Hellwig E (1997) Microscopic studies of accessory canals in primary molar furcations. *Journal of Dentistry for Children* **67**, 118–22.

176. Wright FAC, Widmer RP (1979) Pulpal therapy in primary molar teeth: a retrospective study. *Journal of Pedodontics* **3**, 195–206.

177. Yacobi R, Kenny DJ, Judd PL, Johnston DH (1991) Evolving primary pulp therapy techniques. *Journal of the American Dental Association* **122**, 83–5.

178. Zander HA (1939) Reaction of the pulp to calcium hydroxide. *Journal of Dental Research* **18**, 373–9.

179. Zarzar PA, Rosenblatt A, Takahashi CS, Takeuchi PL, Costa LA (2003) Formocresol mutagenicity following primary tooth pulp therapy: an in vivo study. *Journal of Dentistry* **31**, 479–85.

180. Zoremchhingi JT, Varma B, Mungara J (2005) A study of root canal morphology of human primary molars using computerised tomography: An in vitro study. *Indian Society of Pedodontics and Preventive Dentistry* **23**, 7–12.

181. Zürcher E (1925) *The anatomy of the root canals of the teeth of the deciduous dentition and of the first permanent molars*, pp. 171–5. London: J Bale, Sons & Danielsson.

Chapter 10
Treatment of the Exposed Pulp–Dentin Complex

Gunnar Hasselgren

10.1 Introduction

Hundreds of thousands of teeth are prepared daily with rotating instruments and all restorative procedures performed in dentin of vital teeth are in essence performed in dentin and pulp: the pulp–dentin complex. It is essential to perform preparation of dentin, including caries excavation, in such a way that minimal damage is done to the pulp. Even if the clinician can closely inspect the dentin, the condition of the pulp is often elusive. When clinical test results are compared to histopathologic findings in the same teeth, it has been found that it is usually impossible to make a correct diagnosis of the pulp condition based on clinical findings. Groth [59] was the first to demonstrate this as long ago as 1933, and his findings have been corroborated by numerous studies. One reason for this discrepancy is that most inflammation of the pulp and periapical tissues is free from symptoms. However, even when symptoms are present, there can only be speculation about the differences between clinical and histopathological findings. These may be due to differences in the neurophysiological responses, differences in the microflora of carious lesions, or other factors.

The causes of pulp pain are not fully understood; these have been reviewed [61]. It has been suggested that an increased intrapulpal pressure caused by inflammation may trigger nerve endings to fire [157]. However, this does not explain why two pulps with similar histopathological features may show different clinical symptoms. The hydrodynamic theory [16,17,19] proposes that an increased flow in dentinal tubules of exposed dentin will cause a reaction from intrapulpal nerve endings that is registered as pain. Experimental support for the theory, or at least for signals reaching the pulp via dentin tubules, has been obtained in animal experiments [116,117], and also in human experiments, which showed that hydrostatic pressure applied to smear-layer-free dentin cavities triggered pain responses [1]. It is conceivable that an increased osmotic pressure caused by accumulated bacterial products can cause signaling through dentin fluid, thus eliciting firing of pulp nerve endings. However, it is not possible to demonstrate this with histological methods which may explain the discrepancies between clinical and histopathological findings.

Caries is the most common cause of pulp inflammation [46]. Breakdown products from bacteria reach pulp cells via dentin tubules [8,84,139]. The treatment is influenced by the clinical situation and factors such as depth of the cavity following excavation, pulpodentinal response, exposure/nonexposure of the pulp, stage of tooth development, and presence or absence of pain.

It is common to use the duration of pain as a guide for initiating, or not initiating, endodontic treatment after caries removal without pulp exposure in a deep cavity. Lingering pain should mean a more severe pulpal involvement. However, as mentioned earlier, clinical symptoms do not usually reveal the true state of the pulp. In other words, there is basically no scientific evidence for this practice. When bacteria and bacteria-produced irritants have been removed during excavation, and the restoration prevents new bacteria from getting access to the pulp part of the dentin, the inflamed pulp has a great potential for healing. However, it is essential to follow up all teeth with deep restorations to evaluate the vitality of the pulp with cold and electric tests, and with radiographs.

10.2 Treatment of the nonexposed pulp

Cutting of dentin and exposure of tubules result in an outward flow of fluid [15,92,130] owing to the pulp having a higher pressure than most other tissues [66]. This can be markedly exaggerated during operative procedures if the dentin is allowed to be dried out by heat caused by insufficient cooling, or by excessive air spray (Fig. 10.1). Also, increased outward flow can cause an aspiration of odontoblasts into the den-

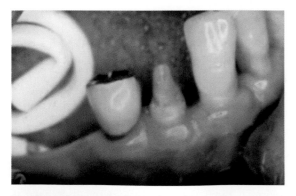

Fig. 10.1 Photograph taken 3 days after crown preparation that was undertaken without sufficient water cooling showing bleeding into dentin has occurred. Later dentin became grey and there was no response to pulp sensitivity testing.

tinal tubules [15,16]. Just as there is a communication from the pulp through the tubules if the dentinal tubules are exposed, products from bacteria can diffuse through them into the pulp and cause an inflammatory response [9]. This is the case in caries, but also if a denuded dentin surface is exposed to oral bacteria. If dentin has been exposed to the oral cavity for a long period of time, bacteria can be found in the dentinal tubules, but very seldom in the pulp [88]. Still there is local pulpal inflammation in the area where the dentinal tubules from the exposed dentin area enter the pulp [9]. In the initial inflammatory response a local accumulation of chronic inflammatory cells can be seen; it is most likely mediated by odontoblasts. At a later stage, dendritic cells become involved and stimulate T-lymphocytes by presenting antigens [46]. During the progress of a carious lesion, the number of chronic inflammatory cells and also dendritic cells in the odontoblast region increases. As the carious process progresses, the dendritic cells aggregate in subodontoblastic regions and later extend into the odontoblast layer. They eventually reach the entrance of dentin tubules beside the odontoblast process [189]. Even if dentin *per se* is a physical barrier against noxious stimuli, the pulp's immune response provides a humoral and cellular defense against invading pathogens. The immune response increases as the carious process advances and titers of T-helper cells, B-lineage cells, macrophages, and neutrophils are directly proportional to the lesion's closeness to the pulp [75].

When dentin has been exposed to the oral cavity for long time periods there is usually no or little inflammation in the pulp [46,88,178]. This shows that the pulp is capable of healing after an initial inflammatory response. It blocks the dentinal tubules to prevent noxious agents from reaching the pulp [9]. The dentin becomes sclerotic and deposition of whitlockite crystals in the tubular lumen is most likely from a stimulation of odontoblasts. Therefore, in the vital tooth, bacteria do not reach the pulp unless the dentin is destroyed by caries [122]. The vital pulp acts as a barrier preventing bacteria from invading the tooth and the periapical tissues. However, in the case of a nonvital tooth bacteria can rapidly grow through the dentinal tubules and reach the pulp cavity [25].

10.2.1 Excavation of caries

When the carious process advances through dentin there is first a demineralization by acids from the bacteria and later a more pronounced breakdown of the hard tissue architecture caused by bacterial enzymatic activity [37]. The demineralized dentin has been referred to as affected dentin and the broken down part has been called infected dentin [95]. It has been proposed that during excavation only the infected carious dentin should be removed and that the affected dentin could be left permanently [95]. However, it has been clearly shown by means of electron microscopy and anaerobic culturing methods that the affected dentin contains bacteria [83]. In spite of this, many clinicians still recommend that the affected dentin can be left in the tooth. It has also been advocated that the affected dentin should be preserved by impregnation with dentin-bonding agents. However, when bonding to sound and to carious dentin was compared, it was found that the bond strength of carious dentin was significantly lower [112]. In other words, an excellent substrate for bacteria will be left under a restoration, which if there were leakage, would pave the way for a new infection close to the pulp.

Clinically, it is difficult to discriminate between the different layers of carious dentin. So, in addition to the scientific evidence that all caries must be removed, from a practical clinical point it is strongly advised to excavate carious dentin until the remaining dentin is sound, that is the remaining dentin feels hard when it is examined with an explorer. Also, sound dentin reflects light and does not have the dull appearance of demineralized dentin. To leave infected material in a cavity under a permanent filling intentionally is like removing all but the deepest layer of plaque during periodontal treatment.

10.2.2 Restorative procedures

In a retrospective study, Felton *et al.* [43] found that 11% of over 1000 teeth followed for a long period of time showed pulp necrosis. During the preparation of a tooth and the placement of a restoration there are many steps during which pulp damage can occur.

Anesthesia

There is an increased risk of pulp necrosis when a vasoconstrictor is added to the anesthetic. The blood flow is temporarily decreased or may even be completely shut down and the pulp cannot regulate its defense towards overheating and subsequent dehydration during preparation. Also, the anesthetic itself may decrease the pulp's sensory nerve regulation of hemodynamic reactions to clinical procedures [121].

Preparation with rotary instruments

During excavation of caries and the subsequent preparation of the cavity, the clinician is likely to be dealing with an inflamed pulp and great care should be taken to avoid further damage to the pulp. Being careful during restorative procedures is a preventive endodontic measure to avoid further endodontic treatment. It is imperative to utilize sufficient water cooling, well-centered burs, and as little pressure as possible to avoid frictional heating of the dentin [10,81,82]. The heat will dehydrate the dentin and indirectly the pulp. The closer the preparation is to the pulp, the greater the risk of pulp damage. In a deep cavity it is possible that the heat can damage the pulp tissue. The healthy pulp responds with increased blood flow as a response to the heating and subsequent dehydration. As mentioned earlier, this may not be possible in a pulp anethetized with the addition of a vasoconstrictor. Still, in most instances the pulp recovers after preparation.

The permeability of dentin markedly increases when the remaining dentin thickness is reduced during preparation as more dentinal tubules are being exposed [128,129]. The fact that dentin is more like a sieve than a solid hard structure, makes it possible for ions and molecules to pass through the tubules from the pulp as well as to the pulp. Therefore, during crown or cavity preparation, it is imperative to keep the remaining dentin as thick as possible to avoid unnecessary pulp damage. Stanley [157] has stated that the remaining dentin thickness is the single most important factor in preventing pulpal insult. It has been shown *in vitro* that 1 mm of remaining dentin reduces the effect of a toxic material to 10% of the original level and a 2 mm dentin thickness basically prevents any pulpal insult from a toxic material [157]. Based on these studies, clinicians know how to restore a tooth while minimizing pulp damage. However, cosmetic dentistry is presently in fashion. Dentin is removed to make space for additional thick layers of composites or porcelain to make matching of the desired tooth color easier. Even veneer preparations are cut deeply into dentin for the same reason, thus increasing the risk of pulp damage [26]. New dental procedures and materials have been introduced that place cosmetic results before pulp protection. This is causing an unnecessary increase in endodontic treatments [27].

Material toxicity and the role of infection

Restorative procedures involve permanent placement of materials on the dentin. The toxic effect of dental materials has been considered a primary cause of pulpal inflammation following restorative procedures [158]. Therefore, methods for testing the biocompatibility of dental materials have been developed and these screening tests are used to weed out harmful materials [6,153–155,184,185]. Dental materials often release toxic substances during the setting phase, but become less toxic when the material has set [3,113,182,183]. Some materials, such as amalgam, corrode and the corrosion products have been shown to be toxic in cell culture experiments [101]. However, the pulp reaction to dental materials is mainly transitory and manifest inflammation only occurs after bacteria, or their byproducts, have been able to reach the pulp [11,17,21,28]. When bacterial contamination can be prevented, favorable pulp responses are seen even to materials with established clinical track records of being harmful to the pulp, such as silicate cement and acrylic resin [20,28]. It is the sealing ability of the restoration that determines its ability to protect the pulp from infection [18]. Modern restorative procedures utilizing bonding techniques are markedly superior to earlier filling methods [56,108–111,163].

A few, or rather too few, controlled studies have evaluated the long-term outcomes of bonded fillings. It has been found that leakage leading to secondary caries is the most common reason for replacement of composite restorations [89,104,136]. When a bonded filling material is inserted, there is a tug-of-war between forces that bond the material to the dental hard tissues and polymerization contraction forces [23]. The polymerization shrinkage as well as the forces caused by the use of the filling, including the stress created when both tooth and filling are loaded, will tend to disrupt the bond to the cavity walls [35]. Therefore, it is still essential to use a cavity sealer to protect the pulp dentin under all types of filling materials.

Dentin and pulp protecting agents (cavity sealers)

The primary function of a cavity sealer is to protect the pulp from bacteria and their products. The secondary function is to protect the pulp from toxic effects during the setting phase of a restorative material [72]. The use of a protective layer between dentin and the restorative material is still highly recommended even if markedly toxic and leaking materials such as silicate cements are no longer being used.

Certain criteria have been established for the use of cavity sealants [96]:

- The whole exposed pulp dentin surface must be covered, to avoid the risk of pulpal injury.
- The material must adhere more to the dentin than to the restorative material which otherwise may pull the cavity sealer from the dentin.
- The material should be applied in a thin layer so that the strength and retention of the filling material is not weakened.
- The material should not dissolve in biological liquids such as saliva, gingival crevicular exudate, and/or dentin fluid.
- The material should be easy to handle.

Traditionally cavity sealers have been divided into varnishes, liners, and base materials [52]. The use of dentin-bonding methods has created an additional group of cavity sealers [70].

Varnish

A varnish is a protective film that coats the freshly cut dentin. The material is dissolved in an organic solvent such as ether, chloroform, or acetone. After application on the dentin surface the solvent evaporates, leaving a coat of the material. Varnishes are commonly used under amalgam restorations to seal the space between the filling and the dentin until corrosion products can fill the gap [5,30]. Natural products such as rosin or copal, or synthetic resins are used as varnishes. Copal varnish reduces dentin permeability by 69% [131]; the effect is increased by the use of two applications [132]. Acceptable retention of crowns has been found after copal varnish application prior to cementation [42].

Liner

A liner is a varnish that contains fillers and additives. It is placed as a thin layer. The additives are intended to have beneficial effects on the pulp and dental hard tissues, e.g., an antibacterial effect or the release of fluoride. One of these commonly used components is calcium hydroxide ($Ca(OH)_2$).

Cavity base

A base material is a thicker sealant that is intended to protect additionally from thermal effects through restorative materials. Zinc phosphate cement was earlier used as a base material. However, its poor sealing ability has been shown to be a major reason for adverse pulp reactions [28]. Zinc oxide/eugenol cements have also been widely used. The pulp protecting ability of zinc oxide/eugenol is most likely due to its antibacterial properties that prevent bacteria from reaching the innermost part of the dentin [126]. On the other hand, it interferes with polymerization of composite resin and normally has poor physical properties [30,41,93]. The use of zinc oxide/eugenol cements should be restricted to temporary restorations.

Calcium hydroxide has also been used for pulp protection. When a thick slurry made with water is placed in a freshly prepared cavity, the pH of the dentin fluid will increase. In the dentin closest to the pulp, this increase will last for up to a week [62,118]. Such an increase may be found under calcium-hydroxide-containing base materials if the hydroxyl ions are not trapped within the set base [169]. This rise in dentin fluid pH may cause a coagulation of proteins which may explain the initial, transient effect of $Ca(OH)_2$ on sensitive dentin [97]. Another possible reason for this is that the $Ca(OH)_2$ particles may protect the pulp by mechanically obturating the dentinal tubules [105].

Setting base materials containing $Ca(OH)_2$ have been quite popular during the past three decades. A major reason for the addition of $Ca(OH)_2$ to the base materials is a desire to stimulate the odontoblasts to increase dentin thickness. Increased dentin formation under cavities lined with $Ca(OH)_2$ has been noted [63,168,170], whereas other investigations have failed to demonstrate this [12,179]. Acids used during acid etching procedures react with $Ca(OH)_2$ thus jeopardizing the protective function of the base material. Calcium-hydroxide-containing base material has less adhesion to dentin than a bonded composite material [55]. The main reasons for using a cavity sealant are to protect the pulp from infection and also from toxic substances from the restorative material especially during the setting phase. Whether additives to obtain additional effects are necessary remains to be elucidated.

Dentin bonding agents

Dentin bonding agents, glass ionomers, and resin cements have been used as cavity sealants to decrease leakage and to provide retention. The latter is obtained by the use of multisubstrate bonding techniques to create a bond between the filling material and the dental hard tissues. Studies using animal models have shown that dentin primers placed on dentin with or without adhesives are well tolerated by the pulp [161,186] and so are glass ionomers [68,119]. However, there are different reports in the literature regarding the benefits of dentin-bonding agents as cavity sealants. Saiku *et al.* [143] demonstrated a marked reduction in marginal leakage when dentin-bonding agents were used. On the other hand Dutton *et al.* [36] found no decrease in leakage. There appears to be agreement that there is marked leakage when cavity margins are placed on cementum [126,167]. Also, dentin-bonding agents are more technique sensitive than for example a varnish [167]. Most studies on dentin bonding are *in vitro* and relatively short term. A more long-term study on bonded amalgam fillings showed breakdown at the restoration interface [143]. The use of bonding agents under amalgam fillings is common. However, since controlled long-term clinical studies are lacking, caution is recommended until the long-term outcome has been assessed [70].

The bond strength is less in the deep part of a cavity compared to superficial dentin [162,165,166]. The closer a cavity is to the pulp the more dentinal tubules are exposed and the ratio between intertubular dentin and tubules decreases [50]. This means a decreased area of intertubular collagen that is necessary for the formation of a hybrid layer [109]. Also, Pashley [129] has demonstrated that immediately adjacent to a dentinal tubule the bond is weaker due to less collagen in the peritubular dentin. All this considered, it is today still advisable to use a base material in the pulpal part of a deep cavity.

10.3 Treatment of the exposed pulp

This consists of a number of different procedures (Fig. 10.2). The goal for treatment of the exposed pulp is healing and preservation of the underlying tissues. This can only be obtained in the absence of infection. Therefore, it is absolutely imperative that all these treatments be performed under aseptic conditions, which among other things includes the use of rubber dam isolation.

The pulp has two healing patterns: a connective tissue scar, like most other tissues, or formation of a hard tissue barrier. Healing with a connective tissue

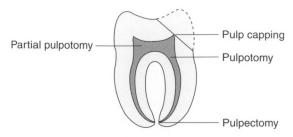

Partial pulpotomy

Pulp capping

Pulpotomy

Pulpectomy

Fig. 10.2   Drawing showing the levels at which pulp capping, partial pulpotomy, pulpotomy, or pulpectomy are performed.

scar can function well if the restoration completely seals the cavity. However, even if adhesive resins render a better seal than earlier filling materials, most, if not all, restorations will leak when adhesion degrades [35,103,104,176]. This means that healing with a hard tissue barrier is necessary as a defense against bacteria entering via microleakage.

10.3.1 Pulp capping

Pulp capping has historically been the name given to two different types of treatment: indirect and direct pulp capping.

Indirect pulp capping usually means a procedure in which the excavation of caries is halted before an anticipated pulp exposure occurs. The deepest layer of caries is then left under a permanent filling. Indirect pulp capping has also been the name used for a procedure in which the excavation of caries is halted before an anticipated exposure and a temporary filling material is placed. The final excavation is done later when – hopefully – new dentin has been formed under the caries.

Direct pulp capping is the covering of exposed pulp tissue with a wound dressing.

10.3.2 Indirect pulp capping

Intentionally leaving caries

This is a form of treatment that unfortunately still is widely practiced. To leave intentionally infected decayed material permanently in the body is unique in the practice of medicine and dentistry. It is easy to understand how this form of treatment originated. Endodontic treatment has been, and still is, time consuming and at many times difficult. Therefore, a halt

is made before reaching the pulp during excavation of caries, with the hope that the pulp will survive and endodontic treatment can be avoided. A successful outcome in common practice is based on the absence of symptoms. As most pulpal inflammations, and definitely pulp necrosis, are free from symptoms, this kind of treatment has become accepted by some dentists. Various antiseptics have been used in attempts to sterilize the remaining caries. Unfortunately, every dentist dealing with endodontic emergencies can testify that cases with pulpal and/or periapical inflammation caused by remaining caries under restorations are quite common. To summarize with the words of the late Professor Birger Nygaard Østby, who emphasized during many a lecture: "To intentionally and permanently leave caries is malpractice and this kind of procedure should be pronounced indirect pulp crapping."

Stepwise excavation

This is a temporary procedure during which the excavation of caries is halted before an expected pulp exposure. The remaining layer of carious dentin is covered with a slurry of $Ca(OH)_2$ and water and a temporary filling is placed [58]. The $Ca(OH)_2$ is used due to its antibacterial effect on the carious dentin [44] and to stimulate further dentin formation [168]. The caries process involves the dissolution as well as reprecipitation of mineral [49] and there is a possibility of the softened dentin remineralizing if the infection is removed and the cavity is sealed off from the oral environment. This has been demonstrated both *in vivo* [39] and *in vitro* [181].

During the next visit, at least 2 months later, the final excavation is performed. If hard dentin is found under the final layer of caries, the tooth is restored with a base material and a permanent filling. If caries has reached the pulp, endodontic treatment is initiated.

Stepwise excavation is commonly used in young patients to reduce the risk of pulp exposure during the final excavation [91]. It is impossible to know if there was an intact layer of dentin present under the remaining caries during the initial excavation or if the intact dentin found during the final step is newly formed. However, in a recent study on permanent molars with deep caries randomly chosen for complete or stepwise excavation, a significantly lower number of pulp exposures were found in the stepwise excavation group [85]. This corroborated the results of an earlier study in deciduous teeth in which it was found that immediate full excavation rendered more exposures than the stepwise approach [91].

10.3.3 Direct pulp capping

The covering of an exposed pulp with a wound dressing is a treatment with old traditions. Many different materials have been advocated for pulp capping during the years. This reflects that no material really worked and the dismal results of this treatment were summarized by Rebel [138]: "the exposed pulp is a doomed organ".

The introduction of $Ca(OH)_2$ as a capping agent [64,65] created new interest. The effects of $Ca(OH)_2$ on exposed pulp tissue has been extensively studied (e.g., [31,33,51,120,148]). It has been clearly shown that the key factor in pulpal healing after exposure is the absence of infection [77]. One of the major reasons for improved pulp capping results following the introduction of $Ca(OH)_2$, is the antibacterial effect of the compound. However, failures, irrespective of capping agent, are caused by infection due to either remaining bacteria or the exposure to new bacteria from leakage. Therefore, pulp capping should be looked upon as a two-step procedure: first the capping of the pulp and then the long-term follow-up [10].

It has been shown that there is a difference in outcome between the capping of an inflamed and a noninflamed pulp. The chance of a successful outcome is markedly higher in the noninflamed pulp exposed by trauma, than in the inflamed pulp exposed during caries excavation [120]. Caries causes pulpal inflammation even if the carious process *per se* has not reached the pulp tissue as bacterial byproducts will reach the pulp via dentinal tubules [8,9,139]. Therefore, pulp capping should not be carried out after carious exposure as well as after accidental exposure following excavation of deep caries. A capping procedure should be carried out only after a relatively fresh traumatic exposure, before a bacterial biofilm is established on the exposed pulp.

Calcium hydroxide has been the dominant material for many years, but mineral trioxide aggregate (MTA; Portland cement) has also shown excellent results in studies [40,100,134,174]. When $Ca(OH)_2$ powder is exposed to air it will react with carbon dioxide and form calcium carbonate which is not useful as a capping agent. In other words, $Ca(OH)_2$ must be fresh or stored in an airtight container to function

as a capping agent. The effect of MTA is most likely due to $Ca(OH)_2$ formed during the setting reaction [22]. The use of MTA gives the benefit of providing nascent $Ca(OH)_2$ in addition to its sealing ability [4,164].

Many other materials, e.g., collagen, cyanoacrylate, and adhesive resins have also been tested as pulp wound dressings [2,29,33,67,78]. There is a great interest in adhesive resins as pulp capping agents. However, most recommendations are based on case reports, e.g., [79,135] or small experimental material [80]. Valid experimental and clinical research is necessary before a material can be recommended for clinical use. Pitt Ford and Roberts [133] carried out an animal study comparing enamel bonding agents to different $Ca(OH)_2$ formulations as pulp capping agents. Most of the teeth with $Ca(OH)_2$ showed bridge formation. On the other hand, less than 25% of the pulps capped with bonding agents demonstrated bridges. Another study compared pulp capping with a dentin bonding agent to capping with Dycal. The Dycal cappings showed more favorable healing and there was no bridge formation in the bonding agent group [160]. Nevertheless, adhesive resins are frequently used in general practice as pulp capping agents. An editorial inadvertently summarized the situation by at the beginning recommending the use of adhesive resins for pulp capping, but at the end admitting that the evidence in the form of long-term studies did not exist [124].

A more biological approach, using growth factors, has been introduced and promising results have been obtained in animal experiments [114,115]. Growth factors are presently being tested worldwide as pulp-capping agents [53,60,73,76,87,140,144,151]. From promising results it is believed that they could become the new generation of pulp wound dressings [173]. Still, it may be too early to introduce them clinically. In a study using human premolars, $Ca(OH)_2$ pulp capping gave more hard tissue barriers than capping with an enamel matrix derivative [125].

Procedure

After anesthesia and the application of rubber dam, the pulp wound and surrounding tooth is cleaned with sterile isotonic saline irrigation. A paste of $Ca(OH)_2$ and water, or a calcium-hydroxide-containing base material, is placed on the exposed pulp tissue. Excess water is removed with sterile cotton pellets. The capping agent is then covered with a cement and the final

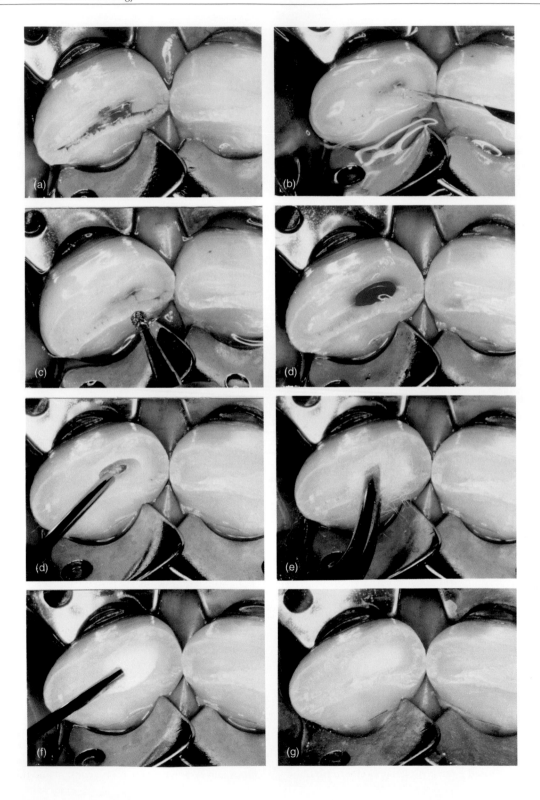

restoration can be placed. Follow-ups should be performed using radiographs, and electric and thermal tests.

10.3.4 Partial pulpotomy

Partial pulpotomy is a procedure in-between pulp capping, that is the placement of a wound dressing on an exposed pulp, and pulpotomy, that is the removal of coronal pulp tissue and the placement of a wound dressing on the canal orifice. Partial pulpotomy was introduced by Cvek [31] and it has been shown to be highly successful in teeth with traumatic pulp exposures [31,32,48].

Procedure

The partial pulpotomy includes surgical removal of the exposed pulp and dentin surrounding the exposure to a depth of 1.5–2 mm (Fig. 10.3). The cutting of the pulp tissue is performed intermittently with a rotating diamond instrument in a high-speed handpiece under copious water spray [57]. The treatment is carried out under aseptic conditions using rubber dam. As an extrapulpal blood clot has been reported to diminish the chances for hard tissue barrier formation [146], the pulp wound is irrigated with sterile isotonic saline until physiological hemostasis is obtained. The pulp wound is then covered with a paste of $Ca(OH)_2$ and sterile water, or a similar commercial product, e.g., Calasept® (Scania Dental, Knivsta, Sweden). The wound dressing is dried with sterile cotton pellets and after that sealed with a suitable material.

The clinical outcome of this treatment has been evaluated in follow-up studies in adolescents (Fig. 10.4) [31,32,48]. In a study by Cvek [32], partial pulpotomy was performed on 178 teeth with crown fractures; the patients were followed for 3–15 years clinically and radiologically. Healing with hard tissue barrier and pulp survival was found in 169 teeth (95%). The majority of these teeth were treated within 72 h following the accident. There was no statistical difference between these teeth and those treated after a longer time interval. Immature and mature teeth also did not show any difference in the frequency of healing. During the follow-up of this clinical material, 126 of the teeth were examined in a special manner. The patients were recalled 3–6 months after the partial pulpotomy. The cavity seal and the wound dressing were removed under aseptic conditions, using rubber dam, to allow for inspection. The hard tissue barriers were found to be continuous when examined with a sharp explorer [32].

The partial pulpotomy has also been utilized in young, posterior, symptom-free teeth with carious exposures (Fig. 10.5) [94,98,190]. Quite high success rates, 91–93%, were found in these studies. These clearly demonstrate that partial pulpotomy rather than direct pulp capping should be the treatment of choice following traumatic exposure, or even carious pulp exposure, in young teeth. Further studies on partial pulpotomy are necessary to evaluate whether the promising results from the treatment of young teeth with carious exposures are also valid for an adult population.

10.3.5 Pulpotomy

This form of treatment encompasses the removal of the coronal pulp tissue and the placement of a wound dressing on the pulp stump(s) at the level of, or just apical to, the orifice of the root canal(s). Pulpotomy is especially indicated in permanent teeth with incomplete root formation to allow for completion of root development [38,145].

Fig. 10.3 Partial pulpotomy technique: (a) maxillary central incisors 8 h after traumatic injury showing limited intrapulpal bleeding in the right incisor. (b) The fractured surfaces are flushed clean with isotonic saline solution. (c)–(h) the superficial layer of the exposed pulp and surrounding dentin are removed to a depth of about 2 mm, using a diamond bur in a high-speed handpiece. This is done intermittently, using short cutting periods with no unnecessary pressure and continuous cooling of the instrument and cutting area with waterspray. The pulp wound is irrigated with isotonic saline until bleeding has ceased; this can be speeded up by applying light pressure to the pulp wound with a sterile cotton pellet. After hemostasis, a thick slurry of $Ca(OH)_2$ and sterile water is applied to the wound surface and adapted with dry, sterile, cotton pellets and light pressure. The cotton pellets are also used to remove water from the paste. Surplus material can be removed with a spoon excavator. It is important that no blood clot is left between the $Ca(OH)_2$ and the cut pulp tissue because this will impair healing. The coronal cavity is then sealed. If the crown is to be restored immediately after treatment with composite resin, the cavity should not be sealed with zinc oxide/eugenol cement as the eugenol may interfere with polymerization. (Courtesy of Dr Miomir Cvek.)

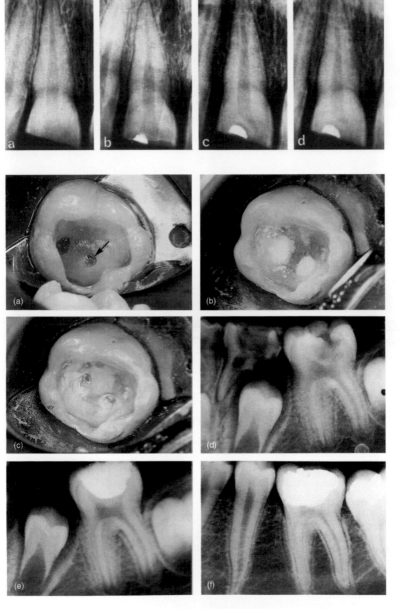

Fig. 10.4 Radiological follow-up of partial pulpotomy: (a) crown fracture and pulp exposure of a maxillary incisor; (b) partial pulpotomy treatment performed 12 h after the accident; (c) after 1 year, there is an intact periapical contour and the tooth responds to vitality testing; (d) after 7 years, there is an intact periapical contour and the tooth responds to vitality testing. Clinical inspection revealed a hard tissue barrier. (Courtesy of Dr Miomir Cvek.)

Fig. 10.5 Partial pulpotomy of first molar pulp exposed during excavation of a deep carious lesion. (a) Partial pulpotomy has been performed at two exposure sites. There is hemostasis in the mesial cavity prepared first (arrowed), and bleeding has ceased in the distal cavity. (b) Pulpal wounds dressed with $Ca(OH)_2$. (c) Appearance of hard tissue barriers 3 months after treatment. (d) Radiograph taken before treatment shows deep carious lesion and normal periapical condition. (e) Radiograph 3 months after treatment. (f) After 8 years complete root development and normal periapical condition are seen. (From Mejàre and Cvek [98] with permission.)

As the outcome for direct pulp capping following carious exposure was considered at best unpredictable [120] pulpotomy was (until the introduction of the partial pulpotomy technique) the treatment of choice especially in immature teeth [145]. Pulpotomy allows for the pulp wound to be placed in a healthier tissue than at the site of exposure. Many different chemical compounds, or combinations of compounds, have been used as wound dressings. Also, the use of different amputation methods such as electrosurgery and laser have been tried, but not evaluated for their long-term outcomes [149,150]. Earlier, wound dressings containing formaldehyde, phenol, creosotes, and other highly toxic materials have been advocated to "mummify" the remaining pulp tissue [14,24]. Histologically, intact pulp tissue has been demonstrated under pulpotomies with formocresol. This has been interpreted as a successful outcome of this treatment form [13]. However, it has later been shown by means of enzyme histochemical methods that this seemingly healthy tissue has been fixed *in vivo* by the formaldehyde component of formocresol [99]. In a 3–5-year follow-up study on pulpotomized primary molars it was found that the pulp tissue reaction to formocresol application was unpredictable [141]. The short-term clinical outcome is usually acceptable which makes the technique still acceptable in primary teeth [74]. On the other hand, it has been shown in a clinical follow-up study on permanent molars with buccal or mesial canals pulpotomized and palatal or distal canals root filled, that with increasing time there is a decreasing success rate following pulpotomy with formaldehyde-containing materials. The root-filled canals in the very same teeth showed a higher long-term success rate [86]. Due to the short lifespan of primary teeth, this form of pulpotomy is still popular in pediatric dentistry.

The use of formocresol pulpotomies has been recommended in permanent teeth with pulp exposures [142], and it has been stated that the plug of fixed tissue can easily be removed later with endodontic instruments [156]. The problem with treating these teeth endodontically years after the pulpotomy procedure is not the removal of a piece of fixed tissue in the coronal part of the canal, but being able to instrument the canal apical to the plug. This part of the canal is often tortuous following appositions, transient resorptions, and calcifications as a response to the toxic material [141]. Also, a high incidence of internal resorption has been demonstrated in formocresol pulpotomized permanent monkey teeth [47].

In pulpotomy, as well as pulp capping, $Ca(OH)_2$ [145] and MTA [107] have been found to render a hard tissue barrier. There are reports on dystrophic calcification or internal resorption following pulpotomy with $Ca(OH)_2$ [90,177]. Studies on healing following pulpotomy have reported that these unwanted treatment results are caused by a blood clot between the wound surface and the $Ca(OH)_2$ [146–148]. When a blood clot was present between the wound surface and the $Ca(OH)_2$, 22% of the teeth showed healing with a continuous hard tissue barrier and an inflammation-free residual pulp. However, a significantly better (76%) healing rate was noted when no blood

clot was present [145–147]. Furthermore, it has been shown that the presence of infection is a prerequisite for internal resorption [180]. It is conceivable that a blood clot between the tissue and capping agent may not only prevent the effect of $Ca(OH)_2$ on the tissue, but it may also serve as a substrate for bacteria if the restoration were to leak.

Procedure

To avoid the formation of a blood clot a gentle pulpotomy technique has been advocated [57]. The coronal pulp tissue is removed with a cutting diamond in a high-speed handpiece under constant irrigation to the level of the canal orifice. Irrigation with sterile isotonic saline is performed until bleeding has stopped. After this a paste of $Ca(OH)_2$ and water or a similar commercial product, e.g., Calasept® (Scania Dental, Knivsta, Sweden) is placed on the pulp wound and then covered with a cement to prevent leakage. The whole procedure is carried out under aseptic conditions using rubber dam. The permanent restoration can be placed during the same visit.

10.3.6 Pulpectomy

Pulpectomy is the removal of the pulp tissue. Following this procedure and the subsequent cleaning and shaping of the root canal, the canal is filled to prevent infection of the periapical tissues. Pulpectomy treatment is described in Chapter 11.

10.3.7 Calcium hydroxide and mineral trioxide aggregate (MTA)

Pulpal healing can be obtained in a sterile environment [29,33,77]. Today's materials for restoration utilizing enamel and dentin bonding techniques render a superior seal compared to traditional materials and techniques [163]. However, the long-term sealing ability of even the best materials is unknown [103,104]. Therefore, it is essential to obtain a continuous hard tissue barrier for protection of the pulp.

Many materials have been tried and tested over the years. Some of them have rendered a barrier, but in most instances this barrier has not been continuous, leaving the pulp open to infection if the restoration were to leak [33]. It appears that presently only the use of calcium hydroxide – $Ca(OH)_2$ *per se* or in the form of MTA – in combination with avoidance of a blood clot will give reasonably predictable healing with a continuous hard tissue barrier (Fig. 10.6) [32].

The mechanism of $Ca(OH)_2$ treatment of exposed pulps has been intensely studied [31,34,51,120,146, 148]. When a paste of $Ca(OH)_2$ and water is placed on a pulp wound surface it causes superficial necrosis. The tissue closest to the wound dressing loses its architecture and under this liquefaction necrosis there is coagulation necrosis [146]. This coagulated necrotic tissue becomes diffusely calcified and under this calcified zone there is subsequent formation of hard tissue [69]. Cox *et al.* [29] have shown in animal experiments that other materials such as silicate cement can in an aseptic environment initiate the formation of a hard tissue barrier. They also concluded that this was caused by low-grade irritation. Investigations have shown that after the formation of a hard tissue zone, underlying pulp cells differentiate into new odontoblasts [45,102,187]. It has been suggested that fibronectin in the initial calcified zone might play a mediating role in the differentiation of pulpal cells

into odontoblasts [188]. Tziafas *et al.* [175] have proposed that $Ca(OH)_2$ might solubilize bioactive molecules from the surrounding dentin matrix thereby signaling progenitor cells to become odontoblasts. It is still not known exactly which cells will become the new odontoblasts. In regular histological sections all fibroblasts look similar, but based on differences in proliferation it is clear that they are not one homogeneous group of cells. Also, based on mineralized nodule formation in pulp cell cultures, many different strains of fibroblasts or fibroblast-like cells have been isolated [106,172]. Initially the hard tissue formed after capping is amorphous, but as the formation continues, it eventually becomes dentin. This process appears similar to the formation of mantle dentin followed by regular dentin during tooth development. Mantle dentin and dentin formation reflect secretory events occurring during odontoblast differentiation [54]. It is conceivable that in a similar manner the odontoblast-to-be produces different-looking hard tissues during its differentiation into an odontoblast.

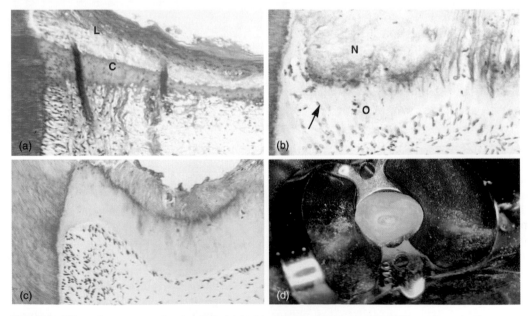

Fig. 10.6   Effect of $Ca(OH)_2$ on the vital pulp. (a) At 6 hours after placement of $Ca(OH)_2$ on the pulp, there is liquefaction necrosis (L) close to the $Ca(OH)_2$ and a coagulation necrosis layer (C) has formed close to the vital tissue. (b) At 3 weeks, a layer of necrotic tissue (N), a darkly stained band of coagulated and later calcified tissue (arrow) are seen. On the pulpal side there is an osteoid-like tissue with lining cells (O). (c) Tissue layers in a completely formed barrier with dentin formation close to the pulp. (d) Clinical appearance of a hard tissue barrier. (Courtesy of Dr Miomir Cvek.)

10.4 Prognosis

10.4.1 Choice of therapy following pulp exposure

The three treatment modalities, pulp capping, partial pulpotomy, and pulpotomy, are similar in principle. The objective is the same: to obtain healing of a pulp wound in order to preserve a vital tooth with a healthy pulp. Pulp capping has a low expectation for success and the number of failures increase with time [7,71]. It has been shown that even if a hard tissue barrier has been formed and there are no clinical symptoms, histologic examination can demonstrate severe pulpal inflammation or necrosis. This is because the hard tissue barrier is often incomplete and leakage under a filling will bring bacteria into direct contact with the pulp tissue [29,120]. Pulpotomy has a higher success expectancy [145], but it is a relatively deep procedure involving the cervical area of a tooth. In developing teeth, it is beneficial to obtain sufficient hard tissue thickness in this area to avoid fracture. Therefore, a more coronal wound surface location is desirable. Based on this, the partial pulpotomy was developed [31]. The pulp wound is placed 1.5–2 mm deeper than the capping level making it easier to get retention for the wound dressing and the covering filling materials. During the direct capping procedure the $Ca(OH)_2$ is placed on a tissue surface which has been exposed to microorganisms and where inflammation is present. The surgical removal of the superficial pulp tissue during partial pulpotomy makes it possible to place the wound dressing on a clean-cut wound surface in a healthier tissue. Nevertheless, the wound surface is situated so far incisally that cervical dentin can be formed. If the procedure should fail it is easier to carry out conventional endodontic treatment in a tooth that has had a partial pulpotomy done than in a pulpotomized tooth which often has canal calcifications. The partial pulpotomy will render hard tissue formation in the crown. This hard tissue can be removed without difficulty with rotating instruments, if root canal retreatment were to become necessary.

Procedures involving the placement of a pulp wound dressing in the coronal part of the tooth (pulp capping, partial pulpotomy, pulpotomy) are carried out in young teeth to allow the root formation to be completed. This has often been referred to as apexogenesis. In the mature tooth, pulpectomy and root filling are the preferred treatment. There are two main reasons for this. Pulpectomy with a subsequent root filling has a high, 90–96%, success rate [152,159]. Also, the wound area is placed apically so that an inflammatory response to infection can be registered early by radiographs. In the pulp-capped or pulpotomized tooth, a persisting inflammation is not noted radiologically until it reaches the periapical tissues. Thus, the current recommendation is to do partial pulp treatment in immature teeth and pulpectomy in fully developed teeth.

10.4.2 Future

The preservation of pulp vitality, not only in the developing but also in the mature tooth, may be beneficial for the patient because loss of vitality also means loss of intradental sensory functions.

It is well known that periodontal receptors not only provide directional information, but they are also important for the control of mastication [171]. Apparently, intradental nerves are also important for the control of masticatory forces. In an experimental study when a force was applied which slightly deformed a cat tooth, activity from pulp nerve endings could be recorded together with an effect on the jaw opening reflex [123]. In a study using human volunteers, it was possible to discriminate by biting between different levels of hardness in test bodies [127]. The conclusion was that the differences were sensed without periodontal assistance by the teeth. Also, in clinical experiments it was possible for a patient to register pressure from loading earlier if the tooth was vital than if the tooth was root-filled [137]. In other words, the nonvital or root-filled tooth can only rely on periodontal ligament nerve endings to register pressure, but there is an intradental registration of pressure in vital teeth. This means that more masticatory load is placed on the root-filled tooth than on the vital and this may at least partially explain why there are more fractures in root-filled teeth [137].

It appears that it would be beneficial to preserve tooth vitality rather than replacing the pulp with a root filling. Among the methods for preservation of vitality of an exposed pulp, the partial pulpotomy has yielded a markedly high success rate in controlled studies [32,94,98]. It is conceivable that the partial pulpotomy method in the future could be used with even more efficient wound dressings containing, e.g., growth factors, in combination with improved local antimicrobial and antiinflammatory methods. This kind of treatment, together with the improved sealing ability of restorative materials, might hopefully change the treatment of vital exposed pulps in the adult population to preserve the intradental sensory functions.

However, the partial pulpotomy is only applicable if the affected part of pulp is not too deep (1.5–2 mm). Usually, young vital teeth with pulp inflammation are treated conventionally with pulpectomy and root filling, resulting in permanent loss of tooth vitality. To harness the natural reparative potential of pulp with the eventual goal of restoring tooth function, a tissue engineering approach utilizing the healing potential of pulp tissue, and perhaps also the use of stem cells, could become a viable form of endodontic treatment. There are, of course, significant challenges to such an approach including: selection of a suitable scaffold to facilitate cell growth; cell source (original pulp cells and/or stem cells); eradication of infection from caries; and "coaching/influencing" the newly formed tissue to form dentin. Still, pulp regeneration could have the potential to become another avenue for endodontic treatment in the future.

10.5 References

1. Ahlquist M, Franzén O, Coffey J, Pashley D (1994) Dental pain evoked by hydrostatic pressures applied to exposed dentin in man: a test of the hydrodynamic theory of dentin sensitivity. *Journal of Endodontics* **29**, 130–4.
2. Albers HK (1981) Histologische Untersuchungen zur direkten Überkappung mit einem Kollagenpräparat (Lyodura) an menschlichen Zähnen. *Deutsche Zahnärztliche Zeitung* **36**, 354–6.
3. Al-Dawood A, Wennberg A (1993) Biocompatibility of dentin bonding agents. *Endodontics and Dental Traumatology* **9**, 1–7.
4. Andelin WE, Browning DF, Hsu GH, Roland DD, Torabinejad M (2002) Microleakage of resected MTA. *Journal of Endodontics* **28**, 573–4.
5. Andrews JT, Hembree JH (1980) Marginal leakage of amalgam alloys with high content of copper: a laboratory study. *Operative Dentistry* **5**, 7–10.
6. Autian J (1974) General toxicity and screening tests for dental materials. *International Dental Journal* **24**, 235–50.
7. Barthel CR, Rosenkranz B, Leuenberg A, Roulet JF (2000) Pulp capping of carious exposures: treatment outcome after 5 and 10 years: a retrospective study. *Journal of Endodontics* **29**, 525–8.
8. Baume LJ (1970) Dental pulp conditions in relation to carious lesions. *International Dental Journal* **20**, 309–16.

9. Bergenholtz G (1977) Effect of bacterial products on inflammatory reactions in the dental pulp. *Scandinavian Journal of Dental Research* **85**, 122–9.
10. Bergenholtz G (1991) Iatrogenic injury to the pulp in dental procedures: aspects on pathogenesis, management, and preventive measures. *International Dental Journal* **41**, 99–110.
11. Bergenholtz G, Cox CF, Loesche WJ, Syed SA (1982) Bacterial leakage around dental restorations: its effect on the dental pulp. *Journal of Oral Pathology* **11**, 439–50.
12. Bergenholtz G, Reit C (1980) Reactions of the dental pulp to microbial provocation of calcium hydroxide treated dentin. *Scandinavian Journal of Dental Research* **88**, 187–92.
13. Berger JE (1965) Pulp tissue reaction to formocresol and zinc oxide–eugenol. *Journal of Dentistry for Children* **32**, 13–28.
14. Berger JE (1972) A review of the erroneously labeled "mummification" techniques of pulp therapy. *Oral Surgery, Oral Medicine, Oral Pathology* **34**, 131–44.
15. Brännström M (1962) Dentinal and pulpal response VI. Some experiments with heat and pressure illustrating the movement of odontoblasts into the dentinal tubules. *Oral Surgery, Oral Medicine, Oral Pathology* **15**, 203–10.
16. Brännström M (1982) *Dentin and pulp in restorative dentistry*. London: Wolfe.
17. Brännström M (1984) Communication between the oral cavity and the dental pulp associated with restorative treatment. *Operative Dentistry* **9**, 57–68.
18. Brännström M (1987) Infection beneath composite resin restorations: can it be avoided? *Operative Dentistry* **12**, 158–63.
19. Brännström M, Åström A (1972) The hydrodynamics of the dentine; its possible relationship to dentinal pain. *International Dental Journal* **22**, 219–27.
20. Brännström M, Vojinovic O (1976) Response of the dental pulp to invasion of bacteria around three filling materials. *Journal of Dentistry for Children* **43**, 83–9.
21. Browne RM, Tobias RS, Crombie IK, Plant CG (1983) Bacterial microleakage and pulpal inflammation in experimental cavities. *International Endodontic Journal* **16**, 147–55.
22. Camilleri J, Montesin FE, Brady K, Sweeney R, Curtis RV, Pitt Ford TR (2005) The constitution of mineral trioxide aggregate. *Dental Materials* **21**, 297–303.
23. Carvalho RM, Pereira JC, Yoshiyama M, Pashley DH (1996) A review of polymerization contraction: the influence of stress development versus stress relief. *Operative Dentistry* **21**, 17–24.
24. Castagnola L (1950) Die Mortalamputation in Lichte Klinischer Röntgen- und Bakteriologischer Untersuchungen an einem Ausgedehnten Statistischen Material. *Schweizerische Monatschrift für Zahnheilkunde* **60**, 332–53.
25. Chirnside IM (1961) Bacterial invasion of non-vital dentin. *Journal of Dental Research* **40**, 134–40.
26. Christensen GJ (2004) What is a veneer? *Journal of the American Dental Association* **135**, 1574–6.
27. Christensen GJ (2005) How to kill a tooth. *Journal of the American Dental Association* **136**, 1711–13.

28. Cox CF, Keall CL, Keall HJ, Ostro E, Bergenholtz G (1987) Biocompatibility of surface-sealed dental materials against exposed pulps. *Journal of Prosthetic Dentistry* **57**, 1–8.

29. Cox CF, Sübay RK, Ostro E, Suzuki S, Suzuki SH (1996) Tunnel defects in dentin bridges: their formation following direct pulp capping. *Operative Dentistry* **21**, 4–11.

30. Craig RG (1993) *Restorative dental materials*, 9th edn. St Louis, MO: Mosby.

31. Cvek M (1978) A clinical report on partial pulpotomy and capping with calcium hydroxide in permanent incisors with complicated crown fracture. *Journal of Endodontics* **4**, 232–7.

32. Cvek M (1993) Partial pulpotomy in crown-fractured incisors – Results 3 to 15 years after treatment. *Acta Stomatologica Croatica* **27**, 167–73.

33. Cvek M, Granath L, Cleaton-Jones P, Austin J (1987) Hard tissue barrier formation in pulpotomized monkey teeth capped with cyanoacrylate or calcium hydroxide for 10 and 60 minutes. *Journal of Dental Research* **66**, 1166–74.

34. Cvek M, Lundberg M (1983) Histological appearance of pulps after exposure by a crown fracture, partial pulpotomy, and clinical diagnosis of healing. *Journal of Endodontics* **9**, 8–11.

35. De Munck, Van Landuyt K, Peumans M, Poitevin A, Lambrechts P, Braem M, Van Meerbeek B (2005) A critical review of the durability of adhesion to tooth tissue: methods and results. *Journal of Dental Research* **84**, 118–32.

36. Dutton FB, Summitt JB, Chan DCN, Garcia-Godoy F (1993) Effect of resin lining and rebonding on the marginal leakage of amalgam restorations. *Journal of Dentistry* **21**, 52–6.

37. Edwardsson S (1974) Bacteriological studies on deep areas of carious dentine. *Odontologisk Revy* **25** (suppl 32), 1–143.

38. Ehrmann EH (1981) Pulpotomies in traumatized and carious permanent teeth using a corticosteroid-antibiotic preparation. *International Endodontic Journal* **14**, 149–55.

39. Eidelman E, Finn SB, Koulourides T (1965) Remineralization of carious dentin treated with calcium hydroxide. *Journal of Dentistry for Children* **32**, 218–25.

40. Faraco IM, Holland R (2004) Histomorphological response of dogs' dental pulp capped with white mineral trioxide aggregate. *Brazilian Dental Journal* **15**, 104–8.

41. Farah JW, Clark AE, Mohsein M, Thomas PA (1983) Effect of cement base thicknesses on MOD amalgam restorations. *Journal of Dental Research* **62**, 109–11.

42. Felton DA, Kanoy BE, White JT (1987) Effect of cavity varnish on retention of cemented cast crowns. *Journal of Prosthetic Dentistry* **57**, 411–16.

43. Felton DA, Madison S, Kanoy E, Kantor M, Mayniuk G (1989) Long term effects of crown preparation on pulp vitality. *Journal of Dental Research* **68**, 1009 (abstract 1139).

44. Fisher FJ (1972) The effect of a calcium hydroxide-water paste on micro-organisms in carious dentine. *British Dental Journal* **133**, 19–21.

45. Fitzgerald M, Chiego DJ, Heys DR (1990) Autoradiographic analysis of odontoblast replacement following pulp exposure in primate teeth. *Archives of Oral Biology* **35**, 707–15.

46. Fouad A, Levin L (2006) Pulpal reactions to caries and dental procedures. In Cohen S, Hargreaves KM, editors. *Pathways of the Pulp*, 9th edn, pp, 514–40. St Louis, MO: Mosby Elsevier.

47. Fuks A, Bimstein E, Bruchim A (1983) Radiographic and histologic evaluation of the effect of two concentrations of formocresol on pulpotomized primary and young permanent teeth in monkeys. *Pediatric Dentistry* **5**, 9–14.

48. Fuks A, Chosak A, Eidelman E (1987) Partial pulpotomy as an alternative treatment for exposed pulps in crown-fractured incisors. *Endodontics and Dental Traumatology* **3**, 100–2.

49. Furseth R (1971) Further observations on the fine structure of orally exposed and carious human cementum. *Archives of Oral Biology* **16**, 71–85.

50. Garberoglio R, Brännström M (1976) Scanning electron microscopic investigation of human dentinal tubules. *Archives of Oral Biology* **21**, 355–62.

51. Glass RL, Zander HA (1949) Pulp healing. *Journal of Dental Research* **28**, 97–102.

52. Going RE (1964) Cavity liners and dentin treatment. *Journal of the American Dental Association* **69**, 415–22.

53. Goldberg M, Six N, Decup F, Buch D, Soheili Majd E, Lasfargues JJ, *et al.* (2001) Application of bioactive molecules in pulp-capping situations. *Advances in Dental Research* **15**, 91–5.

54. Goldberg M, Smith AJ (2004) Cells and extracellular matrices of dentin and pulp: a biological basis for repair and tissue engineering. *Critical Reviews in Oral Biology and Medicine* **15**, 13–27.

55. Goracci G, Mori G (1996) Scanning electron microscopic evaluation of resin–dentin and calcium hydroxide–dentin interface with resin composite restorations. *Quintessence International* **27**, 129–35.

56. Goracci G, Mori G, Casa de'Martinis L (1993) Valutazione della chiusura marginale dei compositi, polimerizzati con due diversi metodi. *Dental Cadmos* **7**, 50–63.

57. Granath LE, Hagman G (1971) Experimental pulpotomy in human bicuspids with reference to cutting technique. *Acta Odontologica Scandinavica* **29**, 155–66.

58. Granath LE, Mejare I, Raadal M (1991) Dental caries; operative procedures. In Koch G, Modéer T, Poulsen S, Rasmussen P, editors. *Pedodontics – a clinical approach*, pp. 164–5. Copenhagen: Munksgaard.

59. Greth H (1933) *Diagnostik der Pulpaerkrankungen*. Berlin: Hermann Meusser.

60. Haddad M, Lefranc G, Aftimos G (2003) Local application of IGF1 on dental pulp mechanically exposed: in vivo study on rabbit. *Bulletin de Groupment International pour la Recherche Scientifique en Stomatologie et Odontologie* **45**, 12–17.

61. Hargreaves KM (2002) Pain mechanisms of the pulpo-dentin complex. In Hargreaves KM, Goodis HE, editors. *Seltzer and Bender's dental pulp*, pp. 181–203. Chicago, IL: Quintessence.

62. Hasselgren G, Kerekes K, Nellestam P (1982) pH changes in calcium hydroxide covered dentin. *Journal of Endodontics* **8**, 502–5.

63. Hasselgren G, Tronstad L (1978) Enzyme activity in the pulp following preparation of cavities and inser-tion of medicaments in cavities in monkey teeth. *Acta Odontologica Scandinavica* **35**, 289–95.

64. Hermann BW (1930) Dentinobliteration der Wurzel-kanäle nach Behandlung mit Calcium. *Zahnärztliche Rundschau* **39**, 888–99.

65. Hermann BW (1936) *Biologische Wurzelbehandlung.* Frankfurt am Main: Kramer.

66. Heyeraas KJ (1985) Pulpal, microvascular, and tissue pressure. *Journal of Dental Research* **64**, 585–9.

67. Heys DR, Fitzgerald RJ, Heys RJ, Chiego DJ (1990) Healing of primate dental pulps capped with Tef-lon. *Oral Surgery, Oral Medicine, Oral Pathology* **69**, 227–37.

68. Heys RJ, Fitzgerald M (1991) Microleakage of three cement bases. *Journal of Dental Research* **70**, 55–8.

69. Higashi T, Okamoto H (1996) Characteristics and effects of calcified degenerative zones on the forma-tion of hard tissue barriers in amputated canine den-tal pulp. *Journal of Endodontics* **22**, 168–72.

70. Hilton TJ (1996) Cavity sealers, liners, and bases: current philosophies and indications for use. *Opera-tive Dentistry* **21**, 134–46.

71. Hørsted P, Søndergaard B, Thylstrup A, El Kattar K, Fejerskov O (1985) A retrospective study of direct pulp capping with calcium hydroxide compounds. *Endodontics and Dental Traumatology* **1**, 29–34.

72. Hørsted-Bindslev P, Mjör IA (1988) Cavity treatment and the use of liners and bases. In Hørslev-Bindslev P, Mjör IA, editors. *Modern concepts in operative den-tistry*, pp. 122–45. Copenhagen: Munksgaard.

73. Hu CC, Zhang C, Qian Q, Tatum NB (1998) Repara-tive dentin formation in rat molars after direct pulp capping with growth factors. *Journal of Endodontics* **24**, 744–51.

74. Huth KC, Paschos E, Hajek-Al-Khatar N, Hollweck R, Crispin A, Hickel R, *et al.* (2005) Effectiveness of 4 pulpotomy techniques – randomized controlled trial. *Journal of Dental Research* **84**, 1144–8.

75. Izumi T, Kobayashi I, Okamura K, Sakai H (1995) Immunohistochemical study on the immuno-compe-tent cells of the pulp in human non-carious and cari-ous teeth. *Archives of Oral Biology* **40**, 609–14.

76. Jepsen S, Albers HK, Fleiner B, Tucker M, Rueger D (1997) Recombinant human osteogenic protein-1 induces dentin formation: an experimental study in miniature swine. *Journal of Endodontics* **23**, 378–82.

77. Kakehashi S, Stanley HR, Fitzgerald RJ (1965) The effect of surgical exposures of dental pulps in germ-free and conventional laboratory rats. *Oral Surgery, Oral Medicine, Oral Pathology* **20**, 340–9.

78. Kanca J (1992) Resin bonding to wet substrate. I. Bonding to dentin. *Quintessence International* **23**, 39–41.

79. Kanca J (1993) Replacement of a fractured incisor fragment over pulpal exposure: a case report. *Quin-tessence International* **24**, 81–4.

80. Kashiwada T, Takagi M (1991) New restoration and direct pulp capping systems using adhesive composite resin. *Bulletin of the Tokyo Medical and Dental Univer-sity* **38**, 45–52.

81. Langeland K (1959) Histologic evaluation of pulp reactions to operative procedures. *Oral Surgery, Oral Medicine, Oral Pathology* **12**, 1357–69.

82. Langeland K (1972) Prevention of pulpal damage. *Dental Clinics of North America* **16**, 709–32.

83. Langeland K (1981) Management of the inflamed pulp associated with deep carious lesions. *Journal of Endodontics* **7**, 169–75.

84. Langeland K (1987) Tissue response to dental caries. *Endodontics and Dental Traumatology* **3**, 249–71.

85. Leksell E, Ridell K, Cvek M, Mejare I (1996) Pulp exposure after stepwise versus direct complete exca-vation of deep carious lesions in young posterior per-manent teeth. *Endodontics and Dental Traumatology* **12**, 192–6.

86. Lindström G (1964) Amputation eller exstirpation? *Svensk Tandläkare Tidskrift* **57**, 807–15.

87. Lovschall H, Fejerskov O, Flyvbjerg A (2001) Pulp-capping with recombinant human insulin-like growth factor I (rhIGF-I) in rat molars. *Advances in Dental Research* **15**, 108–12.

88. Lundy T, Stanley HR (1969) Correlation of pulpal histology and clinical symptoms in human teeth sub-jected to experimental irritation. *Oral Surgery, Oral Medicine, Oral Pathology* **27**, 187–201.

89. MacInnis, WA, Ismail A, Brogan H (1991) Placement and replacement of restorations in a military popula-tion. *Journal of the Canadian Dental Association* **57**, 227–30.

90. Magnusson B (1970) Therapeutic pulpotomy in pri-mary molars – clinical and histological follow-up. I. Calcium hydroxide paste as wound dressing. *Odon-tologisk Revy* **21**, 415–26.

91. Magnusson B, Sundell SO (1977) Stepwise excavation of deep carious lesions in primary molars. *Journal of the International Association for Dentistry for Children* **8**, 36–40.

92. Maita E, Simpson MD, Tao L, Pashley DH (1991) Fluid and protein flux across the pulpodentine com-plex of the dog in vivo. *Archives of Oral Biology* **36**, 102–10.

93. Markowitz K, Moynihan M, Liu MT, Kim S (1992) Biologic properties of eugenol and zinc oxide–euge-nol. A clinically oriented review. *Oral Surgery, Oral Medicine, Oral Pathology* **73**, 729–37.

94. Mass E, Zilberman U (1993) Clinical and radiograph-ic evaluation of partial pulpotomy in carious exposure of permanent molars. *Pediatric Dentistry* **15**, 257–9.

95. Massler M, Pawlak J (1977) The affected and infected pulp. *Oral Surgery, Oral Medicine, Oral Pathology* **43**, 929–47.

96. Mattsson B, Brännström M, Torstensson B (1987) Isolering under kompositer – en kritisk översikt. *Tandläkartidningen* **79**, 813–20.

97. McFall WT (1986) A review of the active agents available for treatment of dentinal hypersensitivity. *Endodontics and Dental Traumatology* **2**, 141–9.

98. Mejàre I, Cvek M (1993) Partial pulpotomy in permanent teeth with deep carious lesions. *Endodontics and Dental Traumatology* **9**, 238–42.

99. Mejàre I, Hasselgren G, Hammarström LE (1975) Effect of formaldehyde-containing drugs on human dental pulp evaluated by enzyme histochemical technique. *Scandinavian Journal of Dental Research* **84**, 29–36.

100. Menezes R, Bramante CM, Letra A, Carvalho VG, Garcia RB (2004) Histologic evaluation of pulpotomies in dog using two types of mineral trioxide aggregate and regular and white Portland cements as wound dressing. *Oral Surgery, Oral Medicine, Oral Pathology, Oral Radiology and Endodontics* **98**, 376–9.

101. Milleding P, Wennberg A, Hasselgren G (1985) Cytotoxicity of corroded and non-corroded dental amalgams. *Scandinavian Journal of Dental Research* **93**, 76–83.

102. Mjör, IA, Dahl E, Cox CF (1991) Healing of pulp exposures: and ultrastructural study. *Journal of Oral Pathology and Medicine* **20**, 496–501.

103. Mjör IA, Gordan VV (2002) Failure, repair, refurbishing and longevity of restorations. *Operative Dentistry* **27**, 528–34.

104. Mjör IA, Shen C, Eliasson ST, Richter S (2002) Placement and replacement of restorations in general practice in Iceland. *Operative Dentistry* **27**, 117–23.

105. Möller B (1975) Reaction of the human dental pulp to silver amalgam restorations. The modifying effect of treatment with calcium hydroxide. *Acta Odontologica Scandinavica* **33**, 233–8.

106. Moule AJ, Li H, Barthold PM (1995) Donor variability in the proliferation of human dental pulp fibroblasts. *Australian Dental Journal* **40**, 110–14.

107 Naik S, Hegde AM (2005) Mineral trioxide aggregate as a pulpotomy agent in primary molars: An in vivo study. *Journal of the Indian Society of Pedodontics and Preventive Dentistry* **23**, 13–16.

108. Nakabayashi N (1992) The hybrid layer: A resin–dentin composite. *Proceedings of the Finnish Dental Society* **88** (suppl 1), 321–9.

109. Nakabayashi N, Ashizawa M, Nakamura M (1992) Identification of a resin-dentin hybrid layer in vital human dentin, created in vivo: durable bonding to vital dentin. *Quintessence International* **23**, 135–41.

110. Nakabayashi N, Kojima K, Masuhara E (1982) The promotion of adhesion by the infiltration of monomers into tooth substrates. *Journal of Biomedical Materials Research* **16**, 265–73.

111. Nakayabashi N, Takarada K (1992) Effect of HEMA on bonding to dentin. *Dental Materials* **8**, 125–30.

112. Nakajima M, Sano B, Burrow MF, *et al.* (1995) Bonding to caries affected dentin. *Journal of Dental Research,* **74**, 36 (Abstract 194).

113. Nakamura M, Kawahara H (1979) Cellular responses to the dispersion amalgams in vitro. *Journal of Dental Research* **58**, 1780–90.

114. Nakashima M (1990) The introduction of reparative dentin in the amputated dental pulp of the dog by bone morphogenic protein. *Archives of Oral Biology* **35**, 493–7.

115. Nakashima M (1994) Induction of dentin formation on canine amputated pulp by recombinant human bone morphogenic proteins (BMP)-2 and -4. *Journal of Dental Research* **73**, 1515–22.

116. Närhi MVO, Hirvonen T (1987) The response of dog intradental nerves to hypertonic solutions of $CaCl_2$ and NaCl, and other stimuli, applied to exposed dentine. *Archives of Oral Biology* **32**, 781–6.

117. Närhi MVO, Kontturi-Närhi T, Hirvonen T, Ngassapa D (1992) Neurophysiological mechanisms of dentin hypersensitivity. *Proceedings of the Finnish Dental Society* **88** (suppl 1), 15–22.

118. Nerwich A, Figdor D, Messer HH (1993) pH changes in root dentin over a 4-week period following root canal dressing with calcium hydroxide. *Journal of Endodontics* **19**, 302–6.

119. Nordenvall KJ, Brännström M, Torstensson B (1979) Pulp reactions and microorganisms under ASPA and Concise composite fillings. *Journal of Dentistry for Children* **46**, 449–53.

120. Nyborg H (1955) Healing processes in the pulp on capping. *Acta Odontologica Scandinavica* **13** (suppl 16), 1–130.

121. Olgart LM (1992) Involvement of sensory nerves in hemodynamic reactions. *Proceedings of the Finnish Dental Society* **88** (suppl 1), 403–10.

122. Olgart L, Brännström M, Johnsson G (1974) Invasion of bacteria into dentinal tubules. Experiments in vivo and in vitro. *Acta Odontologica Scandinavica* **32**, 61–70.

123. Olgart L, Gazelius B, Sundström F (1988) Intra dental nerve activity and jaw-opening reflex in response to mechanical deformation of cat teeth. *Acta Physiologica Scandinavica* **133**, 399–406.

124. Ölmez A (2005) Adhesive resins as pulp-capping agents. Editorial commentary. *Practical Procedures & Aesthetic Dentistry* **17**, 444–6.

125. Olsson H, Davies JR, Holst KE, Schröder U, Petersson K (2005) Dental pulp capping: effect of Emdogain Gel on experimentally exposed human pulps. *International Endodontic Journal* **38**, 186–94.

126. Pameijer CH, Wendt SL (1995) Microleakage of "surface-sealing" materials. *American Journal of Dentistry* **8**, 89–91.

127. Paphangkorakit J, Osborn JW (1998) Discrimination of hardness by human teeth apparently not involving periodontal receptors. *Archives of Oral Biology* **43**, 1–7.

128. Pashley DH (1979) The influence of dentin permeability and pulpal blood flow on pulpal solute concentrations. *Journal of Endodontics* **5**, 355–9.

129. Pashley DH (1991) Clinical considerations of dentin structure and function. *Journal of Prosthetic Dentistry* **66**, 777–81.

130. Pashley DH, Kehl T, Pashley E, Palmer P (1981) Comparison of in vitro and in vivo dog dentin permeability. *Journal of Dental Research* **60**, 763–7.

131. Pashley D, Livingston MJ, Outhwaite WC (1977) Rate of permeation of isotopes through human dentin in vitro. *Journal of Dental Research* **56**, 83–8.

132. Pashley DH, O'Meara JA, Williams EC, Kepler EE (1985) Dentin permeability: effects of cavity varnishes and bases. *Journal of Prosthetic Dentistry* **53**, 511–16.

133. Pitt Ford TR, Roberts GJ (1991) Immediate and delayed pulp capping with the use of a new visible light cured calcium hydroxide preparation. *Oral Surgery, Oral Medicine, Oral Pathology* **71**, 338–42.

134. Pitt Ford TR, Torabinejad M, Abedi HR, Bakland LK, Kariyawasam SP (1996) Using mineral trioxide aggregate as a pulp-capping material. *Journal of the American Dental Association* **127**, 1491–94.

135. Prager M (1994) Pulp capping with the total etch technique. *Dental Economics* **84**, 78–9.

136. Qvist V, Qvist J, Mjör IA (1990) Placement and longevity of tooth-colored restorations in Denmark. *Acta Odontologica Scandinavica* **48**, 305–11.

137. Randow K, Glantz PO (1986) On cantilever loading of vital and non-vital teeth. An experimental clinical study. *Acta Odontologica Scandinavica* **44**, 271–7.

138. Rebel HH (1922) Über die Ausheilung der freigelegten Pulpa. *Deutsche Zahnheilkunde Heft* **55**, 3–83.

139. Reeves R, Stanley HR (1966) The relationship of bacterial penetration and pulpal pathosis in carious teeth. *Oral Surgery, Oral Medicine, Oral Pathology* **22**, 59–65.

140. Ren WH, Yang LJ, Dong SZ (1999) Induction of reparative dentin formation in dogs with combined recombinant human bone morphogenetic protein 2 and fibrin sealant. *Chinese Journal of Dental Research* **2**, 21–4.

141. Rölling I, Hasselgren G, Tronstad L (1976) Morphologic and enzyme histochemical observations on the pulp of human primary molars 3 to 5 years after formocresol treatment. *Oral Surgery, Oral Medicine, Oral Pathology* **42**, 518–28.

142. Rothman MS (1977) Formocresol pulpotomy: a practical procedure for permanent teeth. *General Dentistry* **25**, 29–30.

143. Saiku JM, St Germain HA, Meiers JC (1993) Microleakage of a dental amalgam alloy bonding agent. *Operative Dentistry* **18**, 172–8.

144. Saito T, Ogawa M, Hata Y, Bessho K (2004) Acceleration effect of human recombinant bone morphogenetic protein-2 on differentiation of human pulp cells into odontoblasts. *Journal of Endodontics* **30**, 205–8.

145. Schröder U (1972) Evaluation of healing following experimental pulpotomy of intact human teeth and capping with calcium hydroxide. *Odontologisk Revy* **23**, 329–40.

146. Schröder U (1973) Effect of an extra-pulpal blood clot on healing following experimental pulpotomy and capping with calcium hydroxide. *Odontologisk Revy* **24**, 257–68.

147. Schröder U (1978) A 2-year follow-up of primary molars, pulpotomized with a gentle technique and capped with calcium hydroxide. *Scandinavian Journal of Dental Research* **86**, 273–8.

148. Schröder U, Granath LE (1971) Early reaction of intact human teeth to calcium hydroxide following experimental pulpotomy and its significance to the developing of hard tissue barrier. *Odontologisk Revy* **22**, 379–96.

149. Sheller B, Morton TH (1987) Electrosurgical pulpotomy: a pilot study in humans. *Journal of Endodontics* **13**, 69–76.

150. Shoji S, Nakamura M, Horiuchi H (1985) Histopathological changes in dental pulps irradiated with CO_2 laser: a preliminary report on laser pulpotomy. *Journal of Endodontics* **11**, 379–84.

151. Six N, Lasfargues JJ, Goldberg M (2002) Differential repair responses in the coronal and radicular areas of the exposed rat molar pulp by recombinant human bone morphogenetic protein 7 (osteogenic protein 1). *Archives of Oral Biology* **47**, 177–87.

152. Sjögren U, Hägglund B, Sundqvist G, Wing K (1990) Factors affecting the long-term results of endodontic treatment. *Journal of Endodontics* **16**, 498–504.

153. Spångberg L (1973) Kinetic and quantitative evaluation of material cytotoxicity in vitro. *Oral Surgery, Oral Medicine, Oral Pathology* **35**, 389–401.

154. Spångberg LSW (1978) Correlation of in vivo and in vitro screening tests. *Journal of Endodontics* **4**, 296–9.

155. Spångberg LSW (1990) The study of biological properties of endodontic biomaterials. In Spångberg L, editor. *Experimental endodontics*, pp. 173–210. Boca Raton, FL: CRC Press.

156. Spedding RH (1975) Formocresol pulpotomies for permanent teeth. In Goldman HM *et al*. editors. *Current therapy in dentistry*, pp. 493–9, Vol. 5. St Louis, MO: Mosby.

157. Stanley HR (1981) *Human pulp response to restorative procedures*. Gainesville, FL: Storter Printing.

158. Stanley HR, Going RE, Chauncey HH (1975) Human pulp response to acid preteatment of dentin and to composite restoration. *Journal of the American Dental Association* **91**, 817–25.

159. Strindberg LZ (1956) The dependence of the results of pulp therapy on certain factors. *Acta Odontologica Scandinavica* **14** (suppl 21), 1–175.

160. Subay RK, Demirci M (2005) Pulp tissue reactions to a dentin bonding agent as a direct capping agent. *Journal of Endodontics* **31**, 201–4.

161. Suzuki S, Cox CF, White KC (1994) Pulpal response after complete crown preparation, dentinal sealing, and provisional restoration. *Quintessence International* **25**, 477–85.

162. Suzuki T, Finger WJ (1988) Dentin adhesives: site of dentin vs bonding of composite resins. *Dental Materials* **4**, 379–83.

163. Swift EJ, Perdigao J, Heymann HO (1995) Bonding to enamel and dentin: a brief history and state of the art, 1995. *Quintessence International* **26**, 95–110.

164. Tang HM, Torabinejad M, Kettering JD (2000) Leakage evaluation of root end filling materials using endotoxin. *Journal of Endodontics* **28**, 5–7.

165. Tao L, Pashley DH (1988) Shear bond strengths to dentin: effects of surface treatments, depth and position. *Dental Materials* **4**, 371–8.

166. Tao L, Tagami J, Pashley DH (1991) Pulpal pressure and bond strengths of SuperBond and Gluma. *American Journal of Dentistry* **4**, 73–6.

167. Tay FR, Gwinnett AJ, Pang KM, Wei SH (1995) Variability in microleakage observed in a total-etch

wet-bonding technique under different handling conditions. *Journal of Dental Research* **74**, 1168–78.

168. Torneck CD, Wagner D (1980) The effect of calcium hydroxide liner on early cell division in the pulp subsequent to cavity preparation and restoration. *Journal of Endodontics* **6**, 719–23.

169. Tronstad L, Birkeland JM (1971) In vitro studies on the influence of cements on the alkaline effect of calcium hydroxide. *Scandinavian Journal of Dental Research* **79**, 350–5.

170. Tronstad L, Mjör IA (1972) Pulp reactions to calcium hydroxide-containing materials. *Oral Surgery, Oral Medicine, Oral Pathology* **33**, 961–5.

171. Trulsson M, Johansson R, Olsson KA (1992) Directional sensitivity in human periodontal mechanoreceptive afferents to forces applied to the teeth. *Journal of Physiology* **47**, 373–89.

172. Tsukamoto Y, Fukutani S, Shin-Ike T, Kubota T, Sato S, Suzuki Y, *et al.* (1992) Mineralized nodule formation by cultures of human dental pulp-derived fibroblasts. *Archives of Oral Biology* **37**, 1045–55.

173. Tziafas D (2004) The future role of a molecular approach to pulp-dentinal regeneration. *Caries Research* **38**, 314–20.

174. Tziafas D, Pantelidou O, Alvanou A, Belibasakis G, Papadimitriou S (2002) The dentinogenic effect of mineral trioxide aggregate (MTA) in short-term capping experiments. *International Endodontic Journal* **35**, 245–54.

175. Tziafas D, Smith AJ, Lesot H (2000) Designing new strategies in vital pulp therapy. *Journal of Dentistry* **28**, 77–92.

176. Van Meerbeek B, Perdigao J, Lambrechts P, Vanherle G (1998) The clinical performance of adhesives. *Journal of Dentistry* **26**, 1–20.

177. Via WF (1955) Evaluation of deciduous molars treated by pulpotomy and calcium hydroxide. *Journal of the American Dental Association* **50**, 34–43.

178. Wartvinge J, Bergenholtz G (1986) Healing capacity of human and monkey dental pulps following experimentally-induced pulpitis. *Endodontics and Dental Traumatology* **2**, 256–62.

179. Warfvinge J, Rozell B, Hedström KG (1987) Effect of calcium hydroxide treated dentin on pulpal responses. *International Endodontic Journal* **20**, 183–93.

180. Wedenberg C, Lindskog S (1985) Experimental internal resorption in monkey teeth. *Endodontics and Dental Traumatology* **1**, 221–7.

181. Wei SHY, Kaqueler JC, Massler M (1968) Remineralization of carious dentin. *Journal of Dental Research* **47**, 381–91.

182. Wennberg A (1978) Evaluation of methods for biological screening of dental materials. Dissertation. Lund: University of Lund.

183. Wennberg A, Hasselgren G (198l) Cytotoxicity of temporary filling materials. *International Endodontic Journal* **14**, 121–4.

184. Wennberg A, Hasselgren G, Tronstad L (1978) A method for evaluation of initial tissue response to biomaterials. *Acta Odontologica Scandinavica* **36**, 67–73.

185. Wennberg A, Hasselgren G, Tronstad L (1979) A method for toxicity screening of biomaterials using cells cultured on Millipore filters. *Journal of Biomedical Materials Research* **13**, 109–20.

186. White KC, Cox CF, Kanca J, Dixon DL, Farmer JB, Snuggs HM (1994) Pulpal response to adhesive resin systems applied to acid-etched vital dentin: damp versus dry primer application. *Quintessence International* **25**, 259–68.

187. Yamamura T (1985) Differentiation of pulpal cells and inductive influences of various matrices with reference to pulpal wound healing. *Journal of Dental Research* **64**, 530–40.

188. Yoshiba K, Yoshiba N, Nakamura H, Iwaku M, Ozawa H (1996) Immunolocalization of fibronectin during reparative dentinogenesis in human teeth after pulp capping with calcium hydroxide. *Journal of Dental Research* **75**, 1590–7.

189. Yoshiba N, Yoshiba K, Iwaku M, Ozawa H (1996) Immunohistochemical localization of HLA DR positive cells in unerupted and erupted normal and carious human teeth. *Journal of Dental Research* **75**, 1585–9.

190. Zilberman U, Eliyahu M, Sarnat H (1989) Partial pulpotomy in carious permanent molars. *American Journal of Dentistry* **2**, 147–50.

Chapter 11

Endodontic Treatment of Teeth Without Apical Periodontitis

Larz S.W. Spångberg

11.1 Introduction

Contemporary endodontic treatment offers a variety of treatment options, all with a high degree of success. Biological principles must be honored, however, for best results. Regretfully, instrumentation and root canal filling techniques have come to dominate the debate about treatment. A mechanistic view on the clinical procedures has come to favor the esthetic radiographic appearance of the root canal filling over biological considerations that form the true foundation for endodontic treatment success. Much is said and written about instruments and treatment techniques studied in the laboratory. However, little objec-tive evaluation on their impact on treatment outcome can be found in the scientific literature.

In this chapter, the discussion of clinical procedures will be based on the biological factors that are funda-mental for treatment success. It is well established in the literature that preoperative presence and sever-ity of pulp tissue infection is an excellent indicator of future treatment success and that residual infection or reinfection after completed treatment is the domi-nant cause for endodontic treatment failure [67]. It is also well established that vital dental pulp tissue is not infected. The necrotic surface of the pulp wound may be infected, however. As the necrosis of the pulp tissue advances deeper into the pulp space, the necrotic tissue as well as the surrounding dentin support spread of the infection. The recognition of these differences between infected and noninfected tissues is fundamental for the understanding of endodontic treatment.

This leads to two different treatment approaches:

* *vital pulp treatment* of noninfected pulp tissue when asepsis is the basic principle of the surgical pulp treatment;
* *root canal treatment*, when antisepsis is essential for the elimination of microorganisms in the pulp space and surrounding root canal dentin walls.

11.2 Treatment principles

There are principal differences in the approach to the endodontic treatment of a tooth with a vital pulp and a tooth with a necrotic (infected) pulp.

The vital pulp tissue and the dentin of the surrounding root canal walls are not infected. If these favorable conditions can be maintained during the procedure of removing the pulp tissue and the subsequent covering of the wound, the root canal filling, the most important conditions for successful tissue healing have been met. Pulpectomy should be seen as a microsurgical removal of vital pulp tissue. As such, it requires a high level of asepsis and good surgical skill for optimal result.

In the teeth with pulp necrosis, the pulp space and the dentin of the surrounding root canal walls are frequently infected. Therefore, one of the important tasks during endodontic treatment of a tooth with a necrotic pulp is thorough disinfection of the pulp space and the surrounding dentin. Thus, this treatment of the root canal aims at removing necrotic tissue debris and eliminates the microorganisms that have infected the tissue remnants and invaded the dentin. Although asepsis is important to prevent the introduction of additional strains of bacteria, antisepsis is the fundamental principle of root canal treatment. These antiseptic principles consist of mechanical debridement of the pulp space, removal of infected dentin surrounding the pulp space and the use of antimicrobial agents. It is difficult to remove all bacteria from the infected root canal system. Therefore, this part of the treatment of the necrotic pulp requires that the practitioner focuses on substantially different treatment procedures compared to the procedures important for a successful pulpectomy.

After completion of the pulpectomy or root canal treatment the pulp space must be filled and sealed with a root canal filling material capable of preventing any future reinfection of the apical wound in the root canal by microorganisms originating from the oral cavity. This important implant serves as a wound dressing for the apical connective tissue wound.

11.3 The vital pulp: pulpectomy

Endodontic treatment of the vital pulp is very successful provided the pulpectomy is skillfully performed and that optimal aseptic conditions are maintained.

11.3.1 Pulp inflammation

Pulpectomy is the treatment of choice for all stages of pulp inflammation. Clinically, irreversible pulpitis are either diagnosed clinically in connection with toothache or associated with pulp exposure as a result of deep caries. If the pulp inflammation and subsequent tissue disintegration have advanced to a stage where major parts of the pulp, including the root pulp, are necrotic the root canal dentin may be infected. This condition will severely compromise the principles of aseptic pulp surgery and is a contraindication for pulpectomy. In cases of limited coronal pulp necrosis pulpectomy may still be the optimal treatment choice. The pulp chamber is easily accessible for both mechanical cleaning and chemical disinfection and may therefore be effectively disinfected. Consequently, pulpectomy may still be attempted as long as the root pulp is vital.

11.3.2 Pulp obliteration

A rapid and diffuse calcification of the pulp tissue of the tooth is often the sequel of traumatic injury to a permanent tooth. This calcification, if unchecked, will in many instances lead to a functional obliteration of the pulp space. In one study, total tissue breakdown, resulting in apical periodontitis, occurred in 21% of cases subsequent to pulp tissue calcification [41]. Teeth with extensive pulp tissue calcification, subsequent to trauma, are often impossible to treat by conventional endodontic methods.

To prevent these clinical conditions from occurring, prophylactic pulpectomy may be instituted when, subsequent to trauma, pulp tissue calcification is diagnosed. As the uncomplicated endodontic treatment of a vital and/or uninfected necrotic pulp will result in a higher degree of success than the complex treatment of an infected necrotic pulp in a calcified pulp space with periradicular osteolysis, prophylactic endodontic intervention is the treatment of choice. It is important to differentiate the physiological accelerated apposition of dentin by functioning odontoblasts (Fig. 11.1) from the irregular calcification of a necrobiotic pulp (Fig. 11.2). Physiological apposition stops when the stimuli have ceased, while pathological calcifications tend to lead to total calcification and subsequent tis-

sue breakdown. Physiological apposition will lead to a narrowing of the pulp space, but total obliteration will not occur [57]. In some instances the necrotic pulp is replaced by an ingrowing connective tissue that frequently forms osteodentin (Fig. 11.3) [73,104].

11.3.3 Apexogenesis

Pulp exposure of a tooth with incomplete root formation results in a clinical condition that is challenging to treat successfully. Although the pulp is vital, the

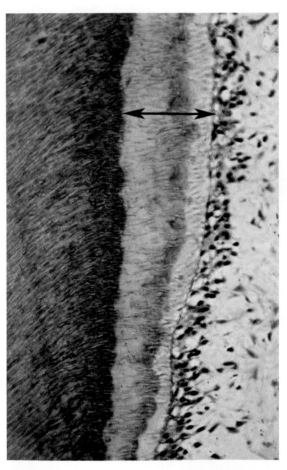

Fig. 11.1 Photomicrograph showing a situation where the odontoblasts have formed irritation dentin in an accelerated fashion after cavity preparation. This extra production of dentin (arrow) will continue as long as the stimulus exists. This mineralization, subsequent to matrix formation by odontoblasts, is a physiological defense mechanism and will not lead to a necrotic pulp or total obliteration of the pulp space.

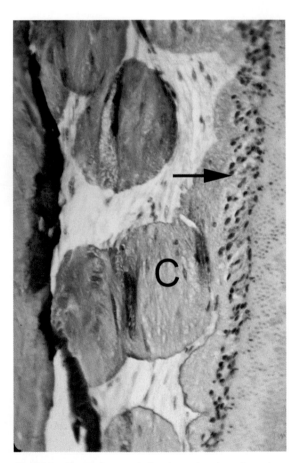

Fig. 11.2 Photomicrograph showing a situation where the dental pulp has calcified. This calcification of the pulp (C), is not associated with odontoblast function, but a sign of poor pulpal health. Note how the odontoblast layer has been included in the calcified tissue (arrow). It will progress in an unpredictable pattern and may lead to pulp necrosis and/or total obliteration of the pulp space.

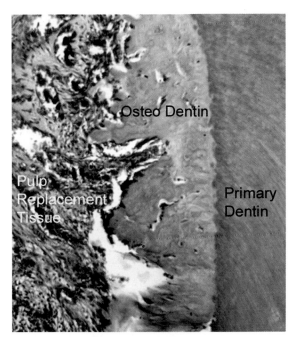

Fig. 11.3 Osteodentin formed in revascularized pulp space. The necrotic pulp has been replaced with fibrous connective tissue. Large amounts of amorphous hard tissue, devoid of dentin tubules, with many cell inclusions have formed.

apical part of the root canal is large with no anatomical constriction in the area of the apical foramen. Furthermore, in very young teeth the root structure is poorly developed and with inadequate strength to provide lifelong support for a coronal reconstruction of the tooth. Thus, the fact that treatment success normally increases with the placement of a more apical wound surface during a pulpectomy must be weighed against the need for continuous apical and lateral root development. This growth can only be achieved if major parts of the pulp tissue remain vital and functional. Therefore, the placement of the wound surface of pulpectomy in immature teeth must be adjusted, in each case, according to the amount of initial tissue destruction (Fig. 11.4).

A pulp capping or pulpotomy is appropriate depending on the amount of initial tissue damage [15]. Superficial pulp surgery procedures, however, carry with them an obligation to undertake frequent clinical evaluations of the pulp healing as successful outcome is less frequent than after conventional pulpectomy and root canal filling. An undiagnosed treatment failure can significantly compromise the survival of the tooth.

As continuous apical and lateral root development is the objective of this treatment, removal of vital pulp tissue to the apex and placement of mineral trioxide as an apical plug may support apical healing with cementum, but it will not allow the completion of root development. A brief period of apparent success will be followed by long-term failure through root fracture. Total removal of vital pulp tissue is absolutely contraindicated.

11.3.4 Iatrogenic pulp injury

Exposure of the vital pulp during preparation of noncarious dentin provides an ideal condition for

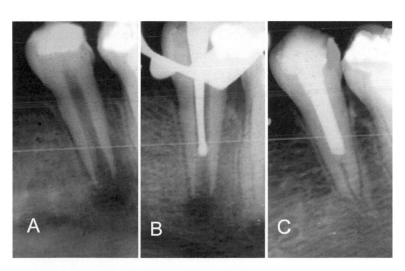

Fig. 11.4 Pulpectomy of tooth with partial necrosis. (A) Occlusal caries with pulp exposure of mandibular premolar in a 10-year-old patient. Incomplete root development.
(B) Vital pulp tissue located 5 mm from root end. Necrotic pulp removed with extended round burs. Multiple dressings with Ca(OH)$_2$.
(C) Completed root formation with apical closure 1 year after start of treatment with Ca(OH)$_2$.

pulpectomy. The chances of maintaining strict asepsis are good if the endodontic treatment is initiated immediately. However, if treatment cannot be started at once, temporization should ideally be done under rubber dam isolation providing good asepsis to reduce bacterial growth on the pulp wound surface until pulpectomy can be undertaken.

The treatment outcome of pulpectomy performed on cases of iatrogenic pulp exposure is superior to pulp capping [27,40]. A failed pulp capping is often first diagnosed as an apical periodontitis on a routine radiograph or as unexpected exacerbation with pain and swelling. In either case the pulp space is now infected. Endodontic treatment of a tooth with infected root dentin is always less successful than a pulpectomy of a vital pulp. Therefore, choosing pulp capping over pulpectomy at the time of original pulp exposure has resulted in a less favorable position for the survival of the tooth when complications occur. Pulpectomy followed by root canal filling always provides a better long-term outcome for the tooth than pulp capping.

11.3.5 Elective pulp surgery

Post placement is sometimes required during the restoration of a tooth that is severely broken down, but where there is no pulp exposure. The pulp in these cases is clinically healthy. Therefore, elective pulpectomy with root canal filling is the treatment of choice.

11.4 The necrotic pulp: root canal treatment

As pulp necrosis advances through the root canal system, bacteria soon establish themselves in the necrotic tissue remnants. In cases of carious pulp exposure this infection is concomitant to the necrosis. In closed pulp spaces the bacterial invasion of the necrotic pulp may take several months or years [8]. The bacteria in the pulp space will subsequently invade the dentin walls of the root canal (Fig. 11.5). This adds the complex problem of disinfection of the dentin and the pulp space to the treatment procedures. Thus, disinfection of the root canals, with involved root canal systems, becomes the main objective of the treatment of the necrotic pulp (see Chapter 12).

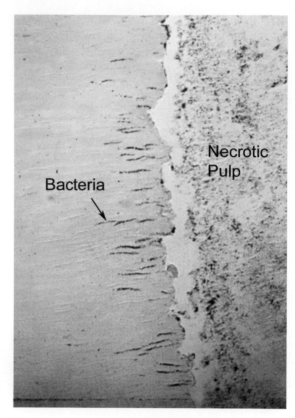

Fig. 11.5 Pulp necrosis with microbial invasion. The microorganisms have invaded the dentin tubules. Brown & Brenn stain.

11.5 Asepsis

Asepsis involves the absence of bacteria and the prevention of adding bacteria to the sterile surgical field. Asepsis in endodontics involves the use of rubber dam, mechanical and chemical preparation of the surgical field as well as the use of sterile instruments.

11.5.1 Rubber dam: purpose and practical application

Rubber dam must be used routinely during endodontic procedures. It is the primary tool for maintaining asepsis during endodontic treatment. It also provides a protective shield preventing small instruments from being aspirated or swallowed during treatment and reduces the risk of chemical injuries. Rubber dams are available in a variety of weights and colors. Of these, the medium weight is most suited for endodontic procedures when a clamp application is used. The conventional rubber dam is made of latex. Nonlatex dental dams are commercially available for use on latex-sensitized patients. The color of the dental dam for endodontic use should be as dark as possible to improve visibility inside the tooth. This allows the pulp space to be the brightest area in the field of vision. A light-colored dam, on the other hand, increases peripheral light that overpowers the eye impairing the ability to visualize details inside the pulp space. Quality rubber dam is strong and the risk of tearing is low if a circular hole for the tooth is made with a sharp and well-centered rubber dam punch.

A rubber dam should be applied only to one tooth at a time to reduce the chances for cross-contamination between teeth. The dam is retained to the tooth with a metal clamp that is available in many different designs. The clamps can easily be modified with diamond burs adapting the clamps better to individual teeth.

In cases with large tooth destruction, where the proper use of a rubber dam and a clamp do not provide adequate isolation, surgical tissue removal is the treatment of choice. This may range from simple removal of soft tissue electrosurgically to periodontal flap surgery and osseous contouring. Tissue removal will allow for good isolation and aseptic working conditions, while also adequately preparing the tooth for subsequent restoration. In certain situations a well-contoured band cemented with glass ionomer cement, after conditioning of the dentin, may provide sufficient support for rubber dam isolation.

11.5.2 Mechanical preparation of the surgical field

The importance of the mechanical cleaning of the external tooth surfaces is often overlooked in isolation of the tooth. This cleaning will reduce the amount of bacteria that may contaminate the field and resist disinfection. All hard deposits should be removed with appropriate scaler after which the tooth surface is polished with pumice or similar mild abrasive [66].

Gross caries must be excavated before the rubber dam is applied to reduce contamination of the surgical field. The pulp space should, however, not be entered unnecessarily during caries removal. Mechanical preparation also includes the removal of restorations as margins of most fillings are of sufficient size to harbor a large number of bacteria. Cervical restorations, not in contact with the access opening, may be retained in cases where their removal will severely complicate the

application of a rubber dam. However, special consideration should be given to these restorations during endodontic treatment as they are a potential source of microbial contamination.

Cast restorations are also a concern in the preparation of the surgical field due to the financial implication of their removal. It must be considered, however, that most cast restorations leak [32,54] and that the endodontic access opening will communicate fully with these leaks. Thus, asepsis is one important reason to remove cast restorations before starting endodontic treatment. In situations where the casting is retained, measures must be taken to minimize leakage. Thus, inside the access cavity the casting–dentin margin may be cleaned carefully with a small inverted cone bur and sealed with zinc oxide/eugenol cement. All intervisit temporary restorations should be placed well below the casting–tooth margins. Due to the compromised conditions associated with treatment through an artificial crown, the treatment sequence for a pulpectomy should be planned so that the entire treatment can be completed in one session.

11.5.3 Disinfection of the surgical field

When the tooth has been cleaned and rubber dam applied, the established surgical field must be thoroughly disinfected. In cases where caries-free dentin is covering the pulp in the path of the access, it is sufficient to disinfect this dentin surface once. In cases where caries has reached the pulp space, the disinfection process becomes more complex.

Functioning vital pulp tissue is not infiltrated with large numbers of microorganisms. If exposed to the oral environment, however, the necrotic surface layer of the vital pulp will be contaminated and/or infected. This is the case when caries has penetrated to the pulp space. Thus, the pulp tissue proper is sterile providing ideal conditions for aseptic pulp surgery; the surface of the pulp is, however, grossly contaminated by microorganisms. Great care must be taken not to transport the surface bacteria down to the apical wound site during the treatment; this can be achieved by systematic disinfection which is done in two steps:

• First, all caries is removed, but the vital coronal pulp tissue is not entered. The cavity and pulp wound are carefully disinfected. The contaminated burs are put aside.
• Secondly, with new sterile burs, the coronal part of the pulp is removed to the root canal orifice. The

cavity and pulp wound are once again carefully disinfected.

The initial tooth surface disinfection is with 30% hydrogen peroxide and 5% tincture of iodine. It has been well demonstrated that the surface treatment with hydrogen peroxide is essential for successful disinfection [66]. The cleaning of the tooth surface with 30% hydrogen peroxide followed by disinfection with 5% tincture of iodine effectively disinfected the tooth crown in 98.4% of cases. Iodine alone was only effective in 43.5% of the cases. The difference was even greater in the cervical junction between tooth and rubber dam; in this area, hydrogen peroxide combined with iodine was effective in 79.8% of cases when only 4.8% was successfully disinfected with iodine alone.

The purpose of the treatment with hydrogen peroxide is to remove all debris that may prevent the subsequent disinfectant from effectively reaching the microbes on the tooth surface. Hydrogen peroxide is not needed on the rubber dam or inside the access cavity during progressive disinfection; its value is in the cleaning of external tooth surfaces. High concentrations of hydrogen peroxide must never be used in dentin cavities of vital teeth that are not scheduled for pulpectomy as they will cause severe pulp injury.

Iodine tincture is a proven effective surface disinfectant with few substitutes. A tincture of chlorhexidine (0.5%) is equally effective. Iodine is practical to use as it is easy to see what areas of tooth and rubber dam have been treated. After applying the disinfectant it should be allowed to dry on the surface.

11.5.4 Instrument sterility

Endodontic procedures are a form of delicate microsurgery that requires a high degree of asepsis to achieve optimal treatment outcome. Therefore, it is important that all instruments used are not only clean and decontaminated, but also sterile. Contamination of instruments with debris is often a detail overlooked in the discussion of sterility. Not only is it difficult to sterilize successfully instruments that have debris attached to their surface, but pulp tissue may detach from the instruments during treatment. This could introduce a foreign body reaction in the pulp or periapical tissues and delay healing or potentially transmit or cause other health problems (e.g., prion disease).

Sterility is defined as the absence of living microorganisms. This stage is reached through various methods to sterilize and rid instruments of living microorganisms. The proof of sterility is based on the ability to demonstrate growth. This uncertainty is today mostly limited to prions and some viral contaminants as there may still be viruses that cannot be isolated. Reliable sterilization can be achieved by dry heat or steam (under pressure: autoclave) sterilization. Chemiclave may also be used if the resulting vapors are properly filtered or ventilated to the outside air. Ethylene oxide sterilization is not a practical alternative for sterilization of endodontic instruments and materials in a dental office as it requires a very long time.

The bead (glass or coarse salt) sterilizer has been used extensively in the past for chairside sterilization of instruments. Sometimes even molted metal (tin/lead mixture) was used. The use of bead sterilizers is an unreliable sterilization method [24]. It has sometimes been suggested that the use of this chairside "sterilization" method during treatment would be a valuable supplement for instrument sterilization. This is not needed, however, if pre-sterilized instruments are used. The antimicrobial irrigation fluid normally used during treatment will maintain clean aseptic files.

Dry heat sterilization of instruments is time consuming as it requires 90 min at 180°C. One of the advantages of this method is its low cost. The high temperature, however, means that linen and plastic items cannot be sterilized by dry heat. Contrary to often cited views, dry heat does not damage sharp root canal instruments [107].

Autoclaves are very effective sterilizers if properly maintained. Various sterilizing pressures with corresponding temperature increases can be selected for most autoclaves. Thus, at very high pressures (133°C) sterilization of unwrapped instruments can be achieved in 4–5 min and in 7–8 min when wrapped. Normal sterilizing time of wrapped instruments in a conventional, small autoclave is 20 min at 121°C and 15 pounds pressure. An effective and reliable autoclave should have an initial vacuum cycle to enhance the penetration of superheated steam to all packaged material. Chemiclave ("Harvey Sterilizer") works at 126°C and 20 pounds pressure. In this sterilizer, most of the steam has been replaced with a mixture of chemical vapors (mainly formaldehyde). This sterilizing method is less effective than the steam autoclave and may release formaldehyde to the clinical environment. Effective ventilation must be maintained as many people are very sensitive to formaldehyde.

Heat sterilization is the only decontamination process that can be easily and reliably checked to assure that the sterilization process works properly. This check of dry heat, steam, and chemical sterilizers should be done weekly. Two different procedures may be used. The easiest technique involves the use of a process indicator. This is usually a tape or crayon that changes color when exposed to a certain temperature. This only shows that the desired temperature has been reached. A process indicator should be used for every load being sterilized. A more exact test of a sterilizer is done with a spore test. This is a test to find whether sterility is achieved. Spore packages for this test can be purchased from various laboratories. For dry heat sterilizers, packages of *Bacillus subtilis* var. *niger* are suitable. For steam and chemical sterilizers, packages of *Bacillus stearothermophilus* should be used. These packages may be mailed to a laboratory for analysis, but can also easily be checked in a special small inexpensive incubator that is commercially available (Fig. 11.6). In contemporary practice, instruments are normally sterilized in pouches that incorporate the process indicator in the print of the bag. These sterilizing bags are also designed to maintain sterility of the contents after processing.

11.6 Tissue removal

11.6.1 Instrumentation

Endodontic instruments have undergone many changes through the history of dentistry. In recent years this evolution has progressed with increasing speed. The focus for instrument development has mostly been on mechanical properties and the ability to cut and machine dentin. Although this is a very important aspect, there are other properties that improve the instruments' use as surgical tools. Thus, little attention has been given to the need to develop instruments adapted to the special biological problems associated with the treatment of the root canal system. This need for special considerations is especially true for instruments intended for (partial) vital pulpectomy. Such an instrument, a pulp knife, was discussed 80 years ago [20]. Later, a Hedström file with the tip cut to a blunt end was suggested as a pulpectomy instrument [63]. Several other different instrument types have been evaluated regarding their suitability for vital pulpectomy [63,69,70]. These studies suggested that none of the instruments explored

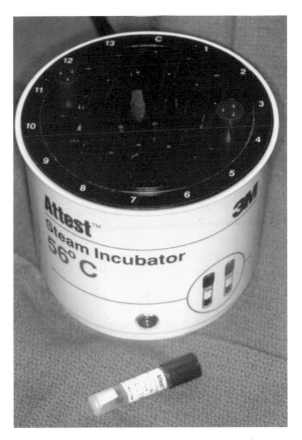

Fig. 11.6 Small incubator for processing spore test for sterilizers. The spore test sample is in front of the incubator.

was superior in preserving the pulp remnants within the root canal. In the majority of cases the pulp remnants were severely damaged and the most common injury was twisting of the remaining pulp. As there is still no ideal instrument for pulp excision, the pulp remnants should not be left longer than a couple of millimeters during pulpectomy procedures. Doing so could in many cases leave a substantial amount of twisted pulp residue in the form of necrotic tissue in the root canal. In clinical studies of vital pulpectomy, however, it was suggested that the level of pulpectomy did not seem to affect the treatment outcome when judged histologically [28,71]. It was also observed that the length of the pulp remaining in the root canals in most cases was shorter than suggested by the working length radiograph [28,71].

The issue of suitable instrument for partial pulpectomy is still unresolved. Therefore, clinical treatment

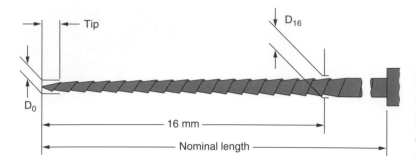

Fig. 11.7 Schematic drawing identifying some key measuring points for instrument standards. D_0 is the projected diameter of the instrument in the plane of the tip. D_{16} is the diameter 16 mm from the tip. Taper is $(D_{16} - D_0)/16$.

discussions must always be modulated by the fact that the endodontic clinician lacks an efficient and atraumatic surgical instrument for the controlled removal of vital pulp tissue from the root canal system.

There are national and international standards for dimensions of K-type and Hedström-type instruments (Fig. 11.7). Most standards are similar, requiring the nominal length of the instrument to be 21, 25, or 31 mm. The working part that is fluted should be at least 16 mm with a taper of 0.02 mm/mm of the length (2%). The size of the file is determined by the projected diameter of the tapered instrument at the tip. This measurement is called D_0. The size of the instrument represents the imaginary diameter in increments of 0.01 mm. The tolerance is allowed to be ±0.02 mm. Thus, a size 030 instrument will have a diameter of 0.30 ± 0.02 mm. The tip length of a Hedström file must be less than twice D_0. The tip of a K-type file must have a tip angle within 75° ± 15°. The shape of the tip is optional. The handle of the instrument must be imprinted with the size number. Coloring of the handles is not mandatory, but, if used, the color must follow a standardized scheme. Often, however, these standard specifications are not carefully followed [108]. Samples of 20 different brands of files failed to show one single group that totally maintained standard size; K-type files usually complied better than other types of instruments. In recent years some manufacturers have produced instruments in "half sizes", e.g., sizes 012.5, 015, 017.5. This is a rather irrational step as long as the regular sizes of the files are allowed to have a tolerance of ±2 number units. Manufacturers already seem unable to follow such a liberal requirement [108]. Thus, if "half sizes" are used, a size 012.5 instrument will in many instances be similar to either a size 010 or 015 instrument.

Endodontic instruments that earlier were limited to carbon steel K-type and Hedström files have been modified dramatically during the past 30 years.

Although K-type and Hedström files made from carbon or stainless steel are the only types recognized in many national standardization protocols, several new nonstandardized instruments are available today.

The K-type instrument represents an instrument that is normally fabricated from a tapered ground blank that has been twisted. The abrasive effect depends on how tight the instrument has been twisted (Fig. 11.8). The cross-section of these blanks may be square, triangular, or rhomboid. The rhomboid

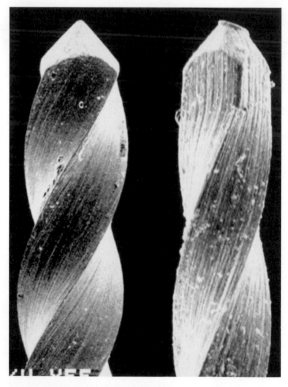

Fig. 11.8 K-files, (left) by Maillefer and (right) by Kerr. Note the difference between these two K-files in number of spirals per unit length.

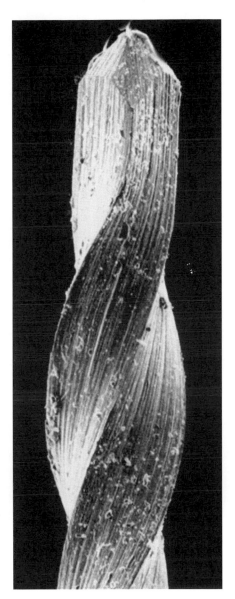

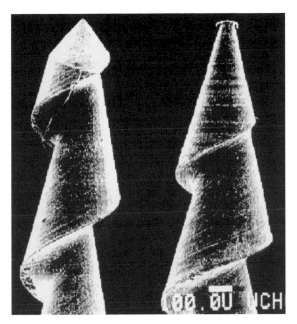

Fig. 11.10 Hedstrom files (left) by Maillefer and (right) by Antaeos. Note the difference in tip design between instruments; the tip of the Antaeos file has been blunted during manufacturing.

Fig. 11.9 K-Flex file (Kerr). The instrument has wide and narrow areas due to the rhomboid cross-section of the original blank.

cross-section has a long diagonal that will provide the dimension resulting in the size of the instrument and a short diagonal that provides increased flexibility (Fig. 11.9). The blanks are twisted counterclockwise to produce the file. The reamers normally have fewer flutes per length unit than files. The tip of the instrument is then ground to a desired form. Much techni-

cal effort has gone into the design of the file tip, but no scientific proof has been given that one is superior over another. The Hedström-type instruments are ground from a round blank (Fig. 11.10). Through computer-assisted manufacturing (CAM) there is today a great freedom to develop instruments with variable configurations. By changing the number and pitch, flutes or core thickness along the length of the instrument, its flexibility can also be controlled during manufacturing. The introduction of the CAM process now allows the manufacturing of K-type instruments through a grinding process instead of twisting. There are also many variations on the classic Hedström file. The double helix instead of the single helix found on the classic Hedström file is common (Fig. 11.11).

There are also substantial variations in the effectiveness in dentin removal between brands and also within the same brand [46]. Dentin is very damaging to the cutting edges of root canal instruments, and the sharpness of the instruments decreases rapidly when used on dentin. Table 11.1 shows a comparison of machining efficiency of some stainless-steel files and the wear of these files when removing dentin. Some instruments may lose as much as 55% of their machin-

Table 11.1 Machining of stainless steel and nickel–titanium endodontic hand files on dentin substrate. Instruments listed in order of initial machining efficiency and a comparison of effectiveness is listed as "relative removal". The nickel–titanium instruments wear less than stainless-steel instruments [46,47]

Brand	Dentin removal[a] (mm^2)	Relative removal (%)	Wear[b] (%)
Stainless steel			
H-file (Sjödings)	0.56 ± 0.32	100	54.8
H-file (Maillefer)	0.37 ± 0.17	66.1	27.0
K-Flex (Kerr)	0.35 ± 0.17	62.5	38.0
S-file (Sjödings)	0.31 ± 0.10	55.4	41.6
K-file (Maillefer)	0.31 ± 0.06	55.3	21.8
Flex-R (Union Broach)	0.29 ± 0.14	51.8	35.1
K-file (Sjödings)	0.29 ± 0.09	51.8	38.3
Nickel–titanium			
Hyflex-X (Hygenic)	0.60 ± 0.16	100	22.2
Mity-H (JS Dental)	0.55 ± 0.18	91.7	22.0
K-file (Maillefer)	0.51 ± 0.20	85.0	17.4
H-file (Texceed)	0.44 ± 0.17	73.3	18.0
Naviflex-H (Brasseler)	0.35 ± 0.16	58.3	11.1
Mity-K (JS Dental)	0.32 ± 0.06	53.3	16.8
K-file (Texceed)	0.31 ± 0.07	51.7	9.0
Mity Turbo (JS Dental)	0.19 ± 0.12	31.7	18.7

[a] Amount removed after 300 push–pull strokes on dentin.
[b] Reduction in efficiency after 300 push–pull strokes on dentin.

ing efficiency after 300 strokes on dentin. Therefore, it may be rational to consider these files as disposable to ensure that each file is performing optimally when used [46].

Nickel–titanium (NiTi) hand instruments are now available from practically all major manufacturers and in most configurations (Figs 11.11 and 11.12). The advantage of NiTi is the increased flexibility it gives to the instruments. NiTi root canal instruments are very flexible and these instruments are therefore useful when negotiating curved root canals. Due to these qualities, NiTi rotary instruments have also been developed. It is important to understand the characteristics of NiTi instruments, however, as the alloy is not without problems. NiTi is a shape memory alloy appearing in two crystal forms: austenite and martensite. It undergoes thermoelastic martensitic transformation due to stress or temperature. During endodontic use the transformation is due to stress. The transformation from the austenitic to martensitic phase is reversible [51,52]. Therefore, it is important to maintain an even strain on the instrument during use as rapid changes will alter the transformation stages. The alloy breaks easily during phase trans-

formation. A sudden change in rotational speed or resistance causes phase transformation in the alloy. Therefore, an electric motor with speed and torque control is essential for the maintenance of a constant speed when using rotary instruments. Under the best circumstances, rotary NiTi instruments must only be used for a limited number of preparations to reduce the risk for instrument separation. The NiTi alloy is work-hardened during the manufacturing of rotary instruments. This results in surface cracks, which during stress on the instrument may propagate and cause instrument breakage. Electropolishing is one method applied after manufacturing to reduce the number of surface cracks. The effects of surface cracks and temperature changes during use are still factors not well understood in the clinical use of NiTi rotary instruments. However, an experienced operator will have few instrument fractures if basic principles are respected. A (glide) path to at least a size 15 hand instrument must always be established before initiating rotary instrumentation. Although NiTi instruments are very flexible, curvatures >45° should be negotiated with great care. Double curvature is a serious problem. Therefore, straight access into the

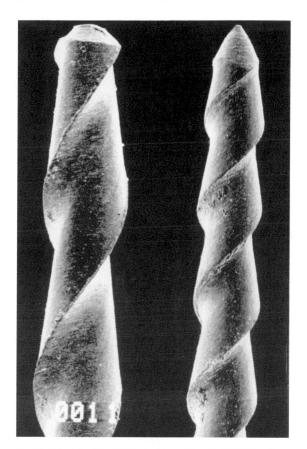

Fig. 11.11   Modified NiTi Hedstrom files, (left) HyFlex file by Hygenic, and (right) Mity Turbo file by JS Dental. Note the instruments have two spiral cutting edges opposite each other (double helix), and also the difference in number of flutes and tip design.

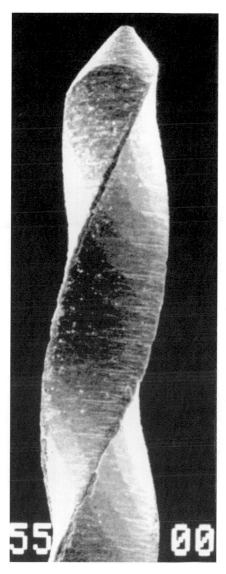

Fig. 11.12   Modified NiTi K-files, UltraFlex file by Texceed. Note how this K-type file has been ground from a wire and not twisted like an original K-file (Fig. 11.8).

root canal to eliminate the first curvature is mandatory when instrumenting posterior teeth. Although it may be wise to consider rotary NiTi instruments disposable, they may be reused a few times. A practical measure is to limit each instrument to approximately 500 rotations during normal use; at 500 rpm this is 1 min of use. The introduction of NiTi has made it possible to develop engine driven root canal instruments that are clinically very useful. The originally introduced NiTi rotary instruments were designed to prevent binding. Therefore, the sharp flutes that characterize regular root canal files were replaced by flat surface called "lands". The more common early rotary instruments are ProFile (Tulsa Dental) and Quantec (Sybron) (Fig. 11.13). Because of their relative lack of cutting they grind the dentin surfaces. Due

to high friction generated during this grinding action these early instruments operated at high torque. The rotating speed used is normally around 300 rpm. The LightSpeed (LightSpeed Technology) (Fig. 11.14) instrument is also designed with lands instead of sharp cutting edges. Due to the relatively small working surface of these instruments they operate with low friction. LightSpeed is normally used at 1500–2000 rpm. K3 (Sybron) is an instrument with great similarity to

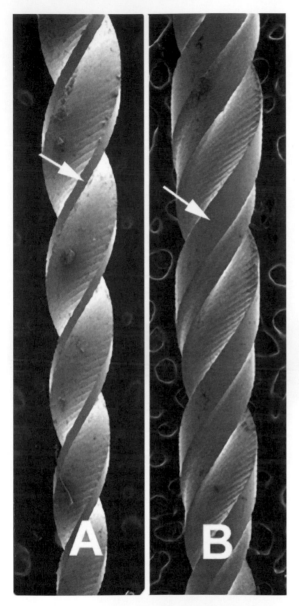

Fig. 11.13   ProFile GT (A, Tulsa Dental) (left) and Quantec (B, Sybron) (right) rotary NiTi instruments. Note well-defined flat surfaces (lands – white arrows) on the ridges of both the instruments that assure a smooth machining process without binding and cutting into the root canal walls.

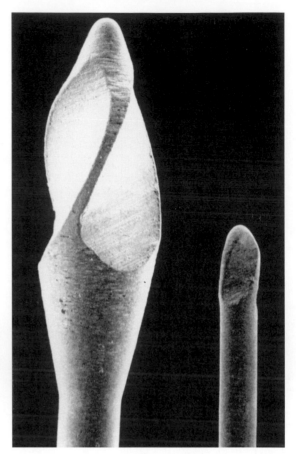

Fig. 11.14   LightSpeed rotary NiTi instrument (LightSpeed Technologies) (left) size 90 and (right) size 20. Note how the fine size instrument lacks edge definition, but the larger instrument has well-defined lands similar to the Profile instrument shown in Fig. 11.13.

Quantec (Sybron) (Fig. 11.15). However, it has a third sharp helix which provides some cutting qualities. This makes the instrument more aggressive than Quantec. All machining of the root canal walls creates smear. It appears that instruments that are less sharp tend to compress smear deeper into the dentin tubules during work compared to instruments with sharper edges (Fig. 11.16) [53]. In recent years even sharper instruments have been brought to the market and some typical instruments are HERO 642 (MicroMega), ProTaper (Tulsa Dental), RaCe (Brasseler), Sequence (Brasseler), and V-Taper (Guidance) (Fig. 11.17). These instruments have sharp cutting edges and they are operated at speeds around 500–600 rpm. Due to their sharpness, friction is low and these instruments are known as low-torque instruments. To prevent binding of these sharp instruments different variations on taper and helical angles are being used.

NiTi hand files are more abrasive and last longer than a similar stainless-steel file (Table 11.1) [47], This

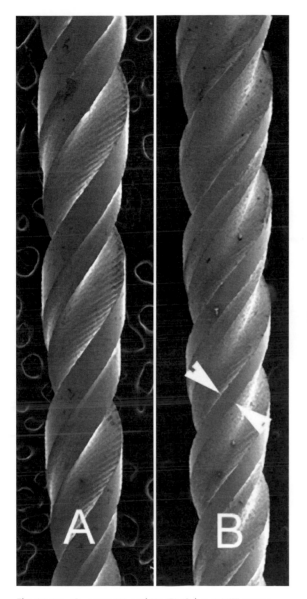

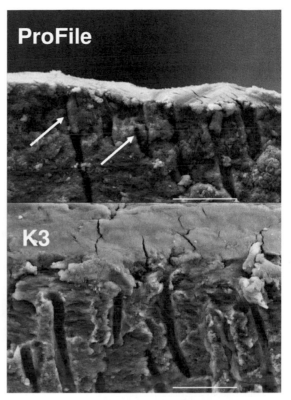

Fig. 11.16 Cross-sections of root canal walls that have been prepared with ProFile and K3 rotary NiTi instruments. Note how the ProFile instrument has compacted smear into the dentin tubules (arrows). The dentin prepared with K3 has less compaction. (Courtesy of Kum *et al.* [53].) Scale bar = 10 μm.

Fig. 11.15 Quantec (A) and K3 (B) (Sybron) NiTi rotary instruments. Note how K3 has a third helix (arrowheads) with a sharp cutting edge.

of the rotary instrument brands are also available as hand instruments for the negotiations of very curved and complex root canal configurations.

11.6.2 Wound surface: working length

The questions related to the working length, or more correctly the wound surface level, have been debated to a great extent. The optimal wound surface in necrotic infected cases is as close as possible to the apical foramen of the root canal [48,95,97]. It is difficult to determine the endpoint for apical preparation of the root canal in many clinical cases as this point often varies relative to the apex [71,28]. This is especially difficult as roots associated with an ongoing resorbing apical periodontitis nearly always lack a distinguishable apical constriction. With the use of a reliable apex locator this guesswork is reduced

may to some extent compensate for the high price of NiTi files. It is also technically more difficult to manufacture instruments in NiTi compared to steel. With the advent of very efficient NiTi rotary instruments for the major bulk of canal preparation, there is little advantage of NiTi files over stainless-steel hand instruments for remaining instrumentation. Several

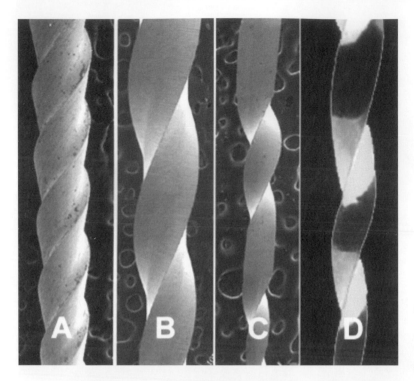

Fig. 11.17   Contemporary low torque NiTi rotary instruments. HERO 642 (A) (MicroMega), ProTaper (B) (Tulsa Dental), RaCe (C) (Brasseler), and Sequence (D) (Brasseler).

[33,50]. In most cases where the pulp is necrotic and infected the wound (apical limit) should be placed within 1 mm of the radiographic apex [95].

The major concern in necrotic cases is related to the elimination of all infected soft and hard tissues from the apical part of the root canal. Disinfection of the most apical part of an infected pulp space is difficult, as it often has branching of the main canal (Fig. 11.18), and extensive apposition of cementum. These anatomical variations make mechanical debridement less effective. Furthermore, conventional antimicrobial solutions, if used in too low concentrations, may be diluted to nonbactericidal levels or inhibited by tissue fluids in this area [76]. Consequently, great efforts must be spent on the most apical part of the root canal when treating infected pulp canals (Fig. 11.5). The need for close apical preparation of teeth with necrotic pulp has been confirmed in several clinical treatment outcome studies [48,97].

The placement of the wound surface in vital teeth is guided by concerns other than those for treating infected root canals. The optimal wound level in teeth with vital pulp appears to be 1–2 mm from the radiographic apex [27,48,49]. When the pulp is vital there is no concern about initial hard or soft tissue infection. The main treatment objective is to opti-

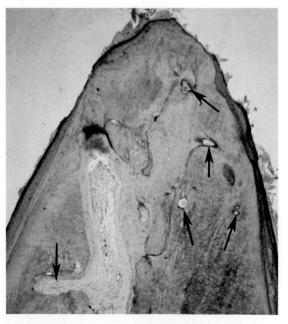

Fig. 11.18   Apical part of human maxillary cuspid. Note the large number of apical ramifications of the pulp (arrows).

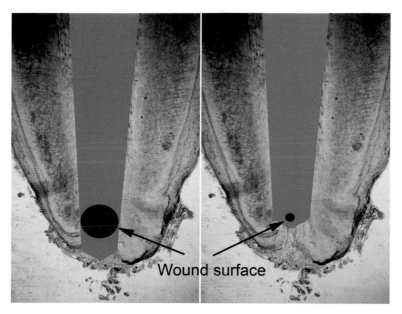

Fig. 11.19 The effect on wound surface size (red circles) as a result of instrumentation technique. The figure illustrates how the resulting wound surface increases very much if the instrumentation is extended through the apical foramen (left). If the instrumentation is kept short of the apical foramen the wound surface can never exceed the cross section of the pulp tissue (right). A smaller wound surface normally heals with fewer complications.

mize the technique of aseptic and atraumatic pulp surgery. When the pulp wound is left well inside the root canal the cross-section of the wound surface will never exceed the cross-section size of the pulp tissue, even if the root canal preparation is made very large (Fig. 11.19). As conventional root canal filling materials are all tissue irritating to some degree, the surface area of root canal filling material exposed to the tissue should be kept as small as possible in order to optimize the chances for the interface of filling material and periapical tissue to heal without complication. If the pulp remnant left in the root canal is more than 2 mm long, the risk of pulp necrosis is high due to amputation injuries. It is crucial for the outcome of vital pulp treatment that the remaining pulp remains vital after the surgery. If the length of the remaining pulp is short, the chances for revascularization are higher than if the pulp stump is long as the ratio between remaining pulp length and size of apical constriction is small [21,73]. The higher this ratio, the more unlikely it is that complete revascularization will occur. It has been demonstrated, however, that if the pulp is removed completely when strict asepsis is maintained, healing will occur even if the root canal filling is placed 2–4 mm short of the working length [39,72]. The observation was also made that the size of the apical foramen is of little consequence as the apical foramen may be opened by a resorptive process during the initial stage of healing.

11.6.3 Chemical adjuncts

Antimicrobial agents are used during the preparation of the pulp space and the removal of pulp tissue. Decalcifying agents, alcohol, and chloroform or similar solvents are additional adjuncts used for various endodontic procedures.

The need for decalcifying agents during endodontic treatment is not clear. The most common decalcifying preparation is ethylenediamine tetraacetic acid (EDTA) [119]. Sodium hypochlorite (NaOCl) is a common irrigation fluid during mechanical instrumentation of the root canal. Properly applied this is a potent agent for the elimination of necrotic pulp tissue from the pulp space. At the completion of the mechanical preparation of the pulp space, however, the root canal walls are covered by a firmly attached mixed smear of organic and inorganic materials of dentin and pulp origin. This smear layer can be removed easily with EDTA or with a weak acid such as citric acid. It appears that when the smear layer is removed before root canal filling, some sealers with small particle sizes may penetrate the dentin tubules better than if the smear is allowed to remain on the root canal walls [74,90,121,122]. EDTA has little beneficial effect on the disinfection of infected root canals when used in combination with NaOCl during instrumentation [11]. There is no unequivocal documentation in the literature to suggest that the outcome of endodontic treatment is improved by removal of the dentin smear.

To aid in the instrumentation of very narrow calcified root canals EDTA may also be used. The decalcifying effect of EDTA is self-limiting [119]. It decalcifies approximately 30 μm of the dentin surface within 5 min. If left in the pulp space for 24 hours, it will reach a depth of 50 μm. Although seemingly an unimportant amount, counting all walls, this will account for 100 μm of decalcification in a root canal. This is the size of the tip diameter of an ISO size 010 file. Frequent irrigation with EDTA and instrumentation will therefore continuously remove dentin and be very useful for the initial opening of a canal orifice smaller than fine files [36]. Despite its effectiveness it must be kept in mind, however, that EDTA will not *find* root canals. It only works where a canal has been located, and has very limited use as an aid in the removal of dentin during routine instrumentation. Its decalcifying effect is much less than the abrasive effect of root canal files and rasps. EDTAC is a mixture of EDTA and a quaternary ammonium compound. This adds some antimicrobial qualities to the chelator. RC-Prep is a combination of EDTA and urea peroxide in carbowax [109]. This preparation, that is not water soluble, is used in combination with NaOCl where the peroxide releases gas that may help remove debris out of the root canal. However, RC-Prep is not proven to be superior to EDTA and may, due to its lack of water solubility, leave residues in the root canals. The effectiveness of NaOCl is inhibited by EDTA when they are mixed together, and therefore their simultaneous use should be avoided [34].

Recently 1-hydroxyethylidene-1,1-bisphosphonate (HEBP) has been suggested as a replacement for EDTA [31]; HEBP does not appear to inhibit the effectiveness of NaOCl when used simultaneously [126].

On the assumption that smear layer removal is a desirable endpoint during root canal debridement a product called MTAD (BioPure MTAD Cleanser, Tulsa Dental, Tulsa, OK) has been developed. The composition of MTAD is a mixture of doxycycline (tetracycline isomer), citric acid, and Tween 80. The combination of citric acid with a detergent provides good cleaning effectiveness. The antimicrobial effect is provided by doxycycline. It is unclear, however, if this provides any enhanced antimicrobial effectiveness under clinical conditions. An antibiotic is difficult to inhibit during clinical trials and so may prevent objective bacterial culturing procedures. The effectiveness of MTAD in removing dentin smear is similar to EDTA [118]; MTAD has similar effect on the strength of dentine as EDTA [58].

Many endodontic sealers do not attach well to wet dentin. To improve the function of these sealers the root canal may be irrigated with 99% ethanol immediately before filling. Ethanol used for a brief rinse will not cause irreversible damage to the tissue wound as its toxicity is low compared to most antimicrobial agents used for endodontic treatment. A 1% solution of NaOCl is four times more cytotoxic *in vitro* than pure ethanol [29,101].

Chloroform (trichloromethane) is often used during endodontic procedures. There are several filling methods where chloroform softening of the gutta-percha is practiced as well as the use of resin chloroform for sealing purposes [1,123]. Chloroform is also one of the more efficient solvents for the softening of gutta-percha and sealers during endodontic retreatment [86]. Chloroform used in large amounts as an anesthetic has been shown to be hepatotoxic. Concerns about liver damage have meant that substitutes such as halothane and rectified white turpentine oil have been suggested as gutta-percha solvents. In a study *in vitro* it was shown that both halothane and rectified turpentine oil have toxic characteristics that are as serious as chloroform [5]. Rectified turpentine oil maintains its toxicity for an extended period of time and turpentine allergy has been demonstrated [77]. Halothane is clinically less effective than chloroform and hepatotoxicity to halothane has also been discussed in the literature [56,60]. It is doubtful, however, that the very minimal amounts of chloroform used for endodontic treatment will cause liver damage. With the use of high-speed evacuation and the dispensing of chloroform through a syringe, little chloroform will evaporate to the ambient air in the dental office. Therefore, it seems that with careful use there is no clinical need to use the clinically less effective halothane or turpentine oil as substitutes for chloroform when a gutta-percha solvent is needed.

11.7 Antisepsis

11.7.1 Irrigation fluids

Irrigation and suction are used for the removal of tissue remnants and dentin debris during the mechanical instrumentation of the root canal. There is much controversy regarding the effectiveness of irrigation and the proper delivery system. Despite such academic debate, irrigation and suctioning is presently the best method available for removing debris created during pulp space instrumentation. Most instrumented root canals are too narrow to allow even a very fine irrigation needle to pass all the way to the apical part of the canal. This reduces the efficacy of irrigation. Therefore, all attempts to irrigate debris out of the root canal must be done in several steps with intermittent agitation of the root canal content with small files. This time-consuming procedure is necessary to prevent root canal contents from settling in the apical parts of the root canal system. Frequent irrigation and agitation are very important to enhance the chances of maintaining a clean pulp space during instrumentation.

Various fluids have been suggested for irrigation. Sterile water or saline has been used for removal of pulp tissue debris. This may seem an excellent solution from a biological point of view and may be sufficient in cases of elective vital pulp removal where there is no contamination by bacteria. However, there are several drawbacks: saline or water have no cleansing effects, have a high surface tension, and do not have any antimicrobial effects [9]. Thus, saline or water have no additional value over being transport vehicles.

Antimicrobial detergents and NaOCl have been popular irrigation solutions. Examples of the first category are benzalkonium chloride sold under the brand name Zephiran. This is a quaternary ammonium compound that has very low surface tension. It has been used in endodontics at 0.1% and 1% concentrations. Besides being antibacterial, it also aids in the cleaning of the root canal, through its effect as a detergent, by removing fatty necrotic deposits in the pulp space. Quaternary ammonium compounds are, however, poor antimicrobial agents with a rather limited spectrum [29,30,102]. They also impair tissue healing and cause tissue injury [7,78,79]. Therefore, cationic antimicrobial compounds are not ideal for use as an endodontic irrigation solution. Anionic detergents have also been applied as endodontic irrigation solutions in combination with a saturated $Ca(OH)_2$ aqueous solution [4].

Sodium hypochlorite is the most universally used irrigation solution. The modern use of hypochlorite as a wound cleansing compound has its origin from the trench warfare in the First World War [16,17]. The original "Dakin's solution" contained 0.5% NaOCl. In endodontics, however, it was for many years applied

at 10 times that concentration and it was usually dispensed from household bleach. This commercially available version is very caustic with a pH of about 12 [78,102]. The toxicity, *in vivo*, of NaOCl compared to other antiseptics used for irrigation has been well described elsewhere [78,103]. It was elegantly demonstrated in clinical studies that the cleaning and disinfection effect is not significantly improved at 5% compared to 0.5% [10,12,14]. The tissue-dissolving effect, if a contributing factor *in vivo*, is dependent on the amount of free chlorine available in the solution. Therefore, to maintain the effectiveness, as the concentration of the solution is lowered, the volume should be increased. The tissue dissolving objectives may be achieved and the tissue properly protected by increasing the irrigation volume and using NaOCl at a concentration of 0.5–1.0 % [100]. If household bleach is used as the stock material, the dilution is best done with 1% sodium bicarbonate. Besides diluting the bleach, the bicarbonate will also lower the pH from over 12 to approximately 8.5. This does not change the tissue dissolving effect, but alters the caustic effect of a pH of 12 [125]. Sodium hypochlorite concentrations at 3% and above also deplete the dentin of important organic components resulting in an increased permeability and lowering of the flexural strength and elastic modulus [35].

11.7.2 Antibacterial agents

Endodontic treatment of the vital pulp should be done in one treatment session. If proper asepsis is maintained during the treatment there should not be any concerns for further need to treat the pulp space with an antimicrobial agent. The continuous treatment of these cases from start to the application of the wound dressing in one session also reduces the very obvious risk for leakage around a temporary restoration [26,44]. Time permitting, the only true contraindication to a one visit treatment of a tooth with a vital pulp is apical tissue hemorrhage that cannot be fully controlled. Hemostasis is absolutely necessary for satisfactory application of the wound dressing as most endodontic sealers bond poorly to wet dentin. In cases where hemostasis cannot be fully controlled, it has also been suggested that good results can be obtained by placing the root canal filling 2–4 mm short of the wound surface [39].

In cases where the pulp tissue is necrotic, dentin infection must always be suspected even when no periapical bone lesion has yet developed or is diagnosable on a radiograph. Although the presence of bacteria in the pulp space is required for the development of an apical bone lesion, the temporal relationship is always such that the pulp space first becomes infected, then a more complex microflora develops after which a bone lesion will appear [110]. On rare occasions this process may take years to develop [8].

Despite careful mechanical instrumentation and the use of rather strong antimicrobial irrigation fluids, infections of the pulp space have been difficult to eradicate predictably in one clinical treatment session [9–12]. Therefore, the treatment of a tooth with a necrotic pulp should always be performed in at least two distinct treatment sessions. The purpose with this extended treatment is to deposit an antimicrobial agent in the pulp space during the intervisit period in order to kill the remaining bacteria. The proper antimicrobial agent may also eliminate the byproducts of the bacteria that are capable of inducing damage to the periapical tissues. This intervisit antimicrobial agent is normally called an "intracanal medication" or "deposit" antiseptic. There are several types of antimicrobial "deposit" antiseptics. The classical antimicrobial agents are phenol and phenol-derivatives such as paramonochlorophenol, cresol, and cresatine. The phenol antiseptics work by indiscriminately denaturing cellular proteins; therefore, they are very toxic and incompatible with a biological approach to endodontic treatment [102,103]. Consequently, phenol and its derivatives should no longer be used in biological-based contemporary endodontic practice.

Antimicrobial agents belonging to the halogen group, such as iodine and chlorine, are strong oxidizing agents able to inhibit cellular enzyme systems and thereby inactivate the bacterial cell. Therefore, this group of antiseptics is very effective and less damaging to connective tissues [78,103]. Iodine compounds such as iodine potassium iodide (Table 11.2) and chlorine compounds such as chloramines are modern alternatives for liquid deposit antiseptics. Iodine potassium iodide has been proposed as a useful water

base for enhancing the antimicrobial effectiveness of $Ca(OH)_2$ [94]. The antimicrobial effect of iodine potassium iodide is limited to only a few hours [25].

11.7.3 Calcium hydroxide

Calcium hydroxide slurry has been used for endodontic procedures since it was first described in 1920 as an endodontic adjunct [37,38]. It has since been used for a number of different applications in endodontics; some of the more successful have been as a pulp capping and pulpotomy wound dressing, and intracanal medication for both vital and necrotic pulps. In a water suspension at body temperature, only 0.17% of the $Ca(OH)_2$ is hydrolyzed into Ca^{2+} and OH^- ions; thus, most $Ca(OH)_2$ in the paste or slurry is not in solution. Therefore the $Ca(OH)_2$ slurry has a large reserve of $Ca(OH)_2$ allowing intracanal deposits to be effective for a long period of time. The best vehicle for $Ca(OH)_2$ is an aqueous solution as the $Ca(OH)_2$ needs water to hydrolyze and provide the active ions. Calcium hydroxide is less antimicrobial in other vehicles such as glycerin [84,85]. Mixing the $Ca(OH)_2$ powder with phenol derivatives, as is often suggested, reduces the amount of free OH^- ions. Mixed with paramonochlorophenol it forms calcium parachlorophenolate; and with cresatine, calcium cresylate and acetic acid are formed. Calcium hydroxide slowly forms calcium carbonate in contact with air; this process may take years. Calcium carbonate has very low solubility and is easily recognized by the granular carbonate in contrast to the normally smooth $Ca(OH)_2$.

The benefits of $Ca(OH)_2$ dressing of superficial pulp wounds are well described in the literature [68,87]. There is no direct evidence, however, that $Ca(OH)_2$ is hard-tissue inducing when successfully used for "apexification" or "apexogenesis" procedures. The beneficial effect is more likely associated with the mild but effective antimicrobial effect of $Ca(OH)_2$ [11,80,81]. In addition to its antimicrobial properties, $Ca(OH)_2$ has been shown to hydrolyze effectively the lipid moiety of bacterial lipopolysaccharide (LPS) from Gram-negative bacteria [42,82,83]. With the antimicrobial effect and LPS inactivation by $Ca(OH)_2$, apical healing, in the form of continuous root formation or apical hard tissue closing, is most likely the natural healing process that can take place when microbial irritants have been eliminated.

Calcium hydroxide slurry is a slow acting antimicrobial agent, and at least a day is required *in vitro* for full effect [81]. Clinically, following a stringent

Table 11.2 Iodine potassium iodide is an effective disinfectant. It is easily prepared by mixing iodine with potassium iodide and then adding distilled water

	2% Solution	5% Solution
Iodine	2 g	5 g
Potassium iodide	4 g	10 g
Distilled water	94 g	85 g

treatment protocol, a week of $Ca(OH)_2$ dressing is sufficient for effective reliable disinfection of most cases with a necrotic pulp [96]. Calcium hydroxide is an effective antimicrobial agent due to the high pH environment that it establishes. However, *Enterococcus* spp. and *Candida* are rather tolerant of high pH conditions and they are therefore somewhat resistant to $Ca(OH)_2$ treatment. These microorganisms were previously considered less important and infrequent in endodontic infections. Recent research has shown that they may appear much more frequently in previously treated and filled root canals than in initial pulp space infections. Recent studies with molecular identification techniques suggests that *Enterococcus* spp. may have a more common presence in initial infections than earlier believed but due to low cell count could not be cultured. How often *Enterococcus* spp. can be found in previously root-filled teeth is still not clear as published studies vary from none to over 70%. It also appears that *Enterococcus* spp. may have a common presence in the pulp space of endodontically treated teeth regardless of whether a periapical lesion is present or not [43]. Thus, it is unclear if *Enterococcus* spp. are important for the development of apical periodontitis or if they are just opportunistically present in root-filled teeth. However, recent findings of *Enterococcus* spp. have led to extensive speculation regarding the value of $Ca(OH)_2$ as a deposit antiseptic in the retreatment of failed endodontic cases. Various other combinations of antimicrobial agents have been proposed, the most common being a mixture of $Ca(OH)_2$ with chlorhexidine. Aqueous solutions of chlorhexidine appear to provide the ideal combination to combine the broad effectiveness of $Ca(OH)_2$ slurry with the proven effectiveness of chlorhexidine against *Enterococcus* spp. and *Candida*. The pH of this mixture reaches over 12, well over what is considered lethal for these microorganisms [94]. Chlorhexidine gluconate is a cationic bisbiguanide solution that is most stable within a pH range of 5–8. Chlorhexidine, which is insoluble in water, precipitates out of chlorhexidine gluconate solution at pH levels higher than 8; at pH levels above that, chlorhexidine gluconate becomes ineffective [127]. Therefore $Ca(OH)_2$ should not be mixed with chlorhexidine. If chlorhexidine is used as a disinfectant during endodontic treatment it should be used separately from $Ca(OH)_2$.

Iodine potassium iodide may be a more promising water-based antimicrobial agent suitable for mixture with $Ca(OH)_2$. No clinical study of such a mixture is yet available, but laboratory studies appear promising [94].

Attempts to mix antibiotics with $Ca(OH)_2$ have been unsuccessful. A mixture of tetracycline or erythromycin with $Ca(OH)_2$ failed to enhance effectiveness against *Enterococcus* spp. [64].

Candida albicans has been found in treatment-resistant endodontic cases. It is also somewhat resistant to $Ca(OH)_2$ treatment, although a highly toxic mixture of camphorated paramonochlorophenol and $Ca(OH)_2$ in glycerin may be effective as an intracanal dressing [93]. It appears, however, that irrigation with EDTA is very effective in eliminating *Candida* in root canals [3].

A thick mix of $Ca(OH)_2$ is best introduced into the root canal with a Lentulo spiral. The slurry must be carried all the way to the wound surface after which it should be carefully compacted. A completely filled canal with most fluid condensed out of the slurry is essential for good disinfection. Although $Ca(OH)_2$ is important for root canal disinfection there are significant concerns over using it for long-term intracanal dressing. The strength of dentin is adversely affected by $Ca(OH)_2$; the flexural strength of dentin is significantly lowered when submerged in $Ca(OH)_2$ [35] The strength of root dentin decreases if $Ca(OH)_2$ dressings are extended over a month [2,23].

11.8 Root canal filling

11.8.1 Function

After the pulp tissue has been removed and the pulp space has been properly disinfected and prepared, the wound in the apical part of the root canal must be protected from further external insults. In the case of vital pulpectomy the wound surface consists of pulp tissue. When necrotic pulp has been removed, the wound surface is either established in granulation tissue within the root canal or ingrowing periodontal tissues. Neither of these tissues can heal with epithelial cover. Thus, a permanent dressing must be placed to protect the tissue wound. This wound dressing is called a root canal filling. The root canal filling functions as an implant and materials used must therefore fulfill the basic biological requirements of an implant material.

11.8.2 Seal

Another, most important function of the root canal filling implant is to protect the underlying tissue from bacterial invasion and subsequent infection and inflammation as the oral cavity harbors a large variety of bacteria known to be pathogens. Thus, a root canal filling material must have such characteristics that it permanently and reliably seals off the apical wound from the oral cavity. Bacteria are the major cause of apical periodontitis. The bacterial cell, however, is not required to bypass the seal of the root canal filling material as many bacterial metabolic byproducts have the same inflammatory effect as the cell itself. Consequently, very small imperfections in the adhesion of the root canal filling material to the root canal walls may allow potent bacterial byproducts in the coronal part of the root to reach the periapical tissues.

Many studies have been published on the subject of root canal leakage after filling. Most of these studies have not been well controlled [45,105,124]. The summary, however, of all the information available, is that even under the best circumstances the hydraulic seal of all parts of the root canal is, in most cases, impossible to achieve. Despite this apparent lack in seal at various levels of the root canal, the combined seal along the root canal between the oral cavity and the periapical tissues is good enough to block communication effectively and reduce microbial leakage to a level that can be managed by the immune system (Fig. 11.20) [18]. The presence of less effective seal at various levels of the root canal, however, must be considered when discussing the effect on treatment outcome of post retention in the root canal. Therefore, every time root canal filling material must be removed from the root canal the potential exists for reinfection of the apical wound. Consequently, all work in the root canal for post retention should be done under rubber dam isolation [19]. As most coronal restorations leak, the importance, for long-term prognosis, of a reliable root canal filling cannot be overemphasized [75]. There are several reports on the risks of coronal leakage when leaving teeth unprotected after the filling. There are examples of studies *in vitro*, using bacteria and artificial saliva as challenge, where bacterial acidic products have penetrated root canals in less than a month [117]. Although impressive, this effect is most likely not the result of initial inherent voids in the filling but rather the effect of the acids produced by the bacteria used. Even rather weak acids are effective in dissolving zinc oxide (ZnO), a

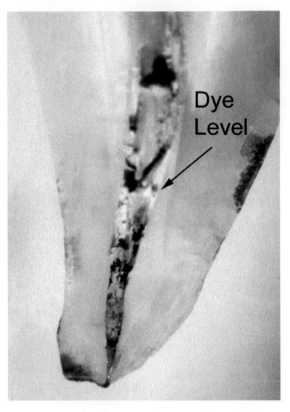

Fig. 11.20 Tooth obturated with gutta-percha and AH26 using lateral condensation. Using a proven dye penetration challenge test [18] penetration of dye could be traced 6 mm into the root canal where the first level of reliable seal appeared.

major component in both gutta-percha and most sealers. It is unknown if sufficient bacterial concentration and substrate will be available in most clinical situations to allow for such acidic penetration. Clinically, poorly sealed access cavities may, however, allow for the build-up of plaque bacteria capable of initiating dissolution of ZnO. Another factor during clinical function of teeth is the deformation of the tooth structure, including the roots, from masticatory forces. Gutta-percha is initially flexible but becomes brittle with time. Most sealers sets hard and brittle and do not bond well to dentin or gutta-percha [120]. In combination these factors will assure that in the long term defects will develop in the coronal–apical filling [59].

11.8.3 Methods

There are, in principle, two basic methods to fill root canals. The root canal may be filled with a solid material that is formed into a tapered rod and fitted to the root canal. This rod is then cemented into the pulp space with a sealer/cement. The other method uses either a soft paste-like material that will set to the form of the root canal or a plasticized material that will harden after placement.

An example of the first method is the use of a solid core made out of gutta-percha that is cemented into the root canal with a sealer/cement. This may be performed as a single cone technique where an attempt is made to prepare the root canal to the same size as the core point or with lateral compaction of more gutta-percha into the canal space to completely fill the root canal space.

Examples of the second method are the use of endodontic sealers like AH26 and Ketac-Endo. These materials, normally used as a sealer in the solid core technique, may also be used as the sole filling material as they are capable of permanently filling the root canal space. Gutta-percha may also be plasticized with a solvent or through heating to better fit the pulp space. Both methods result in a slight shrinkage of approximately 2% when the gutta-percha has solidified [62,123].

The search for simplification and increased proficiency in combination with more efficient methods to shape the pulp space has led to the development of many new hybrid root canal filling techniques and materials. Most hybrid methods practiced today are based on gutta-percha. With the advent of new man-made polymer materials, however, the hybrid methods are also being adapted to these new materials. The differences focus on alternative methods to introduce the core material into the root canal system with maintained control. The methods presently in use are either techniques of injecting heat plasticized core materials or use of core materials attached to a more rigid skeleton for better handling. Most hybrid filling methods require modification in the outline of the root canal preparation. Therefore, before attempting hybrid filling methods it is important to consider and implement technique variations required for optimal results.

Plasticized gutta-percha may either be in the form of rods that are packed into the root canal and subsequently heated inside the root canal, or gutta-percha that is heated in special devices and subsequently injected into the root canal system. Ultrafil/Successfil (Hygenic) is a system where the modified heated (70°C) gutta-percha is injected, under pressure, into the prepared root canal, sometimes with the additional application of a core point. Similar systems, Obtura (Obtura Spartan) and Calamus Flow Obturation Delivery System (Tulsa Dental), dispense a heavier form of gutta-percha heated to a higher temperature (150°C). The Ultrafil system is intended as an obturation system while Obtura and Calamus are primarily delivery systems for gutta-percha. Plasticized gutta-percha is often used with the warm vertical condensation techniques.

There are now also systems marketed where the gutta-percha is loaded on a mechanical compactor that heats the gutta-percha through frictional heat (Quick-Fil, JS Dental, Microseal, Analytic Technologies, EZ-Fill, EndoSolutions).

Thermafil (Tulsa Dental), Densfil (Caulk), and Soft-Core (Septodont) are devices that combine the features of filling with a master cone and the use of heat plasticized gutta-percha. In this system the gutta-percha is attached to a metal or plastic carrier device. After heating in a special oven, the prefitted device is inserted into the root canal to the working length. A different carrier system, SimpliFill has been developed by LightSpeed Endodontics. Here a short gutta-percha cone is attached to the end of a smooth, file-like rod. After choosing the appropriate size the gutta-percha section can be placed in the apically prepared root canal. This requires a coronal backfill with plasticized gutta-percha.

11.8.4 Core material

Gutta-percha has for many years been the dominant root canal filling material. Pure silver has been used, but is rarely applied today. Core materials require the use of a sealer/cement as they, even under the best circumstances, are unable to seal against the root canal dentin as they lack adhesive properties.

Gutta-percha is the dried juice of the thebaine tree (*Isonandra percha*). It was first introduced to the Royal Asiatic Society of England in 1843 by Sir José D'Almeida. It has been used in dentistry since the late 1800s. It occurs naturally as 1,4-polyisoprene and is harder, more brittle and less elastic than natural rubber. A linear crystalline polymer like gutta-percha will melt at a set temperature, and a random but distinct change in structure will result. The crystalline phase appears in two forms, α-phase and β-phase. They differ only in the molecular repeat distance and single bond form. The α-form is the material that comes from the natural tree product. The processed form, called β-form, is the gutta-percha used for root canal fillings. When heated, gutta-percha undergoes phase transitions. Thus when the temperature increases there is a transition from β-phase to α-phase at around 47°C. This then changes to an amorphous phase at 57°C. When cooled very slowly (0.5°C/hr), it crystallizes to the α-phase. Normal cooling returns the gutta-percha to the β-phase. The β-form softens and melts at a temperature above 64°C. It can easily be dissolved in chloroform and halothane.

Recently, polymer materials (Resilon/Epiphany and Resilon, Resilon Research LLC, Madison, CT; Epiphany, Pentron Clinical Technologies) and polymer coated gutta-percha cones (EndoREZ, Ultradent, Salt Lake City, UT) have become popular for bonded root canal fillings. These core materials are bonded to the root canal dentin walls with a resin sealer. Similarly glass ionomer coated gutta-percha (ActiV GP, Brasseler, Savanna, GA) is available for cementation with glass ionomer cements. All these techniques claim the formation of "monobloc" root canal fillings where the core is firmly bonded to the root canal dentin walls. Resilon is a thermoplastic biodegradable polyester (polycaprolactone) resin composite with bioactive glass and radiopaque fillers designed for root canal filling. Epiphany is a dual-cure resin cement sealer used for the bonding of Resilon to the root canal walls. It has been suggested that it provides a better root canal seal than available gutta-percha sealer fillings [91]. It has also been proposed that a root canal filling with Resilon/Epiphany will strengthen the root after root canal filling [116]. There are still concerns about the quality of the seal with the Resilon/Epiphany system as it appears equivalent to gutta-percha fillings when using resin sealer [112]. Complete bonding in a root canal is exceedingly difficult due to the lack of stress relief during polymerization. This will result in areas of debonding in the root canal during polymerization [113]. Polylactone is biodegradable and the issue has been raised that in addition to enzyme hydrolysis, microorganisms may degrade the Resilon [114,115]. Resilon may be a promising material, but much more laboratory and clinical research must still be done before it can routinely replace gutta-percha. Resilon can be used in heat delivery systems giving it wider use than EndoREZ and ActiV GP, which in principle can only be used for single-cone filling techniques. There is no convincing research showing that root canal fillings with EndoREZ and ActiV GP materials can result in a bonded monobloc.

Gutta-percha and its replacing polymers are normally applied in root canals with some form of condensation pressure. It has been shown, however, that compression of these materials is practically impossible. Thus, cold pressure on these materials during root canal filling procedures cannot be expected to compress the material. It will instead, if done correctly, laterally dislodge the points to fill as much as possible of available space within the root canal. Modern gutta-percha cones for root canal fillings contain only about 20% gutta-percha. The major component is ZnO that constitutes 60–70% of endodontic gutta-percha. The ZnO provides a major part of the radiopacity of endodontic gutta-percha. The remaining 10% is not normally specified as it is proprietary information but consists of a mixture of resins, waxes, and metal sulfates.

Silver cones for root canal filling are rarely used. Most endodontic silver cones contain small amounts of other trace metals (0.1–0.2%) such as copper and nickel. This adds to the corrosive characteristic of silver cones that is a very common complication in old clinical cases. Other reasons for the corrosion of silver *in situ* are the presence of metal restorations and posts that may be used in the area and are therefore contributing to the galvanic corrosion taking place (Fig. 11.21). The silver corrosion products are highly toxic and may in themselves cause severe tissue injury [89]. Stainless-steel files are far less corrodible and therefore a better alternative material in cases where a metal core is deemed necessary.

Like instruments, gutta-percha cones are regulated in many national and international standards. In

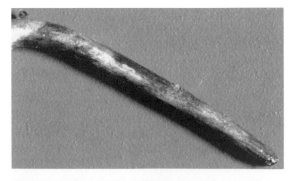

Fig. 11.21 Silver cone root filling removed from maxillary molar. The silver is covered by large areas of corrosion (dark areas).

addition to standards for core material there is also a standard for gutta-percha accessory cones. The sizing of core material is similar to the files but there is one very important difference. The size tolerance for files is ±0.02 mm, but ±0.05 mm for the silver and gutta-percha cones. Thus, there is not an exact match between file sizes and the dimensions of the filling material. The sizes for accessory cones are not related to file sizes. They are also more tapered than the core material. Accessory cones come in sizes such as "fine", "fine-medium", and "medium".

11.8.5 Endodontic sealers

There are a variety of sealers from which to choose. Many are simply zinc oxide/eugenol cements which have been modified for endodontic use. The liquid for these materials is eugenol. The powder contains ZnO that is finely sifted to enhance the flow of the cement. Setting time is adjusted to allow for adequate working time. These cements easily lend themselves to the addition of chemicals, and paraformaldehyde has often been added for antimicrobial and mummifying effects, germicides for antiseptic action, rosin or Canada balsam for greater dentin adhesion, and corticosteroids for suppression of inflammation. Zinc oxide is a valuable component in the sealer. It is effective as an antimicrobial agent and has been shown to provide cytoprotection to tissue cells. The incorporation of rosins in sealers may initially have been for the adhesive properties. Rosins (colophony), which are derived from a variety of conifers, are composed of approximatively 90% resin acids. The remaining parts are volatile and nonvolatile compounds such as terpene alcohol, aldehydes, and hydrocarbons. Resin acids are monobasic carboxylic acids with the basic molecular formula $C_{20}H_{30}O_2$. Resin acids are amphiphilic with the carbon group being lipophilic affecting the lipids in the cell membranes. This way the resin acids have a strong antimicrobial effect, which on mammalian cells is expressed as cytotoxicity. The resin acids work similarly to quaternary ammonium compounds by increasing the cell membrane permeability of the affected cell. Although toxic, the combination of ZnO and resin acids may be beneficial overall. The antimicrobial effect of ZnO in both gutta-percha cones as well as in many sealers will bring a low level of long-lasting antimicrobial effect. The resin acids are both antimicrobial and cytotoxic, but the combination with ZnO exerts a significant level of cytoprotection. Resin acids may under certain conditions react with zinc,

forming resonates; this matrix-stabilized zinc resinate is only slightly soluble in water [61,98].

The setting of zinc oxide/eugenol cements is a chemical process combined with physical embedding of ZnO in a matrix of zinc eugenolate. Particle size of ZnO, pH, and the presence of water regulate the setting, as well as other additives that might be included in special formulations. The formation of eugenolate constitutes the hardening of the cement. Free eugenol will always remain in the mass and act as an irritant. Some common zinc oxide/eugenol sealers are Rickert's sealer (Kerr), Proco-Sol (Star Dental), Grossman's sealer (Sultan Chemists), Wach's sealer (Sultan Chemists), Tubli-Seal (Kerr). Zinc oxide/eugenol sealers will lose some volume with time due to dissolution in tissues with the release of eugenol and ZnO. It can be expected that the addition of resin acids to the zinc oxide/eugenol cement significantly reduces this dissolution [61].

For a long time it has been common to mix formaldehyde into endodontic sealers. The most common combinations have been zinc oxide/eugenol sealers mixed with formaldehyde [Endométhasone (Septodont), and N2 (Agsa)]. This is an undesirable additive to any sealer as it will only add to the already toxic effect of eugenol and prevent or delay healing. The reason why it has been popular to use endodontic materials containing formaldehyde is because formaldehyde necrotizes the nerve endings in the tissue area thereby masking inflammatory processes that may cause pain. Thus, despite the necrotic effect of formaldehyde, patients have few symptoms.

Chloropercha (Moyco) is another type of sealer that has been in use for many years. It is made by mixing gutta-percha with chloroform. This will allow a gutta-percha root canal filling to fit better in the canal. It is important to recognize, however, that chloropercha has no adhesive properties. Another commercial form of chloropercha, called Kloroperka N-Ø (N-Ø Therapeutics), contains resins and Canada balsam thereby providing better adhesive properties. The general problem with most chloropercha products is their shrinkage during the evaporation/disappearance of the chloroform. Some brands, like the Kloroperka N-Ø, contain filler particles such as ZnO to reduce the shrinkage. ZnO also increases radiopacity. Another technique is to use a mixture of 5–8% of rosins in chloroform [1,13]. A rosin–chloroform wash of the root canal leaves a very adhesive residue. This residue in combination with dipping of the gutta-percha cone in resin chloroform provides the sealer

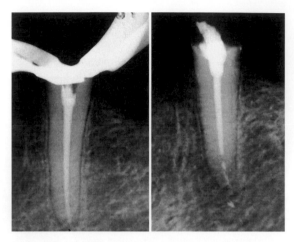

Fig. 11.22 Mandibular premolar root filled with gutta-percha and rosin chloroform: radiograph taken immediately after completion of filling shows good result (left); radiograph taken 2 weeks later shows how excess chloroform has evaporated leaving large voids in the pulp space (right). Softened gutta-percha has flowed into the periradicular tissues.

in this technique. Chloroform techniques for filling require that the operator has good basic skills with various filling techniques as it is very sensitive to manipulation (Fig. 11.22). When correctly used the shrinkage is not greater than when gutta-percha is plasticized by heat [123].

The use of chloroform has been sharply curtailed in recent years due to its toxicity. In endodontics, however, the amounts used are normally insignificant and cause no health hazard. One must, however, take prudent steps to reduce the vaporization during use as chloroform is highly volatile. Thus, when used for softening of gutta-percha during revision of old root canal fillings, the chloroform should be dispensed through a syringe and hypodermic needle. For other uses the exposure time, amounts used, and chloroform surface exposed should all be minimized. There are some chloroform substitutes in use such as halothane and turpentine. Halothane is less effective in softening gutta-percha than chloroform, is hepatotoxic like chloroform and has a higher local toxicity than chloroform. Therefore, halothane is not a good substitute. Turpentine is not carcinogenic but may easily cause allergies; it has high local toxicity and dissolves gutta-percha poorly. Therefore, there are no good substitutes for the use of chloroform in endodontic treatment procedures. With careful workplace proto-

col and hygiene there is little risk associated with the use of chloroform in endodontics [4].

Several Ca(OH)$_2$-based sealers have been marketed. Examples of such sealers are Sealapex (Kerr), CRCS (Hygenic), and Apexit (Vivadent). These sealers are promoted as having therapeutic effect due to the Ca(OH)$_2$ content. No such convincing results from scientific trials have been shown. Calcium hydroxide must be dissociated into Ca^{2+} and OH$^-$ to be therapeutically effective. Therefore, to be therapeutic, an endodontic sealer based on Ca(OH)$_2$ must dissolve and consequently lose volume [111]. Thus, one major concern is that the Ca(OH)$_2$ content may dissolve and leave voids. These sealers also have poor cohesive strength [120]. There is no objective proof that a Ca(OH)$_2$ sealer provides any advantage for root canal filling.

Several sealers are polymers. The more common brands are Endofill (Lee Pharmaceuticals), AH26 and AH Plus (DeTrey), Diaket (ESPE), Epiphany, and EndoREZ. The AH products are epoxy resins initially developed to serve as a sole filler material [106]. Due to its good handling characteristics it has been extensively used as a sealer. It has a good flow, seals well to dentin walls, and has sufficient working time [55]. Ketac-Endo (ESPE), glass ionomer cement, has also been produced for endodontic procedures; it may also be used as the sole filling material. Glass ionomer cement is also used with the ActiV GP system recently marketed. AH26 appears to have good sealing qualities whereas there are questions about the quality of the seal with Ketac-Endo due to dentin–sealer adhesive failures [22,99]. Because of the difficulty in retreating such an epoxy or glass ionomer filling it would always be prudent to use a gutta-perch master cone even if lateral condensation is not practiced [65].

11.9 Tissue responses

Remaining vital pulp tissue or the periapical tissues will respond to pulp canal manipulations in a variety of ways. Pulpectomy or the removal of necrotic pulp tissue is a surgical procedure that under the best circumstances will result in transient surgical tissue inflammation. Clinical experimentation has suggested that surgical skills, instrument choice, wound level, choice of wound dressing and asepsis play very important roles in the sequel to this initial surgical inflammation. It is important for optimal healing that

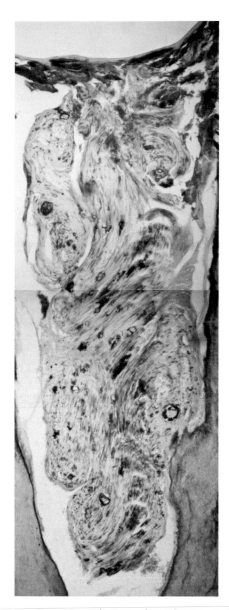

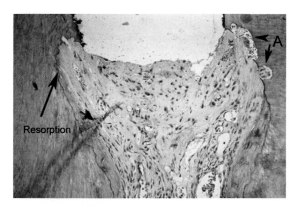

Fig. 11.24 Tissue in the apical 2–3 mm of a root canal subsequent to pulpectomy. The lateral walls of the root canal have undergone resorption on a broad front (arrow) and in localized areas (A); no inflammatory cell infiltrate can be seen.

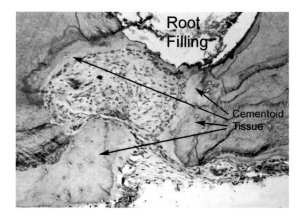

Fig. 11.25 Tissue in apical 2–3 mm of root canal after pulpectomy and root canal filling. After the initial dentin and cementum resorption following pulpectomy (Fig. 11.24), the tissue has undergone repair. Apposition of cementum-like tissue can be seen around the entire pulp space (arrows).

Fig. 11.23 Remaining pulp tissue after pulpectomy with a root canal reamer. The pulp tissue was twisted all the way to the apical foramen. (Courtesy of Dr H. Nyborg.)

all these various tissue manipulations are adjusted to promote healing.

The major issues to consider are tissue injuries as a result of the surgical procedure and chemical injuries as a result of the use of antimicrobial agents as well as root canal filling materials.

11.9.1 Instrumentation

The effect of instrument choice on the remaining apical tissues has been studied for a century [6,20]. It is difficult, however, to study the long-term effect of these manipulations as wound dressings, asepsis, antisepsis, and coronal seal will play an important role in the post-surgical healing. It has been well documented that there is no best instrument with which to sever the apical pulp tissue when partial pulp removal is intended [70,71,88,92]. Thus, the development of an accurate pulp knife is still awaited (Fig. 11.23).

The initial inflammation is normally followed by a resorption and apposition process in the apical hard tissues. The intensity and direction of this rebuilding of the apical area of the root canal depends on the access microorganisms may have. If the wound is placed within the root canal, in a vital pulp, studies of treatment outcome suggest that the highest level of success is reached if the pulp wound is placed 1–2 mm from the radiographic apex [27,49]. Most histological studies tend to support these findings [28,49] while there are studies in humans suggesting that the pulp remnant may be left longer without impaired healing [71].

The apical part of the pulp and surrounding periodontal tissues have a great ability to resist non-infectious tissue damage. This normally takes place through a process where initially the apical root dentin and cement is resorbed (Fig. 11.24) providing access to the narrowly enclosed apical pulp that is usually severely damaged during pulpectomy [70]. The pulp that may survive will form an osteodentin wall that will close off the vital pulp tissue from the root canal filling implant. In most instances the damaged pulp tissue is revascularized and a fibrous connective tissue replaces the pulp. If the pulp were initially necrotic, it would be replaced by periodontal connective tissue. When the apical resorption is arrested, cementum will form and replace the lost dentin and further close off the pulp space (Fig. 11.25) [28,71]. Studies suggest that over-instrumentation will heal with apical repair provided the root canal is obturated properly after the pulpectomy [6,39]. If root canals are left empty after pulpectomy, chronic inflammation will dominate with no subsequent repair [30,92]. It has been suggested that apical repair after pulpectomy may be improved if the pulp is completely removed and the root canal filling placed several millimeters short of the instrumentation leaving an apical blood clot in the root canal [72]. It appears that healing of the apical wound after instrumentation has a high degree of regenerative strength provided bacteria are not allowed to settle in the wound area.

11.10 References

1. Andersson K, Jonsson M, Sjögren U (1986) Metoder och material vid endodontibehandling. *Tandläkartidningen* **78**, 940–4.
2. Andreasen JO, Farik B, Munksgaard EC (2002) Long-term calcium hydroxide as a root canal dressing may increase risk of root fracture. *Dental Traumatology* **18**, 134–7.
3. Ates M, Akdeniz BG, Sen BH (2005) The effect of calcium chelating or binding agents on *Candida albicans*. *Oral Surgery, Oral Medicine, Oral Pathology, Oral Radiology, Endodontics* **100**, 626–30.
4. Barbosa SV, Spångberg LSW, Almeida D (1994) Low surface tension calcium hydroxide solution is an effective antiseptic. *International Endodontic Journal* **27**, 6–10.
5. Barbosa SV, Burkard DH, Spångberg LSW (1994) Cytotoxic effects of gutta-percha solvents. *Journal of Endodontics* **20**, 6–8.
6. Benatti O, Valdrighi L, Biral RR, Pupo J (1995) A histological study of the effect of diameter enlargement of the apical portion of the root canal. *Journal of Endodontics* **11**, 428–34.
7. Bengmark S, Rydberg B (1968) Cytotoxic action of cationic detergents on tissue growth in vitro. *Acta Chirurgica Scandinavica* **134**, 1–5.
8. Bergenholtz G (1974) Micro-organisms from necrotic pulp of traumatized teeth. *Odontologisk Revy* **25**, 347–58.
9. Byström A, Sundqvist G (1981) Bacteriological evaluation of the efficacy of mechanical root canal instrumentation in endodontic therapy. *Scandinavian Journal of Dental Research* **89**, 321–8.
10. Byström A, Sundqvist G (1983) Bacteriological evaluation of the effect of 0.5 percent sodium hypochlorite in endodontic therapy. *Oral Surgery, Oral Medicine, Oral Pathology* **55**, 307–12.
11. Byström A, Claesson R, Sundqvist G (1985) The antibacterial effect of camphorated paramonochlorphenol, camphorated phenol and calcium hydroxide in the treatment of infected root canals. *Endodontics and Dental Traumatology* **1**, 170–5.
12. Byström A, Sundqvist G (1985) The antibacterial action of sodium hypochlorite and EDTA in 60 cases of endodontic therapy. *International Endodontic Journal* **18**, 35–40.
13. Callahan JR (1914) Rosin solution for the sealing of the dentinal tubuli and as an adjuvant in the filling of root canals. *Journal of Allied Dental Society* **9**, 53–7.
14. Cvek M, Nord CE, Hollender L (1976) Antimicrobial effect of root canal debridement in teeth with immature root. A clinical and microbiologic study. *Odontologisk Revy* **27**, 1–10.
15. Cvek M (1978) A clinical report on partial pulpotomy and capping with calcium hydroxide in permanent incisors with complicated crown fracture. *Journal of Endodontics* **4**, 232–41.
16. Dakin HD (1915) The antiseptic action of hypochlorites: The ancient history of the 'new antiseptic'. *British Medical Journal* **2**, 809–10.
17. Dakin HD (1915) On the use of certain antiseptic substances in treatment of infected wounds. *British Medical Journal* **2**, 318–20.
18. Dalat DM, Spångberg LSW (1994) Comparison of apical leakage in root canals obturated with various gutta-percha techniques using a dye vacuum tracing method. *Journal of Endodontics* **20**, 315–19.

19. Dalat DM, Spångberg LSW (1994) Effect of post preparation on the apical seal of teeth obturated with plastic Thermafil obturators. *Oral Surgery, Oral Medicine, Oral Pathology* **76**, 760–5.

20. Davis WC (1922) Partial pulpectomy. *Dental Items of Interest* **44**, 801–9.

21. Davis MS, Joseph SW, Bucher JF (1971) Periapical and intracanal healing following incomplete root canal fillings in dogs. *Oral Surgery, Oral Medicine, Oral Pathology* **31**, 662–75.

22. DeGee AJ, Wu MK, Wesselink PR (1994) Sealing properties of Ketac-Endo glass ionomer cement and AH26 root canal sealer. *International Endodontic Journal* **27**, 239–44.

23. Doyon GE, Dumsha T, von Fraunhofer JA (2005) Fracture resistance of human root dentin exposed to intracanal calcium hydroxide. *Journal of Endodontics* **31**, 895–7.

24. Engelhardt JP, Grün L, Dahl HJ (1984) Factors affecting sterilization in glass bead sterilizers. *Journal of Endodontics* **10**, 465–70.

25. Engström B (1958) Om den antibacteriella effectens varaktighet hos några antiseptika använda som rotkanalsinlägg. *Svensk Tandläkaretidskrift* **51**, 1–6.

26. Engström B, Lundberg M (1966) The frequency and causes of reversal from negative to positive bacteriological tests in root canal therapy. *Odontologisk Tidskrift* **74**, 189–95.

27. Engström B, Lundberg M (1965) The correlation between positive culture and the prognosis of root canal therapy after pulpectomy. *Odontologisk Revy* **16**, 194–203.

28. Engström B, Spångberg L (1967) Wound healing after partial pulpectomy. A histological study performed on contralateral tooth pairs. *Odontologisk Tidskrift* **75**, 5–18.

29. Engström B, Spångberg L (1967) Studies on root canal medicaments. I. Cytotoxic effect of root canal antiseptics. *Acta Odontologica Scandinavica* **25**, 77–81.

30. Engström B, Spångberg L (1969) Toxic and antimicrobial effects of antiseptics *in vitro*. *Svensk Tandläkaretidskrift* **62**, 543–9.

31. Girard S, Paqué F, Badertscher M, Sener B, Zehnder M (2005) Assessment of a gel-type chelating preparation containing 1-hydroxyethylidene-1,1-bisphosphonate *International Endodontic Journal* **38**, 810–16.

32. Goldman M, Laosonthorn P, White RR (1992) Microleakage – full crowns and the dental pulp. *Journal of Endodontics* **18**, 473–5.

33. Gordon MP, Chandler NP (2004) Electronic apex locators. *International Endodontic Journal* **37**, 425–37.

34. Grawehr M, Sener B, Waltimo T, Zehnder M. (2003) Interactions of ethylenediamine tetraacetic acid with sodium hypochlorite in aqueous solutions. *International Endodontic Journal* **36**, 411–17.

35. Grigoratos D, Knowles J, Ng YL, Gulabivala K (2001) Effect of exposing dentine to sodium hypochlorite and calcium hydroxide on its flexural strength and elastic modulus. *International Endodontic Journal* **34**, 113–19.

36. Heling B, Shapiro S, Sciaky I (1965) An in vitro comparison of the amount of calcium removed by the disodium salt of EDTA and hydrochloric acid during

37. Hermann BW (1920) Calciumhydroxyd als Mittel zum Behandel und Füllen von Zahnwurzelkanälen. Würzburg, Med. Dissertation.

38. Hermann BW (1930) Dentinobliteration der Wurzelkanäle nach Behandlung mit Calcium. *Zahnärtzliche Rundschau* **39**, 888–9.

39. Hørsted P, Nygaard-Östby B (1978) Tissue formation in the root canal after total pulpectomy and partial root filling. *Oral Surgery, Oral Medicine, Oral Pathology* **46**, 275–82.

40. Hørsted-Bindslev P, Bergenholtz G (1995) Endodontisk behandling af den vitale pulpa. *Journal of the Swedish Dental Association* **87**, 95–105.

41. Jacobsen I, Kerekes K (1977) Long-term prognosis of traumatized permanent anterior teeth showing calcifying processes in the pulp cavity. *Scandinavian Journal of Dental Research* **85**, 588–98.

42. Jiang J, Zuo J, Holliday LS (2003) Calcium hydroxide reduces lipopolysaccharide-stimulated osteoclast formation. *Oral Surgery, Oral Medicine, Oral Pathology, Oral Radiology, Endodontics* **95**, 156–62.

43. Kaufman B, Spångberg L, Barry J, Fouad AF (2005) *Enterococcus* Spp. in endodontically treated teeth with or without periradicular lesions. *Journal of Endodontics* **31**, 851–7.

44. Kazemi RB, Safavi KE, Spångberg LSW (1994) Assessment of marginal stability and permeability of an interim restorative endodontic material. *Oral Surgery, Oral Medicine, Oral Pathology* **78**, 788–96.

45. Kazemi RB, Spångberg LSW (1995) Effect of reduced air pressure on dye penetration in standardized voids. *Oral Surgery, Oral Medicine, Oral Pathology, Oral Radiology, Endodontics* **80**, 720–5.

46. Kazemi RB, Stenman E, Spångberg LSW (1995) The endodontic file is a disposable instrument. *Journal of Endodontics* **21**, 451–5.

47. Kazemi RB, Stenman E, Spångberg LSW (1996) Machining efficiency and wear resistance of nickel-titanium endodontic files. *Oral Surgery, Oral Medicine, Oral Pathology, Oral Radiology, Endodontics* **81**, 596–602.

48. Kerekes K, Tronstad L (1979) Long-term results of endodontic treatment performed with a standardized technique. *Journal of Endodontics* **5**, 83–90.

49. Ketterl W (1965) Kriterien für den Erfolg der Vitalexstirpation. *Deutsche Zahnärztliche Zeitschrift* **20**, 407–16.

50. Kobayashi C, Suda H (1994) New electronic canal measuring device based on the ratio method. *Journal of Endodontics* **20**, 111–14.

51. Kuhn G, Tavernier B, Jordan L (2001) Influence of structure on nickel-titanium endodontic instruments failure. *Journal of Endodontics* **27**, 516–20.

52. Kuhn G, Jordan L (2002) Fatigue and mechanical properties of nickel-titanium endodontic instruments. *Journal of Endodontics* **28**, 716–20.

53. Kum KY, Kazemi RB, Cha BY, Zhu Q (2006) Smear layer production of K3 and ProFile Ni-Ti rotary instruments in curved root canals: A comparative SEM study. *Oral Surgery, Oral Medicine, Oral Pathology, Oral Radiology, Endodontics* **101**, 536–41.

54. Kydd WL, Nicholls JI, Harrington G, Freeman M (1996) Marginal leakage of cast gold crowns luted with zinc phosphate cement: An in vivo study. *Journal of Prosthetic Dentistry* **75**, 9–13.

55. Limkangwalmongkol S, Burtscher P, Abbott PV, Sandler AB, Bishop BM (1991) A comparative study of the apical leakage of four root canal sealers and laterally condensed gutta-percha. *Journal of Endodontics* **17**, 495–9.

56. Lunam CA, Hall PM, Cousins MJ (1989) The pathology of halothane hepatotoxicity in a guinea-pig model: a comparison with human halothane hepatitis. *British Journal of Experimental Pathology* **70**, 533–41.

57. Lundberg M, Cvek M (1980) A light microscopic study of pulps from traumatized permanent incisors with reduced pulpal lumen. *Acta Odontologica Scandinavica* **38**, 89–94.

58. Machnick TK, Torabinejad M, Munoz CA, Shabahang S (2003) Effect of MTAD on flexural strength and modulus of elasticity of dentin. *Journal of Endodontics*. **29**, 747–50.

59. Madison S, Wilcox LR (1988) An evaluation of coronal microleakage in endodontically treated teeth. Part III. In vivo study. *Journal of Endodontics* **14**, 455–8.

60. Malledant Y, Sirpoudhis L, Tanguy M (1990) Effects of halothane on human and rat hepatocyte cultures. *Anesthesiology* **72**, 526–34.

61. Matsuya Y, Matsuya S (1994) Effect of abietic acid and poly(methyl methacrylate) on the dissolution process of zinc oxide-eugenol cement. *Biomaterials* **15**, 307–14.

62. McElroy DL (1955) Physical properties of root canal filling materials. *Journal of the American Dental Association* **50**, 433–40.

63. Mejàre B, Nyborg H, Palmkvist E (1970) Amputation instruments for partial pulp extirpation. III. A comparison between the efficiency of the Hedström file with cut tip and an experimental instrument. *Odontologisk Revy* **21**, 63–9.

64. Molander A, Dahlen G (2003) Evaluation of the antimicrobial potential of tetracycline and erythromycin mixed with calcium hydroxide as intracanal dressing against *Enterococcus faecalis* in vivo. *Oral Surgery, Oral Medicine, Oral Pathology, Oral Radiology, Endodontics* **96**, 744–50.

65. Moshonov J, Trope M, Friedman S (1994) Retreatment efficacy 3 months after obturation using glass ionomer cement, zinc oxide-eugenol, and epoxy resin sealers. *Journal of Endodontics* **20**, 90–2.

66. Möller ÅJR (1966) Microbiological examination of root canals and periapical tissues of human teeth. (Thesis) *Odontologisk Tidskrift* **74**, 1–380.

67. Nair PNR (2004) Pathogenesis of apical periodontitis and the causes of endodontic failures. *Critical Reviews in Oral Biology and Medicine* **15**, 348–81.

68. Nyborg H (1955) Healing processes in the pulp on capping. *Acta Odontologica Scandinavica* **13**, (Suppl 16) 1–130.

69. Nyborg H (1960) Försök med amputationsinstrument för partiell pulpaexstirpation. *Odontologisk Revy* **11**, 247–54.

70. Nyborg H, Halling A (1963) Amputation instruments for partial pulp extirpation. II. A comparison between the efficiency of the Antheos root canal reamer and the Hedström file with cut tip. *Odontologisk Tidskrift* **71**, 277–83.

71. Nyborg H, Tullin B (1965) Healing processes after vital extirpation. An experimental study of 17 teeth. *Odontologisk Tidskrift* **73**, 430–46.

72. Nygaard-Östby B, Hjortdal O (1971) Tissue formation in the root canal following pulp removal. *Scandinavian Journal of Dental Research* **79**, 333–49.

73. Öhman A (1965) Healing and sensitivity to pain in young replanted human teeth. *Odontologisk Tidskrift* **73**, 168–227.

74. Okşan T, Aktener BO, Şen BH, Tezel H (1993) The penetration of root canal sealers into dentinal tubules. A scanning electron microscopic study. *International Endodontic Journal* **26**, 301–5.

75. Orahood JP, Cochran MA, Swartz M, Newton CW (1986) In vitro study of marginal leakage between temporary sealing materials and recently placed restorative materials. *Journal of Endodontics* **12**, 523–7.

76. Portenier I, Haapasalo H, Rye A, Waltimo T, Ørstavik D, Haapasalo M (2001) Inactivation of root canal medicaments by dentine, hydroxylapatite and bovine serum albumin. *International Endodontic Journal* **34**, 184–8.

77. Rudzki E, Berova N, Czernielewski A (1991) Contact allergy to oil of turpentine: a 10-year retrospective view. *Contact Dermatitis* **24**, 317–18.

78. Rutberg M, Spångberg E, Spångberg L (1977) Evaluation of enhanced vascular permeability of endodontic medicaments in vivo. *Journal of Endodontics* **3**, 347–51.

79. Rydberg G, Zederfeldt B (1968) Influence of cationic detergents on tensile strength of healing skin wounds in the rat. *Acta Chirurgica Scandinavica* **134**, 317–20.

80. Safavi KE, Dowden WE, Introcaso JH, Langeland K (1985) A comparison of antimicrobial effects of calcium hydroxide and iodine potassium iodide. *Journal of Endodontics* **11**, 454–6.

81. Safavi KE, Spångberg LSW, Langeland K (1990) Root canal dentinal tubule disinfection. *Journal of Endodontics* **16**, 207–10.

82. Safavi KE, Nichols FC (1993) Effect of calcium hydroxide on bacterial lipopolysaccharide. *Journal of Endodontics* **19**, 76–8.

83. Safavi KE, Nichols FC (1994) Alteration of biological properties of bacterial lipopolysaccharide by calcium hydroxide treatment. *Journal of Endodontics* **20**, 127–9.

84. Safavi, K, Perry E (1995) The influence of mixing vehicle on antimicrobial effects of calcium hydroxide. *Journal of Endodontics* **21** (Abstract RS64), 231.

85. Safavi K, Nakayama TA (2000) Influence of mixing vehicle on dissociation of calcium hydroxide in solution. *Journal of Endodontics* **26**, 649–51.

86. Schäfer E, Zandbiglari T (2002) A comparison of the effectiveness of chloroform and eucalyptus oil in dissolving root canal sealers. *Oral Surgery, Oral Medicine, Oral Pathology, Oral Radiology, Endodontics* **93**, 611–16.

87. Schröder U (1973) Reaction of human dental pulp to experimental pulpotomy and capping with calcium hydroxide. *Odontologisk Revy* **24**, Suppl 25.

88. Seltzer S, Soltanoff W, Sinai I, Goldenberg A, Bender IB (1968) Biologic aspects of endodontics. Part III. Periapical tissue reactions to root canal instrumentation. *Oral Surgery, Oral Medicine, Oral Pathology* **26**, 534–46.

89. Seltzer S, Green DB, Weiner N, DeRenzis F (1972) A scanning electron microscope examination of silver cones removed from endodontically treated teeth. *Oral Surgery, Oral Medicine, Oral Pathology* **33**, 589–605.

90. Şen BH, Pişkin B, Baran N (1996) The effect of tubular penetration of root canal sealers on dye microleakage. *International Endodontic Journal* **29**, 23–8.

91. Shipper G, Ørstavik D, Teixeira FB, Trope M (2004) An evaluation of microbial leakage in roots filled with a thermoplastic synthetic polymer-based root canal filling material (Resilon). *Journal of Endodontics* **30**, 342–7.

92. Sinai I, Seltzer S, Soltanoff W, Goldenberg A, Bender IB (1967) Biologic aspects of endodontics. Part II. Periapical tissue reaction to pulp extirpation. *Oral Surgery, Oral Medicine, Oral Pathology* **23**, 664–79.

93. Siqueira JF, Rôças IN, Lopes HP, Magalhães FAC, Uzeda M (2003) Elimination of *Candida albicans* infection of the radicular dentin by intracanal medications. *Journal of Endodontics* **29**, 501–4.

94. Sirén EK, Haapasalo MPP, Waltimo TMT, Ørstavik D (2004) In vitro antibacterial effect of calcium hydroxide combined with chlorhexidine or iodine potassium iodide on *Enterococcus faecalis*. *European Journal of Oral Sciences* **112**, 326–31

95. Sjögren U, Hägglund B, Sundqvist G, Wing K (1990) Factors affecting the long term results of endodontic treatment. *Journal of Endodontics* **16**, 498–504.

96. Sjögren U, Figdor D, Spångberg L, Sundqvist G (1991) The antimicrobial effect of calcium hydroxide as a short term intracanal dressing. *International Endodontic Journal* **24**, 119–25.

97. Sjögren U (1996) Success and failure in endodontics. Odontological Dissertation No. 60. Umeå: Umeå University.

98. Soltes EDJ, Zinkel DF (1989) Chemistry of rosin. In Zinkel DF and Russell J, editors. *Naval stores; production, chemistry, utilization*, pp. 262–331. New York: Pulp Chemical Association.

99. Smith MA, Steinman HR (1994) An in vitro evaluation of microleakage of two new and two old root canal sealers. *Journal of Endodontics* **20**, 18–21.

100. Spanó JCE, Barbin EL, Santos TC, Guimarães LF, Pécora JD (2001) Solvent action of sodium hypochlorite on bovine pulp and physico-chemical properties of resulting liquid. *Brazilian Dental Journal* **12**, 154–7.

101. Spångberg L, Engström B (1967) Studies on root canal medicaments. II. Cytotoxic effect of medicaments used in root filling. *Acta Odontologica Scandinavica* **25**, 183–6.

102. Spångberg L, Engström B, Langeland K (1973) Biological effect of dental materials. 3. Toxic and antimicrobial effects of endodontic antiseptics *in vitro*. *Oral Surgery, Oral Medicine, Oral Pathology* **36**, 856–71.

103. Spångberg L, Rutberg M, Rydinge E (1979) Biological effects of endodontic antimicrobial agents. *Journal of Endodontics* **5**, 166–75.

104. Spångberg L, Hellden L, Roberson PB, Levy BM (1982) Pulpal effects of electrosurgery involving based and unbased cervical restorations. *Oral Surgery, Oral Medicine, Oral Pathology* **54**, 678–85.

105. Spångberg LSW, Acierno TG, Cha BY (1989) Influence of entrapped air on the accuracy of leakage studies using dye penetration methods. *Journal of Endodontics* **15**, 548–51.

106. Spångberg LSW, Barbosa SV, Lavigne GD (1993) AH26 releases formaldehyde. *Journal of Endodontics* **19**, 596–8.

107. Stenman E (1977) Effects of sterilization and endodontic medicaments on mechanical properties of root canal instruments. Odontological Dissertation No. 8. Umeå: Umeå University.

108. Stenman E, Spångberg LSW (1993) Root canal instruments are poorly standardized. *Journal of Endodontics* **19**, 327–34.

109. Stewart G, Kapsimalis P, Rappaport H (1969) EDTA and urea peroxide for root canal preparation. *Journal of the American Dental Association* **78**, 335–40.

110. Sundqvist G (1976) Bacteriological studies of necrotic dental pulps. Odontological Dissertation No. 7. Umeå: Umeå University.

111. Tagger M, Tagger E, Kfir A (1988) Release of calcium and hydroxyl ions from set endodontic sealers containing calcium hydroxide. *Journal of Endodontics* **14**, 588–91.

112. Tay FR, Loushine RJ, Weller RN, Kimbrough WF, Pashley DH, Mak YF, *et al.* (2005) Ultrastructural evaluation of the apical seal in roots filled with a polycaprolactone-based root canal filling material. *Journal of Endodontics* **31**, 514–19.

113. Tay FR, Loushine RJ, Lambrechts P, Weller RN, Pashley DH (2005) Geometric factors affecting dentin bonding in root canals: a theoretical modeling approach. *Journal of Endodontics* **31**, 584–9.

114. Tay FR, Pashley DH, Williams MC, Raina R, Loushine RJ, Weller RN, *et al.* (2005) Susceptibility of a polycaprolactone-based root canal filling material to degradation. I. Alkaline hydrolysis. *Journal of Endodontics* **31**, 593–8.

115. Tay FR, Pashley DH, Yiu CKY, Yau JYY, Yiu-fai M, Loushine RJ, *et al.* (2005) Susceptibility of a polycaprolactone-based root canal filling material to degradation. II Gravimetric evaluation of enzymatic hydrolysis. *Journal of Endodontics* **31**, 737–41.

116. Teixeira FB, Teixeira ECN, Thompson JY, Trope M (2004) Fracture resistance of roots endodontically treated with a new resin filling material. *Journal of the American Dental Association* **135**, 646–52.

117. Torabinejad M, Ung B, Kettering JD (1990) In vitro bacterial penetration of coronally unsealed endodontically treated teeth. *Journal of Endodontics* **16**, 566–9.

118. Torabinejad M, Cho Y, Khademi AA, Bakland LK, Shabahang S (2003) The effect of various concentrations of sodium hypochlorite on the ability of MTAD to remove the smear layer. *Journal of Endodontics* **29**, 233–9.

119. von der Fehr FR, Nygaard-Östby B (1963) Effect of EDTAC and sulfuric acid on root canal dentine. *Oral Surgery, Oral Medicine, Oral Pathology* **16**, 199–205.

120. Wennberg A, Ørstavik D (1990) Adhesion of root canal sealers to bovine dentine and gutta-percha. *International Endodontic Journal* **23**, 13–19.

121. White RR, Goldman M, Lin PS (1984) The influence of the smeared layer upon dentinal tubule penetration by plastic filling materials. *Journal of Endodontics* **10**, 558–62.

122. White RR, Goldman M, Lin PS (1987) The influence of the smeared layer upon dentinal tubule penetration by plastic filling materials. Part II. *Journal of Endodontics* **13**, 369–74.

123. Wong M, Peters DD, Lorton L, Bernier WE (1982) Comparison of gutta-percha filling techniques: three chloroform-gutta-percha filling techniques, part 2. *Journal of Endodontics* **8**, 4–9.

124. Wu MK, Wesselink PR (1993) Endodontic leakage studies reconsidered. Part 1. Methodology, application and relevance. *International Endodontic Journal* **26**, 37–43.

125. Zehnder M, Kosicki D, Luder H, Sener B, Waltimo T (2002) Tissue-dissolving capacity and antibacterial effect of buffered and unbuffered hypochlorite solutions. *Oral Surgery, Oral Medicine, Oral Pathology, Oral Radiology, Endodontics* **94**, 756–62.

126. Zehnder M, Schmidlin P, Sener B, Waltimo T (2005) Chelation in root canal therapy reconsidered. *Journal of Endodontics* **31**, 817–20.

127. Zerella JA, Fouad AF, Spångberg LSW (2005) Effectiveness of a calcium hydroxide and chlorhexidine digluconate mixture as disinfectant during retreatment of failed endodontic cases. *Oral Surgery, Oral Medicine, Oral Pathology, Oral Radiology, Endodontics* **100**, 756–61.

Chapter 12
Endodontic Treatment of Apical Periodontitis

Martin Trope and Gilberto Debelian

12.1 Introduction

Apical periodontitis is caused by the communication of root canal microbes and/or their byproducts with the surrounding periodontal structures (Fig. 12.1). This occurs primarily through the apical foramina, but can occur through accessory or lateral canals. Treatment strategies are directed at removal of these microbes and their byproducts from the root canal system and thus eliminating the stimuli to the periodontal structures that sustain or cause apical periodontitis. Once maximal microbial control is achieved, the root and top filling are placed to ensure that remaining microbes are separated from the periodontal structures and that new microbes cannot enter the canal space.

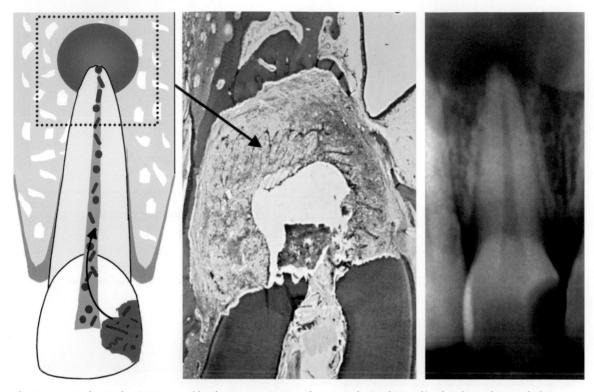

Fig. 12.1 Apical periodontitis is caused by the communication of root canal microbes and/or their byproducts with the surrounding periodontal structures (left). It presents histologically as a cyst or granuloma (center) and radiographically as a radiolucency (right).

12.2 Microbes as the cause of apical periodontitis

The classical study of Kakehashi *et al.* [116] demonstrated that in germ-free rats pulp canals left open did not result in appreciable pulpal or periodontal disease. Rats with normal oral bacterial profiles developed pulpal necrosis and periapical destruction. Möller *et al.* [164] showed that devitalized pulps required infection before periapical disease would develop. Bergenholtz in 1974 [21] and Sundqvist in 1976 [251] showed in humans that pulps that were necrotic due to trauma required bacteria before apical periodontitis developed. These studies also refuted the previously held view that the necrotic pulp alone was enough of a stimulus for the development of apical periodontitis. Möller *et al.* [164] showed in monkey teeth that devitalized pulps required microorganisms for the development of apical periodontitis and confirmed

that a necrotic pulp in the absence of infection will not induce periradicular inflammation.

The unique environment of the necrotic pulp canal results in a "natural" selection or climax community reducing more than 700 microbial species inhabiting the oral cavity, to 20–40 species in the canal [64,65]. Morphologically, the root canal microbiota consists of cocci, rods, filaments, and spirochetes [256]. Fungal cells can also be sporadically found [287]. Some of the endodontic microbiota remains suspended in the fluid phase of the main root canal [139]; in addition, dense bacterial aggregates or coaggregates can be seen adhered to the root canal walls, sometimes forming multilayered bacterial condensations that resemble biofilm-like communities [97,129,134,257,290]. Bacteria forming dense accumulations on the root canal walls are often seen penetrating the dentinal tubules [96,139,148,183]. The diameter of dentinal tubules is large enough to permit penetration of most oral bacteria. It has been reported that dentinal tubule infection can occur in about 50–80% of the teeth with apical periodontitis lesions [77,84,95,97,139,166,167, 230]. Although a shallow penetration is more common, bacterial cells can be observed reaching approximately 300 μm, and in some teeth permeating the entire span of the tubules, reaching the cementum of the periodontal ligament from the dentin side [97,283]. Treatment may fail due to persistence of microorganisms after primary root canal treatment, or due to microbes that enter the root canal after the completion of root treatment [86,158,192,196,232,233,254, 256]. The microbiota associated with persistent infections is usually different from that in primary infections [96,233]. Persistent and secondary infections are clinically indistinguishable and as such are treated with a similar protocol.

Enterococcus faecalis has created a large amount of interest in conjunction with failed root canal therapy [192]. It is a facultative anaerobic Gram-positive coccus that can be a normal inhabitant of the oral cavity. It is found in a much higher incidence in failed root treatment cases compared to primary infections [86,158,192,196,232,233,254,256].

Of special interest is its ability to survive in a higher pH than most microbes, making it relatively resistant to $Ca(OH)_2$, the current most popular intracanal medicament used in endodontics [50,62,84,94,117,159,190].

12.2.1 Anatomic location of the microbes

Intraradicular infection

Most of the microorganisms are found in the fluid phase in the main root canal (Fig. 12.2) [257]. Microbes can also be found in a thick aggregate on the canal wall as a biofilm (Fig. 12.3) and they then usually penetrate the dentinal tubules extending to varying depths into dentin (Fig. 12.4) [77,95,166,167]. In addition, the bacteria are found in lateral and accessory canals as well as in isthmuses between the main canals (Fig. 12.5) [139,230].

Extraradicular infection

It has also been shown that in some cases bacteria may be found outside the root canal system itself (extraradicularly), mainly as a biofilm on the external surface of the root [3,79,113,247–250,271–273,277,294] (Fig. 12.6), but also sometimes as independent aggregates in the periradicular tissues (Figs 12.6 and 12.7). When one appreciates the irregularities of the root

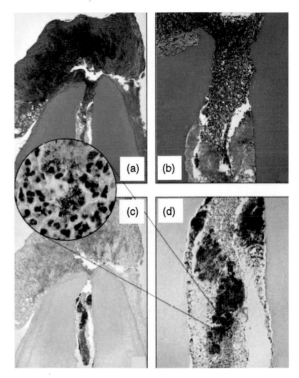

Fig. 12.2 Microorganisms in the fluid phase in the main root canal. (Reproduced with permission from [194].)

canal system and the uniformity and relatively simple shape of endodontic instruments it becomes clear that although our armamentarium will allow us to remove most intracanal bacteria, the superficial biofilm and the microbes in the tubules close to the pulp canal, it is unrealistic to expect that the infected root canal system can be completely disinfected [97].

12.2.2 Infection in endodontically treated teeth

When root canal treatment fails to prevent or eliminate apical periodontitis it is assumed that the cause is failure to seal the root canal after the microbial control phase allowing new microbes in the liquid phase, canal wall biofilm or superficial tubules [139,257]. Alternatively the primary treatment may have failed to remove these microbes in the first place. Another possible cause of persistent apical periodontitis is that the microbes were inaccessible and thus not susceptible to standard treatment protocols. This may be the case with deep tubular microbes, microbes

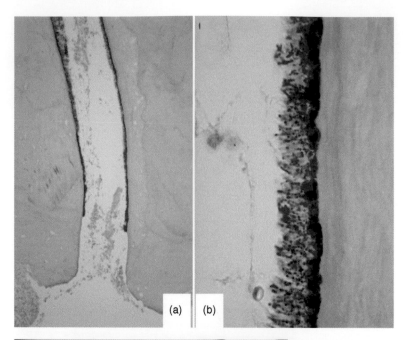

Fig. 12.3 Microbes in a thick aggregate on the canal wall as a biofilm at low (a) and higher magnification (b). (Reproduced with permission from [257].)

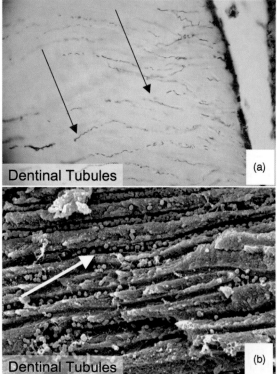

Fig. 12.4 Microbes penetrating the dentinal tubules observed by light microscopy (a) and scanning electron microscopy (b). (Courtesy of Drs JF Siqueira Jr and IN Rocas.)

in canal isthmuses or extraradicular microbes [257]. Finally, a foreign body reaction should be considered [124,169].

12.3 The significance of apical periodontitis in the outcome of endodontic treatment

It has become abundantly clear that the treatment outcome of infected teeth with apical periodontitis is poorer than the treatment outcome after preventative treatment of initially vital teeth [121,211,235,246] (see Chapter 14). Almost all studies that have assessed endodontic treatment outcome have shown a clearly poorer outcome for those where radiolucencies are present before treatment [33,34,48,72,160,235,236, 246,177] (Table 12.1).

Since the main difference between a tooth with or without an apical radiolucency is that the root canal system is infected in the former, it may be assumed that the presence of pulp space bacteria negatively affects the outcome of endodontic treatment [20,33,57,235,309]. This assumption is strengthened when one looks at the studies comparing treatment outcomes where bacterial cultures were taken at the

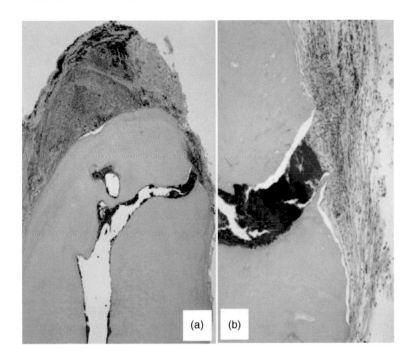

(a)   (b)

Fig. 12.5   Microbes in the dentinal tubules and an accessory canal. (Reproduced with permission.)

end of the microbial control phase of treatment and before the root filling was performed [121,211,235,246] (Table 12.2). These studies have clearly shown that the treatment results are better in teeth without cultivable bacteria at the time of root canal filling.

12.4 The significance of filling the canal without and with cultivable bacteria

The importance of bacterial elimination is further documented by an often overlooked finding: the outcome of treating teeth with *apical periodontitis* when filled without cultivable bacteria is excellent and matches that with vital teeth or teeth with necrotic pulps but without apical periodontitis [235,237].

Byström *et al.* in the 1980s performed a series of studies evaluating the antibacterial effectiveness of various procedures in endodontics [29,32,33]. When they followed those teeth that were filled after a negative culture was reached, a successful outcome was found in more than 90% of cases. The high success rate of teeth filled after a negative culture was again demonstrated in the prospective study of Sjögren *et al.* [237], where they took cultures just before filling teeth that were treated in one visit. When the teeth were examined for healing, a distinct difference in

healing outcomes was found between those teeth that were filled where bacteria could be cultured (68%) and those that were filled without cultivable bacteria (94%) (Table 12.2). Recently Waltimo *et al.* [288] again demonstrated the high success rates if a negative culture was obtained before filling the root canal. While it is readily conceded that the culturing techniques used in most of these studies will not detect all remaining bacteria in the canal and that radiographic success may still miss histological inflammation, these experiments have demonstrated that, if a treatment protocol is used that will result in minimal bacteria within the canal before filling of the canal, a very high success rate by currently accepted criteria can be achieved. In fact we should expect an outcome similar to vital (noninfected) teeth. While culturing may not be mandatory for clinical practice, the practitioner should choose a treatment protocol that has been shown in controlled studies to result in a predictably low microbial count before filling the canal.

12.5 Microbial control phase: infection control of the root canal

In the following section each step within the microbial control phase of treatment of roots with apical

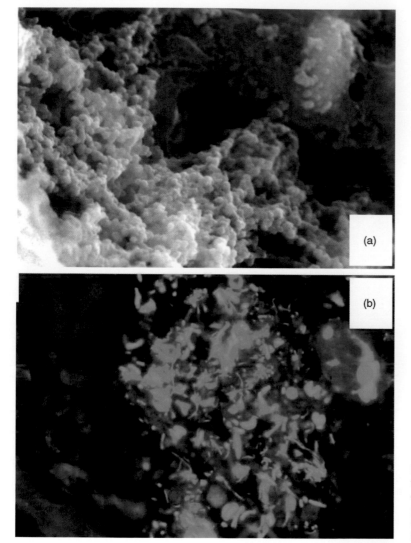

Fig. 12.6 Microbes as a biofilm on the external root surface (scanning electron microscopy, a) and in the periapical tissues (FISH technique, b). (Reproduced with permission from [250].)

periodontitis is evaluated with the aim of selecting a treatment protocol that will result in a predictable negative culture before filling the canal. If this is achieved, the clinician should expect a high probability of success for teeth with apical periodontitis, similar to that expected for teeth without apical periodontitis.

12.5.1 Controlling the infection by mechanical instrumentation

Mechanical instrumentation is a critical step in the microbial control phase of root canal treatment. In terms of bacterial numbers, instrumentation even without disinfectant reduces the volume of microbial flora more than 90% [29,52]. Furthermore, as the size of file used in the apical third of the canal increases there is a significant reduction in the number of remaining bacteria [52,175,222,228]. The use of files that actively engage the root canal wall (adequate apical sizes) is in line with the recent focus on the biofilm on the root canal wall. Logically the most effective means of eliminating this biofilm is to "scrape" the canal wall with root canal files.

Dalton *et al.* [52] using saline in conjunction with the files thus evaluated the anti-bacterial effect of

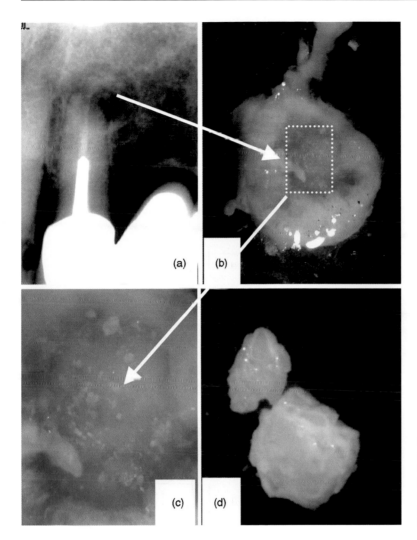

Fig. 12.7 Extraradicular infection by microbes in granules in the periapical tissues. Radiographic appearance (a); the whole granule in macroscopic view (b); inner view of capsule (c) and granules extracted from the inner part of the lesion (d).

mechanical instrumentation without the addition of an anti-bacterial irrigant (Fig. 12.8). Increased instrumentation reduced the remaining bacteria significantly. However even in the relatively small mesiobuccal canal of a mandibular molar it was found that apical size #25 resulted in only 20% of the canals being free of any cultivable bacteria. At an apical size of #35 the remaining cultivable bacteria were reduced to 60% of the tested canals. Clearly, too many canals had abundant remaining bacteria to recommend moving to the filling phase at this stage. Another important finding in this study was that it made no difference for the number of remaining bacteria whether the instrumen-

tation was performed with stainless-steel files used in a predominantly apical to coronal direction or with nickel–titanium files of variable taper used with a crown-down technique.

The study of Dalton *et al.* [52] confirmed the studies of Byström *et al.* [29] from the previous decade. In the Byström studies only stainless-steel files were used. The more recent Dalton study reinforced the point that the use of nickel–titanium files has no additional effect on the infection when apical instrument sizes were similar: it is the final shape of the instrumented canal rather than the tools used to obtain it that matters.

Table 12.1 Treatment outcomes and preoperative pulpal status. There is a clearly lower probability of success if a radiolucency is present pre-operatively

	Preoperative status	
Reference	No radiolucency	Radiolucency
Strindberg (1956) [246]	89%	68%
Seltzer *et al.* (1963) [211]	92%	76%
Kerekes and Tronstad (1979) [121]	94%	84%
Sjögren *et al.* (1990) [235]	96%	86%

Table 12.2 Treatment outcomes where bacterial cultures were taken at the end of the microbial control phase of treatment and before the root filling was performed. Results are better in teeth without cultivable bacteria at the time of root canal filling

	Culture results	
Reference	Positive culture	Negative culture
Zeldow and Ingle (1963) [309]	83%	93%
Engström *et al.* (1964) [57]	76%	89%
Byström *et al.* (1987) [33]		95%
Sjögren *et al.* (1997) [237]	68%	94%

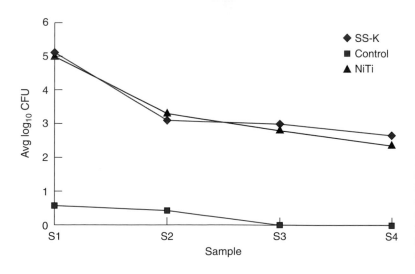

Fig. 12.8 Increased reduction of canal bacteria with increasing apical file sizes. At an apical size of #25 (S2) only 20% of the canals cultured negative; at an apical size of #35 (S4) the remaining uncultivable bacteria increased to 40% of the tested canals. (Data from [52].)

12.5.2 Controlling the infection by antimicrobial irrigation

Traditionally an irrigant is used in conjunction with mechanical instrumentation in order to aid in the cutting efficiency of the instrument and to facilitate the removal of cut dentin [17,90,91,125,238,308].

However, the most important property of the irrigant is its antimicrobial property. Sodium hypochlorite is the most commonly used endodontic irrigant [7,31,46,51, 71,102]. It has been used and tested at strengths ranging from 0.5% to 6% [30,31,109,161,181,214, 231,234,308].

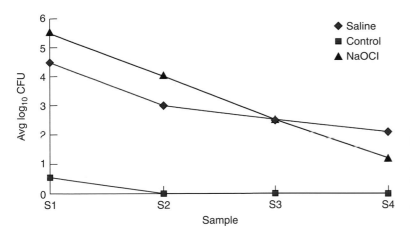

Fig. 12.9 Added effect of sodium hypochlorite on bacterial reduction in infected canals. At an apical size of #30 (S3), no added benefit of NaOCl was found; only at an apical size of #35 did NaOCl significantly reduce the microbial load (S4). (Data from [222].)

Sodium hypochlorite

Sodium hypochlorite has a potent antibacterial effect and the ability to dissolve necrotic organic matter [30,31,90,109,161,181,199,229,234,305]. When added to mechanical instrumentation it further reduces the number of infected roots to approximately 40–50% [31,265]. In the study of Shuping *et al.* [222] there was no beneficial effect for the NaOCl when used at an apical size of #30. Only when the apical size of #35 was attained did the use of the NaOCl irrigant significantly reduce the microbial load (Fig. 12.9). When comparing the results from recent studies where crown-down nickel-titanium instrumentation was used with those from older studies using stainless-steel files only, there is no appreciable difference between the methods [31,52,151,265]. Again, it seems as if the preparation shape rather than the technical aids to obtain the desired shape is the critical factor.

Some clinicians have claimed that increasing the strength and exposure time of the NaOCl would reduce the bacterial load in the canal to levels that will allow filling the root canal immediately after instrumentation with optimal outcomes [27,28,90,165,208]. However, previous studies comparing the antibacterial effectiveness of different strengths of NaOCl have not found a substantial increase in potency with increased concentration [31,229]. Moreover, a recent study by McGurkin-Smith *et al.* [151] using 5.25% NaOCl and ethylenediamine tetraacetic acid (EDTA) replaced every 5 min and for a total of 30 min did not show any increase in the antibacterial effectiveness.

Thus, it is clear that when typical apical sizes (#35 for a mesiobuccal root in a mandibular molar) are used in conjunction with various strengths of NaOCl

irrigation, it is not possible to attain predictably bacteria-free canals by conventional culturing techniques, a status that is required for root filling with optimal outcomes (Fig. 12.10).

EDTA

EDTA was introduced to endodontics in 1957 by Nygaard Østby [171]. EDTA is a chelating agent that is able to soften the root canal dentin to depths of 20–50 μm [171]. It is used primarily for its ability to remove the smear layer created by mechanical instrumentation and to facilitate the removal of dentin debris from the canal [16,42,50,55,81,109,110,137, 138,140,171,182,186,207,244,245,266,302,306,307]. An alternate flush with NaOCl and EDTA has been shown to effectively remove both organic and inorganic matter from the root canal [97,306,307], but EDTA by itself has little if any antibacterial effect [182,300,307].

Chlorhexidine

Chlorhexidine gluconate of varying concentrations has been introduced as an alternative irrigant and intracanal dressing [53,63,69,83,84,85,88,114,227,260, 285,296,304]. It is prepared in either liquid or gel form. Chlorhexidine is a cationic bisbiguanide with optimal antimicrobial action over the pH range 5.5–7.0, and acts by adsorbing onto the cell walls of microorganisms causing leakage of intracellular components [84,107,135]. It has a strong antibacterial activity against a wide range of Gram-positive, Gram-negative, facultative anaerobic, and aerobic bacteria

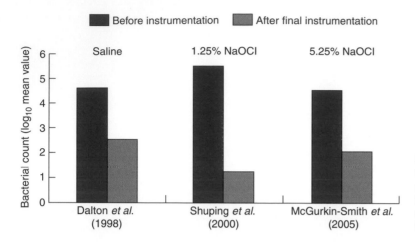

Fig. 12.10 Bacterial reduction in mesiobuccal canals of mandibular molars instrumented with various irrigants. Predictably bacteria-free canals could not be obtained. (Data from [52,151,222].)

as well as yeasts [243,286]. *In vitro* studies have consistently shown that chlorhexidine is superior to NaOCl in killing of *E. faecalis* [174,213]. Ercan *et al.* [59] showed that 2% chlorhexidine solution is more effective than 5.25% NaOCl in disinfecting root canals in a clinical study.

There may be several advantages of chlorhexidine as an intracanal irrigant or as a dressing: (a) it can retain its antimicrobial effect up to 12 weeks after the treatment, (b) it is less cytotoxic than NaOCl, and (c) it is effective against microorganisms resistant to $Ca(OH)_2$ such as *E. feacalis* [84]. Its one major disadvantage is that it does not break down proteins and necrotic tissue as does NaOCl [165,190,191]. An *in vivo* study by Zamany *et al.* [304] showed that 92% of the roots treated with a final rinse of 2% chlorhexidine did not culture bacteria while those roots rinsed with the saline control grew bacteria in 58% of the specimens. A comparative clinical study on the antimicrobial efficacy of chlorhexidine and NaOCl showed favorable results for chlorhexidine. These studies point to a potential for chlorhexidine as an irrigant in endodontics with possible improvement relative to NaOCl.

MTAD

MTAD (Biopure, Tulsa Dentsply, Tulsa, OK, USA) is a mixture of doxycycline, citric acid, and the detergent Tween-80 [18,19,218,219,261,267,268,310]. It has a pH in the range of 2.5. The idea behind this product is to "gently" remove the smear layer while enhancing intracanal bacterial killing. Antibacterial effectiveness studies have been contradictory [18]. In addition

isolated cases with discoloration presumably from the tetracycline have been reported.

Principles of biomechanical instrumentation

Combining large apical sizes and antibacterial irrigation is crucial for maximum disinfection effect. The introduction of nickel–titanium files with variable taper provided a potential to attain much larger apical preparations that were not previously possible with stainless-steel files. If the canal is prepared with a crown down technique with each file that reaches deeper into the canal having a decreasing taper it is possible to instrument the apical third of the canal with a parallel or 0.02 tapered instrument without touching (and thus over preparing) the more coronal part of the canal. Card *et al.* [37] evaluated the antibacterial effectiveness of large apical sizes and NaOCl and found in single rooted mandibular premolars that 100% of the tested roots were bacteria-free and in 91% of the mesiobuccal roots of mandibular molars the roots were culture negative. Therefore, if large apical sizes are used in combination with greater coronal taper to create a canal preparation design previously unattainable with stainless-steel files, a case can be made for a single-visit approach where no further steps are needed to remove additional bacteria before filling the canal.

12.5.3 Controlling the infection by intracanal medication

Mechanical instrumentation and irrigation significantly reduce the number of bacteria within the root canal. However, when conventional, small apical sizes are used in conjunction with NaOCl as the irrigant approximately 50% of canals will still harbor bacteria [222]. Given space and nutrition these remaining bacteria can increase in number close to that which was present in the root canal before treatment. Thus, a canal should not be left empty after initial instrumentation and between visits. Since root filling canals which have a 50% chance of still having bacteria will result in a lower success, the question remains if the addition of an intracanal medication before filling the root canal can predictably lower the bacterial count.

Calcium hydroxide

Calcium hydroxide has been widely utilized in endodontic therapy as an intracanal dressing [32,38,58,103, 130,201,202,203,226,236,269]. At saturation, the substance has a high pH (12.5–12.8), and its dental use relates chiefly to its ability to facilitate mineralization [155], its antibacterial properties [32], and its tissue-dissolving capability [106]. It may seem that $Ca(OH)_2$ has a unique potential to induce mineralization, even in tissues that have not been programmed to mineralize [24,156]. In cases of trauma, its use appears to be successful in arresting inflammatory root resorption, although the mechanism by which $Ca(OH)_2$ initiates the reparative process is unclear [281].

Most of the desirable properties of $Ca(OH)_2$ may be attributed to its bactericidal effects [47,70,123]. This is attributed to the alkaline effects of hydroxyl ions, producing a pH over 11, which prevents the growth and survival of oral bacteria [32,46]. Calcium hydroxide also alters the biological properties of bacterial lipopolysaccharides [203]; and, by inactivating enzymes in bacterial membranes, it also upsets membrane transportation mechanisms, resulting in cell toxicity [61]. It has a nonspecific bactericidal action within the confines of the root canal, alkalis in general having a pronounced destructive effect on cell membranes and protein structure. Although most microorganisms are destroyed at pH 9.5, a few can survive at pH 11 or higher [108]. Therefore, to act as an effective antimicrobial dressing its pH has to be high both in the canal and some distance into the dentinal tubules.

The ability to maintain a high pH in the dentin is related to its diffusion capacity through dentine tubules. It appears that the hydroxyl ions derived from $Ca(OH)_2$ diffuse faster and reach higher levels in cervical root dentin than in more apical levels of the root [60,170,181].

Wang and Hume [293] measured hydroxyl ion diffusion across the dentin between an occlusal cavity containing $Ca(OH)_2$ and a saline-filled pulp chamber over 16 days, using a pH meter. By taking ground dentin (subsequently mixed with saline) from various depths, they demonstrated a gradient of pH values from the cavity layer decreasing to the middle and pulpal layers, indicating a slow movement of the hydroxyl ion through the dentin. Importantly, they showed in series of experiments that dentin has the capacity to buffer hydroxyl ions as these ions diffuse through dentine. Haapasalo *et al.* [94] showed that dentin powder had an inhibitory effect on some endodontic medicaments. They used saturated $Ca(OH)_2$ solution, 1% solution hypochlorite, 0.5% and 0.05% chlorhexidine acetate and 2/4%, and 0.2/0.4% iodine potassium iodide; with *E. faecalis* as a test organism. The effect of $Ca(OH)_2$ on *E. faecalis* was totally abolished by the presence of dentine powder.

The method of the $Ca(OH)_2$ medicament insertion could be an important determinant of the pH of the dentin inside the canal and at distant dentinal sites. Peters *et al.* [184] reported that a reduction in the number of microbes was not accomplished by insertion of $Ca(OH)_2$ into the root canal. In these studies the medicament was plugged into the canals with the blunt end of a sterile paper point. However, in most studies where it was reported that $Ca(OH)_2$ was beneficial in reducing culturable bacteria it was placed using a spiral filler [32,222,236].

In a recent *in vitro* study by Teixeira *et al.* [264] it was found that placement of the $Ca(OH)_2$ paste with a spiral and plugging with the blunt end of a sterile paper point resulted in higher pH values on the canal walls and in the inner dentin than placement with paper points only. When the $Ca(OH)_2$ was placed with the spiral filler the highest pH values were obtained at 7 days. Although not directly shown, there was an indication of effective buffering of the alkalinity of $Ca(OH)_2$ by dentine when the various sites on the root wall were analyzed and compared.

Most studies have confirmed that $Ca(OH)_2$ mixed into a toothpaste consistency and placed into the canal with a lentulospiral instrument is effective in further reducing the bacterial load in the root canal (Table 12.3). Byström *et al.* [32] found that 97% of canals were without cultivable bacteria after a month with $Ca(OH)_2$. Sjögren *et al.* [236] found similar results after a 7-day application of $Ca(OH)_2$, whereas

Table 12.3   Effectiveness of calcium hydroxide as an intracanal medicament

Reference	Duration of medication (days)	Number of teeth	Percentage bacteria-free after Ca(OH)$_2$ treatment
Byström et al. (1985) [32]	30	35	95
Molander et al. (1988) [158]	14	35	77
Sjögren et al. (1991) [236]	7	18	100
Yared et al. (1994) [301]	7	60	68
Barbosa et al. (1997) [12]	7	45	73
Shuping et al. (2000) [222]	7	42	92.5
McGurkin-Smith et al. (2005) [151]	28	40	86
Average			85.2

a 10-min application of the medicament was found insufficient. Thus, the results showing the effectiveness of Ca(OH)$_2$ have been confirmed in numerous clinical studies [228].

Other medicaments used for intracanal medication

Phenol derivatives. Camphorated paramonochlorophenol (CMCP), camphorated phenol and formocreosol have been used as intracanal medicaments [32]. The use of these medicaments, in liquid or vapor form, has become outdated since their effectiveness has been shown to be limited [276]. These medicaments have a very short duration of action, are toxic and inefficient as antimicrobial agents [270].

Iodine. A case has been made for a short-term (5-min) dressing with iodine–potassium iodide at the end of a treatment session with conventional instrumentation with NaOCl. The number of residual bacteria was reduced and approached or surpassed the antibacterial efficacy of a 1-week dressing with Ca(OH)$_2$ [128].

Ledermix. Ledermix® is a water-soluble paste containing 1% triamcinolone and 3% demeclocycline. It is proposed as a root canal dressing and may be applied in trauma cases where control of root resorption is important [188,189]. Triamcinolone is a highly active steroid providing potent antiinflammatory action and demeclocycline is a broad-spectrum antibiotic effective against a wide range of Gram-positive and Gram-negative bacteria. The active agents in Ledermix have a rapid initial release followed by a slow steady release. Components in Ledermix can diffuse through dentin, and levels of triamcinolone sufficient for antiinflammatory action have been recorded in the periradicular area. However, there may be little benefit for intracanal Ledermix in reducing post-treatment pain [278]. This may be due to the pain being produced by inflammation outside the canal inaccessible to the corticosteroid, or to rapid removal by the tissue fluids of corticosteroid penetrating into the tissues.

Other concepts. The use of interim dressings without antibacterial potency, or leaving the canal open or unfilled is contraindicated. There are a number of clinical studies that have shown regrowth or ingrowth of bacteria in canals where no medicament has been present between appointments [32,280].

Chlorhexidine. Chlorhexidine is adsorbed to hard tissues and thus has the ability to kill bacteria long after its placement in the root canal. It has been applied alone as a gel, or in combination with Ca(OH)$_2$ or other medicaments (CMCP) [53,63,69, 83,84,85,88,114,227,260,285,296,304]. Its potential as root canal medicament also stems from its relative efficacy towards *E. faecalis* [174,213].

12.5.4 Controlling the infection in one and multiple visits

Studies comparing outcomes of treatments performed in one visit (root filled at the first visit without an intracanal medicaments) with an intracanal dressing with Ca(OH)$_2$ have been inconclusive [66,75,173,185,237, 279,280,295]. This is primarily due to limited sample sizes in these studies. Some studies have shown about a 10% increase in success with the use of $Ca(OH)_2$ [75, 280] while others have shown no difference [185,295]. None of the studies showed statistically significant differences. The question of differences in treatment outcomes for teeth treated in one visit vs $Ca(OH)_2$ as an intracanal medication, highlights the difficulty of using a strictly evidence-based approach for treatment strategies in endodontics. Sathorn *et al.* in 2005 [204] attempted to perform a systematic review of the available literature dealing with this issue. However, when the strict criteria required for this type of study were utilized only three articles qualified, and the data available for analysis did not permit any conclusions on the suitability of one method over the other. Therefore, we must use data also from animal and laboratory experiments, and clinical case collections and reports, in order to apply the principles of best available evidence to formulate a treatment protocol for apical periodontitis.

12.5.5 Special considerations in root canal disinfection

Ultrasonics

Ultrasonic instruments have been adapted for use in endodontics [43,44,45,146,147]. They were originally introduced as cutting instruments, but lost favor primarily because of their aggressive cutting which increased the potential for procedural errors [140,150,152,210].

The use of ultrasonics as an adjunct in disinfection of the root canal was first proposed by Martin [146,147]. Studies have suggested that the ultrasonic has an energizing effect on the irrigant and the files [146,239], thus enhancing disinfection. It has been found for example that if EDTA is used with ultrasonics after NaOCl irrigation, the removal of the smear layer was enhanced [35,36,92]. In a study comparing remaining canal bacteria after passive ultrasonic irrigation it was shown that bacterial counts were lower when ultrasonics was used [239]. Ultrasonics appears to exert its antimicrobial effect in conjunction with irrigants, perhaps via the physical mechanism of cavitation and acoustic streaming and by moving the irrigant into areas of complex anatomy [35,36,92,97, 146,149,200]. The ultrasonic movement of the file causes streaming patterns in the irrigant. Biologic material that enters these streaming fields will be subjected to shear stresses and may be damaged. In addition, the ultrasonic energy may enhance the movement of the irrigant into irregularities in the canal. Also it is possible that the irrigant is warmed, which in the case of NaOCl makes it more effective in breaking down organic material [234]. It appears important that the ultrasonic device is loose in the root canal since contact with the canal wall causes most of the ultrasonic energy to be absorbed by the dentin.

Lasers

The effectiveness of various lasers in disinfecting the root canal has been studied by many authors [6,11,25, 87,93,115,122,131,133,142,153,209,259]. Results are contradictory, but most studies find little advantage over NaOCl [25,26,97,163]; however, the technology is steadily improving, and applications for endodontic purposes show improving potential for application. The synergistic effect of a traditional irrigating solution energized by laser energy has yet to be studied in detail.

Antibiotics

MTAD. Applied as an irrigation solution (see above), this product contains a derivative of tetracycline, minocycline, as the active, antibacterial ingredient. Tetracyclines exhibit substantivity to dental hard tissues [18,19,54,218,219,240,241,261,267,268,310]. The proposed benefits of MTAD are linked to this property, and the concept for treatment with MTAD is that the antibiotic remains in the root canal for a long time and exerts a lasting effect on microbes that might have survived the biomechanical instrumentation procedures.

Ledermix. From a theoretical point of view Ledermix, with its demeclocycline content also has the potential to reduce remaining bacteria in the canal and dentinal tubules through diffusion of the antibiotic [262]. However, an improved antibacterial efficacy relative to $Ca(OH)_2$ has not been documented.

Triple antibiotic paste. The bactericidal efficacy of topical antibiotics against oral pathogens has been the subject of many investigations. Metronidazole, demonstrated by Ingham *et al.* [111] to have a broad spectrum of activity against oral obligate anaerobes, has shown much promise in the disinfection of carious dentin. In a study by Hoshino *et al.* [105], metronidazole caused effective disinfection of carious dentin when applied in an α-tricalcium phosphate cement containing 5% metronidazole. However, metronidazole, even at concentrations of 100 µg/ml could not kill all of the bacteria, indicating that additional drugs may be necessary to disinfect the lesions.

Sato *et al.* [205] demonstrated the effectiveness of an antibiotic paste consisting of ciprofloxacin, metronidazole, and minocycline at concentrations of 100 µg/ml in the disinfection of carious lesions, necrotic pulps, and infected root dentin of deciduous teeth *in situ*. This drug combination did not result in any pathological changes when placed on vital pulp tissue [8,106]. Whereas none of the drugs resulted in complete elimination of bacteria when tested alone, the combination of metronidazole, ciprofloxacin, and minocycline at concentrations of 25–50 µg/ml consistently disinfected all samples. In a further study, Sato *et al.* [206] investigated the ability of this drug combination to kill bacteria in the deep layers of root canal dentin *in situ*. Extracted teeth were decoronated followed by the placement of 0.5 mg of each drug into the root canal space. Cell suspensions of *Escherichia coli* were placed into cavities prepared adjacent to the root canals, and bacteria were sampled from the cavities at intervals up to 48 hours. Bacterial recovery decreased at each time period, with no recovery after 48 hours.

Thus, the combination of ciprofloxacin, metronidazole, and minocycline appears to be very effective at bacterial reduction *in vitro* and *in situ*. A similar combination was used in the report by Iwaya *et al.* [112] that demonstrated pulp revascularization after infection. If this triple antibiotic paste could consistently disinfect the canals of immature teeth, revascularization should be possible.

In a recent study by Windley *et al.* [298] the disinfection potential of this triple antibiotic paste was tested in infected dog roots. The number of bacteria in the canals was measured before (S1) and after (S2) irrigation with 1.25% NaOCl, and after dressing with a triple antibiotic paste consisting of metronidazole, ciprofloxacin, and minocycline (S3). No mechanical instrumentation was performed since these were immature teeth. At S1, 100% of the samples cultured positive for bacteria with a mean colony-forming unit (CFU) count of 1.7×10^8. At S2, 13% of the samples were bacteria-free, and the mean CFU count was down to 1.4×10^4. At S3, 70% of the samples were bacteria-free, and the mean CFU count was only 26.

One disadvantage of this medicament is the potential for the minocycline to stain the crown of the teeth. Great care needs to be taken to remove all medicament from the access cavity after the medicament has been placed.

Exacerbations

Exacerbations after the microbial phase of the treatment of apical periodontitis have been reported to range from less than 3% [13,279,289] up to 85% [172]. The incidence of exacerbations depends on many factors including definition (any postoperative pain vs the need for an unscheduled visit), treatment technique, state of the pulp (vital vs necrotic; root filled), and the use of adjunctive therapy. The causes of exacerbations are not clear. A number of possible causes have been discussed alone or in combination; these include:

Mechanical irritation. Instrumentation through the apical foramen will cause physical damage to the periapical tissues resulting in the release of both tissue and plasma mediators of pain [212]. The addition of microbes to this condition increases the chance of a post-treatment exacerbation as evidenced by the much higher incidence of exacerbations in teeth with apical periodontitis compared to vital teeth [13,279,289]. Anaerobes in mixed infections were thought to play an important role in these exacerbations [89,251,252].

Underinstrumentation. If the root canal is not adequately instrumented, particularly in the apical third of the canal, and an intracanal medicament is not used or is ineffective, remaining bacteria may proliferate and initiate acute exacerbations [211].

Immunological factors. Immunological factors may play a role in acute exacerbations [212].

Psychological factors. It has been reported that some patients are more susceptible to pain due to psychological factors. Thus, the psychological profile of the patient is important in predicting an exacerbation. The threshold of pain is different in different ethnic groups [99], and the tolerance to pain decreases when it is an unexpected consequence to treatment. Thus informing the patient of what to expect after treatment is important so as to limit the psychological reaction to inconsequential postoperative pain.

Other possible contributing factors include the effect of the introduction of oxygen into the canal during treatment [212] with associated changes in the microbial ecology [253,256], changes in periapical tissue pressure [157], or psychological, adaptive mechanisms (e.g., the local adaptation theory of Seyle [215]).

12.6 Root filling phase

According to current concepts of endodontic practice, the ideal root filling should be inert with little, if any, tissue-damaging effect. It follows that current materials for filling also claim no antimicrobial properties. Rather, the root filling is considered a second phase of treatment with the aim of sealing the canal space in order to prevent reinfection of the canal and to separate any remaining bacteria from a food source or communicating with the surrounding periodontal ligament [179]. The treatment aim for teeth with apical periodontitis is to remove as many microbes from the root canal as possible with instrumentation, irrigation, and medication: the microbial control phase. When this phase is completed, the canal should be filled so as to minimize regrowth and reinfection: the filling phase.

The root filling has three primary functions: (a) to prevent periapical fluids from tracking into the canal to feed remaining bacteria; (b) to entomb remaining bacteria, thus stopping the inflammatory stimulators from communicating with the surrounding periodontal tissues; and (c) to inhibit coronal leakage of oral bacteria [255].

For the past few decades most filling materials have included a gutta-percha core material with cement as the filler between this core and the dentin wall [179]. Studies over the decades have shown conclusively that many root fillings fail to consistently seal the root canal [15,143,144,193,258,274], and the quality and timeliness of the coronal restoration is therefore believed to be critical for long-term success after root filling [193,274]. Today it is accepted that the coronal restoration should be placed as soon as possible after the root filling. Newer filling materials using bonding technology show some promise in improving the seal of the root canal [221,222,263,292,297]. Future filling materials may seal well enough to make the coronal restoration less critical for successful treatment of apical periodontitis, and, possibly, effectively assist the microbial control phase [221,222,263,292].

12.7 Clinical procedures for the treatment of primary apical periodontitis

12.7.1 Diagnosis of an infected canal

Since the vital tooth should not contain microbes in the root canal, the focus of treatment of this category of teeth is asepsis (once a diagnosis has been made) [23,80]. In the vast majority of cases a nonvital tooth or a tooth with radiographic signs or clinical symptoms of apical periodontitis will contain microbes in the root canal space. These must be treated with a disinfection protocol aimed at reducing the bacteria to a minimum. This should ensure a high probability of successful treatment also of infected cases, which otherwise are associated with a high incidence of persistent infection and inflammation.

Teeth in the diagnostic categories of: (a) vital pulp with acute apical periodontitis (AAP); (b) necrotic pulp with chronic apical periodontitis (CAP); (c) necrotic pulp with acute excacerbation of CAP; (d) necrotic pulp with abscess; and (e) necrotic pulp with sinus tract are all treated with the disinfection protocol for infected root canals.

12.7.2 Asepsis

One of the most overlooked aspects of root canal therapy is the importance of working with an aseptic technique. It is absolutely critical that no microbial contaminants enter the root canal during the treatment procedure. In order to ensure that contamination does not occur, the following general principles should be followed.

Leaky restorations and caries are removed and the access cavity preparation is performed before the placement of the rubber dam. Once the access cavity has been prepared the rubber dam is placed and adequately sealed from saliva contamination. A solution of 2% chlorhexidine or betadine is then placed in the access cavity and used to wash the field of at least 3 cm diameter around the tooth on the rubber dam and for at least 1 min. Sterile instruments must be separated from those that have entered the root canal and become contaminated with bacteria. If an instrument has been contaminated it must be disinfected chemically or by heat before it again enters the infected root canal. Strict asepsis is used when handling the endodontic files. At no time should the files be touched by the operator or assistant before entering the root canal system.

12.7.3 Working length

It is clear from available evidence that the best probability of success is achieved when the mechanical instrumentation and root filling is kept within the root canal. A root filling ending 0–2 mm short of the radiographic apex seems to be optimal (94% success), while underfilling more than 2 mm will give a 68% success rate, and overfilling a 76% probability of successful healing of apical periodontitis [235]. More recently, it has been suggested that 0.5 mm short of the radiographic apex is the length that provides the best prognosis and that for every millimeter short of this length there is a 14% decrease in success rate [39,40]. Most studies report that root filling long lowers the success rate [22,39,40,56,176,235,246,303].

12.7.4 Instrumentation size of the apical third

It is not possible to physically clean or create enough space for effective irrigation if a step-back shape (i.e.,

apical sizes of #25) is used. Conceptually it is best to instrument the apical third of the canal as large as possible without weakening or perforating the root.

Figure 12.11 shows suggested minimum sizes for effective disinfection of the canal for each tooth type [78,118,119,120,162,197,299]. The sizes displayed are norms and should serve as a guideline when instrumentation is started. However, clinical judgment must be exercised when each individual tooth is treated, with some canals requiring larger and some smaller apical sizes.

While a skilled operator is able to achieve similar disinfection efficiency with both stainless-steel and nickel–titanium files [52], the latter may offer an additional degree of safety in achieving larger apical sizes. In addition, the use of nickel–titanium files alone will result in less straightening and almost entirely eliminate procedural errors even when used by novice practitioners [187]. Moreover, the larger apical file sizes may facilitate improved disinfection of the canal by the irrigating solution [37].

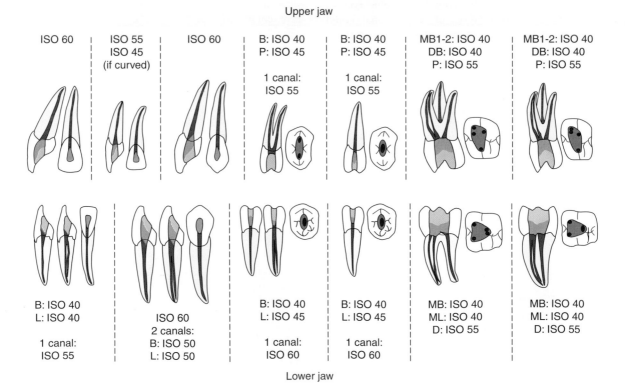

Upper jaw

| ISO 60 | ISO 55 ISO 45 (if curved) | ISO 60 | B: ISO 40 P: ISO 45 1 canal: ISO 55 | B: ISO 40 P: ISO 45 1 canal: ISO 55 | MB1-2: ISO 40 DB: ISO 40 P: ISO 55 | MB1-2: ISO 40 DB: ISO 40 P: ISO 55 |

| B: ISO 40 L: ISO 40 1 canal: ISO 55 | ISO 60 2 canals: B: ISO 50 L: ISO 50 | B: ISO 40 L: ISO 45 1 canal: ISO 60 | B: ISO 40 L: ISO 45 1 canal: ISO 60 | MB: ISO 40 ML: ISO 40 D: ISO 55 | MB: ISO 40 ML: ISO 40 D: ISO 55 |

Lower jaw

Fig. 12.11 Normative apical sizes for safe and effective disinfection in permanent teeth. The clinician must use his or her clinical judgment in choosing apical sizes for each individual tooth.

Most current instrumentation techniques are crown down using decreasing taper of the instruments in order to preserve tooth structure (Fig. 12.12a, b). Once working length is achieved the apical third is enlarged by using files with increasing tip sizes at a taper that is smaller than the file that achieved the working length (Fig. 12.12c).

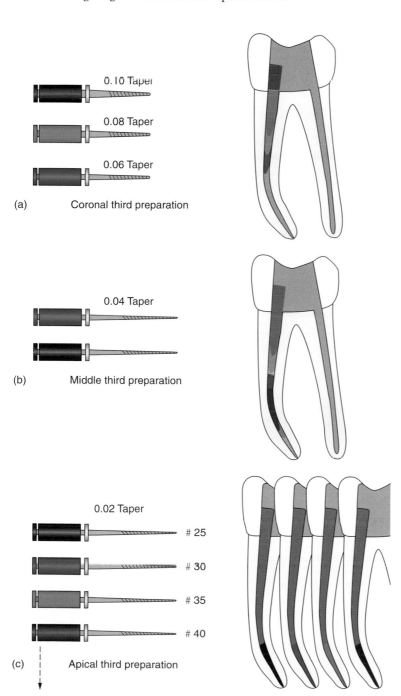

(a)   Coronal third preparation

0.10 Taper

0.08 Taper

0.06 Taper

(b)   Middle third preparation

0.04 Taper

(c)   Apical third preparation

0.02 Taper

\# 25

\# 30

\# 35

\# 40

Fig. 12.12 Most nickel–titanium techniques start crown down using instruments of decreasing taper in order to preserve tooth structure. Files of high, but decreasing taper are used to instrument the coronal third (a); the middle third is instrumented typically with files of medium taper (b), and the apical third with files of small taper and increasing tip size (c).

12.7.5 Irrigation

As shown by a number of studies, the addition of NaOCl as an irrigating solution will significantly reduce the bacterial load in the root canal [222]. Apparently this action is achieved by direct killing of bacteria and by breaking down necrotic tissue [308]. Interestingly, the volume of NaOCl appears to be more important than its strength for bacterial reduction [151].

Also, as mentioned above, the antibacterial effectiveness of NaOCl increases as the apical third is widened [37]. This seems logical as an increased volume will reach the apex as the canal size increases. Soaking the canal for extended time periods or warming the NaOCl has not been shown to be beneficial *in vivo* [151].

Thus, 0.5–1% NaOCl should be used with the emphasis on increased volume of irrigation. Needle sizes and designs that bring the irrigant to the apical area are a logical corollary to this concept. It is important to flush the canal with abundant irrigant after each file.

EDTA is used as an adjunct to NaOCl as an irrigating solution. Its ability to soften dentin for 20–50 μm can make instrumentation easier, and in the case of rotary instruments, the potential for instrument separation lower. In addition, its ability to remove the smear layer may aid in the removal of bacteria; it allows medicaments access to the dentinal tubules; and it may prepare the root canal wall for bonded-filling techniques.

As reviewed above, the use of NaOCl, with or without the addition of EDTA, does not eliminate enough bacteria to attain a predictable negative culture at the end of the first visit [282]. Therefore, this irrigation protocol will not provide a biologically acceptable reason for filling the root canal on the first visit.

Recently numerous irrigants/short-term medicaments have been tested in order to further lower the bacterial count of the root canal and to attain the elusive, predictable negative culture. Iodine–potassium iodide, MTAD, chlorhexidine, and ultrasonic agitation, all have shown promise in further reducing the bacterial count at the first visit. They have been tested *in vitro*, and to some extent *in vivo*, alone or in combination with NaOCl and/or EDTA.

Chlorhexidine is readily available to dentists and is relatively cheap. The use of 2% chlorhexidine may potentially make an intracanal medicament unnecessary; moreover, a 2% chlorhexidine gel may replace NaOCl as the irrigant of choice in teeth with api-cal periodontitis [291,304]. Of particular interest is the use of chlorhexidine as an alternating irrigant with NaOCl [127] or as a final soaking of the canal (>1 min). This would seem well founded on the clinical experiments performed and on the numerous *in vitro* studies that have documented antibacterial activity, ability to kill *E. faecalis*, and substantivity of chlorhexidine [53,63,69,83–85,88,114,227,240,241, 260,286,296,304]. Based on available evidence, copious irrigation with 0.5–1% NaOCl during instrumentation remains the irrigating fluid of choice. After complete instrumentation the canal is rinsed with EDTA in order to remove the smear layer. The effect of the EDTA may be improved with passive (not contacting the canal wall) ultrasonics, which will act to maximize the distribution of the liquid in the root canal system. A final soak of 2% chlorhexidine is left in the canal for at least 1 minute and up to 5 min before placement of an intracanal medicament or final filling.

12.7.6 Intracanal medication

Instrumentation and irrigation by current standard protocols bring the proportion of infected canals from 100 down to 25–50%. The placement of a $Ca(OH)_2$ paste as a medicament for at least 7 days further decreases the incidence of bacteria-positive canals by some 20% [222,236]. Thus, the addition of $Ca(OH)_2$ will result in negative cultures in 80–95% of canals [222]. It is therefore possible, with this protocol, to have a treatment outcome that is similar to what is expected from the vital tooth.

Other antibacterial protocols, such as those discussed in the section above, need to be studied in depth and to be shown as effective as, or better than, $Ca(OH)_2$ in decreasing intracanal bacteria. Until then, current evidence favors the now well established practice of applying a slurry of $Ca(OH)_2$ with a spiral instrument and leaving it for at least 7 days before filling the root canal [283] (Fig. 12.13).

12.7.7 Root canal filling and coronal seal

The function of the root filling is to maintain the environment in the root canal at the time the microbial control phase is completed. This is achieved by filling as much of the empty space as possible thus limiting the leakage of periapical tissue fluids, coronal bacteria or the growth and movement of bacteria left inside the canal. In this way the periapical disease will heal and be maintained in a healthy state. Since the filled

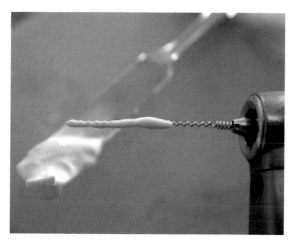

Fig. 12.13 Calcium hydroxide is mixed with sterile saline to a creamy mix and placed into the canal with a spiral paste carrier.

root canal is our final "snapshot" of the quality of our treatment, its role in the success for root canal treatment may have been over-emphasized. However, while successful treatment depends on a number of steps, all aimed at removing microbes from the root canal and keeping those microbes from communicating with the periradicular tissues, the root filling itself is the key to permanent exclusion of root canal infection.

A great number of root filling techniques have been proposed, including lateral condensation, vertical condensation of heat softened core material, chemically softened core material with a chloroform–rosin sealer, and thermomechanical compaction of core material heated by friction with rotating compaction [273,297].

Each technique has proponents that claim superiority of their technique over others. However, there is little scientific evidence to support such claims. In fact many studies show no difference among the techniques [2,74,220,305].

Scientific evaluation strongly indicates that a sealer must coat the core material; that the canal should appear radiographically to contain a dense fill; and that the fill should be about 0–1 mm short of the radiographic apex. Not least importantly, the root filling should be covered by a tightly fitting coronal restoration [193,220,274,305].

12.8 Treatment of exacerbations

While some postoperative pain is to be expected after the microbial control phase of treatment of a tooth with apical periodontitis, pain sufficient to require an unscheduled visit for evaluation is rare. This occurs in approximately 3–5% of primary cases and 15% of refractory cases [13,279,289]. If the theoretical causes of exacerbations are taken into account, these reactions can be decreased. Thus, periapical mechanical irritation is prevented by meticulously adjusting the working length so as not to instrument or push debris through the apical foramen. Unless technically impossible, the canal should be fully instrumented to adequate sizes at the first visit and the canal filled with an intracanal medicament or filling material so as to remove additional microbes and/or to limit space and nutrition for the proliferation of additional microbes.

Postoperative pain can be decreased by giving the patient a loading dose of nonsteroidal antiinflammatory agents before the treatment commences, to be continued every 4–6 hours after treatment as needed [100,104,154]. Pre-operative loading with antibiotics, however, does not decrease the incidence of postoperative exacerbations. The psychological aspects of pain should not be overlooked. A patient will tolerate moderate pain much more readily if he or she has been warned in advance that some pain is to be expected. Some patients may be somewhat disorientated after root canal therapy, and it may be wise to give them written instructions that mild to moderate pain is to be expected. Persistent or increasing pain may indicate an infection which should be treated separately. If there is no swelling, the patient is not febrile and the pain is elicited mainly by touching the tooth, the pain is most likely of mechanical origin and should be treated by relieving the occlusion and with systemic administration of nonsteroidal analgesics. Narcotic analgesics should be avoided if possible as they offer little if any additional effectiveness against the pain and the side-effects are considerable. If it is determined that the patient's psychological reaction to the pain is playing a part in intensifying the pain, an anti-anxiety medication can be given separately from the analgesics.

If the patient shows signs of an active infection (swelling, fever), measures aimed at removing the infection should be taken. If the pain is severe and an apical abscess is suspected, one may consider opening the tooth and gently passing a small file through the apical foramen in order to get drainage. If a fluctuant swelling is present and drainage through the tooth is not successful, an incision and drainage procedure with or without a drain should be considered. Penicillin VK in high doses for 7–10 days is still considered the antibiotic of choice. If in 48 hours the patient does not show signs of improvement, metronidazole can be administered in addition to the penicillin. For patients allergic to penicillin, clindamycin is a good alternative.

Once the symptoms have been controlled the patient should be brought back to the office for assessment of the cause of the exacerbation. The working lengths should be reevaluated, additional canals should be carefully looked for and the final sizes of instrumentation reassessed. Generally, if the incidence of exacerbations over an extended period is higher than the norm (~5%), aseptic techniques, sterilization methods and treatment techniques must be thoroughly reassessed.

12.9 Treatment of refractory or recurrent apical periodontitis

When apical periodontitis does not heal, either following long-term medication or after root filling, a state of refractory or recurrent apical periodontitis exists. It is apparent that the conventional treatment strategy suitable for primary apical periodontitis is inadequate in these cases.

Treatment of a tooth with apical periodontitis that has had prior root canal treatment is a special challenge. Retreatments show a relatively poor prognosis [74]. The low success rate may be a reflection of the technical difficulty of removing all the previous filling and infectious material from the pulp canal system. It may also be a result of the presence of a microbial community refractory to disinfection by the conventional approach for teeth with apical periodontitis. Another reason for failure may be that the microorganisms are located extraradicularly [247–250,271–277]. *Actinomyces israelii* and *Propionibacterium propionicum* are known to be able to survive in the soft tissues in periapical lesions [277] (Fig. 12.7). In addition, oral microorganisms may organize in an extraradicular plaque on the external root surface in long-standing canal infections [249,250,277] (Fig. 12.6b). Foreign-body reaction to the excess filling material may also be a cause of persistent periapical tissue inflammation [124]. This would explain why it is not possible to grow bacteria in some cases of persistent apical periodontitis. Another possible cause of refractory disease is the presence of a "true" cyst dissociated from the root apex [168,223,224]. There is, however, no means of diagnosing such a cyst or predicting whether or not they may heal after root canal therapy.

12.9.1 Intraradicular refractory infection

Infection of a filled root canal system, as well as that of root canals subjected to long-term medication, poses many additional problems compared with the infection in primary apical periodontitis. The microbial flora is different in refractory cases, with *E. faecalis* of special interest [192]. *E. faecalis* is relatively tolerant of standard root canal antibacterial agents like NaOCl and Ca(OH)$_2$ [50,53,117,190–192,225]. In addition, dentine, root filling materials, and other canal components can neutralize and block the movement of the antibacterial agents.

A primary consideration for the retreatment strategy is whether it will be possible to improve on the previous root filling taking into account the canal contents (e.g., posts) and the position of the previous instrumentation and filling (e.g., ledging, perforations, etc.). Obstructions to the root canal must be eliminated, and the old filling removed with the aid of a solvent and friction heat from rotary endodontic instruments. If not endangering the integrity of the root, it should be instrumented to considerably larger sizes than previously. Full strength (5%) NaOCl is used as irrigant alternating with buffered EDTA. The tissue-dissolving effect of NaOCl may be better at this high concentration [41]. Energizing the irrigation with passive (the ultrasonic file does not contact the canal walls) ultrasonic energy will strengthen the antimicrobial efforts, and a final soak with 2% chlorhexidine or 5% iodine–potassium iodide for at least 60 s may be advantageous [128]. A creamy mix of Ca(OH)$_2$ is meticulously placed and capped with a 4-mm deep temporary restoration for 7–30 days. The above procedures would ensure that all intracanal, antibacterial efforts have been applied to the case, and if the patient is comfortable and the canal dry, the root canal should be filled at the second visit.

However, if it is determined at the outset that retreatment will not improve on the previous root canal or removal of posts or other obstacles contraindicates conservative retreatment, a surgical approach to treatment should be considered (see below and Chapter 13).

12.9.2 *Extraradicular refractory infection*

Extraradicular infections present particular problems for the anti-infective measures in treatment [277]. Thus, if an extraradicular infection exists, the primary, intracanal application of root canal medicaments will not reach the infecting microbes and the treatment will not succeed [275,277]. Repeating futile efforts by conservative retreatment procedures also obviously will not help.

The challenge is to identify if the persistent apical periodontitis is a true extraradicular infection. This is particularly difficult because the limitations of radiographs may make an inadequate root filling appear satisfactory radiographically. On the other hand, a perfectly well-treated canal may become infected due to breakdown of the coronal restoration and the poor seal of many traditional root filling materials.

Two strategies exist for the treatment of extraradicular infections: antibiotics and surgery. In either case, treatment should be preceded by the placement or replacement of an optimal intracanal filling.

Antibiotics. Since the bacteria involved are facing soft tissues with adequate blood supply, they should in theory be exposed to adequate concentrations of systemic antibiotics when administered in high doses [1]. However, they may form plaques on the root surface or microcommunities in the tissues with the characteristics of biofilms, which may make the infection robust and resist even high serum concentrations of antibiotics [249,277] (see Chapter 5). An intracanal exudate may be useful in characterizing the bacteria and provide a susceptibility profile of the infecting organisms, and systemic antibiotics (see Chapter 7) may be applied successfully in selected clinical cases.

Surgical endodontics. A surgical approach to refractory apical periodontitis should always be considered [249,277]. If the surgical approach is selected, the principles include removal of all extraradicular diseased tissue, removal of complex anatomy by root resection, and the placement of a 4-mm plug to obturate the end of the root thus trapping any remaining bacteria in the root canal system. Whether using the retrofilling or plug, the aim of treatment is that bacteria trapped inside the root canal system can no longer communicate with the surrounding periradicular tissues and induce or sustain periapical inflammation [275,277] (see Chapter 13).

The introduction of the operating microscope, ultrasonic preparation instruments, and improved retrofilling materials have considerably improved the probability of success for surgical endodontic treatment [98,198,239]. This approach is indicated when an extraradicular infection is suspected or when conditions within the root canal system make conventional retreatment dangerous.

12.10 Treatment of immature permanent teeth with apical periodontitis

12.10.1 Apexification

The immature permanent tooth with apical periodontitis presents special challenges. The canal is infected, but mechanical instrumentation cannot be aggressive due to the thin dentinal walls, and the apex is open so that even if disinfection is successful it is difficult to adequately fill the root canal without a matrix against which to pack the root filling material. Lastly even if the first two challenges are successfully addressed, the thin walls of the root are always susceptible to root fracture.

Apexification with long-term $Ca(OH)_2$ has for many years been the treatment of choice for these teeth [9,49,275,282] (Fig. 12.14). The canals are disinfected with a combination of light instrumentation, copious irrigation with 5.25% NaOCl, and $Ca(OH)_2$ medication replaced every 3 months until a hard tissue barrier forms as the natural healing response at the apex. When the hard tissue barrier is formed, the root is filled typically with thermoplasticized filling material packed against the apical barrier. The thin dentinal walls are then reinforced with a bonded resin to below the bone level.

There are some disadvantages of the traditional technique: it takes a long time (3–18 months) requiring strict patient compliance [67,68,132]; the long-term $Ca(OH)_2$ treatment may further weaken the thin dentinal walls [4,216,217]; and the length of treatment leaves the root susceptible to fracture for too long before the root can be reinforced internally. However, the probability of success from an endodontic point of view is excellent [14,49,281]. The susceptibility to fracture remains a question unanswered in the literature up to now [73].

In order to shorten the time taken for the procedure a technique using mineral trioxide aggregate (MTA) as a hard barrier has become popular [5,68,

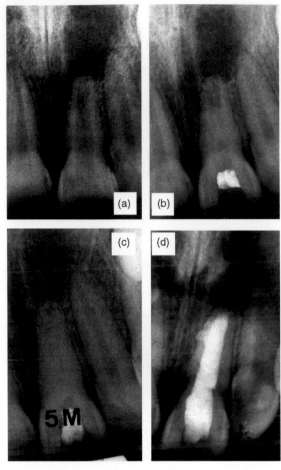

Fig. 12.14 Apexification. Tooth with necrotic infected root canal, thin dentinal walls and an open apex (a). The root canal was disinfected with long-term Ca(OH)$_2$ paste (b, c) and within 12 months a hard tissue barrier had formed which enabled filling of the canal without overfill (d).

82,126,136,145,217,242] (Fig. 12.15). In this procedure the canal is disinfected as before, but 4 mm of MTA is placed at the apex closing off the open apex. When the MTA has set the canal can be root filled and reinforced. This treatment can be performed in a number of weeks rather than months resulting in fewer visits to the dentist for the patient and presumably less susceptibility to fracture for the tooth. While case histories have been presented showing hard tissue formation underneath such MTA barriers, few if any outcome studies have compared this newer procedure with the traditional, long-term Ca(OH)$_2$ apexification technique [68].

12.10.2 Revascularization

Under certain conditions a necrotic immature tooth may revascularize and regain vitality [10]. The critical factors necessary for this to occur are that the canal remain free of microbes and the necrotic pulp can act as a scaffold into which the new vital tissue can grow through the open apex. Hoshino *et al.* [106] successfully used a tri-antibiotic paste to disinfect root canals in immature teeth. The effectiveness of the paste was confirmed in dogs by Windley *et al.* [298]. Preliminary data from studies in dogs indicate that if a blood clot is used as a scaffold after effective disinfection, revascularization is possible. Several case reports have confirmed that revascularization procedures may be applied clinically with clinical and biological success [195,298] (Fig. 12.16).

12.11 Prognosis

University-based studies on endodontic outcome have shown the overall success rate to be around 90% [193,282]. However, cross-sectional, retrospective population studies have revealed success rates of only 60–75% [193,282]. There is a consistent association in the cross-sectional studies between poor quality of the root fillings and the presence of a periapical radiolucency [193,274]. However, several epidemiological studies have demonstrated that many pre-treatment, intra-treatment, and post-treatment factors may influence the prognosis of the root canal treatment (see Chapter 14).

Pre-treatment factors. Of the many pre-treatment, prognostic factors that at times have been considered relevant to treatment of apical periodontitis, only the size of the lesion at start [39] and the presence of deep periodontal pockets [178] are dominant as risk factors for a poor treatment outcome.

Treatment-related factors. Several treatment-related factors may influence the prognosis. These include apical extent of root canal filling, apical enlargement, number of treatment sessions, materials and techniques, and treatment complications. Extrusion of filling materials beyond the root-end generally results in a poorer treatment outcome in cases with periapical inflammation, but not in teeth with a healthy apical periodontium. In infected canals a short filling (2 mm or shorter) results in a poorer healing rate, whereas

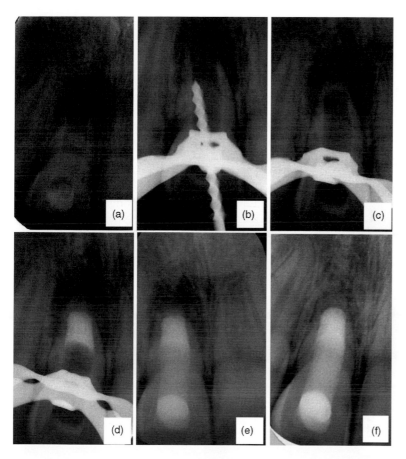

Fig. 12.15 Apexification. The infected canal (a) is cleansed with light instrumentation and copious irrigation and a creamy mix of Ca(OH)$_2$ is placed (b). Calcium sulfate powder is placed through the apex so as to create a barrier (c) against which 4 mm of MTA is packed (d). The canal is filled with Resilon and Epiphany sealer and a bonded resin is placed below the bone level in order to reinforce the tooth and resist fracture (e, and follow-up in f). (Courtesy of Dr Marga Ree.)

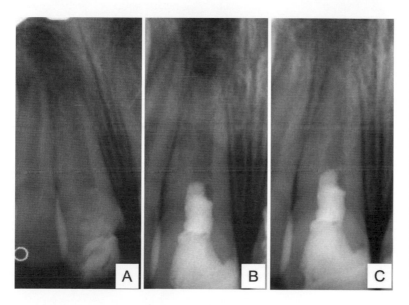

Fig. 12.16 Revascularization. The immature tooth with a necrotic infected canal and apical periodontitis (a) is disinfected with irrigation with NaOCl and the placement of tri-antibiotic paste. After 4 weeks the antibiotic is removed and a blood clot created in the canal space. The access is filled with an MTA base and bonded resin above it. At 7 months the patient is asymptomatic and the apex shows some signs of healing the apical periodontitis and closure of the apex (b). At 12 months apical healing is obvious and root wall thickening has occurred indicating that the root canal has been revascularized and contains vital tissue (c). (Courtesy of Dr B. Thibodeau.)

in noninfected canals filling short does not affect the treatment outcome. Also the use of a $Ca(OH)_2$ intracanal medicament in teeth with apical periodontitis appears to result in a higher incidence of healing. Some studies have demonstrated a high success rate (about 90%) using the modified step-back technique, i.e., larger apical sizes [121]. Also it appears that different sealers may influence the prognosis of the treatment [180]. Treatment complications such as perforations in the furcation area, file separations, and sealer extrusion contribute to a surprisingly small portion (4%) of failures of endodontic treatment [246].

Post-treatment factors. It has become increasingly clear that bacterial penetration along the root filling subsequent to endodontic therapy may lead to root canal infection and consequently to failure. The coronal restoration must protect the root canal filling material and provide an additional barrier to reinfection of the root canal space. In cases where the canal is filled with gutta-percha and sealer the coronal restoration may be as effective (and thus important) as the root filling in stopping coronal leakage of microbes.

Monitoring healing or development of apical periodontitis. Failures following endodontic therapy do occur and clinical–radiographic follow-up examina-tion should take place 12 months after completion of the treatment [178]. The period of observation can be extended up to 4 years for treatment of apical periodontitis, as healing may be very slow in some instances [76].

Clinical studies. In the past 80 years numerous studies have been published on the prognosis and treatment outcome of endodontic therapy. Most of these studies vary considerably in material composition, treatment procedures, and methodology, which makes it difficult to compare them and come to solid conclusions. However, the information accumulated from these studies provides a general insight into the outcome of endodontic therapy. It is apparent from the studies that the prognosis of treatment of apical periodontitis is very good when properly performed under optimal conditions.

Endodontic treatment of teeth in the presence of apical periodontitis has a success rate 10–25% lower than when it is not present preoperatively. The poorer outcome of treatment in teeth with apical periodontitis highlights the difference between prevention (which is a challenge of asepsis) and treatment (which is a challenge of disinfection) of an established disease. The poorer outcome may reflect a lack of understand-ing of the importance of disinfection of the root canal

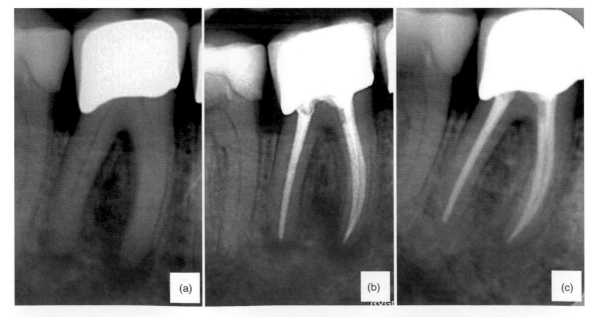

Fig. 12.17   Healing of apical periodontitis following treatment with the proposed disinfection and filling protocol.

before it is filled. In retreatment cases, pretreatment apical periodontitis is even more detrimental to the treatment outcome, highlighting the difficulty in disinfecting the root canals of previously treated canals. The protocol suggested in this chapter is based on extensive clinical documentation [30–33,37,151,222,236,237,254,255] and when followed will ensure that the prognosis of teeth with pretreatment apical periodontitis will approach that of teeth without (Fig. 12.17).

12.12 References

1. Abbott PV, Hume WR, Pearman JW (1990) Antibiotics and endodontics. *Australian Dental Journal* **35**, 50–60.
2. Abitbol S (2001) Outcome of non-surgical endodontic treatment. MSc Dissertation. Toronto: University of Toronto.
3. Abou-Rass M, Bogen G. (1998) Microorganisms in closed periapical lesions. *International Endodontic Journal* **31**, 39–47.
4. Andreasen JO, Farik B, Munksgaard EC (2002) Long-term calcium hydroxide as a root canal dressing may increase risk of root fracture. *Dental Traumatology* **18**, 134–7.
5. Andreasen JO, Munksgaard EC, Bakland LK (2006) Comparison of fracture resistance in root canals of immature sheep teeth after filling with calcium hydroxide or MTA. *Dental Traumatology* **22**, 154–6.
6. Arrastia-Jitosho AM, Liaw LH, Lee W, Wilder-Smith P (1988) Effects of a 532 nm Q-switched nanosecond pulsed laser on dentin. *Journal of Endodontics* **24**, 427–31.
7. Austin JH, Taylor HD (1918) Behavior of hypochlorite and of chloramine-T solutions in contact with necrotic and normal tissue in vivo. *Journal of Experimental Medicine* **27**, 627–63.
8. Ayukawa Y (1994) Pulpal response of human teeth to antibacterial biocompatible pulp-capping agent-improvement of mixed drugs. *Japanese Journal of Conservative Dentistry* **37**, 643–51.
9. Bakland L, Andreasen JO (2004) Dental traumatology: essential diagnosis and treatment planning. *Endodontic Topics* **7**, 14–34.
10. Banchs F, Trope M (2004) Revascularization of immature permanent teeth with apical periodontitis: new treatment protocol? *Journal of Endodontics* **30**, 196–200.
11. Barbakow F, Peters O, Havranek L (1999) Effects of Nd:YAG lasers on root canal walls: a light and scanning electron microscopic study. *Quintessence International* **30**, 837–45.
12. Barbosa CA, Goncalves RB, Siqueira JF Jr, DeUzeda M (1997) Evaluation of the antimicrobial activities of calcium hydroxide, chlorhexidine, and camphorated paramonochlorophenol as an intracanal medicament. A clinical and laboratory study. *Journal of Endodontics* **23**, 297–300.
13. Barnett F, Tronstad L (1989) The incidence of flare-ups following endodontic treatment. *Journal of Dental Research* **68**, 1253.
14. Barnett F (2002) The role of endodontics in the treatment of luxated permanent teeth. *Dental Traumatology* **18**, 47–56.
15. Barthel CR, Moshonov J, Shuping G, Ørstavik D (1999) Bacterial leakage versus dye leakage in obturated root canals. *International Endodontic Journal* **32**, 370–5.
16. Baumgartner JC, Ibay AC (1987) The chemical reactions of irrigants used for root canal debridement. *Journal of Endodontics* **13**, 47–51.
17. Baumgartner JC, Mader CL (1987) A scanning electron microscopic evaluation of four root canal irrigation regimens. *Journal of Endodontics* **13**,147–57.
18. Baumgartner JC, Johal S, Marshall JG (2007) Comparison of the antimicrobial efficacy of 1.3% NaOCl/BioPure MTAD to 5.25% NaOCl/15% EDTA for root canal irrigation. *Journal of Endodontics* **33**, 48–51.
19. Beltz RE, Torabinejad M, Pouresmail M (2003) Quantitative analysis of the solubilizing action of MTAD, sodium hypochlorite, and EDTA on bovine pulp and dentin. *Journal of Endodontics* **29**, 334–7.
20. Bender IB, Seltzer S, Turkenkopf S (1964) To culture or not to culture? *Oral Surgery, Oral Medicine, Oral Pathology* **18**, 527–40.
21. Bergenholtz G (1974) Micro-organisms from necrotic pulp of traumatized teeth. *Odontologisk Revy* **25**, 347–58.
22. Bergenholtz G, Lekholm U, Milthon R, Engström B (1979) Influence of apical overinstrumentation and overfilling on retreated root canals. *Journal of Endodontics* **5**, 310–14.
23. Bergenholtz G (1990) Pathogenic mechanisms in pulpal disease. *Journal of Endodontics* **16**, 98–101.
24. Bergenholtz G, Dahlén G. (2004) Advances in the study of endodontic infection: introduction. *Endodontic Topics* 9,1–4.
25. Blum JY, Abadie MJ (1997). Study of the Nd:YAP laser. Effect on canal cleanliness. *Journal of Endodontics* **23**, 669–75.
26. Blum JY, Michailesco P, Abadie MJ (1997) An evaluation of the bactericidal effect of the Nd:YAP laser. *Journal of Endodontics* **23**, 583–5.
27. Buchanan LS (1999) The standardized-taper root canal preparation, part I: Concepts for variably tapered shaping instruments. *Dentistry Today* **18**, 78–86.
28. Buchanan LS (1999) The standardized-taper root canal preparation, part II: GT file selection and safe handpiece-driven file use. *Dentistry Today* **18**, 68–70, 72 6.
29. Byström A, Sundqvist G (1981) Bacteriologic evaluation of the efficacy of mechanical root canal instrumentation in endodontic therapy. *Scandinavian Journal of Dental Research* **89**, 321–8.
30. Byström A, Sundqvist G (1983) Bacteriologic evaluation of the effect of 0.5 percent sodium hypochlorite in endodontic therapy. *Oral Surgery, Oral Medicine, Oral Pathology* **55**, 307–12.
31. Byström A, Sundqvist G (1985) The antibacterial action of sodium hypochlorite and EDTA in 60 cases of

endodontic therapy. *International Endodontic Journal* **18**, 35–40.

32. Byström A, Claesson R, Sundqvist G (1985) The antibacterial effect of camphorated paramonochlorophenol, camphorated phenol and calcium hydroxide in the treatment of infected root canals. *Endodontics and Dental Traumatology* **1**, 170–5.

33. Byström A, Happonen R, Sjögren U, Sundqvist G (1987) Healing of periapical lesions of pulpless teeth after endodontic treatment with controlled asepsis. *Endodontics and Dental Traumatology* **3**, 58–63.

34. Caliskan MK, Sen BH (1986) Endodontic treatment of teeth with apical periodontitis using calcium hydroxide: a long term study. *Endodontics and Dental Traumatology* **12**, 215–21.

35. Cameron JA (1995) Factors affecting the clinical efficiency of ultrasonic endodontics: a scanning electron microscopy study. *International Endodontic Journal* **28**, 47–53.

36. Cameron JA (1995) The choice of irrigant during hand instrumentation and ultrasonic irrigation of the root canal: a scanning electron microscope study. *Australian Dental Journal* **40**, 85–90.

37. Card SJ, Sigurdsson A, Ørstavik D, Trope M (2002) The effectiveness of increased apical enlargement in reducing intracanal bacteria. *Journal of Endodontics* **28**, 779–83.

38. Chance K, Lin L, Shovlin FE, Skribner J (1987) Clinical trial of intracanal corticosteroid in root canal therapy. *Journal of Endodontics* **13**, 466–8.

39. Chugal NM, Clive JM, Spångberg LSW (2001) A prognostic model for assessment of the outcome of endodontic treatment: effect of biologic and diagnostic variables. *Oral Surgery, Oral Medicine, Oral Pathology, Oral Radiology, and Endodontics* **91**, 342–52.

40. Chugal NM, Clive JM, Spångberg LS (2003) Endodontic infection: Some biologic and treatment factors associated with outcome. *Oral Surgery, Oral Medicine, Oral Pathology, Oral Radiology and Endodontics* **96**, 81–90.

41. Clarkson RM, Moule AJ, Podlich H, Kellaway R, Macfarlane R, Lewis D, *et al.* (2006) Dissolution of porcine incisor pulps in sodium hypochlorite solutions of varying compositions and concentrations. *Australian Dental Journal* **51**, 245–51.

42. Coons D, Dankowski M, Diehl M, *et al.* (1987) Performance in detergents, cleaning agents and personal care products, pp. 197–305. In: Falbe J, editor. *Surfactants in consumer products*. Berlin: Springer.

43. Cunningham W, Martin H, Forrest W (1982) Evaluation of root canal debridement by the endosonic ultrasonic synergistic system. *Oral Surgery, Oral Medicine, Oral Pathology* **53**, 401–4.

44. Cunningham W, Martin H (1982) A scanning electron microscope evaluation of root canal debridement with the endosonic ultrasonic synergistic system. *Oral Surgery, Oral Medicine, Oral Pathology* **53**, 527–31.

45. Cunningham W, Martin H, Pelleu G, Stoops D (1982) A comparison of antimicrobial effectiveness of endosonic and hand root canal therapy. *Oral Surgery, Oral Medicine, Oral Pathology* **54**, 238–41.

46. Cvek M, Nord CE, Hollender L (1976) Antimicrobial effect of root canal debridement in teeth with immature root. A clinical and microbiologic study. *Odontologisk Revy* **27**, 1–10.

47. Cvek M, Hollender L, Nord C-E (1976) Treatment of non-vital permanent incisors with calcium hydroxide. VI. A clinical, microbiological and radiological evaluation of treatment in one sitting with mature or immature root. *Odontologisk Revy* **27**, 93–108.

48. Cvek M, Granath L, Lundberg M (1983) Failures and healing in endodontically treated non-vital anterior teeth with posttraumatically reduced pulpal lumen. *Acta Odontologica Scandinavica* **40**, 223–8.

49. Cvek M (1994) Endodontic management of traumatized teeth. In Andreassen JO, Andreassen FM, editors. *Textbook and color atlas of traumatic injuries to the teeth*, pp. 517–86, 3rd edn. Copenhagen: Munksgaard.

50. Dahlén G, Samuelsson W, Molander A, Reit C (2000) Identification and antimicrobial susceptibility of enterococci isolated from the root canal. *Oral Microbiology and Immunology* **15**, 309–12.

51. Dakin HD (1915) On the use of certain antiseptic substances in treatment of infected wounds. *British Medical Journal* **2**, 318–20.

52. Dalton BC, Ørstavik D, Phillips C, Pettiette M, Trope M (1998) Bacterial reduction with nickel–titanium rotary instrumentation. *Journal of Endodontics* **24**, 763–7.

53. Dametto FR, Ferraz CCR, Gomes BPFA, Zaia AA, Teixeira FB, Souza-Filho FJ (2005) In vitro assessment of the immediate and prolonged antimicrobial action of chlorhexidine gel as an endodontic irrigant against *Enterococcus faecalis*. *Oral Surgery, Oral Medicine, Oral Pathology, Oral Radiology and Endodontics* **99**, 768–72.

54. Demirel K, Baer PN, McNamara TF (1991) Topical application of doxycycline on periodontally involved root surfaces in vitro: comparative analysis of substantivity on cementum and dentin. *Journal of Periodontology* **62**, 312–16.

55. Di Lenarda R, Cadenaro M, Sbaizero O (2000) Effectiveness of 1 mol L^{-1} citric acid and 15% EDTA irrigation on smear layer removal. *International Endodontic Journal* **33**, 46–52.

56. Engström B, Hård af Segerstad L, Ramstrom G, Frostell G (1964) Correlation of positive cultures with the prognosis for root canal treatment. *Odontologisk Revy* **15**, 257–70.

57. Engström B, Lundberg M (1965) The correlation between positive culture and the prognosis of root canal therapy after pulpectomy. *Odontologisk Revy* **16**, 193–203.

58. Engström B, Spångberg L (1967) Wound healing after partial pulpectomy. A histological study performed on contralateral tooth pairs. *Odontologisk Tidskrift* **75**, 5–18.

59. Ercan E, Ozekinci T, Atakul F, Gül K (2004) Antibacterial activity of 2% chlorhexidine gluconate and 5.25% sodium hypochlorite in infected root canal: in vivo study. *Journal of Endodontics* **30**, 84–7.

60. Esberard RM, Carnes DL, del Rio CE (1996) pH changes at the surface of root dentin when using root canal sealers containing calcium hydroxide. *Journal of Endodontics* **22**, 399–401.

61. Estrela C, Pimenta FC, Ito II, Bammann LL (1988) In vitro determination of direct antimicrobial effect of calcium hydroxide. *Journal of Endodontics* **24**, 15–17.

62. Estrela C, Bammann LL, Pimenta FC, Pecora JD (2001) Control of microorganisms in vitro by calcium hydroxide pastes. *International Endodontic Journal* **34**, 341–5.

63. Evans MD, Baumgartner CJ, Khemaleelakul S, Xia T (2003) Efficacy of calcium hydroxide: chlorhexidine paste as an intracanal medication in bovine dentin. *Journal of Endodontics* **29**, 338–9.

64. Fabricius L, Dahlén G, Holm SE, Möller AJR (1982) Influence of combinations of oral bacteria on periapical tissues of monkeys. *Scandinavian Journal of Dental Research* **90**, 200–6.

65. Fabricius L (1982) Oral bacteria and apial periodontitis: an experimental study in monkeys. Thesis. Göteborg: University of Göteborg.

66. Farzaneh M, Abitbol S, Lawrence HP, Friedman S (2004) Treatment outcome in endodontics – the Toronto study. Phase II: initial treatment. *Journal of Endodontics* **30**, 302–9.

67. Felippe MCS, Felippe WT, Marques MM, Antoniazzi JH (2005) The effect of renewal of calcium hydroxide paste on the apexification and periapical healing of teeth with incomplete root formation. *International Endodontic Journal* **38**, 436–42.

68. Felippe WT, Felippe MCS, Rocha MJC (2006) The effect of mineral trioxide aggregate on the apexification and periapical healing of teeth with incomplete root formation. *International Endodontic Journal* **39**, 2–9.

69. Ferraz CCR, de Almeida Gomes BPF, Zaia AA, Teixeira FB, de Souza-Filho FJ (2001) In vitro assessment of the antimicrobial action and the mechanical ability of chlorhexidine gel as an endodontic irrigant. *Journal of Endodontics* **27**, 452–5.

70. Fisher FJ (1972) The effect of calcium hydroxide/water paste on micro-organisms in carious dentine. *British Dental Journal* **133**, 19–21.

71. Frais S, Ng YL, Gulabivala K (2001) Some factors affecting the concentration of available chlorine in commercial sources of sodium hypochlorite. *International Endodontic Journal* **34**, 206–15.

72. Friedman S, Löst C, Zarrabian M, Trope M (1985) Evaluation of success and failure after endodontic therapy glass ionomer cement sealer. *Journal of Endodontics* **21**, 384–90.

73. Friedman S, Moshonov J, Trope M (1993) Resistance to vertical fracture of roots, previously fractured and bonded with glass ionomer cement, composite resin and cyanoacrylate cement. *Dental Traumatology* **9**, 101–5.

74. Friedman S (2002) Considerations and concepts of case selection in the management of post-treatment endodontic disease (treatment failure). *Endodontic Topics* **1**, 54–78.

75. Friedman S, Abitbol S, Lawrence HP (2003) Treatment outcome in endodontics: the Toronto study. Phase 1: initial treatment. *Journal of Endodontics* **29**, 787–93.

76. Fristad I, Molven O, Halse A (2004) Nonsurgically retreated root filled teeth – radiographic findings after 20–27 years. *International Endodontic Journal* **37**, 1–12.

77. Fukushima H, Yamamoto K, Hirohata K, Sagawa H, Leung K-P, Walker CB (1990) Localization and identification of root canal bacteria in clinically asymptomatic periapical pathosis. *Journal of Endodontics* **16**, 534–8.

78. Gani O, Visvisian C (1999) Apical canal diameter in the first upper molar at various ages. *Journal of Endodontics* **25**, 689–91.

79. Gatti JJ, Dobeck JM, Smith C, White RR, Socransky SS, Skobe Z (2000) Bacteria of asymptomatic periradicular endodontic lesions identified by DNA–DNA hybridization. *Endodontics and Dental Traumatology* **16**, 197–204.

80. Gesi A, Bergenholtz G (2003). Pulpectomy – studies on outcome. *Endodontic Topics* **5**, 57–70.

81. Girard S, Paqué F, Badertscher M, Sener B, Zehnder M (2005) Assessment of a gel-type chelating preparation containing 1-hydroxyethylidene-1,1-bisphosphonate. *International Endodontic Journal* **38**, 810–16.

82. Giuliani V, Baccetti T, Pace R, Pagavino G (2002) The use of MTA in teeth with necrotic pulps and open apices. *Dental Traumatology* **18**, 217–21.

83. Gomes BP, Ferraz CC, Vianna ME, Berber VB, Teixeira FB, Souza-Filho FJ (2001) In vitro antimicrobial activity of several concentrations of sodium hypochlorite and chlorhexidine gluconate in the elimination of *Enterococcus faecalis*. *International Endodontic Journal* **34**, 424–8.

84. Gomes BP, Souza SF, Ferraz CC, Teixeira FB, Zaia AA, Valdrighi L, *et al.* (2003) Effectiveness of 2% chlorhexidine gel and calcium hydroxide against *Enterococcus faecalis* in bovine root dentine in vitro. *International Endodontic Journal* **36**, 267–75.

85. Gomes BPFA, Sato E, Ferraz CCR, Teixeira FB, Zaia AA, Souza-Filho FJ (2003) Evaluation of time required for recontamination of coronally sealed canals medicated with calcium hydroxide and chlorhexidine. *International Endodontic Journal* **36**, 604–9.

86. Gomes BPFA, Pinheiro ET, Gade-Neto CR, Sousa ELR, Ferraz CCR, Zaia AA, *et al.* (2004) Microbiological examination of infected dental root canals. *Oral Microbiology and Immunology* **24**, 71–81.

87. Goodis HE, White JM, Marshall SJ, Marshall GW Jr (1993) Scanning electron microscopic examination of intracanal wall dentin: hand versus laser treatment. *Scanning Microscopy* **7**, 979–87.

88. Greenstein G, Berman C, Jaffen R (1986) Chlorhexidine an adjunct to periodontal therapy. *Journal of Periodontology* **57**, 370–6.

89. Griffee MB, Patterson SS, Miller CH, Kafrawy AH, Newton CW (1980) The relationship of *Bacteroides melaninogenicus* to symptoms associated with pulpal necrosis. *Oral Surgery* **50**, 457–61.

90. Grossman LI, Meiman BW (1941) Solution of pulp tissue by chemical agents. *Journal of the American Dental Association* **28**, 223–5.

91. Grossman LI (1943) Irrigation of root canals. *Journal of the American Dental Association* **30**, 1915–17.

92. Guerisoli DMZ, Marchesan MA, Walmsley AD, Lumley PJ, Pecora JD (2002) Evaluation of smear layer removal by EDTAC and sodium hypochlorite with

ultrasonic agitation. *International Endodontic Journal* **35**, 418–21.

93. Gutknecht N, Nuebler-Moritz M, Burghardt SF, Lampert F (1997) The efficiency of root canal disinfection using a holmium:yttrium–aluminum–garnet laser in vitro. *Journal of Clinical Laser Medicine and Surgery* **15**, 75–8.

94. Haapasalo HK, Sirén EK, Waltimo TM, Ørstavik D, Haapasalo MP (2000) Inactivation of local root canal medicaments by dentine: an in vitro study. *International Endodontic Journal* **33**, 126–31.

95. Haapasalo M, Ørstavik D (1987) In vitro infection and disinfection of dentinal tubules. *Journal of Dental Research* **66**, 1375–9.

96. Haapasalo M, Udnæs T, Endal U (2003) Persistent, recurrent and acquired infection of the root canal system post-treatment. *Endodontic Topics* **6**, 29–56.

97. Haapasalo M, Endal U, Zand H, Coil JR (2005) Eradication of endodontic infection by instrumentation and irrigation solutions *Endodontic Topics* **10**, 77–102.

98. Hoskinson AE (2005) Hard tissue management: osseous access, curettage, biopsy and root isolation. *Endodontic Topics* **11**, 98–113.

99. Hargreaves KM, Seltzer S (2002) Pharmacological control of dental pain. In Hargreaves KM, Goodis HE, editors. *Seltzer and Bender's dental pulp*, pp. 205–26. Chicago, IL: Quintessence.

100. Hargreaves K, Keiser K (2002) Building effective strategies for the management of endodontic pain. *Endodontic Topics* **3**, 93–105.

101. Hasselgren G, Olsson B, Cvek M (1988) Effects of calcium hydroxide and sodium hypochlorite on the dissolution of necrotic porcine muscle tissue. *Journal of Endodontics* **14**, 125–7.

102. Heling I, Rotstein I, Dinur T, Szwec-Levine Y, Steinberg D (2001) Bactericidal and cytotoxic effects of sodium hypochlorite and sodium dichloroisocyanurate solutions in vitro. *Journal of Endodontics* **27**, 278–80.

103. Hermann BW (1920) Calciumhydroxide als Mittel zum Behandel und Füllungen von Zahnwurzelkanälen. Medical dissertation. Würzburg: V. Würzburg.

104. Holstein A, Hargreaves KM, Niederman R (2002). Evaluation of NSAIDs for treating post-endodontic pain. *Endodontic Topics* **3**, 3–13.

105. Hoshino E, Kota K, Sato M, Iwaku M (1988) Bactericidal efficacy of metronidazole against bacteria of human carious dentin. *Caries Research* **22**, 280–2.

106. Hoshino E, Kurihara-Ando N, Sato I, *et al.* (1996) In vitro antimicrobial susceptibility of bacteria taken from infected root dentine to a mixture of ciprofloxacin, metronidazole and minocycline. *International Endodontic Journal* **29**, 125–30.

107. Hugo WB, Longworth AR (1964) Some aspects of the mode of action of chlrorhexidine. *Journal of Pharmacy and Pharmacology* **16**, 665–72.

108. Hugo WB, Russel AD (1998) *Pharmaceutical microbiology*, 6th edn. Oxford: Blackwell.

109. Hülsmann M, Hahn W (2000) Complications during root canal irrigation – literature review and case reports. *International Endodontic Journal* **33**, 186–93.

110. Hülsmann M, Heckendorff M, Lennon A (2003) Chelating agents in root canal treatment (mode of action and indications for their use). *International Endodontic Journal* **36**, 810–30.

111. Ingham HR, Selkon JB, Hale JH (1975) The antibacterial activity of metronidazole. *Journal of Antimicrobial Chemotherapy* **1**, 355–61.

112. Iwaya S, Ikawa M, Kubota M (2001) Revascularization of an immature permanent tooth with apical periodontitis and sinus tract. *Dental Traumatology* **17**, 185–7.

113. Iwy C, Macfarlane TW, Mackenzie D, Stenhouse D (1990) The microbiology of periapical granulomas. *Oral Surgery, Oral Medicine, Oral Pathology* **69**, 502–5.

114. Jeansonne MJ, White RR (1994) A comparison of 2.0% chlorhexidine gluconate and 5.25% sodium hypochlorite as antimicrobial endodontic irrigants. *Journal of Endodontics* **20**, 276–8.

115. Kaitsas V, Signore A, Fonzi L, Benedicenti S, Barone M (2001) Effects of Nd:YAG laser irradiation on the root canal wall dentin of human teeth: a SEM study. *Bulletin du Groupement International pour la Recherche Scientifique en Stomatologie & Odontologie* **43**, 87–92.

116. Kakehashi S, Stanley HR, Fitzgerald RJ (1965) The effects of surgical exposures of dental pulps in germ-free and conventional laboratory rats. *Oral Surgery, Oral Medicine, Oral Pathology* **18**, 340–8.

117. Kayaoglu G, Ørstavik D (2004) Virulence factors of *Enterococcus faecalis*: relationship to endodontic disease. *Critical Reviews in Oral Biology and Medicine* **15**, 308–20.

118. Kerekes K, Tronstad L (1977) Morphometric observations on root canals of human anterior teeth. *Journal of Endodontics* **3**, 24–9.

119. Kerekes K, Tronstad L (1977) Morphometric observations on root canals of human premolars. *Journal of Endodontics* **3**, 74–9.

120. Kerekes K, Tronstad L (1977) Morphometric observations on the root canals of human molars. *Journal of Endodontics* **3**, 114–18.

121. Kerekes K, Tronstad L (1979) Long-term results of endodontic treatment performed with a standardized technique. *Journal of Endodontics* **5**, 83–90.

122. Kesler G, Gal R, Kesler A, Koren R (2002) Histological and scanning electron microscope examination of root canal after preparation with Er:YAG laser microprobe: a preliminary in vitro study. *Journal of Clinical Laser Medicine and Surgery* **20**, 269–77.

123. King JB, Crawford JJ, Lindhahl, RL (1965) Indirect pulp capping: a bacteriological study of deep carious dentin in human teeth. *Oral Surgery, Oral Medicine, Oral Pathology* **20**, 663–71.

124. Koppang HS, Koppang R, Solheim T, Aarneals H, Stølen SØ (1989) Cellulose fibers from endodontic paper points as an etiologic factor in postendodontic periapical granulomas and cysts. *Journal of Endodontics* **15**, 369–72.

125. Koskinen KP, Meurman JH, Stenvall H (1980) Appearance of chemically treated root canal walls in the scanning electron microscope. *Scandinavian Journal of Dental Research* **88**, 505–12.

126. Kratchman SI (2004) Perforation repair and one-step apexification procedures. *Dental Clinics of North America* **48**, 291–307.

127. Kuruvilla JR, Kamath MP (1998) Antimicrobial activity of 2.5% sodium hypochlorite and 0.2% chlorhexidine gluconate separately and combined, as endodontic irrigants. *Journal of Endodontics* **24**, 472–6.

128. Kvist T, Molander A, Dahlén G, Reit C (2004) Microbiological evaluation of one- and two-visit endodontic treatment of teeth with apical periodontitis: a randomized, clinical trial, *Journal of Endodontics* **30**, 572–6.

129. Langeland K (1987) Tissue response to dental caries. *Endodontics and Dental Traumatology* **3**, 149–71.

130. Laws AJ (1962) Calcium hydroxide as a possible root filling material. *New Zealand Dental Journal* **58**, 199–215.

131. Le Goff A, Bunetel L, Mouton C, Bonnaure-Mallet M (1997) Evaluation of root canal bacteria and their antimicrobial susceptibility in teeth with necrotic pulp. *Oral Microbiology and Immunology* **12**, 318–22.

132. Leonardo MR, Silva LAB, Leonardo RT, Utrilla LS, Assed S (1993) Histological evaluation of therapy using a calcium hydroxide dressing for teeth with incompletely formed apices and periapical lesions. *Journal of Endodontics* **19**, 348–52.

133. Liesenhoff T, Lenz H, Seiler T (1989) Root canal preparation using Excimer laser beams. *Zahnärztliche Welt, Zahnärztliche Reform* **98**, 1034–9.

134. Lin L, Shovlin F, Skribner J, Langeland K (1984) Pulp biopsies from the teeth associated with periapical radiolucencies. *Journal of Endodontics* **10**, 436–48.

135. Lindskog S, Pierce AM, Blomlöf L (1998) Chlorhexidine as a root canal medicament for treating inflammatory lesions in the periodontal space. *Endodontics and Dental Traumatology* **14**, 186–90.

136. Linsuwanont P (2003) MTA apexification combined with conventional root canal retreatment. *Australian Endodontic Journal* **29**, 45–9.

137. Liolios E, Economides N, Parissis-Messimeris S, Boutsioukis A (1997) The effectiveness of three irrigating solutions on root canal cleaning after hand and mechanical preparation. *International Endodontic Journal* **30**, 51–7.

138. Loel DA (1975) Use of acid cleanser in endodontic therapy. *Journal of the American Dental Association* **90**, 148–51.

139. Love R (2004) Invasion of dentinal tubules by root canal bacteria. *Endodontic Topics* **9**, 52–65.

140. Lumley PJ, Walmsley AD (1992) Effect of precurving on the performance of endosonic files. *Journal of Endodontics* **18**, 232–6.

141. Machado-Silveiro LF, Gonzalez-Lopez S, Gonzalez-Rodriguez MP (2004) Decalcification of root canal dentine by citric acid, EDTA and sodium citrate. *International Endodontic Journal* **37**, 365–9.

142. Machida T, Wilder-Smith P, Arrastia AM, Liaw LH, Berns MW (1995) Root canal preparation using the second harmonic KTP:YAG laser: a thermographic and scanning electron microscopic study. *Journal of Endodontics* **21**, 88–91.

143. Madison S, Swanson K, Chiles SA (1987) An evaluation of coronal microleakage in endodontically treated teeth. Part II. Sealer types. *Journal of Endodontics* **13**, 109–12.

144. Madison S, Wilcox LR (1988) An evaluation of coronal microleakage in endodontically treated teeth. Part III. In vivo study. *Journal of Endodontics* **14**, 455–8.

145. Maroto M, Barbería E, Planells P, Vera V (2003) Treatment of a non-vital immature incisor with mineral trioxide aggregate (MTA). *Dental Traumatology* **19**,165–9.

146. Martin H (1976) Ultrasonic disinfection of the root canal. *Oral Surgery, Oral Medicine, Oral Pathology* **42**, 92–9.

147. Martin H, Cunningham W (1985) Endosonics – the ultrasonic synergistic system of endodontics. *Endodontics and Dental Traumatology* **1**, 201–6.

148. Matsuo T, Shirakami T, Ozaki K, Nakanishi T, Yumoto H, Ebisu S (2003) An immunohistological study of the localization of bacteria invading root pulpal walls of teeth with periapical lesions. *Journal of Endodontics* **29**, 194–200.

149. Mayer BE, Peters OA, Barbakow F (2002) Effects of rotary instruments and ultrasonic irrigation on debris and smear layer scores: a scanning electron microscopic study. *International Endodontic Journal* **35**, 582–9.

150. McCann JT, Keller DL, LaBounty GL (1990) Remaining dentin/cementum thickness after hand or ultrasonic instrumentation. *Journal of Endodontics* **16**, 109–13.

151. McGurkin-Smith R, Trope M, Caplan D, Sigurdsson A (2005) Reduction of intracanal bacteria using GT rotary instrumentation, 5.25% NaOCl, EDTA, and Ca(OH)$_2$. *Journal of Endodontics* **31**, 359–63.

152. McKendry DJ (1990) Comparison of balanced forces, endosonic, and step-back filing instrumentation techniques: quantification of extruded apical debris. *Journal of Endodontics* **16**, 24–7.

153. Mehl A, Folwaczny M, Haffner C, Hickel R (1999) Bactericidal effects of 2.94 microns Er:YAG-laser radiation in dental root canals. *Journal of Endodontics* **25**, 490–3.

154. Menhinick KA, Gutmann JL, Regan JD, Taylor SE, Buschang PH (2004) The efficacy of pain control following nonsurgical root canal treatment using ibuprofen or a combination of ibuprofen and acetaminophen in a randomized, double-blind, placebo-controlled study. *International Endodontic Journal* **37**, 531–41.

155. Mjor A, Furseth R (1968) The inorganic phase of calcium hydroxide- and corticosteroid-covered dentin studied by electron microscopy. *Archives of Oral Biology* **13**, 755–63.

156. Mitchell DF, Shankwalker GD (1958) Osteogenic potential of calcium hydroxide and other materials in soft tissue and bone wounds. *Journal of Dental Research* **37**, 1157–63.

157. Mohorn HW, Dowson J, Blankenship JR (1971) Pressure exerted by odontic periapical lesions. *Oral Surgery, Oral Medicine, Oral Pathology* **31**, 810–18.

158. Molander A, Reit C, Dahlén G, Kvist T (1998) Microbiological status of root-filled teeth with apical periodontitis. *International Endodontic Journal* **31**, 1–7.

159. Molander A, Dahlén G (2003) Evaluation of the antibacterial potential of tetracycline or erythromycin mixed with calcium hydroxide as intracanal dressing against *Enterococcus faecalis* in vivo. *Oral Surgery, Oral*

Medicine, Oral Pathology, Oral Radiology and Endodontology **96**, 744–50.

160. Molven O, Halse A (1988) Success rates for gutta-percha and kloroperka N-Ø root fillings made by undergraduate students: radiographic findings after 10–17 years. *International Endodontic Journal* **21**, 243–50.

161. Moorer WR, Wesseling PR (1982) Factors promoting the tissue dissolving capability of sodium hypochlorite. *International Endodontic Journal* **15**, 187–96.

162. Morfis A, Sykaras SN, Georgopoulou M, Kernani M, Prountzos F (1994) Study of the apices of human permanent teeth with the use of a scanning electron microscope. *Oral Surgery, Oral Medicine, Oral Pathology* **77**, 172–6.

163. Moshonov J, Ørstavik D, Yamauchi S, Pettiette M, Trope M (1995) Nd:YAG laser irradiation in root canal disinfection. *Endodontics and Dental Traumatology* **11**, 220–4.

164. Möller AJR, Fabricius L, Dahlén G, Öhman AE, Heyden G (1981) Influence on periapical tissues of indigenous oral bacteria and necrotic pulp tissue in monkeys. *Scandinavian Journal of Dental Research* **89**, 475–84.

165. Naenni N, Thoma K, Zehnder M (2004) Soft tissue dissolution capacity of currently used and potential endodontic irrigants. *Journal of Endodontics* **30**, 785–7.

166. Nair PNR (1987) Light and electron microscopic studies of root canal flora and periapical lesions. *Journal of Endodontics* **13**, 29–39.

167. Nair PNR, Sjögren U, Krey G, Kahnberg K-E, Sundqvist G (1990) Intraradicular bacteria and fungi in root-filled, asymptomatic human teeth with therapy-resistant periapical lesions: a long-term light and electron microscopic follow-up study. *Journal of Endodontics* **16**, 580–8.

168. Nair PNR (2003) Non-microbial etiology: periapical cysts sustain post-treatment apical periodontitis. *Endodontic Topics* **6**, 96–113.

169. Nair PNR (2003) Non-microbial etiology: foreign body reaction maintaining post-treatment apical periodontitis. *Endodontic Topics* **6**, 114–34.

170. Nerwich A, Figdor D, Messer HM (1993) pH changes in dentine over a four week period following root canal dressing with calcium hydroxide. *Journal of Endodontics* **19**, 302–6.

171. Nygaard Østby B (1957) Chelation in root canal therapy. *Odontologisk Tidskrift* **65**, 3–11.

172. O'Keefe EM (1976) Pain in endodontic therapy: preliminary study. *Journal of Endodontics* **2**, 315–19.

173. Oliet S (1983) Single visit endodontics: a clinical study. *Journal of Endodontics* **9**, 147–53.

174. Onçagö M, Hosgör M, Hilmioglu S, Zekioglu O, Eronat C, Burhanoglu D (2003) Comparison of antibacterial and toxic effects of various root canal irrigants. *International Endodontic Journal* **36**, 423–32.

175. Ørstavik D, Kerekes K, Molven O (1991) Effects of extensive apical reaming and calcium hydroxide dressing on bacterial infection during treatment of apical periodontitis: a pilot study. *International Endodontic Journal* **24**, 1–7.

176. Ørstavik D, Hörsted-Bindslev P (1993) A comparison of endodontic treatment results at two dental schools. *International Endodontic Journal* **26**, 348–54.

177. Ørstavik D (1996) Time-course and risk analyses of the development and healing of chronic apical periodontitis in man. *International Endodontic Journal* **29**, 150–5.

178. Ørstavik D, Qvist K, Stoltze K (2004) A multivariate analysis of the outcome of endodontic treatment. *European Journal of Oral Sciences* **112**, 224.

179. Ørstavik D (2005) Materials used for root canal obturation: technical, biological and clinical testing. *Endodontic Topics* **12**, 25–8.

180. Ørstavik D, Kerekes K, Eriksen HM (1987) Clinical performance of three endodontic sealers. *Endodontics and Dental Traumatology* **3**, 178–86.

181. Pashley EL, Birdsong NL, Bowman K, Pashley DH (1985) Cytotoxic effects of NaOCl on vital tissue. *Journal of Endodontics* **11**, 525–8.

182. Patterson SS (1963) In vivo and in vitro studies of the effect of the disodium salt of ethylenediamine tetra-acetate on human dentine and its endodontic implications. *Oral Surgery, Oral Medicine, Oral Pathology* **16**, 83–103.

183. Peters LB, Wesselink PR, Moorer WR (1995) The fate and the role of bacteria left in root dentinal tubules. *International Endodontic Journal* **28**, 95–9.

184. Peters LB, van Winkelhoff AJ, Buijs JF, Wesselink PR (2002) Effects of instrumentation, irrigation and dressing with calcium hydroxide on infection in pulpless teeth with periapical bone lesions. *International Endodontic Journal* **35**, 13–21.

185. Peters LB, Wesselink PR (2002) Periapical healing of endodontically treated teeth in one and two visits obturated in the presence or absence of detectable microorganisms. *International Endodontic Journal* **35**, 660–7.

186. Peters OA, Boessler C, Zehnder M (2005) Effect of liquid and paste-type lubricants on torque values during simulated rotary root canal instrumentation. *International Endodontic Journal* **38**, 223–9.

187. Pettiette MT, Metzger Z, Phillips C, Trope M (1999) Endodontic complications of root canal therapy performed by dental students with stainless-steel K-files and nickel–titanium hand files. *Journal of Endodontics* **25**, 230–4.

188. Pierce A, Lindskog S (1987) The effect of an antibiotic/corticosteroid paste on inflammatory root resorption in vivo. *Oral Surgery, Oral Medicine and Oral Pathology* **64**, 216–20.

189. Pierce A, Heithersay G, Lindskog S (1988) Evidence for direct inhibition of dentinoclasts by a corticosteroid/antibiotic endodontic paste. *Endodontics and Dental Traumatology* **4**, 44–5.

190. Portenier I, Haapasalo H, Rye A, Waltimo T, Ørstavik D, Haapasalo M (2001) Inactivation of root canal medicaments by dentine, hydroxylapatite and bovine serum albumin. *International Endodontic Journal* **34**, 184–8.

191. Portenier I, Haapasalo H, Ørstavik D, Yamauchi M, Haapasalo M (2002) Inactivation of the antibacterial activity of iodine potassium iodide and chlorhexidine digluconate against *Enterococcus faecalis* by dentin, dentin matrix, type-I collagen, and heat-killed microbial whole cells. *Journal of Endodontics* **28**, 634–7.

192. Portenier I, Waltimo T, Haapasalo M (2003) *Enterococcus faecalis* – the root canal survivor and 'star' in post-treatment disease. *Endodontic Topics* **6**, 135–59.

193. Ray HA, Trope M (1995) Periapical status of endodontically treated teeth in relation to the technical quality of the root filling and the coronal restoration. *International Endodontic Journal* **28**, 12–18.

194. Ricucci D, Bergenholtz G (2004) Histologic features of apical periodontitis in human biopsies. *Endodontic Topics* **8**, 68–87.

195. Ritter ALS, Ritter AV, Murrah V, Sigurdsson A, Trope M (2004) Pulp revascularization of replanted immature dog teeth after treatment with minocycline and doxycycline assessed by laser Doppler flowmetry, radiography, and histology. *Dental Traumatology* **20**, 75–84.

196. Rôças IN, Siqueira Jr JF, Santos KRN (2004) Association of *Enterococcus faecalis* with different forms of periradicular diseases. *Journal of Endodontics* **30**, 315–20.

197. Rollison S, Barnett F, Stevens RH (2002) Efficacy of bacterial removal from instrumented root canals in vitro related to instrumentation technique and size. *Oral Surgery, Oral Medicine, Oral Pathology* **94**, 366–71.

198. Rubinstein R (2005) Magnification and illumination in apical surgery. *Endodontic Topics* **11**, 56–77.

199. Sabala CC, Powell SE (1989) Sodium hypochlorite injection into periapical tissues. *Journal of Endodontics* **15**, 490–2.

200. Sabins RA, Johnson JD, Hellstein JW (2003) A comparison of the cleaning efficacy of short term sonic and ultrasonic passive irrigation after hand instrumentation in molar root canals. *Journal of Endodontics* **29**, 674–8.

201. Safavi KE, Dowden WE, Introcaso JH, Langeland K (1985) A comparison of antimicrobial effects of calcium hydroxide and iodine–potassium iodide. *Journal of Endodontics* **11**, 454–6.

202. Safavi KE, Nichols FC (1993) Effect of calcium hydroxide on bacterial lipopolysaccharide. *Journal of Endodontics* **19**, 76–8.

203. Safavi KE, Nichols FC (1994) Alteration of biological properties of bacterial lipopolysaccharide by calcium hydroxide treatment. *Journal of Endodontics* **20**, 127–9.

204. Sathorn C, Parashos P, Messer HH (2005) Effectiveness of single- versus multiple-visit endodontic treatment of teeth with apical periodontitis: a systematic review and meta-analysis. *International Endodontic Journal* **38**, 347–55.

205. Sato T, Hoshino E, Uematsu H, Kota K, Iwaku M, Noda T (1992) Bactericidal efficacy of a mixture of ciprofloxacin, metronidazole, minocycline and rifampicin against bacteria of carious and endodontic lesions of human deciduous teeth in vitro. *Microbial Ecology in Health and Disease* **5**, 171–7.

206. Sato I, Kurihara-Ando N, Kota K, Iwaku M, Hoshino E (1996) Sterilization of infected root-canal dentine by topical application of a mixture of ciprofloxacin, metronidazole and minocycline in situ. *International Endodontic Journal* **29**, 118–24.

207. Scelza MF, Teixeira AM, Scelza P (2003) Decalcifying effect of EDTA-T, 10% citric acid, and 17% EDTA on root canal dentin. *Oral Surgery, Oral Medicine,*

Oral Pathology, Oral Radiology and Endodontology **95**, 234–6.

208. Schilder H (1974) Cleaning and shaping the root canal. *Dental Clinics of North America* **18**, 269.

209. Schoop U, Moritz A, Kluger W, Patruta S, Goharkhay K, Sperr W, et al. (2002) The Er:YAG laser in endodontics: results of an in vitro study. *Lasers in Surgery and Medicine* **30**, 360–4.

210. Schulz-Bongert U, Weine FS, Schulz-Bongert J (1995) Preparation of curved canals using a combined hand-filing, ultrasonic technique. *Compendium of Continuing Education in Dentistry* **16**, 272–4.

211. Seltzer S, Bender IB, Turkenkopf S (1963) Factors affecting successful repair after root canal therapy. *Journal of the American Dental Association* **67**, 651–62.

212. Seltzer S (1978) *Pain control in dentistry: diagnosis and management*. Philadelphia, PA: Lippincott.

213. Sena NT, Gomes BPFA, Vianna ME, Berber VB, Zaia AA, Ferraz CCR, et al. (2006) In vitro antimicrobial activity of sodium hypochlorite and chlorhexidine against selected single-species biofilms. *International Endodontic Journal* **39**, 878–85.

214. Senia ES, Marshall FJ, Rosen S (1971) The solvent action of sodium hypochlorite on pulp tissue of extracted teeth. *Oral Surgery, Oral Medicine, Oral Pathology* **31**, 96–103.

215. Seyle H (1956) The stress-concept as it presents itself in 1956. *Antibiotics and Chemotherapy* **3**, 1–17.

216. Shabahang S, Torabinejad M, Boyne PP, Abedi H, McMillan P (1999) A comparative study of root-end induction using osteogenic protein-1, calcium hydroxide, and mineral trioxide aggregate in dogs. *Journal of Endodontics* **25**, 1–5.

217. Shabahang S, Torabinejad M (2000) Treatment of teeth with open apices using mineral trioxide aggregate. *Practical Periodontics & Aesthetic Dentistry* **12**, 315–20.

218. Shabahang S, Pouresmail M, Torabinejad M (2003) In vitro antimicrobial efficacy of MTAD and sodium. *Journal of Endodontics* **29**, 450–2.

219. Shabahang S, Torabinejad M (2003) Effect of MTAD on *Enterococcus faecalis* contaminated root canals of extracted human teeth. *Journal of Endodontics* **29**, 576–9.

220. Shipper G, Ørstavik D, Teixeira FB, Trope M (2004) An evaluation of microbial leakage in roots filled with a thermoplastic synthetic polymer-based root canal filling material (Resilon). *Journal of Endodontics* **30**, 342–7.

221. Shipper G, Teixeira FB, Arnold RA, Trope M (2005) Periapical inflammation after coronal microbial inoculation of dog roots filled with gutta-percha or Resilon. *Journal of Endodontics* **31**, 91–6.

222. Shuping GB, Ørstavik D, Sigurdsson A, Trope M (2000) Reduction of intracanal bacteria using nickel–titanium rotary instrumentation and various medications. *Journal of Endodontics* **26**, 751–5.

223. Simon JHS (1980) Incidence of periapical cysts in relation to the root canal. *Journal of Endodontics* **6**, 845–8.

224. Simon JHS, Enciso R, Malfaz JM, Roges R, Bailey-Perry M, Patel A (2006) Differential diagnosis of large periapical lesions using cone-beam computed tomog-

raphy measurements and biopsy. *Journal of Endodontics* **32**, 833-7.

225. Sirén EK, Haapasalo MP, Waltimo TM, Ørstavik D (2004) In vitro antibacterial effect of calcium hydroxide combined with chlorhexidine or iodine potassium iodide on *Enterococcus faecalis*. *European Journal of Oral Sciences* **112**, 326–31.

226. Siqueira JF Jr, de Uzeda M (1996) Disinfection by calcium hydroxide pastes of dentinal tubules infected with two obligate and one facultative anaerobic bacteria. *Journal of Endodontics* **22**, 674–6.

227. Siqueira JF Jr, Uzeda M (1997) Intracanal medicaments: Evaluation of the antibacterial effects of chlorhexidine, metronidazole, and calcium hydroxide associated with three vehicles. *Journal of Endodontics* **3**, 167–9.

228. Siqueira JF Jr, Lima KC, Magalhaes FA, Lopes HP, de Uzeda M (1999) Mechanical reduction of the bacterial population in the root canal by three instrumentation techniques. *Journal of Endodontics* **25**, 332–5.

229. Siqueira JF Jr, Rôças IN, Favieri A, Lima KC (2000) Chemomechanical reduction of the bacterial population in the root canal after instrumentation and irrigation with 1%, 2.5%, and 5.25% sodium hypochlorite. *Journal of Endodontics* **26**, 331–4.

230. Siqueira JF Jr, Lopes HP (2001) Bacteria on the apical root surfaces of untreated teeth with periradicular lesions: a scanning electron microscopy study. *International Endodontic Journal* **34**, 216–20.

231. Siqueira JF Jr, Rocas IN, Santos SR, Lima KC, Magalhaes FA, de Uzeda M (2002) Efficacy of instrumentation techniques and irrigation regimens in reducing the bacterial population within root canals. *Journal of Endodontics* **28**, 181–4.

232. Siqueira J (2003) Taxonomic changes of bacteria associated with endodontic infections. *Journal of Endodontics* **29**, 619–23.

233. Siqueira JF Jr, Rôças IN (2005) Exploiting molecular methods to explore endodontic infections: part 2 – redefining the endodontic microbiota. *Journal of Endodontics* **31**, 488–98.

234. Sirtes G, Waltimo T, Schaetzle M, Zehnder M (2005) The effects of temperature on sodium hypochlorite short-term stability, pulp dissolution capacity, and antimicrobial efficacy. *Journal of Endodontics* **31**, 669–71.

235. Sjögren U, Hägglund B, Sundqvist G, Wing K (1990) Factors affecting the long-term results of endodontic treatment. *Journal of Endodontics* **16**, 498–504.

236. Sjögren U, Figdor D, Spångberg L, Sundqvist G (1991) The antimicrobial effect of calcium hydroxide as a short-term intracanal dressing. *International Endodontic Journal* **24**, 119–25.

237. Sjögren U, Figdor D, Persson S, Sundqvist G (1997) Influence of infection at the time of root filling on the outcome of endodontic treatment of teeth with apical periodontitis. *International Endodontic Journal* **30**, 297–306.

238. Spångberg L, Rutberg M, Rydinge E (1979) Biologic effects of endodontic antimicrobial agents. *Journal of Endodontics* **5**, 166–75.

239. Stropko JJ, Doyon GE, Gutmann JL (2005) Root-end management: resection, cavity preparation, and material placement. *Endodontic Topics* **11**, 131–51.

240. Stabholz A, Kettering J, Aprecio R, Zimmerman G, Baker PJ, Wikesjö UM (1993) Retention of antimicrobial activity by human root surfaces after in situ subgingival irrigation with tetracycline HCl or chlorhexidine. *Journal of Periodontology* **64**, 137–41.

241. Stabholz A, Kettering J, Aprecio R, Zimmerman G, Baker PJ, Wikesjö UM (1993) Antimicrobial properties of human dentin impregnated with tetracycline HCl or chlorhexidine. An in vitro study. *Journal of Clinical Periodontology* **20**, 557–62.

242. Steinig TH, Regan JD, Gutmann JL (2003) The use and predictable placement of Mineral Trioxide Aggregate in one-visit apexification cases. *Australian Endodontic Journal* **29**, 34–42.

243. Steinberg D, Heling I, Daniel I, Ginsburg I (1999) Antibacterial synergistic effect of chlorhexidine and hydrogen peroxide against *Streptococcus sobrinus*, *Streptococcus faecalis* and *Staphylococcus aureus*. *Journal of Oral Rehabilitation* **26**, 151–6.

244. Stewart GG (1961) A study of a new medicament in the chemomechanical preparation of infected root canals. *Journal of the American Dental Association* **63**, 33–7.

245. Stewart GG, Kapsimalas P, Rappaport H (1969) EDTA and urea peroxide for root canal preparation. *Journal of the American Dental Association.* **78**, 335–8.

246. Strindberg LZ (1956) The dependence of the results of pulp therapy on certain factors. An analytic study based on radiographic and clinical follow-up examination. *Acta Odontologica Scandinavica* **14**, suppl 21.

247. Sunde PT, Olsen I, Lind PO, Tronstad L (2000) Extraradicular infection: a methodological study. *Endodontics and Dental Traumatology* **16**, 84–90.

248. Sunde PT, Tronstad L, Eribe ER, Lind PO, Olsen I (2000) Assessment of periradicular microbiota by DNA–DNA hybridization. *Endodontics and Dental Traumatology* **16**, 191–6.

249. Sunde PT, Olsen I, Debelian GJ, Tronstad L (2002) Microbiota of periapical lesions refractory to endodontic therapy. *Journal of Endodontics* **28**, 304–10.

250. Sunde PT, Olsen I, Göbel UB, Theegarten D, Winter S, Debelian GJ, *et al*. Fluorescence in situ hybridization (FISH) for direct visualization of bacteria in periapical lesions of asymptomatic root-filled teeth. *Microbiology* **149**, 1095–102.

251. Sundqvist G (1976) Bacteriological studies of necrotic dental pulps. Dissertation. Umeå: University of Umeå.

252. Sundqvist GK, Eckerbom MI, Larsson AP, Sjögren UF (1979) Capacity of anaerobic bacteria from necrotic dental pulps to induce purulent infections. *Infection and Immunity* **25**, 685.

253. Sundqvist G (1992) Associations between microbial species in dental root canal infections. *Oral Microbiology and Immunology* **7**, 257–62.

254. Sundqvist G, Figdor D, Persson S, Sjögren U (1998) Microbiologic analysis of teeth with failed endodontic treatment and outcome of conservative retreatment. *Oral Surgery, Oral Medicine, Oral Pathology* **85**, 86–93.

255. Sundqvist G, Figdor D (1998) Endodontic treatment of apical periodontitis. In Ørstavik D, Pitt Ford TR, editors. *Essential endodontology: prevention and treatment of apical periodontitis*. Oxford: Blackwell.

256. Sundqvist G, Figdor D (2003) Life as an endodontic pathogen. Etiological differences between untreated and root-filled root canals. *Endodontic Topics* **6**, 3–28.

257. Svensäter G, Bergenholtz G (2004) Biofilms in endodontic infections. *Endodontic Topics* **9**, 27–36.

258. Swanson K, Madison S (1987) An evaluation of coronal microleakage in endodontically treated teeth. Part I. Time periods. *Journal of Endodontics* **13**, 56–9.

259. Takeda FH, Harashima T, Kimura Y, Matsumoto K (1988) Comparative study about the removal of smear layer by three types of laser devices. *Journal of Clinical Laser Medicine and Surgery* **16**, 117–22.

260. Tanomaru Filho M, Leonardo MR, Silva LAB, Anibal EF, Faccioli LH (2002) Inflammatory response to different endodontic irrigating solutions. *International Endodontic Journal* **35**, 735–9.

261. Tay FR, Mazzoni A, Pashley DH, Day TE, Ngoh EC, Breschi L (2006) Potential iatrogenic tetracycline staining of endodontically treated teeth via NaOCl/MTAD irrigation: a preliminary report. *Journal of Endodontics* **32**, 354–8.

262. Taylor MA, Hume WR, Heithersay GS (1989) Some effects of Ledermix paste and Pulpdent paste on mouse fibroblasts and on bacteria in vitro. *Endodontics and Dental Traumatology* **5**, 266–73.

263. Teixeira FB, Teixeira EC, Thompson JY, Trope M (2004) Fracture resistance of roots endodontically treated with a new resin filling material. *Journal of the American Dental Association* **135**, 646–52.

264. Teixeira FB, Levin LG, Trope M (2005) Investigation of pH at different dentinal sites after placement of calcium hydroxide dressing by two methods. *Oral Surgery, Oral Medicine, Oral Pathology, Oral Radiology and Endodontology* **99**, 511–16.

265. Tittle K, Farley J, Linkhart T, Torabinejad M (1996) Apical closure induction using bone growth factors and mineral trioxide aggregate. *Journal of Endodontics* **22**, 198.

266. Torabinejad M, Khademi AA, Babagoli J, Cho Y, Johnson WB, Bozhilov K, *et al.* (2003) A new solution for the removal of the smear layer. *Journal of Endodontics* **29**, 170–5.

267. Torabinejad M, Cho Y, Khademi AA, Bakland LK, Shabahang S (2003) The effect of various concentrations of sodium hypochlorite on the ability of MTAD to remove the smear layer. *Journal of Endodontics* **29**, 233–9.

268. Torabinejad M, Shabahang S, Aprecio RM, Kettering JD (2003) The antimicrobial effect of MTAD: an in vitro investigation. *Journal of Endodontics* **29**, 400–3.

269. Tronstad L, Andreasen JO, Hasselgren G, Kristerson L, Riis I (1980) pH changes in dental tissues after root canal filling with calcium hydroxide. *Journal of Endodontics* **7**, 17–21.

270. Tronstad L, Yang Z-P, Trope M, Barnett F (1985) Controlled release of medicaments in endodontic therapy. *Endodontics and Dental Traumatology* **1**, 130–4.

271. Tronstad L, Barnett F, Riso K, Slots J (1987) Extraradicular endodontic infections. *Endodontics and Dental Traumatology* **3**, 86–90.

272. Tronstad L, Barnett F, Cervone F (1990) Periapical bacterial plaque in teeth refractory to endodontic treatment. *Endodontics and Dental Traumatology* **6**, 73–7.

273. Tronstad L, Kreshtool D, Barnett F (1990) Microbiological monitoring and results of treatment of extraradicular endodontic infection. *Endodontics and Dental Traumatology* **6**, 129–36.

274. Tronstad L, Asbjornsen K, Doving L, Pedersen I, Eriksen HM (2000) Influence of coronal restorations on the periapical health of endodontically treated teeth. *Endodontics and Dental Traumatology* **16**, 218–21.

275. Tronstad L (2003) *Clinical endodontics*, pp. 120–3. 2nd edn. Stuttgart: Thieme.

276. Tronstad L (2003) *Clinical endodontics*, pp. 189–201, 2nd edn. Stuttgart: Thieme.

277. Tronstad L, Sunde PT (2003) The evolving new understanding of endodontic infections. *Endodontic Topics* **6**, 57–77.

278. Trope M (1990) Relationship of intracanal medicaments to endodontic flare-ups. *Endodontics and Dental Traumatology* **6**, 226–9.

279. Trope M (1991) Flare-up rate of single-visit endodontics. *International Endodontic Journal* **24**, 24–7.

280. Trope M, Delano E, Ørstavik D (1999) Endodontic treatment of teeth with apical periodontitis: single vs multivisit treatment. *Journal of Endodontics* **25**, 345–50.

281. Trope M (2002) Clinical management of the avulsed tooth: present strategies and future directions. *Dental Traumatology* **18**, 1–11.

282. Trope M, Bergenholtz G (2002) Microbiological basis for endodontic treatment: can a maximal outcome be achieved in one visit? *Endodontic Topics* **1**, 40–53.

283. Trope M, Debelian G (2005) *Endodontics manual for the general dentist*, p. 57. London: Quintessence.

284. Valderhaug J (1972) A histologic study of experimentally induced radicular cysts. *International Journal of Oral Surgery* **1**, 137–47.

285. Vianna ME, Gomes BP, Berber VB, Zaia AA, Ferraz CC, de Souza-Filho FJ (2004) In vitro evaluation of the antimicrobial activity of chlorhexidine and sodium hypochlorite. *Oral Surgery, Oral Medicine, Oral Pathology, Oral Radiology and Endodontics* **97**, 79–84

286. Wåler SM (1990) Further in vitro studies on the plaque inhibiting effect of chlorhexidine and its binding mechanism. *Scandinavian Journal of Dental Research* **98**, 422–7.

287. Waltimo T, Haapasalo M, Zehnder M, Meyer J (2004) Clinical aspects related to endodontic yeast infections. *Endodontic Topics* **9**, 66–78.

288. Waltimo T, Trope M, Haapasalo M, Ørstavik D (2005) Clinical efficacy of treatment procedures in endodontic infection control and one year follow-up of periapical healing. *Journal of Endodontics* **31**, 863–6.

289. Walton R, Fouad A (1992) Endodontic interappointment flare-ups: a prospective study of incidence and related factors. *Journal of Endodontics* **18**, 172–7.

290. Walton RE, Ardjmand K (1992) Histological evaluation of the presence of bacteria in induced periapical lesions in monkeys. *Journal of Endodontics* **18**, 216–27.

291. Weber CD, McClanahan SB, Miller GA, Diener-West M, Johnson JD (2003) The effect of passive ultrasonic activation of 2% chlorhexidine or 5.25% sodium hypochlorite irrigant on residual antimicrobial activity in root canals. *Journal of Endodontics* **29**, 562–4.

292. Wang CS, Debelian GJ, Teixeira FB (2006) Effect of intracanal medicament on the sealing ability of root canals filled with Resilon. *Journal of Endodontics* **32**, 532–6.

293. Wang JD, Hume WR (1988) Diffusion of hydrogen ion and hydroxyl ion from various sources through dentine. *International Endodontic Journal* **21**, 17–26.

294. Wayman BE, Murata SM, Almeida RJ, Fowler CB (1992) A bacteriological and histological evaluation of 58 periapical lesions. *Journal of Endodontics* **18**, 152–5.

295. Weiger R, Rosendahl R, Löst C (2000) Influence of calcium hydroxide intracanal dressings on the prognosis of teeth with endodontically induced periapical lesions. *International Endodontic Journal* **33**, 219–26.

296. White RR, Hays GL, Janer LR (1997) Residual antimicrobial activity after canal irrigation with chlorhexidine. *Journal of Endodontics* **23**, 229–31.

297. Whitworth J (2005) Methods of filling root canals: principles and practice. *Endodontic Topics* **12**, 2–24.

298. Windley W III, Teixeira F, Levin L, Sigurdsson A, Trope M (2005) Disinfection of immature teeth with a triple antibiotic paste. *Journal of Endodontics* **31**, 439–43.

299. Wu MK, Barkis D, Roris A, Wesselink PR (2002) Does the first file to bind correspond to the diameter of the canal in the apical region? *International Endodontic Journal* **35**, 264–7.

300. Yamaguchi M, Yoshida K, Suzuki R, Nakamura H (1996) Root canal irrigation with citric acid solution. *Journal of Endodontics* **22**, 27–9.

301. Yared GM, Bou Dagher FE (1994) Influence of apical enlargement on bacterial infection during treatment of apical periodontitis. *Journal of Endodontics* **20**, 535–7.

302. Yoshida T, Shibata T, Shinohara T, Gomyo S, Sekine I (1995) Clinical evaluation of the efficacy of EDTA solution as an endodontic irrigant. *Journal of Endodontics* **21**, 592–3.

303. Yusuf H (1982) The significance of the presence of foreign material periapically as a cause of failure of root treatment. *Oral Surgery, Oral Medicine, Oral Pathology* **54**, 566–74.

304. Zamany A, Safavi K, Spångberg LS (2003) The effect of chlorhexidine as an endodontic disinfectant. *Oral Surgery, Oral Medicine, Oral Pathology, Oral Radiology and Endodontology* **96**, 578–81.

305. Zehnder M, Kosicki D, Luder H, Sener B, Waltimo T (2002) Tissue-dissolving capacity and antibacterial effect of buffered and unbuffered hypochlorite solutions. *Oral Surgery, Oral Medicine, Oral Pathology, Oral Radiology and Endodontology* **94**, 756–76.

306. Zehnder M, Schicht O, Sener B, Schmidlin P (2005) Reducing surface tension in endodontic chelator solutions has no effect on their ability to remove calcium from instrumented root canals. *Journal of Endodontics* **31**, 590–2.

307. Zehnder M, Schmidlin P, Sener B, Waltimo T (2005) Chelation in root canal therapy reconsidered. *Journal of Endodontics* **31**, 817–20.

308. Zehnder M (2006) Root canal irrigants. *Journal of Endodontics* **32**, 389–98.

309. Zeldow BJ, Ingle JI (1963) Correlation of the positive culture to the prognosis of endodontically treated teeth. A clinical study. *Journal of the American Dental Association* **66**, 9.

310. Zhang W, Torabinejad M, Li Y (2003) Evaluation of cytotoxicity of MTAD using the MTT-tetrazolium method. *Journal of Endodontics* **29**, 654–7.

Chapter 13
Surgical Treatment of Apical Periodontitis

Thomas Pitt Ford

13.1 Introduction, including history

Surgical management of teeth with apical periodontitis has been practiced for hundreds of years, although surgical resection of roots did not become commonplace until the 1880s [11,23,49], when the main concern was to remove the necrotic apex. At about the same time curettage was performed to remove diseased tissue around the apex, without necessarily addressing the source of the infection inside the root canal [154]. Root-end resection was developed in Germany in the 1890s [132–134], and this led to its widespread practice during the early part of the twentieth century in central Europe [50]. Root-end cavity preparation and filling with amalgam received attention at about the same time [29,103,156,196].

In the 1930s indications for surgical endodontics were proposed [140], and these influenced clinical practice for many decades. Surgical endodontic treatment has historically often been considered as an alternative to root canal treatment, or the preferred choice when root canal treatment is difficult or impossible. Much surgical endodontic treatment has been carried out with a poor outcome because clinicians have failed to appreciate the biological basis. Careful review of some clinical studies has shown that the success rates are so low as to question the value of the treatment [2,55]. More recently, experimental research has investigated the reasons for failure, and a major cause has been found to be continuing infection from the root canal. Unless the root canal space is effectively cleaned, shaped and filled during preliminary root canal treatment and/or root-end preparation, it remains as a source of infection that may allow inflammation to continue after surgical endodontics. Root-end resection may in fact create more avenues of communication between an infected root canal system and the tissues than previously existed, by opening up a large number of dentinal tubules that had naturally been sealed by cementum. It has also been realized that root-end fillings often do not provide the intended seal.

The current view is that root-end resection should be avoided where possible as root canal treatment, or retreatment, is likely to have a better outcome, and to be preferred by the patient [2,68]. Where root-end resection is indicated, beveling of the root end should be avoided because it opens up more dentinal tubules [35]. Second, root-end cavity preparation should be carried out with ultrasonic instruments to limit damage and achieve better canal cleaning [28,180]. Third, amalgam should not be used as the root-end filling material [144,193]. Fourth, it is essential to use magnification to see the root end during treatment [28,159].

13.2 Procedures

The various surgical procedures that will be reviewed are:

- curettage;
- root-end resection;
- perforation repair;
- replantation;
- root amputation, hemisection.

These will be considered in turn; these procedures may be carried out separately or in combination.

13.3 Indications

Apical periodontitis is a prerequisite for surgical endodontics. A surgical approach may be employed to establish drainage of an acute infection, to remove a lesion of apical periodontitis, or to place a filling in the root end to stop endodontic infection causing recurrent apical periodontitis. Historically, a large number of indications for surgical endodontics have been proposed [60,140], although the current view is that indications should be more limited, as root canal retreatment has a better outcome than surgery, particularly with improvements of techniques in root canal treatment [2,68].

Periapical granuloma

The presence of a periapical granuloma is not now considered an indication for surgical endodontics, but rather for the provision of good quality root canal treatment. Many studies have reported good healing of periapical lesions following root canal treatment [16,17,173,178] (this is covered in detail in Chapter 14).

Periapical cyst

The equating of a well-defined radiolucency with a cyst cannot now be supported [155], and many lesions considered cystic will heal following root canal treatment alone [119].

Horizontal root fracture

This condition is rarely an indication for surgical removal of the apex. In most instances, the pulp in the apical fragment remains vital, even if the pulp in the coronal fragment becomes necrotic [81].

Foreign material periapically

The mere presence of foreign material (usually root canal filling material) is not of itself an indication for its removal [68], unless it is toxic, has caused a foreign body response [118], or is associated with infection [117].

Perforation

The majority of root perforations can be managed conservatively [95], however the outcome is poor if the perforation is infected [110,122,149]. Some root perforations may require surgical repair; the prognosis is better when the perforation is near the apex, and surgically accessible. In addition to filling the perforation defect, the apical part of the root canal must be cleaned, shaped and filled to prevent failure. The majority of reports refer to limited numbers of cases; and long-term breakdown has been common, particularly when amalgam has been used, or the site is close to the gingival sulcus [122].

Broken instrument

Most root canal instruments are made from corrosion resistant alloys, therefore their removal on the grounds of irritancy is unjustified. In many instances, the instrument may be removed from the root canal by ultrasonics [116] or special extractors; in others it may be bypassed to allow the root canal to be cleaned and a root canal filling to be placed [54]. Where an instrument in the apical part of the canal cannot be removed or bypassed, it may need to be removed surgically if it is associated with infection in the uncleaned part of the canal [54].

Failed root canal treatment

This is generally best managed by root canal retreatment, particularly if there are technical deficiencies in the root canal filling [2]. Surgical endodontics might be considered as an alternative if the tooth has a post crown and supports a large fixed prosthesis, or if there is a high risk that the root might split during post removal.

Inaccessible root canal

With improved skills in root canal treatment, there are now relatively few canal systems that are inaccessible, so surgical endodontics is rarely indicated [68]. For a tooth with apical periodontitis where the pulp canal has been obliterated by calcification following trauma, and the root canal system is not negotiable, root-end resection and filling is indicated.

Biopsy

If there is significant concern that a lesion might be malignant then it should be biopsied [68].

Persisting radiolucency

If a radiolucency persists following root canal retreatment that is of good quality technically, curettage may be indicated to remove a lesion that has walled itself off from the body's defenses. However, if there is any doubt about the quality of the root canal treatment, root canal retreatment should be undertaken first.

Investigative surgery

On occasions surgery is required to investigate the possible presence of a longitudinal root fracture, or in the case of a perforation to assess its position and accessibility for repair [68].

13.4 Contraindications

Inadequate periodontal support

Root-end resection is contraindicated where the root is short, or there is extensive gingival recession, or extensive marginal periodontitis.

Nonrestorable tooth

If the tooth is carious, broken down or cracked in the floor of the pulp chamber, then it is essential to ascertain that it can be restored before undertaking surgical endodontics.

Poor access

If surgical access is severely restricted, it may not be possible to carry out surgical endodontics. This may occur because the patient has a small mouth, the apex is angled away from the access, or other anatomical structures are in the way or at too high risk of damage.

Medical conditions

These may require the patient to be prepared for the surgical procedure. Patients at risk of endocarditis require antibiotic cover; those with bleeding disorders require appropriate preparation by their hematologist; those on steroid therapy require an adjustment of dose prior to surgery. The medical condition becomes more significant if it is intended to use sedation or general anesthesia. Where the medical condition is complicated, there should be discussion with the patient's medical practitioner and/or specialist.

13.5 Anesthesia

Most surgical endodontics is carried out under local anesthesia, which must provide profound analgesia for patient comfort. The presence of a vasoconstrictor prolongs anesthesia and also provides a relatively bloodless field. A higher concentration of adrenalin in the local anesthetic reduces bleeding [65,208] if injected into the adjacent submucosa. Injections into the surrounding muscle should be avoided [208] otherwise bleeding may be increased.

13.6 Surgical anatomy

This will be considered first in general terms relating to the soft tissues and bone, and then in relation to specific structures which may be damaged during surgery, or which may restrict access.

13.6.1 General soft tissue anatomy

Surgical access to all roots apart from the palatal root in maxillary molars and occasionally in maxillary premolars is from the buccal aspect. On the buccal side there are three types of mucosa, namely, alveolar mucosa, attached gingiva, and marginal gingiva.

Alveolar mucosa

The mucosa in the sulcus is termed the alveolar mucosa. It is loosely attached to the underlying tissue and can be stretched as the lip is pulled. It has a thin non-keratinized epithelial covering, a fibrous underlayer

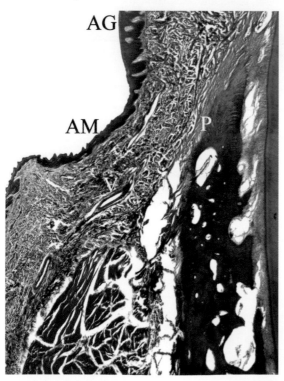

Fig. 13.1 Buccopalatal section through the alveolar mucosa (AM) and attached gingiva (AG) of a dog incisor. Note the vertical vessel (V) above the periosteum (P). (Original magnification ×100, Masson's trichrome stain.)

known as the lamina propria, and a loose connective tissue submucosa. The mucogingival junction separates the alveolar mucosa from the attached gingiva.

Attached gingiva

The attached gingiva has a thicker and keratinized epithelial layer than the alveolar mucosa (Fig. 13.1), and the lamina propria is bound down by fibers directly to the periosteum with the absence of a submucosa. The vasculature to both the alveolar mucosa and attached gingiva runs in a vertical direction, therefore horizontal incisions should preferably be avoided in order to reduce bleeding and so as not to compromise the blood supply to the remaining attached gingiva [91,101].

When a full thickness mucoperiosteal flap of attached gingiva is lifted, its vasculature is retained on its underside allowing the tissue to maintain a good blood supply and hence its vitality, so that rapid healing may occur afterwards.

13.6.2 Incisions

A number of incisions have been employed over the years. These have been reviewed [142,199,200].

Intrasulcular

This incision extends along the gingival sulcus of the tooth being treated and usually adjacent ones. There is normally a vertical incision at each end (Fig. 13.2), but one may be omitted if sufficient access to the root end is available. This flap was first reported in the 1930s [79], and provides good surgical access particularly to a large periradicular lesion; and the blood supply to the flap is kept intact [68]. Subsequent flap reapproximation is straightforward, and healing is normally by primary intention because all incision lines were placed on bone; the attached gingiva is stuck back by a very thin layer of fibrin to bone, therefore subsequent displacement is avoided, and epithelization across the incision wound can occur rapidly. There is little opportunity for the blood clot in the bony cavity to become infected [74]. Postoperative sequelae of pain and swelling are usually minimal, but a high level of oral hygiene postoperatively is essential [68]. A disadvantage of this traditional flap is that slight gingival recession may occur to expose a crown margin which had previously been in the gingival sulcus [94]; this is normally only a problem in the maxillary

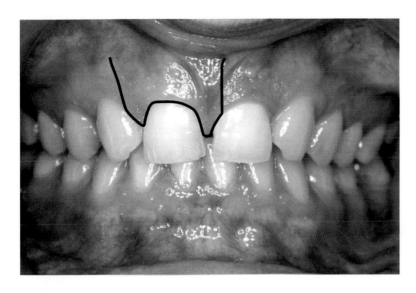

Fig. 13.2 Diagram to show incision line for an intrasulcular mucoperiosteal flap to allow surgery on a maxillary central incisor.

anterior region where the existing artificial crown is to be retained. Damage to the interdental papillae has been reported [62,198]. The papilla base incision was proposed to prevent loss of interdental papilla height [197], by leaving the papilla *in situ*. Data after 1 year showed significantly less recession with this type of incision [198].

Palatal flaps are usually only raised to treat palatal roots of molars or premolars. An incision is normally made along the gingival sulcus of several teeth, and a relieving incision placed in the premolar/canine region, where there are no underlying vessels of significance. The palatal mucosa resembles buccal attached gingiva, but has a submucosa. The need to be aware of the palatine neurovascular bundle is covered in a later section.

Submarginal

This flap, also known as the Luebke-Ochsenbein, is made in attached gingiva and follows the gingival contour, so taking on a scalloped outline, and at each end has a short vertical incision (Fig. 13.3) [104]. It appears to have been first proposed in the 1920s [121]. Of necessity it requires a wide attached gingiva, which may not always be present, so that a minimum of 3 mm is left between the base of the gingival sulcus and the incision, to prevent ischemia of the remaining attached gingiva. This flap often cannot be used in the mandible because of the restricted width of the attached gingiva. The overriding reason for selecting this flap design is to leave the gingival tissues

undisturbed [62], particularly adjacent to crowns. Disadvantages are that surgical access is limited if there is a large periradicular lesion, and that the blood supply to the remaining attached mucosa may be compromised. Because the free margin of the flap is in attached gingiva, it is much easier to suture back than a flap entirely in alveolar mucosa, and the attached gingiva is more resistant to tearing by sutures than alveolar mucosa. Postoperative scarring has sometimes been a problem [94].

Semilunar

This is the oldest type of flap design and dates back 100 years [22,68,133,135]; it consists of an incision entirely in alveolar mucosa and is typically curved apically at its ends (Fig. 13.4). It is not now widely practiced because it provides limited surgical access to a large periradicular lesion, as well as causing disruption to the blood supply, flap shrinkage, difficulty with reapproximation, more postoperative swelling and pain, slower healing because of exposed granulation tissue, and more scarring than any of the other designs (Fig. 13.5) [30,64,68,94]. There is a lack of systematic evidence on its suitability.

Vertical incision

This is a single vertical incision in the alveolar mucosa over the root, and the tissues are retracted laterally to reveal the bone over the apex [24,205]. It has

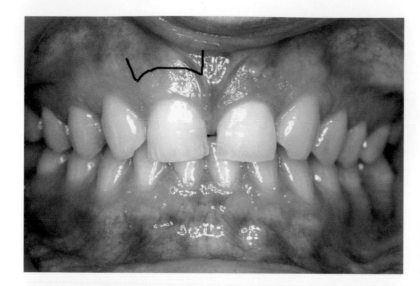

Fig. 13.3 Diagram to show incision line for a submarginal mucoperiosteal flap to allow surgery on a maxillary central incisor.

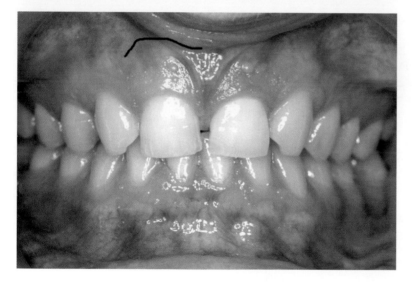

Fig. 13.4 Diagram to show incision line for a semilunar flap to allow limited surgery at the apex of a maxillary central incisor.

advantages over the semilunar flap of not cutting across vessels, and ease of reapproximation of the tissue. It is best suited to the maxillary anterior region, and to teeth with long roots. Disadvantages are limited access to a large periradicular lesion, and risk of postoperative infection because the incision may lie directly over the blood clot.

13.6.3 General osseous anatomy

After reflection of the mucoperiosteal flap, the lesion of apical periodontitis may on occasions be visible through a perforation in the cortical plate. The perforation is a guide for removal of surrounding bone and locating the apex. Quite often the cortical plate is intact but thin; it can be perforated with a sharp instrument to reveal the underlying periradicular lesion. Where the cortical plate has not been thinned, it is necessary to go through it with a bur. Care must be taken not to damage the underlying root which is often very close, nor to damage adjacent apices.

Bone removal is best achieved with a round bur using adequate coolant to avoid damaging osteocytes [20,177]. Sufficient bone should be removed to allow

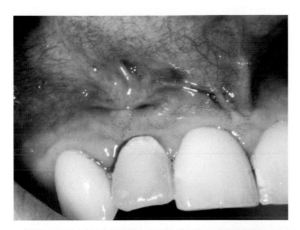

Fig. 13.5   Scarring following healing of a semilunar flap incision.

adequate access. Best practice dictates that the coolant is sterile and isotonic.

In the mandibular molar region where there is a thick cortical plate, a technique of bony lid removal has been performed [88]. In this technique a piece of the cortical plate over the apices is isolated by drilling a series of holes to allow the cortical plate to be prized off and placed in isotonic saline. After root-end surgery, the bone is replaced. In one clinical study a low incidence of postoperative complications was reported [88]. It is essential to avoid damage to the underlying roots from burs when this technique is used, since this may initiate inflammatory resorption in endodontically treated teeth that harbor any infection.

13.6.4 Specific anatomy

Maxillary sinus

The sinus is close to the root apices of the maxillary premolar and molar teeth, and the proximity varies among patients [3]. This relationship has been reviewed [76]. Prior to surgery the distance between the sinus and the root apices, as well as tooth length, should be determined from the preoperative radiograph; the use of tomography provides additional information [200]. When the maxillary sinus is in close proximity, it may be necessary to cut off a specific amount of the apex, rather than use a shaving technique which progressively removes dentin starting at the apex, in order to avoid penetrating the sinus. Sometimes perforation of the antral lining occurs, and consequently

the patient may become aware of cooling solution entering the nose. It is essential to avoid debris or the resected apex being forced into the maxillary sinus to prevent sinusitis [98]. After surgery the mucoperiosteal flap provides an effective seal from the mouth, and so an oro-antral fistula is a rare complication; in such instances healing is normally uneventful and it is unnecessary to prescribe antibiotics and antihistamines. There have been reports of performing palatal root surgery via an approach through the maxillary sinus [3,204]. This radical approach is in contrast to the usually conservative avoidance of the sinus, but minimal complications have been reported.

Palatine neurovascular bundle

The greater palatine neurovascular bundle emerges from the greater palatine foramen palatal to the second/third molar, and runs forward approximately midway between the midline of the palate and the gingival margin. With palatal flap surgery a vertical relieving incision should not be made in the molar region, to avoid damaging this neurovascular bundle. However, a relieving incision can be made in the premolar/canine region without risk of bleeding [67,68]. When the mucoperiosteal flap is raised, care must be taken to avoid damaging the bundle.

Inferior dental neurovascular bundle

This neurovascular bundle is at potential risk during surgery on mandibular molars and premolars. Careful assessment of the preoperative radiograph will indicate the proximity of the inferior dental canal. Usually the neurovascular bundle is inferior and lingual to the apices. Where the neurovascular bundle is in close proximity, it is usual to cut through the root to remove the apex rather than risk damage by using a shaving technique. Curettage inferior to the apex must necessarily be done with caution.

Mental neurovascular bundle

The position of the mental foramen should be identified on a preoperative radiograph as its position is variable. This neurovascular bundle is at risk, first with vertical incisions in the mandibular premolar region, secondly with bone removal, thirdly with root-end resection, and fourthly from crushing with a retractor [68]. Two alternative strategies have been employed: one is to find the neurovascular bundle and then protect it with a retractor [67,68], or secondly to keep well away. With the latter approach damage may occur if the operator is disorientated.

13.7 Curettage

Curettage is essentially removal of the soft tissue lesion of apical periodontitis from around the root end; it may be carried out with or without root-end resection. In the past many indications have been proposed but the indications for curettage alone are now limited, since most lesions of apical periodontitis will resolve following well-executed root canal treatment. Furthermore, as many lesions develop as a response to infection within the tooth, removal of the lesion will not effect a permanent cure [78], unless the root canal system is cleaned, shaped and filled. Curettage is now only undertaken to remove those lesions that do not respond to root canal treatment or retreatment, to remove excess filling material, or to biopsy a suspicious lesion.

The importance of understanding the type of lesion of apical periodontitis is often underestimated. A periapical granuloma would be expected to resolve following root canal treatment. A true cyst would not necessarily be expected to resolve following root canal treatment [119]. Most abscesses will heal following root canal treatment, but a few may persist. Most sinus tracts resolve following root canal treatment, but a few may persist. Surgical curettage may be indicated for management of persisting lesions; provided that the root canal system is well filled, root-end resection is not normally indicated.

There has been some discussion about the necessity to remove the entire lesion [22,99,123,160,163]. Healing of a periapical granuloma would be expected whether or not the lesion was removed in its entirety at surgery. A cyst might persist if curettage were incomplete. Abscesses would be expected to heal following root-end filling even if curettage were incomplete. There is a risk that persisting extraradicular infection (e.g., periapical actinomycosis) might persist if curettage were incomplete.

Most lesions of apical periodontitis can be dissected away from the bony cavity. Greater effort may be required to dissect the lesion from the root surface. The lesion should be carefully lifted out of the bony cavity with tissue forceps, and placed in transport medium or fixative for histopathological examination. If the lesion fragments during removal, then it is necessary to remove it in several pieces. Care must be taken not to compromise the blood supply to the adjacent teeth when the lesion is large, or to damage anatomical structures, e.g., the inferior dental neurovascular bundle.

13.8 Root-end resection

This is the most frequently performed surgical endodontic procedure, and usually includes root-end cavity preparation and filling. This has recently been reviewed [179].

Many of the historical reasons proposed for root-end resection have been questioned, particularly when root canal treatment can be performed carefully and thoroughly. Complex canal anatomical form can be managed satisfactorily by skilled root canal treatment. There has been a tendency by some to regard the periradicular inflammatory lesion as the reason for needing surgery, but that is invariably addressing the effect rather than the cause. The purpose of root-end resection is to allow access to the infection in the root canal so that it may be eliminated and the canal space thoroughly filled. Achieving this aim surgically is harder than it first appears, because of restricted access.

Root ends may be resected either by shaving away the apex with a long-tapered fissure bur and reducing the root length as far as is considered appropriate, or alternatively a predetermined amount of the root end may be cut off in one cut through the root. Both methods have their strengths and weaknesses. With the shaving approach there is a risk of damage to other anatomical structures, e.g., inferior dental neurovascular bundle. With the cutting-through approach it is possible to become disorientated and misjudge tooth position and angulation, thus removing more of the root than was intended, create more bevel than planned, or risk damage to an adjacent root.

Traditionally the root face has been beveled to improve mechanical and visual access to the root canal(s) [28,67,160]. Recent evidence has shown that bevels have a deleterious effect on healing because more dentinal tubules are opened [35,59,183]; therefore the current recommendation is to make as little bevel as possible although this compromises access. The reduction in access can be compensated for by use of specially designed ultrasonic surgical tips and use of surgical mirrors [28,159]. Where the root is angled or curves away from the surgical access, then

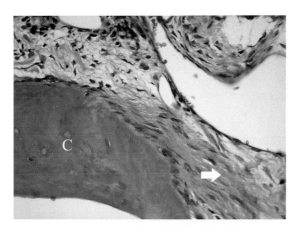

Fig. 13.6 Deposition of a layer of new cementum (C) on resected dentine. Note the new periodontal fibers (arrowed) (original magnification ×200, hematoxylin & eosin stain) (from Torabinejad *et al.* [193]).

the placing of a bevel may be unavoidable. Histological evidence has shown that in those teeth where the root canal is thoroughly cleaned and filled then cementum can be expected to reform over the dentin of the resected root end (Fig. 13.6) [6,7,148,193].

The resected root should be kept as long as possible to give the tooth maximum support in the long term. Resection of the root to the base of a large periradicular lesion [25] is now regarded as unnecessary [67,68]. A reduction of the root length by 3 mm is often cited to remove a high number of accessory foramina [68]. It is also important to preserve as much bone as possible over the buccal aspect of the root to reduce the chance of marginal periodontal breakdown. The type of bur and speed of rotation required to carry out the resection appear to be relatively unimportant. Adequate cooling with sterile isotonic saline is essential to prevent damage to the tissues and disruption to the root canal filling material [69]. The resected root surface is best smoothed with a plain-cut tungsten-carbide or fine-grit diamond bur.

13.8.1 Need for root-end preparation

If there is excessive bleeding from the bony cavity, it may be controlled by packing the cavity with gauze, or cotton wool, soaked in local anesthetic containing 1:50,000 epinephrin (or 1:80,000) or even epinephrin solution and left for several minutes [90,202]. It is rarely necessary to use more potent hemostatic

agents or bone wax, which may have potential adverse effects on healing [208]. The resected root face must be examined carefully for the main root canal, but also just as importantly for secondary and accessory root canals as well as joining isthmuses. If the main canal is offcenter, then the root face must be carefully explored for a secondary canal which could otherwise be overlooked. If the root face has been cut with a steep bevel, then canal orifices will appear elongated. Further, if the apex of a tooth with a curved canal is resected, it is possible to enter the canal laterally and to leave the apical foramen intact, particularly if a shaving technique has been used, because the operator is often disorientated to the long axis of the root. When it is difficult to observe the canal orifice, dye may be applied to the resected root face to stain the canal [69]. The use of magnification aids detection of canal orifices or an anastomosis. In some roots two canals may be joined by a fine isthmus (Fig. 13.7), which must be included in the root-end cavity preparation [109].

If the resected root face has readily visible canal orifices which are very well filled with gutta-percha and no evidence of any isthmus, then there may be little benefit in removing some of the gutta-percha to replace it by a root-end filling material, particularly amalgam. Indeed, in two clinical studies the success rate was higher for gutta-percha filled teeth than for teeth root-end filled with amalgam [9,163]. There is evidence from a recent clinical study to show that insertion of currently available root-end filling materials in contemporary preparations yields a very good outcome [33].

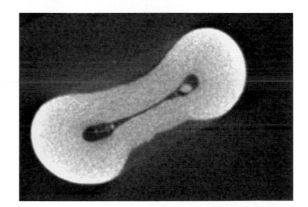

Fig. 13.7 Microcomputed tomographic horizontal section of a mesial root of a mandibular molar showing the isthmus between the two main canals (from Mannocci *et al.* [109]).

13.8.2 Root-end preparation

Root-end preparation is undertaken because the quality of the existing root canal filling is often unsatisfactory either due to insufficiency of sealer between laterally condensed gutta-percha points or anastomoses between main canals. Traditionally root-end preparation has been carried out with burs, but the problem of limited access frequently results in the preparation not being centered on the canal but mainly in the palatal wall, and even perforating the palatal root into the periodontal ligament (Fig. 13.8). A further often unrecognized problem is the risk of leaving infected material on the buccal aspect of the root-end cavity, i.e., under the dentinal tubules of the buccal bevel; this remaining infection will subsequently cause inflammation adjacent to the cut dentin [35].

Special tips have been produced for ultrasonic handpieces, and because of their angled design they allow preparation to be carried out in the long axis of the root canal. Furthermore the entire preparation can be more conservative because dentin removal is slower and more controlled [70,180,211]. Ultrasonic preparation is able to clean root-end preparations of bacteria significantly better than burs [70], or hand filing [180]; irrigating the cavity with a syringe is little better than doing nothing [180]. There is some controversial evidence that ultrasonic preparation of root-end cavities may cause cracks in the root [56,97], but this has not been substantiated [12,87]; the type of tip appears to have some effect. The clinical significance of cracks remains unknown. Sonic handpieces have also been investigated for root-end cavity preparation [53,87,102]. After preparation, the root-end cavity must be dried and inspected using magnification and surgical mirrors to ensure all aspects are clean. The shape of an ultrasonic preparation normally has sufficient retention for a root-end filling. There is no need to create specific undercut retention, as was formerly recommended for bur preparations.

It is essential not to leave uncleaned space in the root canal system, therefore the preparation should extend to well-condensed gutta-percha or to the apical end of a post. If this necessitates a very deep preparation then it may be possible to clean and shape the apical end of the root canal with files held in hemostats [152,175,207] or by use of a suitably modified ultrasonic root canal file [180]. If it is noted at the treatment planning stage that there would be a large distance between the resected root end and the end of a post, root canal retreatment should be considered as the first line of treatment because the prognosis of surgery is better when the canal is well filled [148,163].

Procedures to cover the resected root end with filling material were first advocated for amalgam [29,157], but have more recently been in favor for

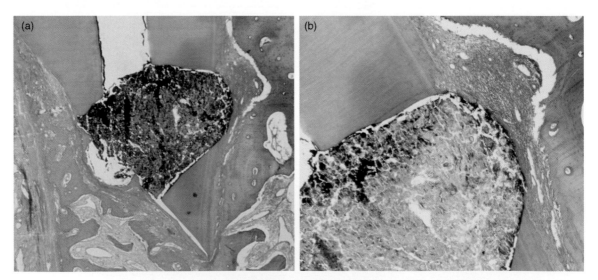

Fig. 13.8 (a) Buccolingual section through a resected root-end filled root of a dog mandibular premolar to show the hazard of perforation of the lingual wall of the root. The misdirection of the root-end cavity using burs has also resulted in canal debris remaining on the inner aspect of the buccal wall to cause failure via the beveled dentinal tubules (original magnification ×25). (b) There is inflammation adjacent to the perforation (original magnification ×100, hematoxylin & eosin stain).

adhesive materials [37,165,166]. A good outcome has been achieved where the root end has been saucered with a large round bur and composite resin placed with dentin bonding agent. The covering of a large surface area with composite resin achieves a good bond and also seals open tubules [165-168]. A method of covering the bevelled root end with glass ionomer cement has shown promising results *in vitro* and experimentally *in vivo* [34,35,37].

13.8.3 Root-end filling

The purpose of the root-end filling material is to fill the apical canal space and achieve a seal, preventing access to periapical tissues by microbial products from the root canal system, thus allowing tissue repair to occur. The root-end filling material should be biocompatible, easy to use, radiopaque, adhesive, antibacterial, insoluble, and unaffected by moisture. Very few materials possess all these properties. A very wide range of materials have been investigated [84,192] and used; these include: amalgam, gutta-percha, zinc oxide/eugenol cement, glass ionomer cement, composite resin, Cavit, Diaket, mineral trioxide aggregate (MTA), and others. Root-end filling materials have recently been reviewed [32].

Amalgam

This has been the most widely used material for many years [19,57,68,196], because dentists have been familiar with its handling and because it is radiopaque. In recent years, its continued use has been questioned for a number of reasons: leakage, lack of biocompatibility, corrosion and staining, and poor performance [32,45,144,193].

Leakage. A large number of studies have assessed the sealing ability of amalgam root-end fillings in laboratory studies. The majority have involved suspending filled roots in dye and assessing passive dye penetration [36,57,127]. A small number have used changes in air pressure to overcome the effect of entrapped air [176,209]. The current consensus is that changes in air pressure only make a small difference, and it is an unnatural condition to which to subject teeth [141,156]. The conclusion is that amalgam root-end fillings allow leakage to occur [38,57,68,194]. Leakage of amalgam root-end fillings has also been assessed by use of bacteria [38,185], and the leakage was found

to be greater than that for other materials, whichever method of assessing leakage was chosen [38].

Biocompatibility. Use of amalgam as a restorative material has come under increasing criticism because of the mercury hazard [47]. The tissue response to amalgam root-end fillings has been shown to be unfavorable and associated with inflammation [10,35,144,187,193]. Histological staining for mercury has shown traces of amalgam in the tissue at some distance from the root end; these amalgam particles were also associated with inflammation [144]. These particles were considered to have migrated from the surface of the root-end filling, rather than being debris scattered by the procedure as all the roots were filled extraorally [144]. In histological studies of root-end fillings, amalgam has always been associated with the most severe and extensive inflammation of all the materials tested (Fig. 13.9) [35,144,146,187,193].

Corrosion and staining. Amalgam is known to undergo corrosion intraorally, and will also do so at the root end. There is no evidence of improved sealing of root-end fillings as corrosion occurs. It is unclear where the corrosion products go, but they appear to be responsible for the presence of inflammatory cells at the root end [144,193]. Furthermore, some patients have developed discoloration of the oral mucosa as a result of corrosion of amalgam root-end fillings [72]; the discoloration may be primarily as a result of the presence of silver salts, since discoloration has also been observed with extruded silver points.

Poor clinical performance. A number of studies have shown that the successful outcome of teeth with amalgam root-end fillings is disappointing when using stringent criteria, in approximately two out of every three cases [2,45,51,83,131].

Gutta-percha

The use of gutta-percha to fill root-end preparations has been described [124,137], but there is limited clinical reporting of its effectiveness [152]. In this technique, files held in artery forceps were used to prepare the apical root canal [5,152,207]. This requires excellent surgical access, and therefore cases must be carefully selected, so that the root end is close to the buccal cortical plate; it is very difficult to use this technique on palatally inclined roots. Gutta-percha with scaler may be cold condensed [207], or chloroform softened

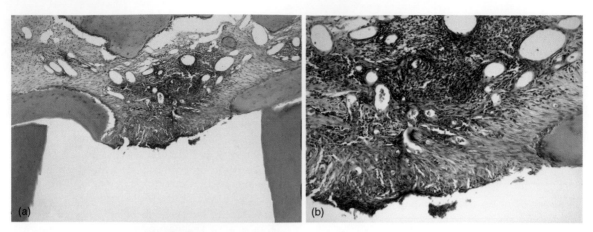

Fig. 13.9   Tissue response to an amalgam root-end filling. (a) New cementum has grown over the cut root-end dentin but not over the root-end filling, where there is inflamed connective tissue (original magnification ×40). (b) The connective tissue over the root-end filling has an infiltrate of inflammatory cells (original magnification ×80, hematoxylin & eosin stain) (from Torabinejad *et al.* [193]).

[152]. The tissue response to the latter has not been as favorable as to zinc oxide/eugenol [147]. The introduction of thermoplasticized gutta-percha also led to greater investigation of [180,209], and clinical use of gutta-percha for root-end filling [41,52].

Zinc oxide/eugenol

Zinc oxide/eugenol cements have been recommended for root-end filling by clinicians for many decades [58,123], and one large clinical study [45] showed that root-end filling with two versions of zinc oxide/eugenol had a significantly better outcome than that with amalgam. A recent randomized controlled trial showed a very good outcome with a zinc oxide/eugenol; this improved with time [33]. In a series of histological investigations [144–146], Super-EBA and IRM were found to be more biocompatible than other formulations of zinc oxide/eugenol. These fortified versions also have low solubility [130], good antibacterial action [31,129,190], and exhibit little leakage in dye testing [126,128]. A frequent finding on histological examination has been the presence of giant cells on the surface of the root-end filling material [144–146].

Glass ionomer cement

These cements have been used for root-end filling for a relatively shorter period [77,83,89,213]. Their antibacterial effect is variable [31,44]; their sealing ability when they are used as root-end fillings has been

questioned [36,148], and has been reviewed [42]. An improved sealing ability has been achieved when the material covers the resected root end [37], or a light-cured material is used [38]. The tissue response has been favorable in the absence of infection in the root canal (Fig. 13.10) [27,148,212]. When infection in the canal is present, the tissue response may be unfavorable, because the setting contraction of the material can allow a microspace for bacterial colonization and a communication between the canal and the tissues [148] (Fig. 13.11). The only long-term clinical evidence on glass ionomer root-end fillings predates use of ultrasonic preparation of root-end cavities, but shows a good outcome [83].

Composite resin

Composite resin in conjunction with a dentin bonding agent has been used for root-end filling in a saucer-type preparation; it has achieved good results in clinical studies over both the short and long term [82,166–168]. The success of the technique is dependent on excellent moisture control, otherwise the material will not adhere to the tooth surface [165]. Several studies *in vitro* have reported on the sealing ability of composite resin placed in a root-end cavity [1,106,107].

Cavit

This material (Espe, Seefeld, Germany) has been used for root-end filling in several clinical studies [51,125,139] with mixed results; these predated the

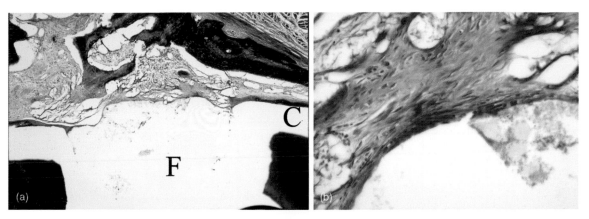

Fig. 13.10   (a) Histological section of root end showing glass ionomer cement root-end filling (F), and a normal connective tissue response. Cementum has grown over dentin but none over the root-end filling (original magnification ×40, hematoxylin & eosin stain). (b) Noninflamed connective tissue abuts the root-end filling material (original magnification ×200, hematoxylin & eosin stain) (from Pitt Ford and Roberts [148]).

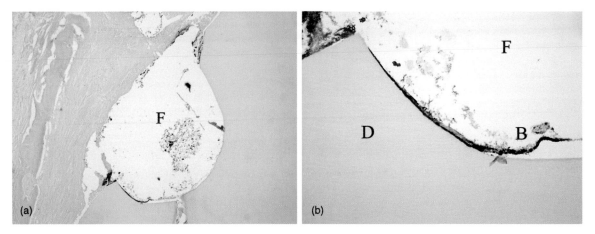

Fig. 13.11   (a) Histological section of root end showing glass ionomer cement root-end filling (F) and bacteria at junction of dentin, tissue and filling (original magnification ×20). (b) Higher magnification shows layer of bacterial biofilm (B) between dentin (D) and filling (original magnification ×80, Brown & Brenn bacterial stain) (from Pitt Ford and Roberts [148]).

use of ultrasonic preparation of root-end cavities. The material is based on zinc oxide and calcium sulfate, and is self-hardening in the presence of moisture. In a recent histological study it had similar biocompatibility to IRM and Super-EBA, displayed no evidence of dissolution, and in common with zinc oxide/eugenol cements demonstrated the presence of giant cells on its surface [146].

Diaket

Diaket is a calcium chelate reinforced with polyvinyl resin, and when mixed to a thicker consistency than

that for use as a root canal sealer, has been advocated as a root-end filling material [182]. The sealing ability of Diaket root-end fillings has also been investigated and found to be superior to amalgam and glass ionomer cement [85], and zinc oxide/eugenol materials [203]. Biocompatibility has been assessed when the material was embedded in bone [120], and also when used for root-end filling in dogs [150,174]; the follow-up period of the root-end fillings was only 2 months, which is considered too short a period to observe the formation of cementum over the root-end filling material [187], but there was a suggestion that a hard tissue matrix had formed. As inflammation was assessed in a different way from that in other studies, direct comparison is not possible; however, the tissue response appeared to demonstrate good healing.

Mineral trioxide aggregate

Mineral trioxide aggregate (MTA) is the most recent material to be proposed for root-end filling, and it has been comprehensively reviewed [32]. It has been subjected to leakage testing [86,181,185,186,194,210], in which it allowed less leakage than amalgam or zinc oxide/eugenol materials. Other properties investigated include antibacterial effects [190], biocompatibility both in cell culture [191] and when embedded in bone [189], and also in histological examinations of root-end fillings in animals [10,150,187,193]. Root-end fillings with MTA were associated with considerably less inflammation than with amalgam, and with all the longer-term specimens the presence of new cementum over the root-end filling material was observed [187,193] (Fig. 13.12). This consistency of response has been unparalleled with other materials. A randomized clinical study demonstrated a very good clinical outcome [33]. In the clinical technique, the cement powder is mixed with water to a stiff consistency and then packed into the root-end cavity with pluggers. Because MTA takes over 3 hours to set [188], it must not be disturbed during the subsequent wound closure procedures.

13.8.4 Wound closure and postoperative care

The bony cavity should be cleaned of any hemostatic agents (e.g., gauze, bone wax) and excess root-end filling material. Traditionally the bony cavity has been syringed out with saline or sterile water. If a non-setting material (e.g. MTA) has been used, then washing out of the bony cavity must be done with consider-

able care to avoid disturbance of the root-end filling. Blood is allowed to fill the bony cavity and the mucoperiosteal flap is then carefully repositioned so that it can be sutured into place. The purpose of the sutures is to hold the tissue flap in close approximation with the underlying bone so that healing occurs by primary intention.

Various materials have been used for suturing, ranging from gut through silk to synthetic fibers [28,68,199]. Silk has traditionally been used, is multifilament that gives good handling, but allows bacteria to colonize the suture intraorally; this infection may be partially counteracted by chlorhexidine mouthwashes. Synthetic fibers (e.g., nylon, polypropylene, PTFE) being monofilaments (or coated multifilaments) are generally preferred [201]. Needle shape, size and curvature are important for the particular procedure. It is important that the needle can be inserted between the teeth, and then after insertion can be pulled through; it therefore needs sufficient length and to be sufficiently thin. Sutures vary in size and there has been a recent tendency to use finer sizes. A number of different stitch types have been used, and probably the final decision rests with operator preference [201]. Interrupted sutures are more widely used than one continuous suture, because the irregular shape of flap lends itself to individual sutures, as opposed to the larger flaps in periodontal surgery where margins may not approximate well because of excision of diseased tissue.

After the flap has been sutured into the correct position, it should be carefully pressed against the underlying bone to make the intervening blood clot as thin as possible, to allow primary healing. The margins must be carefully approximated to reduce

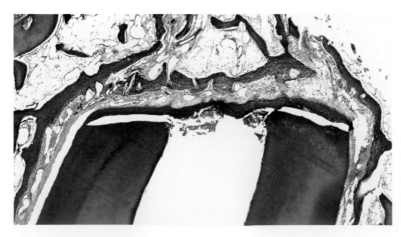

Fig. 13.12 Tissue response to mineral trioxide aggregate root-end filling. New cementum has grown over the cut root-end dentin and over the root-end filling; there is no inflammation in the adjacent connective tissue (original magnification ×20) (from Torabinejad *et al.* [193]).

the risk of infection of the underlying blood clot with associated pain and swelling, together with delayed healing. The patient should be sent home with specific instructions for the first day, to avoid strenuous exercise which could precipitate bleeding, to avoid pulling on the lip which could pull on the sutures, to take analgesics both to prevent and to reduce pain [80], to avoid rinsing which could cause bleeding, and to avoid eating until the effects of the local anesthetic have worn off. Swelling may be prevented by holding an ice pack against the side of the cheek for 20 min, then resting for 20 min, followed by repetition of the cycle for several hours [66,68]. Arrangements should be made so that the patient can contact the surgeon in case of postoperative complications.

From the second day the patient should be instructed to rinse the affected area twice daily with a chlorhexidine mouthwash to prevent bacterial colonization of the wound margins and the sutures. The sutures should be removed several days later. As early as 48 hours has been recommended [68] although 4 days is commonplace [67,199,200]. Sutures should not be left as long as 7 days because infection of the sutures may damage the interdental papillae [62,68,200]. In contrast to periodontal surgical procedures the marginal interdental tissues involved in endodontic surgery are normally healthy, and therefore iatrogenic damage to them must be avoided.

When sutures are removed, the wound should be inspected for satisfactory healing which is to be expected. On the rare occasions when there are signs of infection of the intraosseous blood clot or swelling of the overlying tissues, antibiotics may need to be prescribed. However, there is no indication for routine prescription of antibiotics in surgical endodontics [66].

13.9 Perforation repair

A perforation is an abnormal communication between the pulp space and the periradicular tissues [151]. Most often it is iatrogenic as a result of incorrect instrumentation in seeking the pulp space or a root canal, preparing post space, or by aggressive canal enlargement. Less frequently osteoclasts may resorb the dentin either externally or internally leading to perforation.

The sites of perforation range from the gingival sulcus through subcrestal and midroot to apical. Those in the gingival sulcus can usually be managed by placement of a restoration from within the tooth. Those which are subcrestal, if not treated immediately, are likely to become infected, with a chronic inflammatory response in the adjacent tissues [122,170]. The prognosis of the tooth with marginal periodontal breakdown is reduced if, as frequently occurs, the site is inaccessible to recontouring by periodontal surgery. Perforations in the midroot are usually managed conservatively by careful placement of material from inside the tooth; for those that respond unfavorably to this approach, surgical repair may be considered where access is favorable, but often it is not. Apical perforations are frequently managed by careful placement of material via the root canal, however a surgical approach is indicated for those that respond unfavorably. With perforations close to the apex, the root end may be resected to include the perforation, and then its management is similar to root-end resection described earlier.

There are few studies of the surgical management of perforations, because most perforations are managed nonsurgically [151]. Those studies that have been undertaken have had very small numbers of teeth managed surgically [14,18,95]. There has been a traditional impression amongst clinicians that surgical repair of perforations does not enjoy a good long-term outcome because of periodontal breakdown, however there is no robust scientific evidence. Repair has traditionally been with amalgam [112,172], which is no longer the material of choice. Zinc oxide/eugenol cements have more recently been used, but in view of the formation of cementum over MTA in experimental studies of root-end filling, and conservative internal repair of furcal perforations (Fig. 13.13) [149,193], MTA has become the material of choice [151,184]. The principles of treatment are similar to root-end cavity preparation and filling, except that the cavity is on the side of the root.

13.10 Replantation

Intentional extraction and replantation was performed 300 years ago, and has been practiced by a few dentists ever since. It is not considered the treatment of choice for teeth with apical periodontitis [206], but rather reserved for situations where root canal treatment or root-end resection is impossible [48,68]. This form of treatment has a poorer outcome than replacement by an implant.

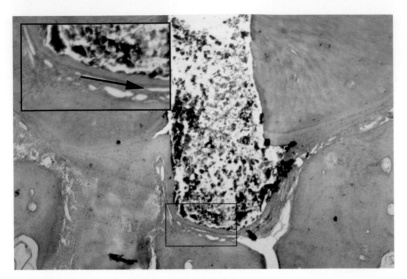

Fig. 13.13   (a) An example of a perforation filled immediately with mineral trioxide aggregate. A layer of continuous new cementum over the excess material is seen (original magnification ×20). (b) Higher magnification (×100) shows a narrow periodontal ligament space (arrowed) between the cementum and bone (hematoxylin & eosin stain) (from Pitt Ford *et al.* [149]).

Although there are many case reports, only a few large clinical studies have been undertaken; comparison of studies is difficult because of the differing methods of treatment and criteria for a successful outcome. In most studies amalgam root-end fillings have been placed [13,43,61], however in a few the root canal system has also been filled [48,92,93]. In one study a successful outcome was defined solely as retention of the tooth with a minimum follow-up period of 6 months [93]. The success rate of studies with strict radiological criteria is disappointingly low ranging from 34% to 67% [43,48,61]. The reasons for unsuccessful outcome are continued radiolucency at the root end or resorption of the tooth [48]. Continued root-end radiolucency may occur because the canal system is infected [144] or canal orifices have not been cleaned and filled. Resorption of the tooth is a consequence of damage to the cementum, during extraction, root-end preparation, or replantation. It may take the form of inflammatory resorption, where the infected dentin stimulates the resorption process through breaches in the cementum; or less commonly replacement resorption, or ankylosis, where there are breaches in the cementum but no infection in the dentin [48]. To prevent damage to the cementum, the tooth should be extracted very carefully, kept out of the socket for as little time as possible, usually less than 15 min [93], and the root surface kept bathed in isotonic saline solution. The root surface must not be handled during root-end procedures. All reported studies have used amalgam as the root-end filling, however current research is investigating zinc oxide/eugenol cement. Meticulous oral hygiene postoperatively combined with chlorhexidine mouthwashes are essential to prevent loss of periodontal attachment. Splinting is not now normally undertaken for molar teeth, in order to facilitate oral hygiene postoperatively; there appear to be no disadvantages. Even with careful technique, resorption has been shown to be a frequent complication at the histological level [144,146,147].

13.11 Root amputation, hemisection

Root amputation is an old established procedure [153,154] that still has a limited place in treatment. Formerly, it was used where root canal treatment was considered too difficult, but now its indications are restricted to multirooted teeth where one or more roots can be saved, while the other cannot. The subject has been thoroughly reviewed [68]. Indications for root amputation are: severe marginal periodontitis, root fracture, cervical resorption, and infected superficial perforation. Contraindications are: deeply placed furcation, or fused roots, inability to restore the remaining tooth, remaining root canals are non-negotiable, or remaining roots are short or have little attachment.

The alternative to root amputation and restoration of the remaining part of the tooth is extraction followed later by replacement with a fixed prosthesis or implant. The decision on which alternative to choose will depend on the importance of the retained tooth, its prognosis, and the cost of treatment relative to that of an alternative.

When root amputation is being considered, it is essential to examine the patient's mouth thoroughly and to carry out a full periodontal assessment, so that an accurate diagnosis is made of attachment loss on each root. Root canal treatment is normally carried out first on the roots to be retained, and a plug of permanent restorative material placed in the coronal part of the root that is to be amputated. Advantages of carrying out root canal treatment prior to surgery are better isolation, and the ability to assess the internal anatomy of the tooth for root fusion and C-shaped canals, before problems are encountered surgically.

The surgical procedure consists of reflecting a full thickness mucoperiosteal flap, sectioning the root with a fine long tapered bur without damaging the root structure that is to be retained, elevating out the root, bony recontouring as required, and repositioning the flap to achieve a good soft tissue contour [68].

In addition to root amputation, part of the crown may also be removed along with the root; this is known as tooth resection. A further procedure that may be performed where there is furcation damage (e.g., perforation) is to divide a mandibular molar through the furcation, and create two separate teeth (bicuspidization); this requires a superficial furcation, and possibly orthodontic separation of the roots. Teeth which have undergone these procedures require crowning to prevent fracture.

The success of these procedures is dependent on good diagnosis, well-executed root canal treatment, carefully performed periodontal surgery, well-contoured crowns, and good oral hygiene by the patient. There have been a few long-term clinical follow-up studies [15,26,46,71,96], and generally the results have been good, with a low incidence of marginal periodontal breakdown.

13.12 Guided tissue regeneration

The use of a membrane to separate bone healing from connective tissue healing has been investigated since the 1950s [100]. An early dento-alveolar application was reported a decade later [21]. The use of a membrane to enhance bone healing following endodontic surgery has been reported in experimental animals [40,108], and in patients [136].

The technique consists of trimming the membrane to shape to fit on the bone surface over the defect. The mucoperiosteal flap is then repositioned and sutured over it. The aim is to allow the bone defect to heal by new bone formation rather than by fibrous connective tissue. Bone healing has been reported to be quicker and more complete when a membrane was used [136]. Exactly how the membrane works is not completely understood [100]: it may prevent fibroblast ingrowth; it may prevent contact inhibition by fibroblasts; it may exclude cell-derived soluble inhibitors; it may allow local concentration of growth factors; and the membrane itself may stimulate bone formation. The membrane may be absorbable or nonabsorbable. In the one clinical study where a membrane was used as part of endodontic surgery, all the membranes were later removed, but no reason was given except in the case of one which became exposed [136]. The use of a membrane allows bone healing to occur, but it can have no influence over the tissue response at the root end, namely reformation of the periodontium, which is dependent on the exclusion of infection from the root canal by effective cleaning, shaping and filling of the root canal system and root-end cavity.

13.13 Surgical retreatment

Conventional surgical endodontics has a reported failure rate (persisting apical periodontitis) of 16% [143]. The most common reason for failure is considered to be insufficient cleaning and filling of the root end either prior to or at the time of surgery; less common reasons are marginal periodontitis, root fracture, and resorption [161,169].

There have been relatively few reports on how to treat a surgical failure [169], or of the outcome of such treatment [143]. Some cases are managed by conventional root canal retreatment without the need for further surgery, a number are retreated surgically, while others are retreated by a combined approach. There appear to be a few studies that have reported on healing following conventional repeat surgical endodontics [125,138,139,161]; in a systematic review [143] the weighted success rate (elimination of apical periodontitis) was low (36%). There are no studies on the outcome of conventional root canal retreatment following previous surgery. With the reduction in indications for surgery and improved surgical technique, it is to be hoped that the need for surgical retreatment will decline, and the outcome will be better. However, the successful outcome of surgical retreatment is never likely to be as high as that of primary treatment, because all the cases are included because of initial treatment failure.

13.14 Modes of healing

The defect in the bone is filled with blood, which clots [68,75]. The clot is protected from infection from the mouth by the epithelium of the repositioned flap. The epithelial cells proliferate to close the incisional wound [74,171,201]. It is therefore essential that the mucoperiosteal flap is not damaged during surgery and is replaced very carefully to minimize exposure of connective tissue or blood clot. In the first week postoperatively, it is important to prevent infection of the connective tissues or blood clot, by use of a suitable antiseptic mouthwash (e.g., chlorhexidine).

13.14.1 Osseous healing

New blood vessels will grow into the margins of the blood clot to form granulation tissue, provided that infection is excluded. In dogs as early as a week after surgery, most if not all of the blood clot is replaced by granulation tissue [34,75]. As the new blood vessels move into the blood clot, so fibroblasts arrive to form a matrix for connective tissue that later mineralizes. This process is most advanced at the bony margins (Fig. 13.14). Under favorable circumstances a very large part of the entire bony cavity will be replaced by woven bone that will mature into normal cancellous bone. This osseous healing occurs independently of dental healing, and is a response to surgical excision of bone or of an inflammatory lesion, rather than a healing response to treatment at the root end.

13.14.2 Dental healing

Similarly, new blood vessels grow from the periodontal ligament into the blood clot to encapsulate the root end. With them come specialized connective tissue cells to reform the periodontium, that is cementum, periodontal ligament and bone (Fig. 13.6). In the absence of infection or irritant materials, cementum will be laid down on the resected dentin [6,7,73,158]. Dental healing occurs at a slower rate than osseous healing. It appears that the process may be accelerated by demineralizing the resected root end with citric acid [39]. Under ideal circumstances cementum will be deposited over the root-end filling; this has rarely been observed with conventional root-end filling materials [158], but has been detected routinely with MTA [187,193]. With most materials a fibrous capsule is formed (Fig. 13.10) [7,73,144,146].

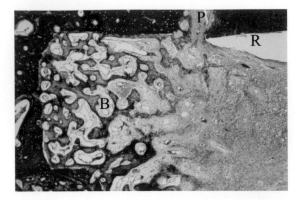

Fig. 13.14   Osseous healing at 2 weeks following surgery in a dog; new bone matrix (B) has formed where a bur cut was made into endosteal bone; (P) periodontal ligament, (R) resected root end (original magnification ×100, Masson's trichrome stain) (from Chong *et al.* [34]).

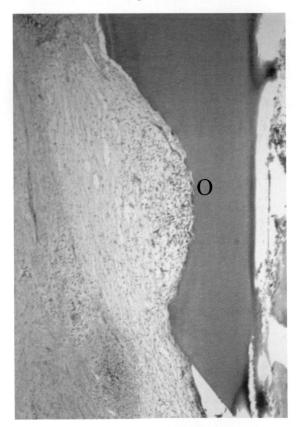

Fig. 13.15   Lateral resorption of the root following beveling and the stimulatory effects of bacteria within the root canal. Osteoclasts (O) are in lacunae on the dentin surface (original magnification ×100, hematoxylin & eosin stain) (from Chong *et al.* [35]).

If the root canal has been infected and root-end preparation or filling has been imperfect, then the desired healing may not occur. Inflammation may be observed adjacent to the root-end filling material and also next to the beveled dentin on the labial side of the root, where the dentinal tubules connect the infected root canal with the tissues [35]. In these circumstances cementum does not form on the resected root end, and osteoclasts may even resorb the dentin (Fig. 13.15). It must be remembered that the healing reported in the absence of infection [73,193] may not be achievable when treating infected root canals [35,144,195]. Mineralization of bone matrix is the slowest part of the healing mechanism, therefore radiological evidence of healing follows after histological signs of matrix formation [73].

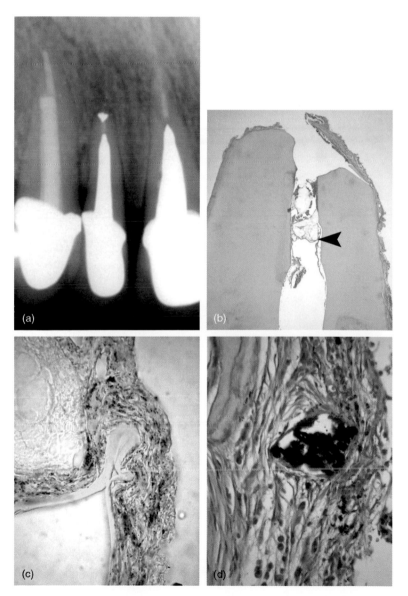

Fig. 13.16 The maxillary incisor had root-end surgery and root-end filling with amalgam 5 years before the tooth fractured. (a) Radiograph shows normal periapical tissues.
(b) Longitudinal section of tooth showing tissue over root end filling and contents of canal (arrowed) (original magnification ×20, hematoxylin and eosin stain).
(c) Arrowed contents of canal contain bacteria, original magnification ×1000, Brown & Brenn bacterial stain). (d) Tissue over root-end filling is chronically inflamed adjacent to metal particles (original magnification ×400, hematoxylin & eosin stain). (Courtesy of Dr D Ricucci.)

13.15 Outcome of surgical endodontics

This is covered in detail in Chapter 14. Many clinical studies have used differing criteria for case selection, period of follow-up and assessment of success. The first comprehensive classification of healing was proposed in 1972 [164], and later refined [113]; healing is graded in four categories: complete healing, incomplete healing (scar), uncertain healing, and failure. This radiological classification is based on good correlation with histological examination [8]. Correlation between radiological and histological examinations is demonstrated in Fig. 13.16. The category of incomplete healing (scar) has been regarded as a stable outcome only after long-term follow-up [115]. With the

advent of high-resolution tomography it is likely that methods for determining outcome will be substantially improved.

The length of the follow-up period is important. Less than a year is too short, since there is inevitably some healing at the periphery of the bone cavity even if there is acute inflammation at the resected root end. A recent study showed improved healing at 2 years compared to that at 1 year (Fig. 13.17) [33]. Two large studies have also shown that a year is too short a period and recommend 4 years when some of the lesions in the uncertain group will have healed [63,162,164]. There is no evidence to support routine radiological follow-up in the period less than a year. The fact that complete healing has

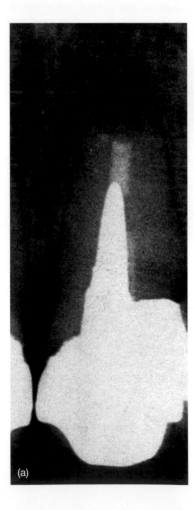 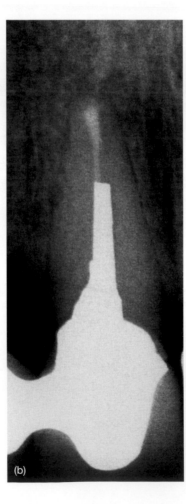

Fig. 13.17 Radiographs of root-end filled maxillary incisors 2 years after placement showing good bony healing. (a) IRM. (b) Mineral trioxide aggregate.

occurred does not mean that failure may not occur later; 42% of teeth initially considered completely healed in one study later failed (12 years) [55]; this is because resistance to infection is a dynamic biological process.

Presence of root canal filling

The presence of a good quality root canal filling is considered essential to the outcome of surgical endodontics [68,114]. This has been supported by clinical studies [78,106,111], and by comparison of conditions in histological studies [35,73,148].

13.16 References

1. Adamo HL, Buruiana R, Schertzer L, Boylan RJ (1999) A comparison of MTA, Super-EBA, composite and amalgam as root-end filling materials using a bacterial microleakage model. *International Endodontic Journal* **32**, 197–203.
2. Allen RK, Newton CW, Brown CE (1989) A statistical analysis of surgical and nonsurgical endodontic retreatment cases. *Journal of Endodontics* **15**, 261–6.
3. Altonen M (1975) Transantral, subperiosteal resection of the palatal root of maxillary molars. *International Journal of Oral Surgery* **4**, 277–83.
4. Altonen M, Mattila K (1976) Follow-up study of apicoectomized molars. *International Journal of Oral Surgery* **5**, 33–40.
5. Amagasa T, Nagase M, Sato T, Shioda S (1989) Apicoectomy with retrograde gutta-percha root filling. *Oral Surgery, Oral Medicine, Oral Pathology* **68**, 339–42.
6. Andreasen JO (1973) Cementum repair after apicoectomy in humans. *Acta Odontologica Scandinavica* **31**, 211–21.
7. Andreasen JO, Rud J (1972) Modes of healing histologically after endodontic surgery in 70 cases. *International Journal of Oral Surgery* **1**, 148–60.
8. Andreasen JO, Rud J (1972) Correlation between histology and radiography in the assessment of healing after endodontic surgery. *International Journal of Oral Surgery* **1**, 161–73.
9. August DS (1996) Long-term, postsurgical results on teeth with periapical radiolucencies. *Journal of Endodontics* **22**, 380–3.
10. Baek SH, Plenk H, Kim S (2005) Periapical tissue responses and cementum regeneration with amalgam, SuperEBA, and MTA as root-end filling materials. *Journal of Endodontics* **31**, 444–9.
11. Beal M (1908) De la résection de l'apex. *Revue de Stomatologie* **15**, 439–46.
12. Beling KL, Marshall JG, Morgan LA, Baumgartner JC (1997) Evaluation for cracks associated with ultrasonic root-end preparation of gutta-percha filled canals. *Journal of Endodontics* **23**, 323–6.
13. Bender IB, Rossman LE (1993) Intentional replantation of endodontically treated teeth. *Oral Surgery, Oral Medicine, Oral Pathology* **76**, 623–30.
14. Benenati FW, Roane JB, Biggs JT, Simon JH (1986) Recall evaluation of iatrogenic root perforations repaired with amalgam and gutta-percha. *Journal of Endodontics* **12**, 161–6.
15. Bergenholtz A (1972) Radectomy of multirooted teeth. *Journal of the American Dental Association* **85**, 870–5.
16. Bergenholtz G, Lekholm U, Milthon R, Engström B (1979) Influence of apical overinstrumentation and overfilling on re-treated root canals. *Journal of Endodontics* **5**, 310–14.
17. Bergenholtz G, Lekholm U, Milthon R, Heden G, Odesjo B, Engström B (1979) Retreatment of endodontic fillings. *Scandinavian Journal of Dental Research* **87**, 217–24.
18. Biggs JT, Benenati FW, Sabala CL (1988) Treatment of iatrogenic root perforations with associated osseous lesions. *Journal of Endodontics* **14**, 620–4.
19. Block RM, Bushell A (1982) Retrograde amalgam procedures for mandibular posterior teeth. *Journal of Endodontics* **8**, 107–12.
20. Boyne P (1966) Histologic response of bone to sectioning by high-speed rotary instruments. *Journal of Dental Research* **45**, 270–6.
21. Boyne PJ (1969) Restoration of osseous defects in maxillofacial casualties. *Journal of the American Dental Association* **78**, 767–76.
22. Brock DO (1961) Minor oral surgery in general practice. VII–Apicectomy. *British Dental Journal* **110**, 216–18.
23. Brophy TW (1880) Caries of the superior maxilla. *Chicago Medical Journal and Examiner* **41**, 582–6.
24. Buckley JP (1911) The rational treatment of chronic dentoalveolar abscess, with root and bone complications. *Dental Review* **25**, 755–76.
25. Buckley JP (1914) Root amputation. *Dental Summary* **34**, 964–5.
26. Buhler H (1988) Evaluation of root-resected teeth. Results after 10 years. *Journal of Periodontology* **59**, 805–10.
27. Callis PD, Santini A (1987) Tissue response to retrograde root fillings in the ferret canine: a comparison of glass ionomer cement and gutta-percha with sealer. *Oral Surgery, Oral Medicine, Oral Pathology* **64**, 475–9.
28. Carr GB (1994) Surgical endodontics. In Cohen S, Burns RC, editors. *Pathways of the pulp*, pp. 531–67, 6th edn. St Louis, MO: Mosby.
29. Castenfelt T (1939) Om retrograd rotfyllning vid radikaloperation av kronisk apikal paradentit. *Svensk Tandlakare Tidskrift* **32**, 227–60.
30. Chindia ML, Valderhaug J (1995) Periodontal status following trapezoidal and semilunar flaps in apicectomy. *East African Medical Journal* **72**, 564–7.
31. Chong BS, Owadally ID, Pitt Ford TR, Wilson RF (1994) Antibacterial activity of potential retrograde root filling materials. *Endodontics and Dental Traumatology* **10**, 66–70.

32. Chong BS, Pitt Ford TR (2005) Root-end filling materials: rationale and tissue response. *Endodontic Topics* **11**, 114–30.

33. Chong BS, Pitt Ford TR, Hudson MB (2003) A prospective clinical study of Mineral Trioxide Aggregate and IRM when used as root-end filling materials in endodontic surgery. *International Endodontic Journal* **36**, 520–6.

34. Chong BS, Pitt Ford TR, Kariyawasam SP (1997) Short-term tissue response to potential root-end filling materials in infected root canals. *International Endodontic Journal* **30**, 240–9.

35. Chong BS, Pitt Ford TR, Kariyawasam SP (1997) Tissue response to potential root-end filling materials in infected root canals. *International Endodontic Journal* **30**, 102–14.

36. Chong BS, Pitt Ford TR, Watson TF (1991) The adaptation and sealing ability of light-cured glass ionomer retrograde fillings. *International Endodontic Journal* **24**, 223–32.

37. Chong BS, Pitt Ford TR, Watson TF (1993) Light-cured glass ionomer cement as a retrograde root seal. *International Endodontic Journal* **26**, 218–24.

38. Chong BS, Pitt Ford TR, Watson TF, Wilson RF (1995) Sealing ability of potential retrograde root filling materials. *Endodontics and Dental Traumatology* **11**, 264–9.

39. Craig KR, Harrison JW (1993) Wound healing following demineralization of resected root ends in periradicular surgery. *Journal of Endodontics* **19**, 339–47.

40. Dahlin C, Gottlow J, Linde A, Nyman S (1990) Healing of maxillary and mandibular bone defects using a membrane technique. An experimental study in monkeys. *Scandinavian Journal of Plastic and Reconstructive Surgery and Hand Surgery* **24**, 13–19.

41. Dawood AJS, Pitt Ford TR (1989) A surgical approach to the obturation of apically flared root canals with thermoplasticized gutta-percha. *International Endodontic Journal* **22**, 138–41.

42. De Bruyne MA, De Moor RJ (2004) The use of glass ionomer cements in both conventional and surgical endodontics. *International Endodontic Journal* **37**, 91–104.

43. Deeb E (1968) Intentional replantation of endodontically treated teeth. *Transactions of the Fourth International Conference on Endodontics*, pp. 147–57. Philadelphia, PA: University of Pennsylvania.

44. DeSchepper EJ, White RR, Von der Lehr W (1989) Antibacterial effects of glass ionomers. *American Journal of Dentistry* **2**, 51–6.

45. Dorn SO, Gartner AH (1990) Retrograde filling materials: a retrospective success-failure study of amalgam, EBA and IRM. *Journal of Endodontics* **16**, 391–3.

46. Eastman JR, Backmeyer J (1986) A review of the periodontal, endodontic, and prosthetic considerations in odontogenous resection procedures. *International Journal of Periodontics and Restorative Dentistry* **6**(2), 34–51.

47. Eley BM, Cox SW (1993) The release, absorption and possible health effects of mercury from dental amalgam: a review of recent findings. *British Dental Journal* **175**, 355–62.

48. Emmertsen E, Andreasen JO (1966) Replantation of extracted molars; a radiographic and histological study. *Acta Odontologica Scandinavica* **24**, 327–46.

49. Farrar JN (1884) Radical and heroic treatment of alveolar abscess by amputation of roots of teeth. *Dental Cosmos* **26**, 79–81.

50. Faulhaber B, Neumann R (1912) *Die chirurgische Behandlung der Wurzelhauterkrankungen*, p. 19. Berlin: Hermann Meusser.

51. Finne K, Nord PG, Persson G, Lennartsson B (1977) Retrograde root filling with amalgam and Cavit. *Oral Surgery, Oral Medicine, Oral Pathology* **43**, 621–6.

52. Flath RK, Hicks ML (1987) Retrograde instrumentation and obturation with new devices. *Journal of Endodontics* **13**, 546–9.

53. Fong CD (1993) A sonic instrument for retrograde preparation. *Journal of Endodontics* **19**, 374–5.

54. Fors UGH, Berg JO (1986) Endodontic treatment of root canals obstructed by foreign objects. *International Endodontic Journal* **19**, 2–10.

55. Frank AL, Glick DH, Patterson SS, Weine FS (1992) Long-term evaluation of surgically placed amalgam fillings. *Journal of Endodontics* **18**, 391–8.

56. Frank RJ, Antrim DD, Bakland LK (1996) Effect of retrograde cavity preparations on root apexes. *Endodontics and Dental Traumatology* **12**, 100–3.

57. Friedman S (1991) Retrograde approaches in endodontic therapy. *Endodontics and Dental Traumatology* **7**, 97–107.

58. Garcia GF (1937) Apicectomia experimental. *Revista Odontologica* **25**, 145–60.

59. Gilheany PA, Figdor D, Tyas MJ (1994) Apical dentin permeability and microleakage associated with root end resection and retrograde filling. *Journal of Endodontics* **20**, 22–6.

60. Grossman LI (1970) Endodontic practice, pp. 378–411, 7th edn. Philadelphia, PA: Lea & Febiger.

61. Grossman LI, Chacker FM (1968) Clinical evaluation and histologic study of intentionally replanted teeth. *Transactions of the Fourth International Conference on Endodontics*, pp. 127–44. Philadelphia, PA: University of Pennsylvania.

62. Grung B (1973) Healing of gingival mucoperiosteal flaps after marginal incision in apicoectomy procedures. *International Journal of Oral Surgery* **2**, 20–5.

63. Grung B, Molven O, Halse A (1990) Periapical surgery in a Norwegian county hospital: follow-up findings of 477 teeth. *Journal of Endodontics* **16**, 411–17.

64. Gutmann JL (1984) Principles of endodontic surgery for the general practitioner. *Dental Clinics of North America* **28**, 895–908.

65. Gutmann JL (1993) Parameters of achieving quality anesthesia and hemostasis in surgical endodontics. *Anesthesia and Pain Control in Dentistry* **2**, 223–6.

66. Gutmann JL (2005) Surgical endodontics: post-surgical care. *Endodontic Topics* **11**, 196–205.

67. Gutmann JL, Harrison JW (1985) Posterior endodontic surgery: anatomical considerations and clinical techniques. *International Endodontic Journal* **18**, 8–34.

68. Gutmann JL, Harrison JW (1991) *Surgical endodontics*. Cambridge, MA: Blackwell.

69. Gutmann JL, Pitt Ford TR (1993) Management of the resected root end: a clinical review. *International Endodontic Journal* **26**, 273–83.

70. Gutmann JL, Saunders WP, Nguyen L, Guo IY, Saunders EM (1994) Ultrasonic root-end preparation: part 1. SEM analysis. *International Endodontic Journal* **27**, 318–24.

71. Hamp SE, Nyman S, Lindhe J (1975) Periodontal treatment of multirooted teeth. Results after 5 years. *Journal of Clinical Periodontology* **2**, 126–35.

72. Harrison JD, Rowley PSA, Peters PD (1977) Amalgam tattoos: light and electron microscopy and electron-probe micro-analysis. *Journal of Pathology* **121**, 83–92.

73. Harrison JW, Johnson SA (1997) Excisional wound healing following the use of IRM as a root-end filling material. *Journal of Endodontics* **23**, 19–27.

74. Harrison JW, Jurosky KA (1991) Wound healing in the tissues of the periodontium following periradicular surgery. I. The incisional wound. *Journal of Endodontics* **17**, 425–35.

75. Harrison JW, Jurosky KA (1992) Wound healing in the tissues of the periodontium following periradicular surgery. III. The osseous excisional wound. *Journal of Endodontics* **18**, 76–81.

76. Hauman CHJ, Chandler NP, Tong DC (2002) Endodontic implications of the maxillary sinus: a review. *International Endodontic Journal* **35**, 127–41.

77. Hickel R (1988) Erste klinische Ergebnisse von retrograden Wurzelfüllungen mit Cermet-Zement. *Deutsche Zahnärztliche Zeitschrift,* **43**, 963–5.

78. Hirsch JM, Ahlström U, Henrikson PA, Heyden G, Peterson LE (1979) Periapical surgery. *International Journal of Oral Surgery* **8**, 173–85.

79. Hofer O (1935) Wurzelspitzenresektion und Zystoperationen. *Zeitschrift für Stomatologie* **32**, 513–33.

80. Jackson DL, Moore PA, Hargreaves KM (1989) Preoperative nonsteroidal anti-inflammatory medication for the prevention of postoperative dental pain. *Journal of the American Dental Association* **119**, 641–7.

81. Jacobsen I, Kerekes K (1980) Diagnosis and treatment of pulp necrosis in permanent anterior teeth with root fracture. *Scandinavian Journal of Dental Research* **88**, 370–6.

82. Jensen SS, Nattestad A, Egdo P, Sewerin I, Munksgaard EC, Schou S (2002) A prospective, randomised, comparative clinical study of resin composite and glass ionomer cement for retrograde root filling. *Clinical Oral Investigation* **6**, 236–43.

83. Jesslén P, Zetterqvist L, Heimdahl A (1995) Long-term results of amalgam versus glass ionomer cement as apical sealant after apicectomy. *Oral Surgery, Oral Medicine, Oral Pathology, Oral Radiology and Endodontics* **79**, 101–3.

84. Johnson BR (1999) Considerations in the selection of a root-end filling material. *Oral Surgery, Oral Medicine, Oral Pathology, Oral Radiology and Endodontics* **87**, 398–404.

85. Kadohiro G (1984) A comparative study of the sealing quality of zinc-free amalgam and Diaket when used as a retrograde filling material. *Hawaii Dental Journal* **15**, 8–9.

86. Keiser K, Johnson CC, Tipton DA (2000) Cytotoxicity of mineral trioxide aggregate using human periodontal ligament fibroblasts. *Journal of Endodontics* **26**, 288–91.

87. Khabbaz MG, Kerezoudis NP, Aroni E, Tsatsas V (2004) Evaluation of different methods for the root-end cavity preparation. *Oral Surgery, Oral Medicine, Oral Pathology, Oral Radiology and Endodontics* **98**, 237–42.

88. Khoury F, Hensher R (1987) The bony lid approach for the apical root resection of lower molars. *International Journal of Oral and Maxillofacial Surgery* **16**, 166–70.

89. Khoury F, Staehle HJ (1987) Retrograde Wurzelfüllungen aus Glasionomerzement. *Deutsche Zeitschrift für Mund-, Kiefer-, und Gesichts-Chirurgie* **11**, 351–5.

90. Kim S, Rethnam S (1997) Hemostasis in endodontic microsurgery. *Dental Clinics of North America* **41**, 499–511.

91. Kindlova M (1965) The blood supply of the marginal periodontium in macaca rhesus. *Archives of Oral Biology* **10**, 869–74.

92. Kingsbury BC, Wiesenbaugh JM (1971) Intentional replantation of mandibular premolars and molars. *Journal of the American Dental Association* **83**, 1053–7.

93. Koenig KH, Nguyen NG, Barkhordar RA (1988) Intentional replantation: a report of 192 cases. *General Dentistry* **36**, 327–31.

94. Kramper BJ, Kaminski EJ, Osetek EM, Heuer MA (1984) A comparative study of the wound healing of three types of flap design used in periapical surgery. *Journal of Endodontics* **10**, 17–25.

95. Kvinnsland I, Oswald RJ, Halse A, Grønningsaeter AG (1989) A clinical and roentgenological study of 55 cases of root perforation. *International Endodontic Journal* **22**, 75–84.

96. Langer B, Stein SD, Wagenberg B (1981) An evaluation of root resections. A ten-year study. *Journal of Periodontology* **52**, 719–22.

97. Layton CA, Marshall JG, Morgan LA, Baumgartner JC (1996) Evaluation of cracks associated with ultrasonic root-end preparation. *Journal of Endodontics* **22**, 157–60.

98. Lin LL, Chance K, Shovlin F, Skribner J, Langeland K (1985) Oroantral communication in periapical surgery of maxillary posterior teeth. *Journal of Endodontics* **11**, 40–4.

99. Lin LM, Gaengler P, Langeland K (1996) Periradicular curettage. *International Endodontic Journal* **29**, 220–7.

100. Linde A, Alberius P, Dahlin C, Bjurstam K, Sundin Y (1993) Osteopromotion: a soft-tissue exclusion principle using a membrane for bone healing and bone neogenesis. *Journal of Periodontology* **64**, 1116–28.

101. Lindhe J, Karring T (1989) The anatomy of the periodontium. In Lindhe J, editor. *Textbook of clinical periodontology*, pp. 19–69, 2nd edn. Copenhagen: Munksgaard.

102. Lloyd A, Jaunberzins A, Dummer PMH, Bryant S (1996) Root-end cavity preparation using the Micro-Mega sonic retro-prep tip. SEM analysis. *International Endodontic Journal* **29**, 295–301.

103. Lucas CD (1916) Root resection and apical canal filling after resection. *Dental Summary* **36**, 201–7.

104. Luebke RG (1974) Surgical endodontics. *Dental Clinics of North America* **18**, 379–91.

105. Lustmann J, Friedman S, Shaharabany V (1991) Relation of pre- and intraoperative factors to prognosis of posterior apical surgery. *Journal of Endodontics* **17**, 239–41.

106. McDonald NJ, Dumsha TC (1990) A comparative retrofill leakage study utilizing a dentin bonding material. *Journal of Endodontics* **13**, 224–7.

107. McDonald NJ, Dumsha TC (1990) An evaluation of the retrograde apical seal using dentine bonding materials. *International Endodontic Journal* **23**, 156–62.

108. Maguire H, Torabinejad M, McKendry D, McMillan P, Simon JH (1998) Effects of resorbable membrane placement and human osteogenic protein-1 on hard tissue healing after periradicular surgery in cats. *Journal of Endodontics* **24**, 720–5.

109. Mannocci F, Peru M, Sherriff M, Cook R, Pitt Ford TR (2005) The isthmuses of the mesial root of mandibular molars: a micro-computed tomographic study. *International Endodontic Journal* **38**, 558–63.

110. Meister F, Lommel TJ, Gerstein H, Davies EE (1979) Endodontic perforations which resulted in alveolar bone loss. *Oral Surgery, Oral Medicine, Oral Pathology* **47**, 463–70.

111. Mikkonen M, Kullaa-Mikkonen A, Kotilainen R (1983) Clinical and radiologic re-examination of apicoectomized teeth. *Oral Surgery, Oral Medicine, Oral Pathology* **55**, 302–6.

112. Mitsis FJ (1970) Flap operation techniques for the treatment of certain endodontic and periodontic problems. *Journal of the British Endodontic Society* **4**, 6–9.

113. Molven O, Halse A, Grung B (1987) Observer strategy and the radiographic classification of healing after endodontic surgery. *International Journal of Oral and Maxillofacial Surgery* **16**, 432–9.

114. Molven O, Halse A, Grung B (1991) Surgical management of endodontic failures: indications and treatment results. *International Dental Journal* **41**, 33–42.

115. Molven O, Halse A, Grung B (1996) Incomplete healing (scar tissue) after periapical surgery – radiographic findings 8 to 12 years after treatment. *Journal of Endodontics* **22**, 264–8.

116. Nagai O, Tagi N, Kayaba Y, Kodama S, Osada T (1986) Ultrasonic removal of broken instruments in root canals. *International Endodontic Journal* **19**, 298–304.

117. Nair PNR (2006) On the causes of persistent apical periodontitis: a review. *International Endodontic Journal* **39**, 249–81.

118. Nair PNR, Sjögren U, Krey G, Sundqvist G (1990) Therapy-resistant foreign-body giant cell granuloma at the periapex of a root-filled human tooth. *Journal of Endodontics* **16**, 589–95.

119. Nair PNR, Pajarola G, Schroeder HE (1996) Types and incidence of human periapical lesions obtained with extracted teeth. *Oral Surgery, Oral Medicine, Oral Pathology, Oral Radiology and Endodontics* **81**, 93–102.

120. Nencka D, Walia HD, Austin BP (1995) Histologic evaluation of the biocompability of Diaket. *Journal of Dental Research* **74**, 101; Abstract 716.

121. Neumann R (1926) *Atlas der radikal-chirurgischen Behandlung der Paradentosen*, p. 14. Berlin: Hermann Meusser.

122. Nicholls E (1962) Treatment of traumatic perforations of the pulp cavity. *Oral Surgery, Oral Medicine, Oral Pathology* **15**, 603–12.

123. Nicholls E (1965) The role of surgery in endodontics. *British Dental Journal* **118**, 59–67.

124. Nygaard-Östby B (1971) Apicectomy, pp. 73–5. In *Introduction to endodontics*. Oslo: Universitetsforlaget.

125. Nord PG (1970) Retrograde rootfilling with Cavit: a clinical and roentgenological study. *Swedish Dental Journal* **63**, 261–73.

126. O'Connor RP, Hutter JW, Roahen JO (1995) Leakage of amalgam and super-EBA root-end fillings using two preparation techniques and surgical microscopy. *Journal of Endodontics* **21**, 74–8.

127. Olson AK, MacPherson MG, Hartwell GR, Weller N, Kulild JC (1990) An in vitro evaluation of injectable thermoplasticized gutta-percha, glass ionomer, and amalgam when used as retrofilling materials. *Journal of Endodontics* **16**, 361–4.

128. Owadally ID, Chong BS, Pitt Ford TR, Watson TF (1993) The sealing ability of IRM with the addition of hydroxyapatite as a retrograde root filling. *Endodontics and Dental Traumatology* **9**, 211–15.

129. Owadally ID, Chong BS, Pitt Ford TR, Wilson RF (1994) Biological properties of IRM with the addition of hydroxyapatite as a retrograde root filling material. *Endodontics and Dental Traumatology* **10**, 228–32.

130. Owadally ID, Pitt Ford TR (1994) Effect of addition of hydroxyapatite on the physical properties of IRM. *International Endodontic Journal* **27**, 227–32.

131. Pantschev A, Carlsson AP, Andersson L (1994) Retrograde root filling with EBA cement or amalgam. A comparative clinical study. *Oral Surgery, Oral Medicine, Oral Pathology* **78**, 101–4.

132. Partsch C (1896) Dritter Bericht der Poliklinik für Zahn- und Mundkrankheiten des zahnärztlichen Instituts der Königl. Universität Breslau. *Deutsche Monatsschrifte fur Zahnheilkunde* **14**, 486–99.

133. Partsch C (1898) Ueber Wurzelresection. *Deutsche Monatsschrift fur Zahnheilkunde* **16**, 80–6.

134. Partsch C (1899) Ueber Wurzelresection. *Deutsche Monatsschrift fur Zahnheilkunde* **17**, 348–67.

135. Partsch C (1908) *Die chronische Wurzelhautenzündung*, pp. 1–55. Leipzig: Thieme.

136. Pecora G, Kim S, Celletti R, Davarpanah M (1995) The guided tissue regeneration principle in endodontic surgery: one-year postoperative results of large periapical lesions. *International Endodontic Journal* **28**, 41–6.

137. Persson G (1964) Efterundersökning av rotamputerade tänder. *Odontologiska Foreningens Tidskrift* **28**, 323–57.

138. Persson G (1973) Prognosis of reoperation after apicectomy. A clinical-radiological investigation. *Svensk Tandlakare Tidskrift* **66**, 49–67.

139. Persson G, Lennartson B, Lundström I (1974) Results of retrograde root-filling with special reference to amalgam and Cavit as root-filling materials. *Swedish Dental Journal* **67**, 123–4.

140. Peter K (1936) *Die Wurzelspitzenresektion der Molaren*, pp. 1–71. Leipzig: Hermann Meusser.

141. Peters LB, Harrison JW (1992) A comparison of leakage of filling materials in demineralized and non-demineralized resected root ends under vacuum and non-vacuum conditions. *International Endodontic Journal* **25**, 273–8.

142. Peters LB, Wesselink PR (1997) Soft tissue management in endodontic surgery. *Dental Clinics of North America* **41**, 513–28.

143. Peterson J, Gutmann JL (2001) The outcome of endodontic resurgery: a systematic review. *International Endodontic Journal* **34**, 169–75.

144. Pitt Ford TR, Andreasen JO, Dorn SO, Kariyawasam SP (1994) Effect of IRM root end fillings on healing after replantation. *Journal of Endodontics* **20**, 381–5.

145. Pitt Ford TR, Andreasen JO, Dorn SO, Kariyawasam SP (1995) Effect of super-EBA as a root end filling on healing after replantation. *Journal of Endodontics* **21**, 13–15.

146. Pitt Ford TR, Andreasen JO, Dorn SO, Kariyawasam SP (1995) Effect of various zinc oxide materials as root-end fillings on healing after replantation. *International Endodontic Journal* **28**, 273–8.

147. Pitt Ford TR, Andreasen JO, Dorn SO, Kariyawasam SP (1996) Effect of various sealers with gutta-percha as root-end fillings on healing after replantation. *Endodontics and Dental Traumatology* **12**, 33–7.

148. Pitt Ford TR, Roberts GJ (1990) Tissue response to glass ionomer retrograde root fillings. *International Endodontic Journal* **23**, 233–8.

149. Pitt Ford TR, Torabinejad T, McKendry DJ, Hong CU, Kariyawasam SP (1995) Use of mineral trioxide aggregate for repair of furcal perforations. *Oral Surgery, Oral Medicine, Oral Pathology, Oral Radiology and Endodontics* **79**, 756–62.

150. Regan JD, Gutmann JL, Witherspoon DE (2002) Comparison of Diaket and MTA when used as root-end filling materials to support regeneration of the periradicular tissues. *International Endodontic Journal* **35**, 840–7.

151. Regan JD, Witherspoon DE, Foyle DM (2005) Surgical repair of root and tooth perforations. *Endodontic Topics* **11**, 152–78.

152. Reit C, Hirsch J (1986) Surgical endodontic retreatment. *International Endodontic Journal* **19**, 107–12.

153. Rhein ML (1890) Amputation of roots as a radical cure in chronic alveolar abscess. *Dental Cosmos* **32**, 904–5.

154. Rhein ML (1897) Cure of acute and chronic alveolar abscess. *Dental Items of Interest* **19**, 688–702.

155. Ricucci D, Mannocci F, Pitt Ford TR (2006) A study of periapical lesions correlating the presence of a radiopaque lamina with histological findings. *Oral Surgery, Oral Medicine, Oral Pathology, Oral Radiology and Endodontics* **101**, 389–94.

156. Roda RS, Gutmann JL (1995) Reliability of reduced air pressure methods used to assess the apical seal. *International Endodontic Journal* **28**, 154–62.

157. Ross WS (1935) Apicectomy in the treatment of dead teeth. *British Dental Journal* **58**, 473–86.

158. Rowe AHR (1967) Postextraction histology of root resections. *Dental Practitioner and Dental Record* **17**, 343–9.

159. Rubinstein R (2005) Magnification and illumination in apical surgery. *Endodontic Topics* **11**, 56–77.

160. Rud J, Andreasen JO (1972) Operative procedures in periapical surgery with contemporaneous root filling. *International Journal of Oral Surgery* **1**, 297–310.

161. Rud J, Andreasen JO (1972) A study of failures after endodontic surgery by radiographic, histologic and stereomicroscopic methods. *International Journal of Oral Surgery* **1**, 311–28.

162. Rud J, Andreasen JO, Möller Jensen JE (1972) A follow-up study of 1,000 cases treated by endodontic surgery. *International Journal of Oral Surgery* **1**, 215–28.

163. Rud J, Andreasen JO, Möller Jensen JE (1972) A multivariate analysis of the influence of various factors upon healing after endodontic surgery. *International Journal of Oral Surgery* **1**, 258–71.

164. Rud J, Andreasen JO, Möller Jensen JE (1972) Radiographic criteria for the assessment of healing after endodontic surgery. *International Journal of Oral Surgery* **1**, 195–214.

165. Rud J, Munksgaard EC, Andreasen JO, Rud V, Asmussen E (1991) Retrograde root filling with composite and a dentin-bonding agent. 1. *Endodontics and Dental Traumatology* **7**, 118–25.

166. Rud J, Munksgaard EC, Andreasen JO, Rud V (1991) Retrograde root filling with composite and a dentin-bonding agent. 2. *Endodontics and Dental Traumatology* **7**, 126–31.

167. Rud J, Rud V, Munksgaard EC (1996) Long-term evaluation of retrograde root filling with dentin-bonded resin. *Journal of Endodontics* **22**, 90–3.

168. Rud J, Rud V, Munksgaard EC (1996) Retrograde root filling with dentin bonded modified resin composite. *Journal of Endodontics* **22**, 477–80.

169. Saunders WP (2005) Considerations in the revision of previous surgical procedures. *Endodontic Topics* **11**, 206–18.

170. Seltzer S, Sinai I, August D (1970) Periodontal effects of root perforations before and during endodontic procedures. *Journal of Dental Research* **49**, 332–9.

171. Selvig KA, Torabinejad M (1996) Wound healing after mucoperiosteal surgery in the cat. *Journal of Endodontics* **22**, 507–15.

172. Sinai IH (1977) Endodontic perforations: their prognosis and treatment. *Journal of the American Dental Association* **95**, 90–5.

173. Sjögren U, Hägglund B, Sundqvist G, Wing K (1990) Factors affecting the long-term results of endodontic treatment. *Journal of Endodontics* **16**, 498–504.

174. Snyder Williams S, Gutmann JL (1996) Periradicular healing in response to Diaket root-end filling material with and without tricalcium phosphate. *International Endodontic Journal* **29**, 84–92.

175. Sommer RF (1946) Essentials for successful root resection. *American Journal of Oral Surgery* **32**, 76–100.

176. Spångberg LSW, Acierno TG, Cha BY (1989) Influence of entrapped air on the accuracy of leakage studies using dye penetration methods. *Journal of Endodontics* **15**, 548–51.

177. Spatz S (1965) Early reaction in bone following the use of burs rotating at conventional and ultra speeds. *Oral Surgery, Oral Medicine, Oral Pathology* **19**, 808–16.

178. Strindberg LZ (1956) The dependence of the results of pulp therapy on certain factors. *Acta Odontologica Scandinavica* **14**, Suppl 21.

179. Stropko JJ, Doyon GE, Gutmann JL (2005) Root-end management: resection, cavity preparation, and material placement. *Endodontic Topics* **11**, 131–51.

180. Sultan M, Pitt Ford TR (1995) Ultrasonic preparation and obturation of root-end cavities. *International Endodontic Journal* **28**, 231–8.

181. Tang HM, Torabinejad M, Kettering JD (2002) Leakage evaluation of root end filling materials using endotoxin. *Journal of Endodontics* **28**, 5–7.

182. Tetsch P (1986) *Wurzelspitzenresektionen*, pp. 96–9. Munich: Hanser.

183. Tidmarsh BG, Arrowsmith MG (1989) Dentinal tubules at the root ends of apicected teeth: a scanning electron microscopic study. *International Endodontic Journal* **22**, 184–9.

184. Torabinejad M, Chivian N (1999) Clinical applications of mineral trioxide aggregate. *Journal of Endodontics* **25**, 197–205.

185. Torabinejad M, Falah Rastegar A, Kettering JD, Pitt Ford TR (1995) Bacterial leakage of Mineral Trioxide Aggregate as a root-end filling material. *Journal of Endodontics* **21**, 109–12.

186. Torabinejad M, Higa RK, McKendry DJ, Pitt Ford TR (1994) Dye leakage of four root end filling materials: effects of blood contamination. *Journal of Endodontics* **20**, 159–63.

187. Torabinejad M, Hong CU, Lee SJ, Monsef M, Pitt Ford TR (1995) Investigation of Mineral Trioxide Aggregate for root-end filling in dogs. *Journal of Endodontics* **21**, 603–8.

188. Torabinejad M, Hong CU, McDonald F, Pitt Ford TR (1995) Physical and chemical properties of a new root-end filling material. *Journal of Endodontics* **21**, 349–53.

189. Torabinejad M, Hong CU, Pitt Ford TR, Kariyawasam SP (1995) Tissue reaction to implanted Super-EBA and Mineral Trioxide Aggregate in the mandible of guinea pigs: a preliminary report. *Journal of Endodontics* **21**, 569–71.

190. Torabinejad M, Hong CU, Pitt Ford TR, Kettering JD (1995) Antibacterial effects of some root end filling materials. *Journal of Endodontics* **21**, 403–6.

191. Torabinejad M, Hong CU, Pitt Ford TR, Kettering JD (1995) Cytotoxicity of four root end filling Materials. *Journal of Endodontics* **21**, 489–92.

192. Torabinejad M, Pitt Ford TR (1996) Root end filling materials: a review. *Endodontics and Dental Traumatology* **12**, 161–78.

193. Torabinejad M, Pitt Ford TR, McKendry DJ, Abedi HR, Miller DA, Kariyawasam SP (1997) Histologic assessment of Mineral Trioxide Aggregate as a root-end filling in monkeys. *Journal of Endodontics* **23**, 225–8.

194. Torabinejad M, Watson TF, Pitt Ford TR (1993) Sealing ability of a mineral trioxide aggregate when used as a root end filling material. *Journal of Endodontics* **19**, 591–5.

195. Trope M, Lost C, Schmitz HJ, Friedman S (1996) Healing of apical periodontitis in dogs after apicoectomy and retrofilling with various filling materials. *Oral Surgery, Oral Medicine, Oral Pathology, Oral Radiology and Endodontics* **81**, 221–8.

196. Von Hippel R (1914) Zur Technik der Granulomoperation. *Deutsche Monatsschrifte fur Zahnheilkunde* **32**, 255–65.

197. Velvart P (2002) Papilla base incision: a new approach to recession-free healing of the interdental papilla after endodontic surgery. *International Endodontic Journal* **35**, 453–80.

198. Velvart P, Ebner-Zimmermann U, Ebner JP (2004) Comparison of long-term papilla healing following sulcular full thickness flap and papilla base flap in endodontic surgery. *International Endodontic Journal* **37**, 687–93.

199. Velvart P, Peters CI (2005) Soft tissue management in endodontic surgery. *Journal of Endodontics* **31**, 4–16.

200. Velvart P, Peters CI, Peters OA (2005) Soft tissue management: flap design, incision, tissue elevation, and tissue retraction. *Endodontic Topics* **11**, 78–97.

201. Velvart P, Peters CI, Peters OA (2005) Soft tissue management: suturing and wound closure. *Endodontic Topics* **11**, 179–95.

202. Vickers FJ, Baumgartner JC, Marshall G (2002) Hemostatic efficacy and cardiovascular effects of agents used during endodontic surgery. *Journal of Endodontics* **28**, 322–3.

203. Walia HD, Newlin S, Austin BP (1995) Electrochemical analysis of retrofilling microleakage in extracted human teeth. *Journal of Dental Research* **74**, 101; Abstract 719.

204. Wallace JA (1996) Transantral endodontic surgery. *Oral Surgery, Oral Medicine, Oral Pathology, Oral Radiology and Endodontics* **82**, 80–4.

205. Weaver SM (1947) Root canal treatment with visual evidence of histologic repair. *Journal of the American Dental Association* **35**, 483–97.

206. Weine FS (1980) The case against intentional replantation. *Journal of the American Dental Association* **100**, 664–8.

207. Weine FS, Gerstein H (1976) Periapical surgery. In Weine FS, editor. *Endodontic therapy*, pp. 287–351, 2nd edn. St Louis, MO: Mosby.

208. Witherspoon DE, Gutmann JL (1996) Haemostasis in periradicular surgery. *International Endodontic Journal* **29**, 135–49.

209. Wu MK, Kean SD, Kersten HW (1990) A quantitative microleakage study on a new retrograde filling technique. *International Endodontic Journal* **23**, 245–9.

210. Wu MK, Kontakiotis EG, Wesselink PR (1998) Long-term seal provided by some root-end filling materials. *Journal of Endodontics* **24**, 557–60.

211. Wuchenich G, Meadows D, Torabinejad M (1994) A comparison between two root end preparation techniques in human cadavers. *Journal of Endodontics* **20**, 279–82.

212. Zetterqvist L, Anneroth G, Nordenram A (1987) Glass-ionomer cement as retrograde filling material: an experimental investigation in monkeys. *International Journal of Oral and Maxillofacial Surgery* **16**, 459–64.

213. Zetterqvist L, Hall G, Holmlund A (1991) Apicectomy: a clinical comparison of amalgam and glass ionomer cement as apical sealants. *Oral Surgery, Oral Medicine, Oral Pathology* **71**, 489–91.

Chapter 14

Expected Outcomes in the Prevention and Treatment of Apical Periodontitis

Shimon Friedman

14.1 The importance of studying the prognosis of apical periodontitis

During the past decade, the concepts of clinical decision-making prevailing in society have gradually shifted. In the past, healthcare professionals, including dentists and endodontists, had been expected to make clinical decisions based on their own knowledge and experience, and to prescribe treatment accordingly for individual patients. They had enjoyed a paternalistic status, and their authority usually overruled the patient's individual preferences. Currently, clinicians are expected to base clinical decisions on evidence derived from clinical trials. Furthermore, they are required to share the evidence-based information with their patients, and to respect the concept of "patient autonomy" [9,116,319,373,460]. Accordingly, patients should be fully informed about the benefits and risks of available treatment alternatives, and allowed to select a specific treatment based on their individual values. In addition to the information obtained from the clinician, patients can readily access information about available treatments via the Internet, and use it to challenge the clinician's recommendations. To be able to function successfully in this new climate, clinicians must be well versed in the evidence that supports the clinical treatment procedures they suggest to patients. A key element of this evidence is the current knowledge about the prognosis and expected outcome of the alternative treatments available.

When used in the context of healthcare, the term "prognosis" is defined as the forecast of the course of disease. In endodontology, this term applies to teeth affected by apical periodontitis; it describes the *time course* and *chances of healing* after endodontic treatment, both nonsurgical and surgical. Because during surgical treatment, the diseased tissue is actually eradicated, the reference to healing applies instead to the surgical wound. Use of similar terms for both the nonsurgical and surgical treatment modalities is particularly helpful when one treatment is to be weighed against the other.

Variations of what comprises contemporary root canal treatment and surgical endodontics have been used clinically for over 100 years. It is not surprising, therefore, that reports describing the outcome of these treatments have been published for nearly a century, including over 90 studies on initial root canal treatment and retreatment, and over 70 studies on surgical endodontics (principally apical surgery). Most of these studies, encompassing data from over 20,000 treated teeth, had been reviewed and comprehensively discussed to summarize the state-of-the-art knowledge at different junctures. Strindberg [405] reviewed studies on nonsurgical treatment reported in the first half of the twentieth century, while Rud *et al.* [355] reviewed studies on surgical endodontics reported up to 1970. In the first edition of this textbook, Friedman *et al.* [125] reviewed studies on both nonsurgical and surgical endodontic treatment reported from 1956 to 1997. These three reviews and subsequent ones [127,130,131,172] have clearly demonstrated that the reported outcomes of nonsurgical and surgical endodontic treatment have been incoherent and, at times, contradictory. Thus, in spite of the vast information available, answers to the main questions related to the prognosis of endodontic treatment have remained obscured by the nonstand-

ardized materials and methods of the many studies. Furthermore, the clinical procedures in endodontics have evolved to such an extent that the results of specific studies are possibly rendered less relevant today than they had been in the past. The methodological and technical variation mentioned above suggests that *indiscriminate review of the many available studies would be futile and potentially misleading.*

It is well established that to answer questions about the prognosis of a disease following state-of-the-art treatment, a review must focus on studies that are selected according to well-defined criteria. The purpose of this chapter is to review reports on the outcome of nonsurgical and surgical endodontic treatment performed for the prevention and treatment of apical periodontitis, and based on selected articles, to define the prognosis of these treatments and to identify predictors of their outcome. The nonsurgical treatment procedures, initial root canal treatment and retreatment, are reviewed first, followed by the surgical treatments.

14.2 The limitations of cross-sectional studies of root-filled teeth in general populations

Data on the prevalence of apical periodontitis is available from many studies published in different countries [4,37,39,41,43,77,78,85,88,90,96,99,100,136, 162,176,179,180,183,191,193,209–212,233,237, 247,293,329,330,332,344,372,376,384,397,439,458]. The epidemiological aspects of these studies are reviewed in Chapter 8. Of interest for this chapter is the information regarding the prevalence of apical periodontitis associated with root-filled teeth (Table 14.1). This prevalence is alarmingly high, ranging from 20% to over 60%, and it should be considered as reflecting the realistic outcome of endodontic treatment in the general population. Paradoxically, the reported prevalence is at the lower end of the range in specific populations where state-of-the-art endodontic treatment has not been readily available; however, in these populations the mean number of teeth in the remaining dentition is lower than in populations of other studies. Smaller remaining dentition suggests that teeth affected by persistent apical periodontitis after endodontic treatment may have been extracted, and thus not accounted for in the respective studies [247].

Table 14.1 Prevalence of apical periodontitis and inadequate root fillings in root–filled teeth, as shown in cross–sectional studies

Study	Country	Subjects	Ages (years)	Apical periodontitis	Inadequate root filling
Hansen and Johansen 1976	Sweden	111	35	20%	–
Hugoson and Koch 1979	Sweden	1000	20–70	22–29%	–
Hugoson et al. 1986	Sweden	1000	20–80	23–44%	–
Allard and Palmqvist 1986	Sweden	500	≥65	27%	69%
Petersson et al. 1986	Sweden	861	20–60	31%	60%
Bergström et al. 1987	Sweden	250	21–60	29%	–
Eckerbom et al. 1987	Sweden	200	20–60+	26%	55%
Eriksen et al. 1988	Norway	141	35	26%	59%
Eckerbom et al. 1989	Sweden	200	20–60+	22%	49%
Petersson et al. 1989	Sweden	567	20–70+	21% [nst]	63%
				65% [st]	
Ödesjö et al. 1990	Sweden	751	20–80+	25%	70%
Eriksen and Bjertness 1991	Norway	119	50	37%	51%
Imfeld 1991	Switzerland	143	66	31%	64%
Eckerbom et al. 1991	Sweden	200	20–60+	26%	–
De Cleen et al. 1993	Netherlands	184	20–60+	39%	51%
Petersson 1993	Sweden	586	20–60	31%	50%
Ray and Trope 1995	USA	985 [teeth]		39%	50%
Buckley and Spångberg 1995	USA	208	–20–80+	31%	58%
Eriksen et al. 1995	Norway	121	35	38%	33%
Soikonen 1995	Finland	133	76, 81, 86	16%	75%
Saunders et al. 1997	UK	340	20–59+	58%	58%
Weiger et al. 1997	Germany	323	12–89	61%	86%
Marques et al. 1998	Portugal	179	30–39	22%	54%
Sidaravicius et al. 1999	Lithuania	147	35–44	35% [a]	87%
De Moor et al. 2000	Belgium	206	18–59	40%	57%
Tronstad et al. 2000	Norway	1001 [teeth]	–	37%	49%
Kirkevang et al. 2000	Denmark	614	20–60+	52%	74%
Kirkevang et al. 2001	Denmark	602	20–60+	51% [c]	73%
				58% [d]	74%
Kirkevang et al. 2001	Denmark	614 [b]	20–60+	52%	–
Boucher et al. 2002	France	208	18–70	30%	79%
Lupi–Pegurier et al. 2002	France	344	33–65	32%	69%
Hommez et al. 2002	Belgium	745 [teeth]	–	33%	66%
Dugas et al. 2003	Canada	610	25–40	45%	61%
Boltacz-Rzepkowska and Pawlicka 2003	Poland	236	15–76	25%	51%
Segura-Egea et al. 2004	Spain	180	31–53	65%	66%
Loftus et al. 2005	Ireland	302	16–98	25%	53%
Georgopolou et al. 2005	Greece	320	16–77	60%	–
Kabak and Abbott 2005	Belarus	1423	15–65+	45%	48%
Kirkevang et al. 2006	Denmark	473 [b]	20–60+	44%	–

[nst] Nonsurgically treated.
[st] Surgically treated.
[a] Pulp amputated teeth excluded.

[b] Repeated sample.
[c] Treated in 1974–5.
[d] Treated in 1997–8.

Other than presenting a "snapshot" picture of the percentage of teeth presenting with periapical radiolucency, the cross-sectional study methodology does not allow collection of all the data pertaining to the treatment histories of the observed root-filled teeth. Therefore, the reported data are subject to interpretation [98]. Some of the teeth may have been captured shortly after treatment and their radiolucency, while definitely present, may have been reduced from its original size. These teeth appear to be associated with apical periodontitis, but their assessment may be premature, and they may even be healing. In fact, when specific populations were re-examined 6–11 years after their first account in a cross-sectional study, a certain percentage of lesions were observed to heal, but a comparable percentage of new lesions had developed [89,209,210,331].

In the past decade attempts have been made to use the cross-sectional data to explore relationships between the outcome of treatment and specific clinical factors, notably the apparent quality of the restoration and root canal filling. One study [344] suggested that the quality of the restoration had a greater impact on the outcome than the quality of the root canal filling, while other studies reported the opposite [436] or no difference in the impact of these two clinical factors [85,176,211,384,439]. These contradictions are not surprising, because the cross-sectional methodology is unsuitable for investigating such relationships [112]. Thus, the outcome impact of the quality of the restoration or the root canal filling cited in these studies may not be valid.

In recent years, there have been attempts to expand the collection of data on the treated teeth examined in cross-sectional studies by interviewing the patients included in the studies and ascertaining that recently treated teeth have been excluded [85,176,384,458]. Nevertheless, essential information on the pretreatment diagnosis and treatment methods is still unavailable even with these methodological improvements. One observation, however, is consistent throughout the cross-sectional studies: the apparent quality of the root canal fillings is poor in the majority of treated teeth (Table 14.1). This poor quality of treatment has been correlated with the poor outcome observed in the studies [211,439].

14.3 The diversity of reported outcomes in follow-up studies on endodontic treatment

Over the years many studies have been published where information can be gleaned on the outcome of initial root canal treatment [2,3,18,19,25,26,31,34, 48–50,63–65,69,71,72,93,94,97,104,107,114,123,129, 145,149,167,169–171,173,177,182,184,192,202,213, 222,246,248,249,265,269–273,275,285,296,297,299, 301,302,304,310,318,326,327,333,367,377,379,382, 391,393,395,399,403,405,418,421,443,454,455,459, 476], root canal retreatment [1,5,36,64,75,76,93,103, 123,132,144,145,219,265,318,334,377,391,405,414, 444], surgical endodontics [5,7,8,20,22,61,62,68,75,76, 81,95,110,113,117,119,134,151,166,174,185,186,189, 190,219,224,227,238,239,245,250,258,266,287–289, 308,322,323,341,343,346,353–355,357,359,361, 363,375,394,407,422,424,448,450,453,456,478,479], and intentional replantation [32,79,92,148,150,194, 198,208,214,468]. As a whole, this extensive body of literature is characterized by great diversity of the reported outcomes. This diversity suggests that indiscriminate summaries and direct comparisons among these studies are inappropriate. The main cause of the diversity of reported outcomes is differences among the studies in the composition of study materials, treatment procedures, and methodology. Some of these differences are highlighted below, with examples for nonsurgical and surgical treatment.

14.3.1 Composition of study materials

Tooth location, number of roots

Relatively few of the studies on nonsurgical endodontic treatment include only anterior or single-rooted teeth [2,31,48,69–72,167,219,222,326,391,393,414,421, 443], whereas the majority pool single- and multi-rooted teeth together. In contrast, the majority of studies on surgical endodontics include primarily anterior or single-rooted teeth. Fewer studies include a substantial proportion of multi-rooted teeth [20,22, 75,95,239,341,343,353,357,359–361,407,424,448,456], whereas only a few studies include primarily multi-rooted teeth [7,119,185,224,323,362,363,450].

Treatment of single- and multi-rooted teeth may present different complexities, and these differences may be reflected in the outcome of treatment. The surgical endodontics procedure in particular, is more complex when performed on a multi-rooted tooth than on a tooth with a single root, and the access to the multi-rooted, posterior teeth is generally more restricted than to the anterior single-rooted tooth.

In studies where each root is evaluated as an independent unit [3,36,64,97,145,192,202,265,273,299,302, 326,391,454], the contribution of multi-rooted teeth to the total study sample is multiplied, as each tooth contributes two or three units, as opposed to the single unit contributed by a single-rooted tooth. Most importantly, when multi-rooted teeth are evaluated as whole units and assessed by the worst appearing root, the risk of observing persistent apical periodontitis after treatment is multiplied [123]. Thus, the outcome recorded is poorer than what would be recorded if each root of the multi-rooted tooth were evaluated independently.

Sample size

The size of the sample included in a clinical study is one of the determinants of the study's internal and external validity [112]. The sample size also determines the power of the statistical analysis, when comparing groups to assess the effect of different variables on the outcome of treatment. The smaller the difference in outcome, the larger is the sample required in each group to achieve sufficient power for significance to be established [112].

The limitations of sample size are demonstrated in the following two examples. Trope *et al.* [443] reported a nonsignificant difference in the outcome of endodontic treatment among 86 teeth with apical periodontitis, treated in one session (64% healed, adjusted calculation) or two sessions (74% healed, adjusted calculation). Their power analysis suggested that 354 teeth would be required in each group to substantiate the 10% difference in healing statistically (with 80% power). Similarly, Wang *et al.* [456] reported a nonsignificant difference in the outcome of surgical endodontics, between 58 teeth with persistent disease after initial root canal treatment (74% healed) and 32 teeth with persistent disease after root canal retreatment (84% healed). They calculated that in order to establish significance between these groups under the conditions of their study (with 80% power and a 5% significance level), 400 teeth would be required in the initial treatment group and 220 teeth in the retreatment group. Thus, in studies with relatively

small samples [3,69,71,219,246,275,326,333,393,414,44 3,459,476], specific variables may not have a significant association with the outcome, whereas in studies with large samples the same variables may emerge as significant outcome predictors.

Case selection criteria

The process of case selection involves the differentiation of potential candidates for treatment according to their prognosis; therefore, it is likely to determine the results of a clinical study [184]. Drastic differences in case selection can be observed among outcome studies, both those on nonsurgical and surgical treatment. Among the former, cases judged to have an unfavorable prognosis or subjects with a compromised immune system were excluded in specific studies [167,182, 270–272,327,443], while one study [3] included only teeth with obstructed canals, in which the ability to fulfill the technical objectives of treatment was doubtful. In other studies [103,104,123,129,248] no exclusion criteria were applied; teeth were included even if they were compromised by advanced marginal periodontitis or procedural errors. Among the surgery studies, teeth with deep periodontal defects, that could impair the prognosis, were frequently excluded [62,134, 189,219,353,479], while one study [394] included only teeth affected by loss of the buccal bone plate. In the majority of studies, consecutive cases were included without specific exclusion criteria. Thus, the reported outcomes in specific studies may have been influenced by inclusion of teeth with poor prognosis.

Proportion of teeth with apical periodontitis

There is wide agreement among studies that the presence of apical periodontitis at the time of treatment has a negative influence on the outcome of nonsurgical endodontic treatment [131]. Therefore, the proportion of teeth affected by apical periodontitis included in any study sample becomes an important consideration. This proportion has ranged among the various studies from less than 30% [3,18,64,94,107, 114,145,149,222,299,304] to 100% [26,48,49,69–71, 97,182,213,219,275,326,382,393,414,443,455,459], while it has not even been specified in many other studies   [173,177,184,270–272,297,302,399,454,476]. Thus, the reported outcomes in specific studies may have been influenced by the proportion of teeth with apical periodontitis; the more such teeth were included, the poorer may have been the overall outcome.

Previous endodontic treatment – initial treatment or retreatment – before surgical endodontics

The majority of teeth included in studies on surgical endodontics have had persistent disease after initial root canal treatment, likely to be sustained by bacteria harbored within the root canal system. The surgical attempt at sealing off the intracanal bacteria may be ineffective; therefore, the treatment outcome may be compromised [128,456]. In one study, however, all the teeth had persistent disease after "at least one non-surgical retreatment to enhance canal debridement" [479], and 91% of them healed. Persistent disease after root canal retreatment is likely to be sustained by bacteria colonizing an inaccessible, possibly extra-radicular site. Because such sites can be eradicated by the surgical procedure, a healing rate in the range of 90% can be expected [128,456]. Thus, the previous treatment history of the teeth included in studies on surgical endodontics is expected to influence the reported outcome; however, the vast majority of the studies do not so characterize their cohorts.

14.3.2 Treatment procedures

Treatment providers

Experienced and skillful operators are less likely to perform procedural errors that might compromise the prognosis [184]; therefore, study results may vary according to the providers of treatment and their expertise. In studies on surgical endodontics a distinction should be made between treatment providers with different qualifications. Surgical endodontics has been predominantly performed by oral surgeons; however, over the years it has gradually become the domain of endodontists. The endodontic community has drastically modified the techniques of surgical endodontics, and now routinely uses operating microscopes and microsurgical instruments, ultrasonic cavity preparation devices, novel materials for root-end filling, and improved strategies for hemostasis and suturing. It appears, however, that oral surgeons have not fully embraced these modified strategies [375], and that their treatment outcomes may have fallen behind those of endodontists [341]. Providers of treatment in the different studies on surgical endodontics included oral surgeons [7,22,61,75, 76,95,110,113,119,151,174,185,186,190,227,238, 239,245,250,258,266,267,287–289,308,321–323,355,

357,359,360,362,363,375,407,424,448,450,478], endodontists [5,20,62,117,119,134,219,238,343,353,354, 479], and specialty trainees [5,189,341,343,456]. In studies on nonsurgical endodontic treatment, providers of treatment varied from undergraduate students [36,48,93,94,97,145,149,169,170,182,184,192,202,213, 265,269,273,299,301,302,391,403,418,454] to endodontists [18,31,49,107,123,132,173,177,184,219,246, 249,270–272,296,297,318,326,327,377,379,399,405, 414,443,459,476]. The reported outcomes in the specific studies are likely to vary accordingly.

Asepsis in studies on nonsurgical endodontic treatment

In at least two of the studies [26,192], treatment was routinely performed without rubber dam. It can be assumed that in these, and several other studies, asepsis was not strictly observed; compromised asepsis would impair the outcome.

Intracanal procedures in studies on nonsurgical endodontic treatment

Specific root canal preparation techniques, such as the serial filing technique [202] and root filling materials, such as Kloroperka N-Ø and rosin–chloroform [265,299], have been associated with poorer prognosis of root canal treatment than other techniques and materials. Several studies [3,48,158,192,202,213,219, 265,391,393,395,399,405,414] have used those reportedly ineffective procedures. In contrast, procedures alleged to be most effective, such as the "Schilder technique", have been used in other studies, exclusively [318] or in part of the sample [103,104,129,248]. The variability with regards to the intracanal procedures is indeed striking; however, the effect of this variability on the outcome is subject to speculation [405].

Also intracanal medicaments used may have been ineffective. Intracanal medication may be critical for controlling root canal infection [44–48,74,383], but not all agents used are effective and beneficial. For example, arsenic and formaldehyde are extremely toxic and no longer used as intracanal medicaments; however, they were used in at least one study [405]. The antimicrobial efficacy of "classical" medications, such as camphorated phenol and paramonochlorophenol, iodine–potassium iodide, and formocresol, is short-lived [102,256,434] and may be insufficient for interappointment disinfection of canals associated with apical periodontitis [46]. These classical medications have been used in many studies [2,25,26,145,167, 169,170,202,270–272,403,421], where they may have compromised the results, while the more effective calcium hydroxide [Ca(OH)$_2$] dressing was used in other studies [48,49,64,97,103,104,123,129,177,182,219,246, 248,299,302,326,327,391,414,443,459]. In contrast, in specific studies [18,107,297,318,393] treatment was invariably completed in one session, without the use of any intracanal medication.

Bacterial culturing in studies on nonsurgical endodontic treatment

In several studies microbiological sampling from canals showing no bacterial growth (negative culture) was a prerequisite for root canal filling [48,93,213,391]. Whenever reliable culturing procedures were used, the negative culture was an indication of effective disinfection; such has been associated with an improved prognosis relative to teeth with a positive culture [93,393,414].

Root-end management in studies on surgical endodontics

The traditional root-end cavity preparation with round burs is inferior to the currently used cavity preparation with ultrasonic tips [55,143,229,254,448, 449,471]. Likewise, root-end filling with amalgam has been shown to be inferior to the currently used materials, IRM and EBA cements or mineral trioxide aggregate [14,338,339,430,442]. In specific studies [189,357–363] none of the above was used, but rather a composite resin "cap" was bonded to the root-end. The reportedly less effective strategies have been used in the majority of studies in the past and in several recent ones [22,75,76,186,219,239,375,424], whereas the current strategies assumed to be more effective have been used in other recent studies [22,62,341,353, 354,407,424,448,450,456,479]. The considerable variability of root-end management procedures is likely to obscure the outcomes of surgical endodontics.

Concurrent root canal and surgical treatment

In a review article, Friedman [118] highlighted the considerable difference in outcome between surgical endodontics performed alone on teeth where disease persisted after previous root canal treatment, and concurrent surgical and root canal treatment, consistent with the historical management of teeth with large

lesions. The latter had been commonly applied in the past, and in fact, represented the majority in many studies [7,68,113,151,166,185,227,258,355]. In those studies, outcomes were often summarized for the entire cohort, resulting in better outcomes reported than what should be expected if only surgical endodontics had been performed [118]. Thus, in many studies the proportion of teeth that received not just apical surgery but also concurrent root canal treatment determined the outcomes.

Preoperative and postoperative restoration

In studies on nonsurgical endodontic treatment the influence of the permanent restoration (type and timing of placement) on the prognosis is vague at best. Occasionally, it is indicated that a proportion of the teeth had not been restored [103,104,169,170,248]. A lacking or compromised restoration may impair the prognosis [103,170,418], and the outcome is likely to be influenced by this factor.

When surgical endodontics is performed, the preoperative restoration is often left in place postoperatively. The outcome of treatment is impaired by lack of a permanent restoration or presence of a defective restoration [341,343,456].

The majority of studies have not provided detailed information about the restorative status of the treated teeth, but it is likely that in many studies the outcomes were influenced by inclusion of teeth with defective or missing restorations.

14.3.3 Methodology

The current emphasis in the healthcare community on evidence-based practice has raised the awareness of the critical role of appropriate methodology in assigning relative importance to clinical studies. Hierarchies of evidence have been developed for differentiating studies, by ranking them according to methodology (see Section 14.5). Among endodontic follow-up studies, there is considerable variability in the methods of collecting, recording, processing and reporting data. Consequently, some studies rank higher than others in the hierarchy of evidence, and they should be assigned more importance.

Study design and availability of detailed data

Retrospective and prospective studies differ, particularly in the possibility of bias influencing the reported outcomes. Furthermore, often the retrospective studies (and occasionally also prospective ones) lack important data on the composition of the material, treatment procedures, and complications. The results of studies where important information is lacking cannot be used as the basis for projecting prognosis.

Similarly, results of specific studies designed to answer one research question, either regarding nonsurgical treatment [101,144,182,219,299,301,326,333, 393,414,443,454,459] or surgical endodontics [62,76, 81,110,134,189,190,219,288,308,322,343,358,478] may not be directly compared with those of other studies with regard to general prognosis.

Recall rate

Availability of the entire study cohort for outcome assessment at the endpoint of the study is subject to population mobility, particularly in long-term studies. When subjects included in the inception cohort are not available for follow-up their treatment outcome is unknown. In the best-case scenario (if all missing patients experienced a favorable outcome) the reported outcome would be better, while in the worst-case scenario (if all missing patients experienced an unfavorable outcome) the reported outcome would be poorer. For example, in a study on surgical endodontics [456] the recall rate was 85%, and 74% of the teeth had healed. The authors calculated that in the best-case scenario 80% of the teeth would have healed, while in the worst-case scenario 57% would have healed. Because the overall "healed" rate is further from the lower value than from the upper one, it would appear to be overestimated [456]. Thus, when a large proportion of the inception cohort is unavailable the results of the study may be considerably skewed and subject to speculation [112,318,405]. The results may be considered invalid unless the unavailable patients are deceased or cannot be reached, suggesting that their absence is not related to the outcome [112,405]. For this reason a recall rate of at least 80% is required for a high level of evidence [80,225,416]. The reported recall rates in the different studies on nonsurgical endodontic treatment have varied from under 20% [64,170,377] to over 90% [49,65,219,275, 296,326,393,414,459]. Similarly, in studies on surgical endodontics the recall rates varied from less than 20% [20] to over 90% [8,68,75,76,95,110,186,190,219, 224,258,322,323,346,357,394,407,448,450,453,478, 479]. Moreover, the recall rate is not even reported in many studies on nonsurgical treatment [2,5,31,69,

71,149,173,399,403,418] and on surgical endodontics [5,61,81,113,117,118,238,266,422]. This may be one reason for the inconsistent outcomes reported among studies.

Interpretation of radiographs

Invariably, radiographs have been used as the principal outcome measure in follow-up studies after endodontic treatment; however, radiographs are poorly standardized, being subject to change in angulation and contrast, and they do not capture subtle inflammatory changes in the periapical tissues [42]. Importantly, interpretation of radiographs is subject to bias [87,141,142,345,475]. These limitations of radiographs may undermine the reliability of the results; therefore, to minimize bias and inconsistency, assessment by blinded examiners who are calibrated for standardized interpretation, is essential [87,157,223,264,299,345, 348]. This requirement has not been fulfilled in the majority of studies, thus the outcomes are likely to reflect differences in radiological interpretation.

Follow-up period

Healing of apical periodontitis after nonsurgical treatment is a dynamic process, requiring sufficient time for completion [48,302,405]. A short-term observation may demonstrate only signs of healing [123,275,302,405]; therefore, short-term studies, particularly those extending a year or shorter [5,123,182,270–272,318, 377,379,418,443], may misrepresent the prognosis and considerably underestimate the healing potential [184,299,347,405]. Although follow-up of at least a year is required to reveal meaningful changes [101,182,302], extension of the follow-up to 3–4 years may be required to record a more stable treatment outcome [48,202,299,302,405]. But changes may occur even at a later time. Indeed, comparing the 4-year and the final follow-up examinations, Strindberg [405] observed a difference in healing rates of 16%, and stated that: "it seems doubtful whether it is possible to establish a practicable upper limit for the observation period beyond which disappearance of rarefaction can be regarded as unlikely". Long-term changes in outcome have also been reported in other studies [132,210,269].

In studies on surgical endodontics a particular concern is recurrence of disease, shown to occur in 5–42% of healed teeth after periods of 4 years or longer [110,117,159,190,219,289,354]. For example, of 45 teeth recorded as healed at the 1-year follow-up, Kvist and Reit[219] reported recurrence of disease in four teeth (9%) at the 4-year follow-up. Thus, short-term studies [5,22,75,76,81,189,224,322,323,353,357,359,375,448, 450,478] may not reflect the true, long-term outcome of surgical endodontics.

Furthermore, because with time, root-filled teeth are subject to adverse effects of periodontal and restorative deterioration, extensive follow-up periods are more likely to reveal the influence of those effects on the outcome. Many studies vary considerably in the extent of follow-up periods; therefore, their reported outcomes are likely to reflect this variability.

Analysis

Statistical analyses are used in treatment outcome studies mainly to investigate associations between the outcome and different variables. This issue can be considerably confused by the nature of the analysis, or the lack thereof. In the vast majority of studies on both nonsurgical and surgical treatment, only bivariate analyses have been used that ignore potential confounding effects of multiple variables [405]. For example, in a study on nonsurgical treatment, Halse and Molven [158] offer two conclusions: (i) teeth in which overfilling occurred have a poorer outcome than teeth filled without overfilling, and (ii) presence of apical periodontitis at the time of treatment has a strong negative influence on the outcome. However, reading through the study reveals that overfilling occurred more frequently in teeth with apical periodontitis. Clearly then, the poorer outcome can be "blamed" on the presence of apical periodontitis, but not necessarily on the overfilling. In studies on surgical endodontics, presence or absence of a root-end filling has often been compared disregarding the fact that some teeth received root canal treatment in conjunction with surgery, while others did not. When concurrent root canal treatment was performed, this had a strong positive impact on the outcome [151,266]. Because root-end fillings were usually absent in these teeth, researchers concluded that teeth without root-end fillings had a better outcome than teeth with root-end fillings [118]. Thus, differences in analyses or use of only bivariate analysis may generate different conclusions in studies regarding the prognostic importance of specific variables.

Unit of evaluation

The outcome of endodontic treatment can be recorded for each root or for each tooth. Considering individual roots as units of evaluation facilitates comparisons among studies; however, this strategy raises concerns in regards to multi-rooted teeth [127]. When roots are counted as units, more weight is assigned to studies with a large proportion of multi-rooted teeth than to studies that include primarily single-rooted teeth. Also, the healing rate becomes higher than if whole teeth are counted as units [93,123,127,270–272,405,418]. This fact is demonstrated clearly in a follow-up study [93], where healing was observed in 78% of teeth and in 83% of roots, and in a cross-sectional study [41] where the prevalence of apical periodontitis was reported separately for root-filled teeth (29.7%) and roots (24.4%) for the same French sub-population. Although the majority of the studies have considered the tooth as the evaluated unit, the individual roots have been evaluated as independent units in many of the studies on nonsurgical treatment [3,36,101,132,145,192,202,265,269,299,302,304,391, 405] and on surgical endodontics [7,119,134,185,238, 359–361,363]. There is a view that the unit of evaluation should be one tooth per patient rather than multiple roots or teeth, to eliminate systemic influences; the evidence for this approach has not been substantiated.

Outcome assessment criteria

The main cause for the diverse outcomes reported in clinical studies in endodontics is the inconsistency of the criteria used to assess the outcome. In many studies on nonsurgical treatment [60,167,169,171, 182,202,213,246,265,275,299,301,302,327,333,377, 379,395,443,454], and in at least one surgical endodontics study [343], the radiological appearance is used as the only outcome measure. This strategy possibly overestimates the "success" rate by not noting teeth that could be radiologically normal, but symptomatic [127]. The rate of success is overestimated to an even greater extent when healed and reduced lesions are grouped together, as has often been the case [31,167,171,249,270–272,377,379,382,395]. This important cause of variability is considered in the following section.

14.4 The assessment and classification of endodontic treatment outcome

The classification of outcome has been inconsistent among follow-up studies on nonsurgical and surgical endodontic treatment [125]. Considerable confusion has been caused by the use of nonspecific, ambiguous terms such as "success" and "failure" to define outcome. The confusion is increased by the frequent lack of calibration of examiners who assess the outcome, and the use of different observer strategies to record radiological findings.

14.4.1 Consistency of assessment

The assessment of radiological images is highly inconsistent [87,141,142,345,475]. To improve the consistency of outcome assessment, specific observer and calibration strategies have been suggested for studies on nonsurgical and surgical endodontic treatment [87, 157,223,264,268,345,348,356]. These strategies have been applied infrequently.

To address concerns of radiological interpretation and outcome definitions, Ørstavik *et al.* [298] introduced the periapical index (PAI) for the radiological appraisal of root-filled teeth. The PAI relies on the comparison of the evaluated radiographs with a set of five radiological images, which represent histologically confirmed periapical conditions [42]. These reference images represent a range of periapical conditions, from a healthy presentation (score 1) to severe apical periodontitis (score 5). To avoid bias, the examiner is calibrated until reaching a level of adequate reproducibility. Each radiograph is then assessed independently in a "blind" manner, and assigned a score according to which of the five reference images it appears to match. By reducing bias associated with the interpretation of radiographs, this method permits reproducible comparisons among different studies [298], and it appears to be more sensitive than a less structured assessment of success/failure [304]. However, it has been used only in a minority of the studies on nonsurgical treatment [103,104,129,182, 246,248,301,302,304,327,443,454,455], and it has not been validated for outcome assessment after surgical endodontics [62]. Nevertheless, the PAI has been used in one recent study on surgical endodontics [456] to assist in unbiased interpretation of the radiographs and to promote comparisons with studies on nonsurgical endodontic treatment by the same group [103,104,129]. Results obtained with the PAI cannot directly be interpreted as measures of success or failure. Originally, the researchers reported on the extent of increase or decrease in mean scores within groups. However, in recent cross-sectional and cohort studies [41,85,103,104,129,182,210,248,327,443,454,455], PAI

scores are dichotomized, with scores 1 and 2 representing "healthy" periapical tissues, and scores of 3 and above representing "disease".

14.4.2 Success/failure: ambiguous terms

The main disparity among studies is between the use of "strict" and "lenient" classifications of a successful outcome, as outlined below.

Strict classification: radiological and clinical normalcy

In the majority of studies a successful outcome is strictly defined by *full normalcy*, comprising both normal *radiological* (absence of radiolucency) and *clinical* (absence of signs, symptoms) presentation. In studies on nonsurgical treatment such full normalcy is most frequently referred to as success. Within this strict definition a small radiolucency is accepted if it appears around extruded filling materials [93,391,393,405,414], but otherwise incomplete healing or any remaining radiolucency is excluded.

In studies on surgical endodontics the full normalcy is often referred to as "complete healing", and occasionally as "success". A typical radiological appearance of a periapical scar, referred to as "incomplete" healing or "cicatrice", is also considered to be a successful outcome [11,12,267,289,356]. Apparently, in studies on surgical endodontics the complete healing category is particularly subject to observer variation [264], and the incomplete healing category has been subject to interpretation errors; in one report [267], one of 24 teeth classified as incomplete healing was later considered as not healed.

Lenient classification: clinical normalcy

In contrast to the strict definition described above, in specific studies on nonsurgical treatment, the researchers define success primarily as the *absence of clinical signs and symptoms*. In the majority of these studies the clinical normalcy is coupled with a decreased size of the radiolucency [249,270–272,310, 333,334,377,379,395] while in a few studies, the radiolucency can even be unchanged, as long as it has not increased [167,382,418].

The confusion is even greater in studies on surgical endodontics, where the category of incomplete healing has often been misused to describe reduced radiolucency rather than the typical scars, but still considered a successful outcome. Furthermore, as in several nonsurgical studies, a successful outcome is occasionally defined primarily by the *normal clinical presentation*, even if it is accompanied by different degrees of residual radiolucency [8,407].

"Uncertain", "questionable", "doubtful", or "improved" categories

These categories have been used to imply uncertainty of outcome, and also improvement, adding to the inconsistency of classification. Several researchers [25,26,64,93,145,177,202,213,405] have used these terms strictly, to describe cases that could not be assessed because of insufficient radiological information. These undetermined cases were neither included in the successful nor the unsuccessful outcome category, usually lowering the success rate somewhat; recalculation of success after elimination of the questionable cases in the relevant studies yields success rates that are approximately 5% higher [64,93,145,202]. However, in other studies on nonsurgical treatment [2,3,49,123,149,192,265,326,459], and in many studies on surgical endodontics [5,60,95,110,224,227,250, 258,289,308,321–323,341,375,448,450,479] these terms have been used to describe decreased radiolucency, and considered either as a successful or uncertain outcome. Using this classification the success rate is not affected, but the failure rate is usually decreased in comparison with the former classification. In other surgical endodontics studies [75,76,113,119,151, 159,239,266,267,355,357,359–363,424,479] uncertain healing represents a decreased radiolucency whose appearance is different from that classified as incomplete healing. In these studies, if uncertain healing persists for 4 years or longer it is considered to be an unsuccessful outcome.

It is important to observe that use of the "lenient" outcome criteria, requiring clinical, but not radiological normalcy, increases the "success" rate in comparison with the "strict" criteria requiring both clinical and radiological normalcy. The difference between these criteria can be demonstrated with the following two examples. In a study on nonsurgical treatment, Friedman *et al.* [123] reported 78% complete healing and 16% incomplete healing; by strict criteria their success rate is 78%, whereas by lenient criteria the success rate is 94%. The discrepancy would be even larger if these researchers included persisting, unchanged radiolucency in the criteria for success. In a study on surgical

endodontics, Wang *et al.* [456] reported that 74% of the teeth healed and a further 15% appeared healing (reduced radiolucency), but only 9% had clinical signs or symptoms. By strict criteria their success rate is 74%, whereas by lenient criteria the success rate is 89% if reduction of the radiolucency is required, or 91% if only clinical normalcy is required.

The main dilemma with the more lenient criteria, however, is the fact that apical periodontitis is frequently asymptomatic, whether it is affecting an untreated tooth or persists after treatment [63,103, 104,114,129,175,177,230,248,318,335,336,459]. With regards to untreated teeth, apical periodontitis is universally considered a disease requiring treatment, regardless of the presence or absence of symptoms. By the same standard, persisting apical periodontitis after treatment cannot be regarded as success only because it is asymptomatic: *it is the same disease that treatment was aiming to cure, and it still requires management.*

As long as different researchers and clinicians continue to use different criteria for its definition, the term "success" will remain ambiguous and its use will continue to confuse communication within the profession and with patients. Because the same term is also used for alternative treatments such as implants, but with a different meaning, the risk exists that indiscriminate use of "success" may mislead patients who are weighing endodontic treatment against replacement of the tooth with an implant. Based on the specific definition of success for single-tooth implants [21,396], that is very different from that used in endodontics, the reported success rates [21,67,156,340,426] are considerably higher than those reported in most studies on endodontic treatment. Being unaware of the differences in the definition of success, the patient is likely to select the treatment alternative that suggests a better chance of success, and give up a tooth that can remain functional for many years.

Another concern is the term "failure" used in many of the endodontic treatment outcome studies to classify an unfavorable outcome. This term is not only ambiguous, as it does not imply the necessity to pursue any course of action, but it also has a negative connotation [419]. According to Ørstavik *et al.* [302], communication with patients can be promoted if the value-laden terms success and failure are replaced with more neutral expressions, such as "chance of healing" and "risk of inflammation". *Thus, it is advisable to avoid using the terms success and failure.*

14.4.3 Healing/disease/function: clear terms

Success is generally defined as "the accomplishment of an aim or purpose" (*Oxford English Dictionary*). The outcome, therefore, *is best defined in direct relation to the specific aim*. The aim of endodontic treatment is to prevent or cure apical periodontitis [303] (in the context of surgical endodontic treatment, the aim is to eradicate the disease and allow healing of the site). Accordingly, in order to promote effective communication within the profession and with patients, the outcome of endodontic treatment should be related to *healing* [48,127,130,131,302]. Indeed, the classification introduced by Rud *et al.* [356] for outcome assessment after surgical endodontics referred to healing (complete, incomplete, uncertain, unsatisfactory), but was construed to represent success and failure [151,189,266,479]. Rather than depending on interpretations of success and failure, the terms healed,

healing, and disease clearly describe the actual observation, as follows:

- *Healed*: a combined clinical (no signs, symptoms) and radiological (no residual radiolucency) normalcy (Fig. 14.1). Included in this classification is the strictly defined typical appearance of a scar after surgical endodontics [11,12,151,264,266,267, 356] (Fig. 14.2).
- *Healing (in progress)*: reduced radiolucency combined with clinical normalcy, in shorter follow-up periods than 4 years (Fig. 14.3). This is consistent with the strict definition of uncertain healing [151,264,266,356].
- *Persistent/recurrent/emerged disease*: presence of radiolucency (new, increased, unchanged, or reduced after observation exceeding 4 years) – an expression of apical periodontitis – with or without clinical signs and symptoms (Fig. 14.4). These terms

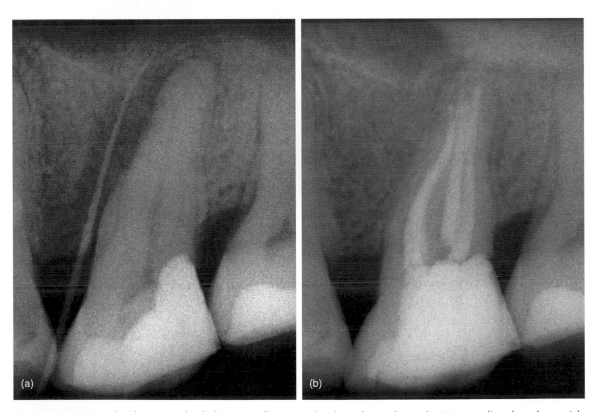

Fig. 14.1 Outcome classification as "healed". (a) Maxillary second molar with apical periodontitis extending along the mesial root surface, and associated sinus tract (traced with a gutta-percha cone). (b) At 1 year, the radiolucency is completely resolved and the tooth is symptom free, indicating it has healed. (Reprinted with permission from Friedman [121].)

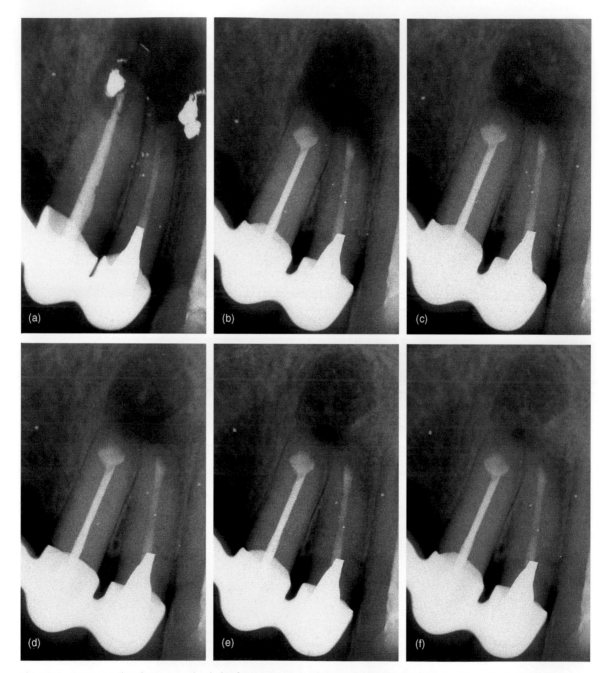

Fig. 14.2 Outcome classification as "healed" after repeat (second-time) surgery. (a) Root-filled and previously surgically-treated maxillary lateral incisor and canine, with poorly placed root-end fillings and persistent apical periodontitis. (b) Completed repeat surgery, including root-end filling with mineral trioxide aggregate. (c–e) After 4, 7, and 13 months, respectively, the lesion is becoming gradually smaller. (f) After 1½ years, the lesion is healed; a small scar is present between the two treated roots. (Reprinted with permission from Friedman [122].)

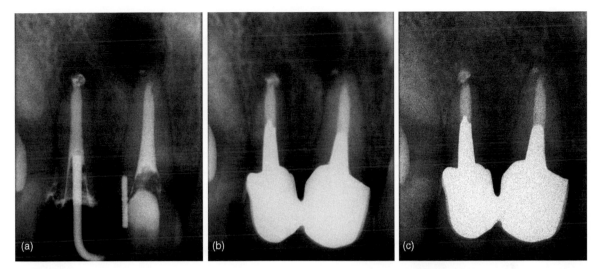

Fig. 14.3 Outcome classification as "healing" or "healed". Extent of the follow-up period. (a) Immediate postoperative radiograph of two maxillary incisors with apical periodontitis. (b) At 9 months, both teeth demonstrate reduced radiolucencies. Termination of a study at this endpoint would result in both teeth being recorded as healing. (c) At 18 months, both teeth are healed. Termination of a study at this endpoint would result in both teeth being recorded as completely healed. (Reprinted with permission from Friedman [121].)

should also be used when symptoms are present, even if the radiological appearance is normal.

For patient autonomy to be respected, clinicians should encourage individual patients to select from treatment alternatives based on their own values [319,373]. Similarly, *patients should be encouraged to articulate their expectations, or aims of treatment, and thus define what outcome should be considered a success.* Although the majority of patients may expect healing as the ultimate outcome, individual patients may only expect the elimination of clinical signs and symptoms. Furthermore, patients who would normally require healing may encounter clinical conditions that compromise the prognosis, such as an extensive loss of supporting bone prior to surgical endodontics [394]. If a patient is still motivated to attempt treatment with the understanding that healing is unlikely to occur, the *retention of the tooth in asymptomatic function* then becomes the aim of treatment, and the outcome defined as follows:

- *Asymptomatic function*: clinical normalcy combined with no or persistent radiolucency, reduced in size or unchanged (Fig. 14.5).

In the review of studies on nonsurgical and surgical endodontic treatment below, the terms healed, heal-

ing, asymptomatic function, and disease are used, in lieu of success and failure. The inconsistencies among studies outlined in previous sections preclude direct comparisons or grouping of studies to calculate average outcomes [127,130,265,395].

14.5 The best evidence for the prognosis of endodontic treatment

When clinicians seek evidence about the course and prognosis of a disease after a specific intervention they are advised to go beyond personal experiences and expert opinions. Rather, they should consult the clinical literature for applicable information [365]. Typically, however, there is much inconsistency among reports on prognosis [365]. Similarly, the reported outcomes of endodontic treatment differ across the many studies, mainly due to inconsistencies in composition, treatment procedures, and methodology (see Section 14.3). This diversity obscures the evidence necessary to estimate the prognosis and thus to support clinical decision-making regarding endodontic treatment. Because of this diversity, the required evidence cannot be derived from indiscriminate browsing of all available studies [10]. Strategies are required, therefore, that would allow the clinician to "navigate" the

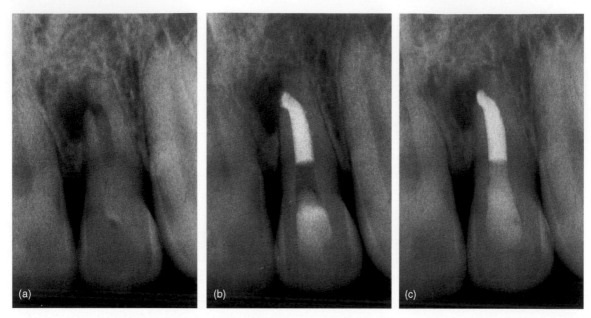

Fig. 14.4 Outcome classification as "disease". (a) Maxillary lateral incisor with apical periodontitis. (b) Immediate postoperative radiograph. (c) At 1 year, the tooth is symptom free, but the radiolucency has not been reduced, indicating persistence of the original disease. (Reprinted with permission from Friedman [121].)

wealth of available literature, and to glean valid and relevant evidence from selected studies. The basis of these strategies is the recognition that *clinical studies vary in the level of evidence they provide*, and the necessity to differentiate clinical studies according to the level of evidence. Therefore, it is necessary to apply an appraisal strategy to identify the studies that provide the best evidence.

14.5.1 Definition of terms

A brief review of the terms used in the appraisal of studies for levels of evidence is appropriate. These definitions differ from one authority to another. One example is the recent series of review articles on evidence-based endodontics [252,307,432,433], where the authors define the "cohort study" as a follow-up of an exposed cohort compared to an unexposed cohort, in contrast to the definition suggested below.

In this chapter the terms used are those defined by the Cochrane Collaboration (http://www.cochrane.dk/cochrane/handbook/hbook.htm), as follows:

* *Prospective study*: "In a prospective study, the study is designed ahead of time, and people are

then recruited and studied according to the study's criteria."
* *Retrospective study*: "In a retrospective study, the outcomes of a group of people are examined in hindsight ('after the event'). Retrospective studies are generally more limited in the data available for analysis, as the data have rarely been collected with the needs of that particular study in mind. This kind of limitation means that a retrospective study is usually less reliable than a prospective study."
* *Clinical trial*: "A clinical trial involves administering a treatment to test it. It is an experiment. Clinical trial is an umbrella term for a variety of health care trials. ... Types include uncontrolled trials, controlled clinical trials (CCT), community trials, and randomized controlled trials (RCT). A randomized controlled trial is always prospective."
* *Observational study*: "A survey or nonexperimental study. The researchers are examining and reporting on what is happening, without deliberately intervening in the course of events."
* *Cohort study*: "A 'cohort' is a group of people clearly identified; a cohort study follows that group over time, and reports on what happens to them. A cohort study is an observational study, and it can be

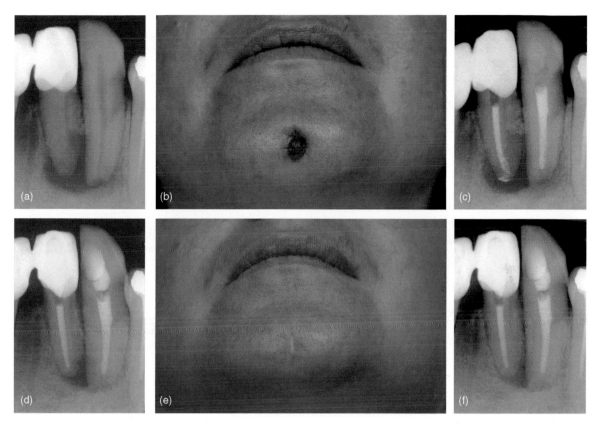

Fig. 14.5 Outcome classification as "functional". (a and b) Mandibular lateral incisor and canine with apical periodontitis associated with an oro-facial fistula. (c) Immediate postoperative radiograph after root canal treatment. (d and e) At 1 year, the radiolucency has become considerably reduced and the fistula has healed with minimal scarring of the skin. (f) At 2 years, no further reduction in the size of the radiolucency is evident. Absence of clinical signs and symptoms allows the teeth to be considered fully functional, even though the periapical tissue is not completely healed. (Reprinted with permission from Friedman [121].)

prospective or retrospective." (A prospective study is also named "concurrent cohort study", while the retrospective study is named "historical cohort study" [112].)

- *Case-control study*: "Compares people with a disease or condition ('cases') to another group of people from the same population who do not have that disease or condition ('controls'). A case-control study can identify risks and trends, and suggest some possible causes for disease, or for particular outcomes. A case-control study is retrospective."
- *Cross-sectional study*: "Also called a prevalence study. It is an observational study. It is like taking a snapshot of a group of people at one point in time and seeing the prevalence of diseases or actions in that population."

- *Case series*: "A case study is a report of a single experience. A case series is a description of a number of 'cases'."

14.5.2 Strategy for appraisal of studies

The design of clinical studies may differ depending on their aim: comparison of the effectiveness of different interventions, assessment of prognosis, or assessment of risk associated with the intervention. Accordingly, there are several strategies for appraising clinical studies to determine their level of evidence and clinical relevance. An important consideration is to differentiate studies designed to assess prognosis or risk; the prognostic factors identified by the former can be different from the risk factors identified by the latter [112].

The most commonly applied criteria are those developed for inclusion/exclusion of studies for systematic reviews of the literature [305]. Taking into account the *research design* and *methodological rigor*, the following hierarchy of evidence has been established, from top to bottom:

- Rigorous randomized controlled trial (RCT); systematic review (SR) or meta-analysis of the same.
- Rigorous cohort study; SR of the same; compromised RCT.
- Rigorous case-control study; SR of the same.
- Compromised cohort or case-control study; cross-sectional study; case series.
- Expert opinion; case report; narrative literature review.

The review process is based on two premises:

- The research design of reviewed studies should be matched to the questions asked [112]. For questions regarding the prognosis the *suggested design is a cohort study,* while for questions regarding the benefits of different treatments the suggested design is an RCT [112,146].
- Evidence-based practice is defined as "… the conscientious, explicit and judicious use of *current best evidence* in making decisions about the care of individual patients" [365]. Thus, reviews should focus on the best evidence available, even if it does not comply with the highest level.

Arguably, the conclusions from structured reviews of *well-designed* observational studies can be consistent with those of systematic reviews or meta-analyses of RCTs [35,66]. Although controversial, this opinion highlights the methodological rigor of a clinical study as a crucial consideration [28]: rigorous cohort studies can outweigh compromised RCTs. Because the primary focus of this chapter is the prognosis of endodontic treatment, and not a comparison of the benefits of endodontic treatment and alternative treatments (e.g., extraction and replacement), the appraisal process includes cohort studies that appear to be methodologically adequate.

Concerns of bias

Appraisal strategies of clinical studies are primarily concerned with validity and relevance [305]. Cohort studies, in particular, are subject to different forms of bias that may distort their conclusions. Because of bias, differences between groups may be demonstrated that do not really exist, while existing differences may be obscured [112]. Bias can potentially occur when the study cohort is assembled (sampling, selection, confounding, or assembly bias). Groups of subjects may differ in regards to prognostic factors other than the studied ones, and these extraneous factors may influence or even determine the outcome of the study [112]. Thus, differences observed at the conclusion of the study may result from inherent differences at the beginning of the study, rather than from the assessed variables. In endodontic cohort studies, assembly bias can occur if subjects differ in preoperative characteristics, such as presence or absence of apical periodontitis in studies on nonsurgical treatment, or prior treatment history before surgical endodontics, i.e., only initial treatment or also retreatment. Similarly, bias occurs if subjects are assembled who have a preferential capacity to benefit from treatment, or are not equally susceptible to the outcome studied. For example, the majority of subjects may be healthy, but some may be affected by compromised systemic health. Specifically in studies on surgical endodontics, teeth are occasionally included that do not have apical periodontitis [341] and therefore have a far greater capacity to heal after surgery than the majority of the teeth that have apical periodontitis. Furthermore, bias can occur when outcomes are assessed (measurement bias) [112]. Subjects may differ in the chance of having a specific outcome detected. For example, in endodontic cohort studies the clinical signs and symptoms may go undetected. Likewise, if the examiners are the same as the providers of treatment their interpretation of follow-up radiographs may be biased towards more favorable assessment [141].

For studies on prognosis the main checklist includes the following questions [80,112,225,365,416]:

- Was the study cohort defined, assembled at the inception of the study, described in detail, entered at a similar point in the course of the disease?
- Was the referral pattern described?
- Were baseline features measured reproducibly?
- Was the follow-up achieved in at least 80% of the inception cohort, the follow-up period described, and long enough for the outcome to occur?
- Were the criteria used for outcome assessment, objective, clinically important, and reproducibly measured?

- Was the outcome assessment blind?
- Was adjustment for extraneous prognostic factors carried out?

The appraisal criteria can be grouped into four general categories.

Cohort, at inception and endpoint of the study

The best evidence is derived from a *prospective* design, with the *inception cohort* defined before the study is initiated, and then observed over time. The cohort should be *clearly characterized* to ascertain unbiased interpretations. The *pattern of referral* of the treated cohort should be described, including types of patients treated and case selection criteria used, to determine the external validity (applicability to the population at large) [112]. At the endpoint of the study at least 80% of the treated subjects should be examined. Importantly, the entire *inception cohort must be accounted for,* identifying "dropouts" (patients who do not present for follow-up at their own volition; their absence may be related to the outcome of interest) and "discontinuers" (patients who are excluded from the study by the investigator for accountable reasons, e.g., death or relocation; their absence is not related to the outcome of interest). Such accounting allows accurate calculation of the recall rate. Finally, the *sample size,* or size of the endpoint cohort, may be required to exceed a certain threshold as determined by the reviewer. For this review a minimum sample size of 45 teeth was required.

Exposure (treatment, intervention)

The *treatment procedures* should be clearly described, to avoid the need for interpretation. The *treatment providers* (students, general dentists, specialty trainees, specialists) should be characterized to establish the external validity of the results [112]. Studies may be excluded if the treatment procedures are considered irrelevant to the review, or otherwise unacceptable. This consideration can be demonstrated with the following two examples. In one study on nonsurgical treatment [270–272], roots associated with apical periodontitis were instrumented "to the approximate center of the lesion", while in one study on surgical endodontics [224], a specific "bony lid approach" has been described; if the review is concerned with typical forms of treatment, both these studies may be excluded.

Outcome assessment

The assessment of outcomes in a study should follow strict rules in order to minimize measurement bias [112]. Outcome dimensions and measures should be *clearly defined*. Bader and Shugars [23] define four dimensions of dental outcomes:

- physical/physiological: disease, pain, and function;
- psychological: perceived aesthetics, level of oral health and satisfaction with oral health status;
- economic: direct and indirect cost;
- longevity/survival: tooth loss and time until repeat treatment for same or new condition.

The endodontic studies of interest usually assess the first, the last, or both of these dimensions. The outcome measures used to assess these dimensions should be as *objective* as possible. To ascertain *consistent assessment* throughout the study, examiners should be *properly calibrated* and their *reliability established*. Outcome assessment should be *blinded or masked*; therefore, the examiner(s) measuring the outcome should be different from the provider(s) of treatment, and direct comparisons of preoperative and follow-up radiographs must be avoided.

The follow-up period should be *long enough* to capture the conclusion of the healing processes in the majority of the study sample. Although a year has been suggested as an adequate follow-up period [151,159,266,302], the chance for delayed healing after nonsurgical treatment [48,132,202,210,269,299, 302,405] and the risk of recurrence of disease in the longer term after surgical endodontics [110,117,159, 190,219,289,354] suggest that the follow-up period should be at least 4 years. For this review a minimum follow-up of a year was required.

Reporting of data and analysis

The reporting of a study should be detailed to the extent that will allow skilled readers to identify potential biases and assess the validity of the study. Thus, all data pertaining to the study cohort, the exposure, outcome assessment, and analysis, should be provided clearly in the report. The statistical analysis should be designed so as to minimize potential bias. The analysis should take into account extraneous factors, and the potential confounding effects of different prognostic factors. In many observational studies the prognostic factors are not controlled by the investigators; at the least they should be observed and recorded, to allow judicious analysis of the outcomes.

14.5.3 Selected studies

Many studies have been published on the outcome of endodontic treatment in the past 50 years. Studies on initial root canal treatment and retreatment are summarized in Tables 14.2–14.5. Studies on surgical endodontics (apical surgery) are summarized in Tables 14.6 and 14.7. Studies on intentional replantation are summarized in Table 14.8. Data related to this chapter are presented. The outcome in all the listed studies is interpreted from that reported by the original authors, as follows:

- Combined clinical and radiological normalcy is classified as healed.
- Whenever the rate of reduced radiolucency combined with clinical normalcy is given, this is classified as healing.
- The rate of teeth without signs and symptoms is classified as functional: for several studies this is simply the sum of healed and healing (when both are available); while for others it includes also teeth where the radiolucency persisted.

True "survival" is not used as an outcome category, because in the majority of studies the outcome is calculated after extracted teeth are excluded from the sample. Data on the long-term survival of teeth after nonsurgical and surgical endodontic treatment are available from several specific studies [6,51,52,60, 187,226,253,369,457]. Typically, the survival rates are lower than the healing and functional rates reported in cohort studies. However, survival analyses of endodontically treated teeth also include a bias, because the "surviving" teeth do not necessarily represent all the teeth with a favourable endodontic treatment outcome [52]. Treatment planning considerations occasionally lead to extraction of functional and periapically healthy teeth, particularly when such teeth require further treatment, i.e., restorative or periodontal, and the patients elect to forego this treatment and extract the tooth [52]. Thus, survival analyses usually underestimate the favourable outcome of endodontic treatment. In recent years researchers have modified the format of survival analyses, by using reviews of either patient charts or electronic databases of dental insurance providers to record untoward events, such as tooth extraction, root canal

retreatment, or surgical endodontics in the long-term after initial root canal treatment [6,226,369]. This type of analysis also is subject to bias, and it appears to overestimate the favourable outcome of endodontic treatment.

The listed studies are related to the general categories of appraisal criteria outlined above, and notation is made of their compliance with those criteria. Insistence on strict compliance with all four criteria would result in a very narrow evidence base. To broaden the evidence base, studies that satisfy any three of the four categories have been selected.

The appraisal process resulted in the selection of 22 studies on initial root canal treatment [48,93,101,104, 129,177,182,202,246,248,299,301,302,304,326,327, 391,393,405,443,455,459] (Table 14.4). Notably, however, the samples of two specific studies [299,443] have been repeated in further studies [97,304,455], and the samples from the Toronto study series have been added up from the first study [129] throughout the successive ones [104,248]. In order to avoid repetition of the same samples only the most recent studies from these three clusters of studies are included in the selected list, reducing the number of studies to 17 (Table 14.4).

In addition to the above, six studies were selected on root canal retreatment [93,103,219,391,405,414] (Table 14.5) and seven studies on surgical endodontics [62,134,189,219,341,456,479] (Table 14.7). All of the above form the *best evidence* for estimating the prognosis after endodontic treatment, and they serve as the reference for defining the expected outcome and its predictors. None of the studies on intentional replantation met the selection criteria, thus the level of evidence to support the prognosis of this specific treatment modality is the lowest.

The selected studies are rather uniform in methodology, but still represent considerable differences in case selection and composition.

14.6 The expected outcome and prognosis after nonsurgical treatment

Initial root canal treatment (Table 14.2) and retreatment (Table 14.3) share the same etiology of disease and basic treatment procedures. It is appropriate, therefore, to put them together into one category – nonsurgical treatment – when reviewing both their prognosis and outcome predictors.

Table 14.2   Follow–up studies on the outcome of initial root canal treatment, appraised for inclusion/exclusion in this chapter review

Study	Examined sample	Follow-up (years)	Cohort	Exposure	Assessment	Analysis	Healed	Healing	Functional*
Strindberg 1956	479	0.5–10	y	y	n	y	90 [d]	–	≥90
Grahnén and Hansson 1961	1277 [c]	4–5	y	n	n	y	86 [d]	–	–
Seltzer *et al.* 1963	2335	0.5	n	n	n	n		84	–
Zeldow et al. 1963	57	≥2	n	n	n	n	86	–	–
Bender *et al.* 1964	706 [b]	2	n	n	n	n	–	82 [f]	–
Grossman *et al.* 1964	432	1–5	n	n	n	n	90	–	–
Engström et al. 1964	306	4–5	y	y	n	y	82 [d]	–	–
Engström and Lundberg 1965	129	3.5–4	y	y	n	n	78 [a,d]	–	–
Oliet and Sorin 1969	398	–	n	n	n	n	79	13	≥92
Storms 1969	158	1	n	n	n	n	81	6	≥87
Harty *et al.* 1970	1139	0.5–2	n	n	n	n	90	–	–
Heling and Tamshe 1970	213	1–5	n	n	n	n	70	–	–
Cvek 1972	55	0.5–2.5	y	y	n	n	91	–	–
Tamse and Heling 1973	122	1–6	n	y	n	n	84	–	–
Lambjerg-Hansen 1974	54	≤1.2	y	y	n	n	80	4	≥84
Selden 1974	504	0.5–1.5	n	n	n	n	–	93 [a]	–
Adenubi and Rule 1976	870	0.5–7	n	n	n	y	88	8	≥96
Cvek *et al.* 1976	131	0.5	y	y	n	n	46	49	≥95
Heling and Shapira 1978	118	1–5	n	y	n	y	78	–	–
Jokinen *et al.* 1978	2459 [c]	2–7	y	n	n	n	53	13	≥66
Soltanoff *et al.* 1978	185	≤20	n	n	n	n	–	86	–
Ashkenaz 1979	145	1–2	n	y	n	n	97	–	–
Kerekes and Tronstad 1979	501 [c]	3–5	y	y	n	y	95 [d]	–	–
Barbakow *et al.* 1980	554	≥1	n	n	n	n	79	11	≥90
Barbakow *et al.* 1981	124 [b]	1–9	n	n	n	y	59	29	≥88
Hession 1981	151 [c]	0.5–20	n	y	n	n	99	–	–
Rudner and Oliet 1981	283	0.5–>2	n	n	n	n	89	–	–
Nelson 1982	299	2–30	n	n	n	n	–	82	–
Cvek *et al.* 1982	54	4	y	n	n	n	88 [e,g,i]	–	–
Oliet 1983	338	≥1.5	n	y	n	n	–	89	–
Klevant and Eggink 1983	336	2	n	n	n	n	48 [f]	15	≥63
Morse *et al.* 1983	220	1	n	n	n	y	–	95	–
Swartz *et al.* 1983	1007	≥1	n	n	n	n	–	88	–
Pekruhn 1986	889	1	n	y	n	n	95	–	–
Halse and Molven 1987	550	10–17	n	n	y	y	85	–	–
Safavi *et al.* 1987	464	0.5–2	n	y	y	n	58	–	–
Byström et al. *1987*	79 [c]	2–5	y	y	y	n	85	9	≥94
Matsumoto *et al.* 1987	85	2–3	n	y	n	n	–	75	–
Ørstavik et al. 1987	546 [c]	1–4	n	y	y	y	87 [i]	–	–
Eriksen et al. 1988	121 [b,c]	3	n	y	y	y	82	9	≥91
Åkerblom and Hasselgren 1988	64 [c]	2–12	n	y	n	n	89 [g]	–	–
Molven and Halse 1988	220 [b,c]	10–17	n	n	y	y	80	–	–
Shah 1988	93	0.5–2	n	n	n	n	–	–	84
Augsburger and Peters 1990	67	0.3–6.5	n	y	n	n	–	97	–

continued

Table 14.2 *Continued*

Study	Examined sample	Follow-up (years)	Cohort	Exposure	Assessment	Analysis	Healed	Healing	Functional*
			Appraisal categories				Outcome (%)		
Sjögren et al. 1990	*849* [c]	*8–10*	y	y	y	y	*91*	–	–
Murphy *et al.* 1991	89	0.3–2	n	n	n	n	46	48	94
Cvek 1992	885	4	y	y	n	n	91	–	–
Ørstavik and Hörsted–Bindslev 1993	282	1–4	n	y	y	y	not interpretable		
Smith *et al.* 1993	821	2–5	n	n	n	y	–	81	–
Ingle 1994	870	2–5	n	n	n	n	–	88	–
Friedman *et al.* 1995	378	0.5–1.5	y	y	n	n	78	16	94
Caliskan and Sen 1996	172	2–5	y	y	n	n	81	8	89
Ørstavik 1996	*599* [b,c]	*4*	n	y	y	y	*90*	*3*	*≥93*
Sjögren et al. 1997	*53*	*≤5*	y	y	y	y	*83*	–	–
Trope et al. 1999	*76*	*1*	n	y	y	y	*80* [h]	–	–
Weiger et al. 2000	*67*	*1–5*	y	y	n	y	*78*	*16*	*94*
Ricucci *et al.* 2000	110	3–15	n	y	n	n	85 [d]	–	–
Waltimo *et al.* 2001	204	1–4	y	y	y	n	72	–	–
Chugal *et al.* 2001	407 [c]	4	n	n	y	y	78	–	–
Peak *et al.* 2001	406	≤1	n	n	n	n	57	28	–
Pettiette *et al.* 2001	40	1	n	y	n	n	60	–	–
Heling *et al.* 2001	319	1–12	n	y	y	n	–	65	–
Molven 2002	265 [b,c]	20–27	y	n	y	n	89	–	–
Benenati 2002	894	0.5–6	n	n	n	n	62	29	–
Peters and Wesselink 2002	*38*	*1–4.5*	y	y	y	y	*76*	*21*	*97*
Hoskinson et al. 2002	*200*	*4–5*	y	y	n	y	*77*	–	*97*
Friedman et al. 2003	*72* [a]	*4–6*	y	n	y	y	*81*	*11*	*97*
Chugal *et al.* 2003	200 [b]	4	n	n	y	y	not reported		
Fouad and Burlesson 2003	540	≥2	n	n	n	n	68	–	–
Huumonen et al. 2003	*156*	*1*	y	y	y	n	*76*	*2*	–
Field *et al.* 2004	223	0.5–4	n	n	n	n	89	–	–
Peters et al. 2004	*233*	*1–3*	y	y	y	y	*87*	–	–
Farzaneh et al. 2004	*242* [b]	*4–6*	y	n	y	y	*85*	*7*	*95*
Ørstavik et al. 2004	*675* [b,c]	*3*	n	y	y	y	*90*	–	–
Caliskan 2004	42	2–10	n	y	y	n	74	10	≥84
Moshonov *et al.* 2005	94	1–5	n	n	n	n	59	–	–
Marending et al. 2005	*66*	*≥2.5*	y	y	y	y	*88*	–	–
Waltimo et al. 2005	*50* [b]	*1*	n	y	y	y	not interpretable		
Chu *et al.* 2005	71	3–4	n	y	n	y	80	–	85
Marquis et al. 2006	*373* [b]	*4–6*	y	n	y	y	*85*	*6*	*95*
Aqrabawi 2006	340	5	n	y	y	n	80	–	–

Studies selected for review are highlighted in italicized font.

* Asymptomatic, without or with residual radiolucency (≥ not reported; rate is sum of healed and healing).
[a] Results recorded at the final observation.
[b] Includes repeated material.
[c] Roots considered as unit of evaluation, rather than teeth.
[d] Recalculated after exclusion of cases classified as "uncertain".
[e] Cases with procedural errors excluded.

[f] Results recorded at 2-year observation.
[g] All canals obliterated to some extent.
[h] Teeth treated in two sessions without intracanal medication excluded.
[i] Results recorded at 4-year observation.
y Satisfies criteria of acceptable quality.
n Does not satisfy criteria of acceptable quality.

Table 14.3 Follow–up studies on the outcome of root canal retreatment, appraised for inclusion/exclusion in this chapter review

Study	Examined sample	Follow-up (years)	Cohort	Exposure	Assessment	Analysis	Healed	Healing	Functional*
Strindberg 1956	187	0.5–10	y	y	n	y	88 [e]	–	–
Grahnén and Hansson 1961	502 [c]	4–5	y	n	n	y	90 [d]	–	–
Engström et al. 1964	180	4–5	y	y	n	y	85	–	–
Selden 1974	52	0.5–1.5	n	n	n	n	–	88 [a]	–
Bergenholtz et al 1979	556 [c]	2	y	y	n	n	75	12	≥87
Pekruhn 1986	36	1	n	y	n	n	83	–	–
Molven and Halse 1988	174 [c]	10–17	n	n	y	y	79 [d]	–	–
Allen et al. 1989	315	≥0.5	n	n	n	n	73	12	≥85
Sjögren et al. 1990	267 [c]	8–10	y	y	y	y	85	–	–
Van Nieuwenhuysen et al. 1994	561 [c]	≥0.5	n	n	n	y	78	–	–
Friedman et al. 1995	128	0.5–1.5	y	y	n	n	70	23	93
Danin et al. 1996	18	1	n	y	n	n	28	28	≥56
Sundqvist et al. 1998	54	4	n	y	y	y	74	–	–
Piatowska et al. 1998	60	–	n	y	n	n	43	42	≥85
Abbott 1999	432	0.3–4	n	n	n	n	98	1	–
Kvist and Reit 1999	47	4	y	y	y	n	58 [f]	–	–
Chugal et al. 2001	85 [c]	4	n	n	y	y	79	–	–
Hoskinson et al. 2002 [g]	76	4–5	n	y	n	y	78	–	–
Farzaneh et al. 2004	103	4–6	y	n	y	y	81	5	93
Gorni et al. 2004	452	2	y	n	n	n	65	4	–
Fristad et al. 2004	112 [b,c]	20–27	n	n	y	y	96	–	–

Studies selected for review are highlighted in italicized font.

* Asymptomatic, without or with residual radiolucency (≥ not reported; rate is sum of healed and healing).
[a] Results recorded at the final observation.
[b] Includes repeated material.
[c] Roots considered as unit of evaluation, rather than teeth.
[d] Cases classified as "uncertain" excluded.

[e] Results recorded at 4-year observation.
[f] Approximate figure deducted from graph.
[g] Study selected for initial treatment, but lacking detail in regards to retreatment.
y Satisfies criteria of acceptable quality.
n Does not satisfy criteria of acceptable quality.

14.6.1 Prevention of apical periodontitis

Teeth that are treated without the presence of apical periodontitis may have a vital pulp that is either intact (elective treatment) or irreversibly inflamed, a necrotic pulp that is not infected, or root-filled canals suspected of harboring bacteria that may become subject to a change in the ecological environment as a result of a restorative procedure. Accordingly, they undergo initial treatment or retreatment. The outcomes of these distinct treatment modalities are reviewed in sequence below.

Several of the selected studies on nonsurgical treatment (Tables 14.4 and 14.5) define distinct groups of teeth without apical periodontitis in their study samples. Although the study methodology and outcome assessment is consistent among the selected studies, their reported outcomes still vary to some extent.

Table 14.4 Methodological characteristics and specific outcomes of selected follow-up studies on the outcome of initial root canal treatment

Study	Recall rate (%)	Proportion of AP (%)	Tooth types	Treatment providers	Root filling	Intracanal medication	Healed (%)	
							without AP	with AP
Strindberg 1956	74	42	mix	en	lc	f	93	88
Engström et al. 1964	72	53	mix	us	–	–	88	76
Kerekes and Tronstad 1979	77	34	mix	us	lc	ct, f	97	91
Byström et al. 1987	56	100	sr	us	lc	ch	–	85
Ørstavik et al. 1987	67	29	mix	us	lc	–	–	–
Eriksen et al. 1988	52	100	mix	us	lc	ch	–	82
Sjögren et al. 1990	46	31	mix	us	lc	ch	97	86
Ørstavik and Hörsted-Bindslev 1993	–	67	mix	us	lc	–	not interpretable	
Ørstavik 1996	82	–	mix	s	lc	ch	94	75
Sjögren et al. 1997	96	100	mix	en	lc	ch, os	–	83
Trope et al. 1999	100 ?	100 ?	sr	en	lc	ch, os	–	80
Weiger et al. 2000	92	100	–	en	lc	ch	–	78
Peters and Wesselink 2002	100	100	sr	en	wl	ch	–	76
Hoskinson et al. 2002	42	70	mix	en	hc, wv	ch, os	88	74
Friedman et al. 2003	sample included in Marquis et al. 2006							
Huumonen et al. 2003	78	100	mix	us, gs, en	lc	ch	–	–
Peters et al. 2004	89	44	mix	en	lc, sb	ch, os	95	76
Farzaneh et al. 2004	sample included in Marquis et al. 2006							
Ørstavik et al. 2004	same sample as Ørstavik et al. 1987						94	79
Marending et al. 2005	79	52	mix	en	lc	ch, os	–	–
Waltimo et al. 2005	same sample as Trope et al. 1999							
Marquis et al. 2006	50	57	mix	gs	lc, wv	ch, os	93	80

mix   All tooth types included.
sr   Single-rooted teeth, or single roots from multi-rooted teeth included.
en   Endodontist(s).
us   Undergraduate students.
gs   Graduate students.
lc   Cold lateral compaction of gutta-percha.

wv   Vertical compaction of warm gutta-percha.
hc   Hybrid thermocompaction of gutta-percha.
wl   Warm lateral compaction of gutta-percha.
f   Formalin (and other medications in fewer cases).
ct   Chloramine T.
ch   Calcium hydroxide.
os   Single-session treatment.

Proportion of healed teeth

The range of reported "healed" rates in the seven selected studies on initial treatment is relatively small, from 88% [93,177] to 97% [391]. The two studies reporting the low healed rate of 88% [93,177] appear to fall considerably below the rates reported in the other five studies (93–97%), and may be considered outliers. The range of reported healed rates in the selected four studies on retreatment is even smaller, from 94% [93] to 98% [391]. Cumulatively, the healed rate range reported in the selected studies is considerably smaller than that observed across all studies (67–97%), as can be expected from the selection of only those studies that satisfy the appraisal criteria. *Thus, the chance of teeth to remain free from apical periodontitis after nonsurgical treatment is 93–98%.*

Proportion of asymptomatic functional teeth

None of the studies on initial treatment or retreatment have specific information on asymptomatic function among teeth treated without apical periodontitis. *Thus, the rate of asymptomatic functional teeth may exceed that of completely healed teeth.*

Table 14.5   Methodological characteristics and specific outcomes of selected follow-up studies on the outcome of root canal retreatment

Study	Recall rate (%)	Proportion of AP (%)	Tooth types	Treatment providers	Root filling	Intracanal medication	Healed (%)	
							without AP	with AP
Strindberg 1956	74	42	mix	en	lc	f	95	84
Engström *et al.* 1964	72	53	mix	us	–	–	93	74
Sjögren *et al.* 1990	46	31	mix	us	lc	ch	98	62
Sundqvist *et al.* 1998	100	100	sr	en	lc	ch	–	74
Kvist and Reit 1999	100	100	sr	en	lc	ch	–	58
Farzaneh *et al.* 2004	34	71	mix	gs	lc, wv	ch	97	78

AP	Apical periodontitis.	gs	Graduate students.
mix	All tooth types included.	lc	Cold lateral compaction of gutta-percha.
sr	Single-rooted teeth (five two-rooted teeth also included).	wv	Vertical compaction of warm gutta-percha.
		f	Formalin (and other medications in fewer cases).
en	Endodontist(s).	ch	Calcium hydroxide.
us	Undergraduate students.		

Dynamics of disease emergence

Emergence of apical periodontitis peaks within the first year after initial root canal treatment [302]. It appears that approximately 75% of the affected teeth demonstrated signs of disease within a year [302]. In the following years the risk of developing disease is not increased [302]. As late emergence of apical periodontitis is infrequent, it has been suggested that observation beyond a year may not be necessary [302]. In selected cases, however, a lesion may develop (up to 4 years after treatment) that later disappears [405], or apical periodontitis may emerge many years after treatment [132,269]. These occurrences, even if they are uncommon, suggest that long-term observation of the treated teeth may be valuable.

14.6.2 Treatment of apical periodontitis

Teeth that present with apical periodontitis may have a primary infection of the pulp and root canal system, or a residual or subsequent infection after root canal treatment. Accordingly, they undergo initial root canal treatment, retreatment, surgical endodontics, intentional replantation, or a combination thereof. The outcomes of the nonsurgical modalities are presented in sequence below, whereas those of the surgical treatment modalities are reviewed separately.

The selected 17 studies on initial treatment [48,93, 177,182,202,246,248,301,302,304,326,327,391,393, 405,443,459], and six studies on retreatment [93,103,

219,391,405,414], form the basis for this section. In spite of their methodological compatibility there is still a considerable variation in their reported treatment outcome of teeth with apical periodontitis (Tables 14.4 and 14.5).

Proportion of healed teeth

The greatest variation among the studies comprising the best evidence is in the healed, or complete healing rate. For initial treatment, the range is from 73% [93] to 90% [202], whereas in the studies on retreatment it is from 56% [219] to 86% (in teeth without perforation) [103]. These ranges are smaller than those observed across all studies on initial treatment (46–97%) and retreatment (28–98%) (Tables 14.2 and 14.3), as can be expected from the selection of only those studies that satisfy the appraisal criteria. Moreover, the lower rates for retreatment of 56% (approximate – the exact rate was not provided) and 62% [219,391], fall considerably below those reported in the other studies, while the higher rate of 90% [202] falls above the reported rates. These unusually low and high rates may be considered as outliers. *Thus, the chance of teeth with apical periodontitis to heal completely after nonsurgical treatment is 73–86%.*

Since, in the selected studies, the criteria for complete healing are usually well defined and rather uniform, the variation in the reported outcomes must be related to other factors (see Section 14.3):

- Different outcomes may have resulted from differences in tooth types, and from the use of the tooth or root as the unit of evaluation [127]. The higher healed rates are reported in studies that either included only single-rooted teeth [48,393] or calculated the outcome for each root [199,391]. Such calculation usually enhances the outcome compared with studies where all tooth types are included and the whole tooth is assessed as the evaluated unit [127]. However, this suggestion is undermined by the fact that in other selected studies roots have been assessed as the evaluated units, and yet the healed rates are lower [97,302,443].
- Different outcomes may have resulted from differences in case selection [184]. In several of the studies [48,93,97,202,391] cases were treated by undergraduate students and are assumed to have been relatively uncomplicated. In contrast, one series of studies [248] occasionally included cases that were complicated by anatomy, advanced marginal periodontitis or procedural errors that occurred before referral for treatment.
- Different outcomes may have resulted from the prerequisite in several of the studies [48,202,391], but not in others, of a no-growth (negative) bacterial culture to be obtained before root canal filling. As shown by Sjögren *et al.* [393] the healed rate in teeth filled after a negative culture was significantly higher than for teeth filled when the culture was positive (94% and 68%, respectively). An even greater difference in the healed rates has been demonstrated in retreated teeth filled after negative cultures (80%) and positive cultures (33%) [414].
- Different outcomes may also have resulted from differences in restoration. In the studies reported by the group from Umeå, Sweden [48,391,393,414] all teeth received a permanent restoration immediately after endodontic treatment, using an antimicrobial layer of zinc oxide/eugenol to seal the canal orifices (personal communication) [393]. Similarly, in the study by Peters *et al.* [326] all the teeth were reportedly well restored. In contrast, in the Toronto study reports [103,248] some 5–10% of the teeth were found lacking permanent restorations at the time of the follow-up examination. In the absence of a permanent restoration microbial ingress into the filled canals can occur [126] and cause persistence of apical periodontitis in some teeth.

Proportion of healing teeth

When reported, the "healing" rates have varied from 9% [48] to 21% [326]. A high proportion of teeth demonstrating incomplete healing is typical of short-term studies where the observation period is insufficient for capturing completion of the healing process [127]. However, this typical pattern is not displayed by the selected studies. *Thus, the chance of teeth with apical periodontitis to demonstrate incomplete healing after nonsurgical treatment is approximately 10–20%.*

Proportion of asymptomatic functional teeth

Six studies on initial treatment [48,97,248,302,326,459] and one study on retreatment [103] have reported a range of teeth that are functional at the follow-up examination, from 88% [302] to 96% [177]. Additional information can be gleaned from the nonselected studies (Tables 14.2 and 14.3). In fact, the functional rates entered in the tables include only teeth where symptoms were absent and the initial radiolucency disappeared (healed) or diminished (healing). It can be assumed that additional teeth were clinically normal without displaying a radiological improvement; however, the numbers of such teeth were not reported in any of the studies. It appears, therefore, that after nonsurgical treatment of teeth with apical periodontitis the rate of asymptomatic functional teeth may approach or even exceed 95%. Even the survival rate of 80% reported after root canal treatment of teeth with apical periodontitis [60] and the 86% general 5-year survival [52] is quite high, while the chart/database reviews have reported survival rates in excess of 93% [6,226,369]. *Thus, the chance of teeth with apical periodontitis to remain functional after nonsurgical treatment may approximate 95%.* This excellent potential for maintained asymptomatic function suggests that for teeth with primary or persistent apical periodontitis and reasonable restorative and periodontal prognosis, *conservative endodontic treatment is definitely justified and should be attempted*. If initial root canal treatment or retreatment is considered feasible and acceptable to the patient, tooth extraction and replacement should not be contemplated.

Dynamics of healing

Healing of apical periodontitis after nonsurgical treatment peaks within the first year [219,347]. By the first year close to 90% of the teeth that heal eventually demonstrate signs of healing [302], and almost 50% are already completely healed [2]. At 2 years, the majority of the teeth are healed [48,299], while the others demonstrate further reduction of the radiolucency [48,213,299,302,391]. The healing process may continue for 4–5 years [2,48,219,299,302,391], or even longer [132,269,405]. Therefore, at 4 years about 13% of the teeth still show reduction of the lesion [302], while closer to 6 years this rate is reduced to under 7% [103,104,248]. Moreover, over 6% of teeth that received initial root canal treatment, and as many as 50% of retreated teeth that were observed to still have disease 10–17 years after treatment, were completely healed a decade later [132,269] resulting in an improved outcome in the long term [132]. The late healing was mainly characteristic of teeth with surplus root filling material [132]. Overall, a continuous reduction of the radiolucency (comparing at least two follow-up examinations) may be considered as a forecast of complete healing at a later time [48].

Reversal of the healing process is believed to be rare [302,405]. For example, no healing reversal was observed within 4 years in one study on retreatment [219]. Based on this observation, it has been suggested that extended follow-up of teeth that demonstrate signs of healing within the first year may be unnecessary [302]. However, it should be taken into account that all root-filled teeth remain constantly challenged by intraoral microorganisms. Thus, recurrence of apical periodontitis in the future remains a possibility for all teeth, even those that have completely healed at one point after treatment. For example, over 1% of teeth observed to be healed 10–17 years after treatment reverted to disease a decade later [269]. Therefore, periodic follow-up of root-filled teeth is advocated.

A different pattern has been observed in teeth that were treated by root-end closure (apexification). About 8% of teeth that had healed during the root-end closure process reverted to disease 2–3 years after permanent root canal filling, while 66% of teeth that had not shown signs of healing during root-end closure, healed after the permanent root canal filling [72].

Healing of apical periodontitis is eventually expected to become complete; therefore, in the long term, a residual radiolucency is interpreted as persistent or recurrent disease [265,347,405]. Seldom, however, healing of very extensive apical periodontitis lesions can be completed without total resolution of the radiolucency. In the few such cases that have

been reported, there was fibrous periapical tissue (apical scar) found, rather than a pathological lesion [38,48,284,320,378].

Persistence of disease

Nonmicrobial etiological factors, including foreign materials and true cysts, have been identified as the cause of persistent apical periodontitis after initial root canal treatment [276,277,282,283]; however, this occurrence may be uncommon. The three specimens where this finding occurred represented one-third of nine teeth subjected to biopsy because of persistent disease after endodontic treatment that employed strict bacteriological monitoring to verify no growth of intracanal bacteria before root canal filling [391]. In routine endodontic treatment, however, bacterial elimination is not commonly confirmed before root canal filling; therefore, the proportion of the nonmicrobial etiology of persistent disease is likely to be much lower than that suggested by Nair *et al.* [282,283].

In contrast, there is consistent evidence that persistent apical periodontitis after root canal treatment is primarily caused by infection [128,388]. The microbial sites can differ, as follows:

- Most frequently the microorganisms are harbored within the root canal system [29,40,59,115,133,155, 161,197,230,231,262,278,281,284,311,312,335, 336,349, 388,414,415,477], after having survived the treatment procedures [393], or invaded the filled canal space after treatment, possibly by way of coronal leakage [126].

- Specific bacteria, particularly *Actinomyces israelii* and *Propionibacterium propionicum*, can become established in the periapical tissues and sustain the infection even after root canal bacteria have been eliminated [108,109,154,163,164,195,279,292,368, 386,390,413,415].

- Recent evidence confirms that other bacterial species can be harbored outside the root canal [135,409–412,440]. They may survive on the root surface in cementum lacunae [280,337], plaque-like microbial biofilms [228,286,387,435,437,438,440], or in dentin debris inadvertently extruded periapically during treatment [474]. However, it has not been established to what extent the recently identified extraradicular bacteria can sustain persistent infection without dependence on bacterial presence in the root canal. This question still requires clarification; *the answer will have an important bearing on treatment strategies for persistent apical periodontitis.* Current knowledge suggests that the dominant cause of persistent apical periodontitis is root canal infection, while exclusive extraradicular infection should be regarded as a less common occurrence [128].

Persistence of apical periodontitis after root canal retreatment may still occur because of bacterial survival in the root canal, despite the repeated attempt to eliminate them during the retreatment procedure [312,414,477]. Nevertheless, the fact that repeated canal disinfection did not result in healing increases the probability that the disease process is sustained by factors other than intracanal infection. The possible etiological factors include foreign body reaction and true cysts [282,283], or extraradicular infection [108,109,135,154,163,164,195,279,280,292,337,368, 386,387,390,409–413,435,437,438,440,474]. To address all these possible factors, surgical endodontics may be considered the treatment of choice for persistent apical periodontitis after root canal retreatment.

14.7 Outcome predictors in nonsurgical endodontic treatment

In the first edition of this book [119] clinical factors were identified that appeared to influence the outcome of treatment without an attempt to differentiate studies according to the level of evidence. Also, no differentiation was made between initial treatment and retreatment. This chapter focuses primarily on selected studies that comprise the best evidence for initial treatment [48,93,177,182,202,246,248,301,302, 304,326,327,391,393,405,443,459] (Table 14.4) and for retreatment [93,103,219,391,405,414] (Table 14.5). Where appropriate, a few studies whose samples are included in other selected ones [101,104,129,299,455] are also cited. The few selected studies on retreatment do not provide an adequate evidence base to assess the influence of many factors on outcome. The similarity between retreatment and initial treatment suggests that the same preoperative, intraoperative, and postoperative factors may be considered as predictors of the outcome in both treatment modalities. However, because teeth subjected to retreatment present with a previous root canal treatment history, characteristics of this history must be addressed as additional preoperative factors. These include the

previous root canal filling, a perforation that may be present in a minority of retreated teeth, and the time elapsed since initial treatment.

For identification in the following section, the references for these selected studies are highlighted in italicized type. The nonselected studies are cited only where selected studies are unavailable. The prognostic factors are divided into preoperative, intraoperative, and postoperative. Because root canal bacteria are critically important as the etiological factor in persistent apical periodontitis, their elimination is reviewed as a separate entity for greater emphasis.

14.7.1 Preoperative factors

The preoperative factors form the basis for projecting the prognosis and the outcome of treatment, and thus the expected benefit that the patient can weigh against those of alternative treatments. Therefore, it is important to recognize the preoperative factors and to take them into account when treatment decisions are formed; this may be critical when selection has to be made between retreatment, surgical endodontics, or extraction and replacement.

Patient's age and gender

Ørstavik *et al.* [*304*] reported a better outcome after initial treatment in older patients; however, in many other initial treatment studies [*177,202,248,301,326, 391*], and in the only retreatment study that examined these factors [*103*], the patients' age and gender have not been significantly associated with outcome. *Thus, age and gender should not be considered as influencing the outcome of nonsurgical endodontic treatment.*

Patient's systemic health

Strindberg [*405*] reported that the patient's health did not influence the outcome. In a recent study, however, Marending *et al.* [*246*] reported that in patients with a compromised nonspecific immune system the prognosis regarding teeth with apical periodontitis was poorer than in healthy patients. A similar observation in diabetic patients was reported in a nonselected study [114]. Thus, a clear relationship between the patient's systemic health and the prognosis of nonsurgical endodontic treatment has not been established; *however, immune-compromised patients, and particularly those with diabetes, may be considered at a greater risk of persistent apical periodontitis after nonsurgical endodontic treatment.* Nevertheless, even if the prognosis may be poorer in teeth with preoperative apical periodontitis, it is not so poor as not to warrant treatment of the affected teeth.

Tooth location

Ørstavik *et al.* [304] observed a better outcome in mandibular than in maxillary teeth. A survival analysis of teeth after endodontic treatment [60] suggested that the chance of survival was significantly lower for mandibular molars than for other teeth. Kerekes and Tronstad [202] observed a better outcome in specific teeth (maxillary canines and second premolars, mandibular canines) than in other teeth, but generally reported a comparable outcome in anterior, posterior, maxillary, and mandibular teeth. Apart from these conflicting findings, no association between the outcome of treatment and tooth location has been shown in other studies on initial treatment [177,248,301,326,459] and retreatment [103]. Although in two studies [93,405] a better outcome was reported in multirooted teeth than in single-rooted teeth, the latter have been shown to have a better outcome in two other studies on nonsurgical treatment [103,248]. However, this finding may merely reflect the use of the whole tooth as the evaluated unit, multiplying the chances of persistent disease by the number of roots [103,248]. *Thus, the location and type of the tooth should not be considered to influence the outcome of nonsurgical endodontic treatment.*

Clinical signs and symptoms

Preoperative symptoms may be a reflection of the bacterial types and numbers in the root canal system [300]. Nevertheless, a comparable treatment outcome has been reported for asymptomatic teeth and for teeth presenting with preoperative symptoms, in studies on initial treatment [48,248,301,304,391,459] and retreatment [103]. *Thus, presence or absence of symptoms should not be considered to influence the outcome of nonsurgical endodontic treatment.*

Status of the pulp: in initial treatment

A better outcome has been reported in teeth with vital rather than necrotic pulps [177,248]. However, because the pulp status is directly associated with the presence or absence of apical periodontitis, this confounding effect must be avoided by assessing teeth without apical periodontitis. In such teeth, the pulp status has not been significantly associated with the outcome of treatment [202,248,304,391]. *Therefore, the pulp status should not be considered to influence the outcome of initial endodontic treatment in teeth without apical periodontitis.*

Presence or absence of apical periodontitis (radiolucency)

The healed rate reported after initial treatment of teeth affected by apical periodontitis, has been significantly (10–15%) lower than in teeth without the disease [93,177,246,248,302,304,327,405]. Similarly, in studies on retreatment this difference is 10–20% [93,103,391,405]. The poorer outcome in teeth with apical periodontitis highlights the difference between prevention and treatment of an established infection. It may reflect difficulties in the repair process of the periradicular tissues, or the limited ability of the endodontic treatment regimen to disinfect the root canal system [405] (see Section 14.7.4). *Thus, preoperative presence of apical periodontitis has a dominant, negative influence on the outcome of nonsurgical endodontic treatment.*

Size of the radiolucent lesion

A better prognosis has been reported in teeth with small lesions, up to 5 mm in diameter, than in teeth with larger lesions after initial root canal treatment [93,177,304,405,459] and retreatment [414]. This was explained by a correlation between the size of the lesion and the number of root canal bacteria [48]. However, statistically nonsignificant differences between small and large lesions have been reported in other studies on initial treatment [48,248,301,326,391,393] and retreatment [103]. *Thus, the size of the radiolucency should not be considered to influence the outcome of nonsurgical endodontic treatment.*

Status of the periodontal supporting tissues

The condition of the marginal periodontal tissues has received little consideration with regard to the prognosis of teeth undergoing nonsurgical endodontic treatment. Ørstavik *et al.* [304] observed a better outcome in teeth with better marginal support; however, according to the few other studies that address this factor [103,248,391], the periodontal status did not influence the prognosis. Friedman *et al.* [129]

observed that of the total of 21 teeth lost within 4–6 years after initial root canal treatment, over 50% had been extracted because of marginal periodontitis. Similarly, in a survival analysis of root-filled teeth with marginal periodontitis, 66% of lost teeth in a period of 9 years were extracted for periodontal reasons. *Clearly, if advanced marginal periodontitis is present at the time of treatment, it is likely to persist during the follow-up period and to advance with time, until tooth loss becomes imminent.*

Apparent quality of the previous root canal filling: in retreatment

Based on the only selected study that addressed this factor [103], the outcome of retreatment in teeth with apical periodontitis was significantly (15% difference) better in teeth where the previous root canal filling appeared to be inadequate in regards to length, density or both, compared to teeth with apparently adequate root canal fillings. The authors speculated that in the teeth with inadequate root canal fillings "the canals constituted the infected sites, which, when retreated, could be effectively disinfected and sealed, leading to healing" [103]. In teeth with adequate root canal fillings, the root canal bacteria may not have been susceptible to routine retreatment procedures, or the disease was sustained by extraradicular infection, cysts or a foreign body, such as would not respond to root canal treatment procedures [103].

One study [144] highlighted the deviation of the previous root canal filling from the pathway of the canal, suggesting that in teeth with altered morphology the prognosis was poorer than in teeth with unaltered morphology. *Thus, in teeth with apical periodontitis undergoing retreatment, the apparent quality of the previous root canal filling may be considered as a significant outcome predictor.*

Previous perforation: in retreatment

Information about the prognosis of teeth in which a root or chamber perforation occurred is scarce. A nonselected study [33] reported 58% healing around perforations repaired with amalgam or gutta-percha. A selected study [103] reported a 36% healed rate in teeth with apical periodontitis where perforations were repaired with resin-modified glass-ionomer cement. The authors speculated that "possibly, the use of MTA [mineral trioxide aggregate] could have been beneficial" [103]. Indeed, in a more recent case-

series study [244] all 16 teeth with MTA-repaired perforations appeared to be healed a year or longer after treatment. *Thus, in teeth undergoing retreatment, the presence of a perforation may be considered as a significant outcome predictor; the impact of the perforation on the prognosis may depend on the material used to seal the perforation.*

Time elapsed from initial treatment to retreatment

One study [103] reported a comparable outcome for teeth retreated within a year or longer after initial treatment. *Thus, the time elapsed since previous treatment should not be considered to influence the outcome of retreatment.*

14.7.2 Intraoperative factors

Intraoperative prognostic factors can be instrumental in maximizing the patient's benefit by improving the outcome of endodontic treatment. Therefore, it is important to recognize intraoperative factors and to take them into account when treatment strategies and techniques are selected. Review of the selected studies clearly reveals the more critical role of these factors in teeth with preoperative apical periodontitis than in teeth without.

Apical extent of treatment

It would be appropriate to distinguish between the apical extent of the canal preparation and that of the root canal filling [93,304,405]; however, the majority of the selected studies refer only to the extent of the root canal filling. This factor has been shown to influence the outcome in five studies on initial treatment [93,301,304,391,405], but not in eight others [48,177, 182,246,248,326,327,459]. Likewise, one retreatment study [103] reported a poorer outcome in teeth with inadequate (both too long and too short) root filling length, whereas two other studies [391,414] did not corroborate this finding. The importance of the apical extent of treatment is, therefore, ambiguous.

Extrusion of filling materials beyond the root-end may impair the prognosis specifically in teeth with preoperative apical periodontitis [93,301,391,405]. Because gutta-percha is well tolerated by the tissue, the impaired prognosis is more likely to result from overinstrumentation and periapical inoculation with infected debris, than from the extrusion of root filling materials *per se* [*391,474*]. Notably, extruded root filling materials can be totally or partially removed during the healing process [*19,158,405*]. Nevertheless, in their presence the healing of apical periodontitis may be slowed down and extend as long as the second or third decade after treatment [*132*].

Sjögren *et al.* [*391*] observed that in teeth with apical periodontitis, inability to instrument the canal to the apical constriction and an excessively short root canal filling (≤2 mm) impaired the prognosis relative to an adequate filling (0–2 mm short); however, this finding was not corroborated in a previous study by the same group of researchers [*48*]. *Thus, the apical extent of the root canal filling should not be considered to influence the outcome of nonsurgical endodontic treatment in teeth without apical periodontitis. In the presence of apical periodontitis, the prognosis may be better if the root canal filling extends 0–2 mm short of the root end.*

Apical enlargement

In teeth with apical periodontitis, the root dentin may be penetrated by intracanal microorganisms [*280,324*] to a depth of 150–250 μm [*152,234,380*], where they may be protected from irrigants and medications [*294*]. Only enlargement of the canal to sizes 300–500 μm larger than its original diameter (e.g., enlargement to ISO size 50–70 if the first file that binds is size 20) could remove the dentin considered to be infected. Therefore, extensive apical enlargement may enhance the removal of infected dentin and disinfection of the apical part of the canal [*53,300,472*], and it should translate into an improved prognosis.

Contrary to this expectation, the extent of apical enlargement has not been significantly associated with the outcome of initial treatment in four studies [*177,202,304,326*], while in the fifth [*405*] the outcome was poorer in teeth with a larger apical preparation. These findings challenge the concept that extensive canal enlargement promotes the prognosis.

Carrying out extensive apical enlargement is frequently associated with canal transportation that may jeopardize canal disinfection and impair prognosis. Clearly, the procedure of extensive apical enlargement is technique sensitive, and requires considerable skill, particularly when performed with stainless-steel hand files. It is possible that the inability to demonstrate differences in prognosis between extensive and minimal apical enlargement is a reflection of the problems associated with each. Extensive apical enlargement,

if not carried out skillfully, may transport the canal, whereas minimal enlargement (actually, no enlargement) may leave infected tissue behind. Both effects would compromise the prognosis to some extent [*127*].

In addition, it should be noted that preoperative canal dimensions have not been recorded in endodontic outcome studies, thus the true extent of apical enlargement cannot be assessed by only noting the size of the last instrument. *Thus, there are insufficient data available to assess the influence of the extent of apical enlargement on the outcome of initial endodontic treatment, and no data at all on the influence of this factor in retreatment.*

No-growth (negative) bacterial culture before root canal filling

The original study that correlated a no-growth (negative) culture obtained before root canal filling with a better prognosis [*93*] utilized microbiological techniques that did not adequately address the anaerobic bacteria that are the major endodontic pathogens [*393*]. Using an advanced anaerobic bacteriological technique during initial treatment, Sjögren *et al.* [*393*] reported that 94% of teeth in which the cultures were negative before root canal filling healed, in contrast to only 68% in teeth with positive cultures. Similarly, in a retreatment study [*414*] 80% of teeth with negative cultures before root canal filling healed, compared to 33% of teeth with positive cultures. In a recent report, Waltimo *et al.* [*455*] observed a better outcome in teeth treated in two sessions, where bacteria could not be recovered at the beginning of the second session compared with teeth where bacteria were recovered. All these findings clearly demonstrate the potential value of using reliable culturing methods to project the prognosis of root canal treatment, even though it is apparently disputed by another recent study [*326*]. Furthermore, it appears that the bacterial species that infect the canal also may influence the prognosis [*393*]. Nevertheless, state-of-the-art culturing techniques are not readily available for use in day-to-day endodontic practice [*393*]. Instead, they should be used for research purposes to assess the efficacy of root canal treatment regimens (see Section 14.7.4). *Thus, results of bacterial cultures obtained from root canals should not be considered as outcome predictors in nonsurgical endodontic treatment.*

Number of treatment sessions

One of the "hottest" questions in endodontics is whether the prognosis differs for treatment in one session or two. Sjögren *et al.* [*393*] have clearly demonstrated that intracanal infection cannot be reliably eliminated in a single treatment session. To maximize disinfection, application of intracanal medication is required [*44–47,261,300,383,472*]. Therefore, a better prognosis is expected when treatment is performed in two sessions and an effective intracanal medication is used in the interim. However, the selected studies on initial treatment [*248,326,443,459*] and retreatment [*103*] do not support this premise. Differences in healing rates reported in the relevant studies for treatment in one or two sessions have been in the range of 10%, inconsistent and statistically nonsignificant. The main reason for the lack of significance is insufficient power of analysis – the differences in healing rates are too small to be substantiated statistically with the limited sample sizes.

When treatment is performed in more than one session the specific number of sessions does not appear to influence the prognosis [*202*]. In a survival analysis [*60*], however, teeth treated in one or two sessions survived longer than teeth treated in three sessions or more. This finding appears to parallel that of Sirén *et al.* [*389*] who suggested that teeth treated in multiple visits were at a greater risk of becoming infected with *Enterococcus faecalis*, and developing persistent apical periodontitis.

Undoubtedly, treatment in one and two sessions can have a good prognosis [*393*], and the biological benefit of multisession treatment has not been supported by clinical evidence [*370*]. *Thus, there are insufficient data available to assess the influence of one or two sessions on the outcome of root canal treatment in teeth with apical periodontitis. However, prolongation of treatment for more than two sessions should be avoided.*

Occurrence of midtreatment flare-up

Several of the initial treatment studies [*48,202,248, 326,391,405*] and one retreatment study [*103*] have reported no significant association between the occurrence of flare-ups in the course of treatment and the outcome of treatment. *Thus, the occurrence of flare-up or pain between treatment sessions should not be considered to influence the prognosis of nonsurgical endodontic treatment.*

Materials and techniques used for treatment

The selected studies offer limited information on the influence of specific treatment regimens on the prognosis. The following aspects of materials and techniques have been addressed:

- *Instrumentation technique*: Kerekes and Tronstad [*202*] suggested that the prognosis might be better using the "standardized" technique than with the "serial" technique; however, none of these techniques are widely used today. Three recent studies have reported no significant associations between the outcome of initial treatment and different aspects of canal preparation, including hand- or engine-driven instruments [*246*], the engine-driven instrument systems [*327*], and the degree of taper [*177*]. *Thus, the instrumentation technique should not be considered to influence the outcome of initial treatment, and by extension, also the outcome of retreatment.*

- *Intracanal medication*: survival analysis has suggested that teeth medicated with $Ca(OH)_2$ have a better chance of survival than teeth that have not been medicated or medicated with other materials [*60*]. *In the absence of any other supporting data, there are insufficient data available to assess the influence of the type of intracanal medication on the outcome of nonsurgical endodontic treatment in teeth with apical periodontitis.*

- *Sealer*: in a study of a large sample of teeth without and with apical periodontitis, Ørstavik *et al.* [*304*] suggested that the choice of sealer might influence the prognosis, but only in teeth without preoperative apical periodontitis. One sealer, Kloroperka N-Ø, was singled out as adversely influencing the outcome. Indeed, in a smaller sample of teeth with apical periodontitis [*97*] and in three subsequent studies of larger populations [*182,301,454*] comparable outcomes for different sealer types have been reported. *Thus, with the exception of Kloroperka N-Ø, the type of sealer should not be considered to influence the outcome of nonsurgical endodontic treatment.*

- *Root canal filling technique*: two recent studies have reported no significant associations between the outcome of initial treatment and different root-filling techniques, including hybrid and vertical compaction [*177*], and lateral and vertical compaction [*327*]. *Thus, the technique used for root canal filling should not be considered to influence the outcome of initial treatment, and by extension, retreatment.*

- *Comprehensive technique*: the reports from the Toronto study [248] have identified a significant difference in outcome in teeth with apical periodontitis treated with two distinct schemes. Use of the classic Schilder technique, including flared canal preparation with ample irrigation and root canal filling with vertically compacted warm gutta-percha, resulted in a significant, 10% improvement in the healed rate compared with teeth treated with step-back or modified step-back instrumentation and lateral compaction of gutta-percha [248]. The Toronto study was not randomized and controlled to assess the influence of an intervention variable on the outcome; therefore, this finding requires validation from an RCT designed to answer this specific research question. Notably, in the retreatment study from the same group [103], the difference in the healed rate between these two techniques was smaller and not significant. Information on other specific treatment techniques for retreatment is not available. *Thus, in spite of the indication of the superiority of the Schilder technique there is insufficient information available to assess the influence of this or other comprehensive treatment techniques on the outcome of nonsurgical endodontic treatment in teeth with apical periodontitis.*

Complications

Overall, midtreatment complications appear to be infrequent [447]. With the exception of one study [304] where midtreatment complications were not significantly associated with the outcome, all perforations of the pulp chamber or root, file breakage that prevents cleaning of the canal, and massive extrusion of filling materials have been reported to impair the prognosis to varying extents [202,248,391,405]. Notably, however, the ability of endodontists to manage these complications successfully has considerably improved in recent years. In contrast to early studies [202,405] that reported poorer outcomes in teeth with broken instruments, a recent review [400] concluded that "in the hands of skilled endodontists prognosis was not significantly affected by the presence of a retained fractured instrument". A recent case-series study [244] on perforations reported complete healing of all 16 teeth in which perforations were repaired with mineral trioxide aggregate. In a recent retreatment study [103] a comparable healed rate was reported in teeth with and without midtreatment complications. *Thus, the adverse influence of midtreatment complications on*

the outcome may be less now than in the past. Nevertheless, the complications listed above should be avoided, as depending on their severity they may adversely affect the outcome of treatment.

14.7.3 Postoperative factors

The only postoperative prognostic factor highlighted below relates to a procedure performed after completion of root canal treatment, in accordance with the common division of labour regarding endodontic treatment. Nevertheless, it is actually an inseparable component of the endodontic treatment continuum [371], and might be considered an intraoperative factor.

Restoration

In an animal study, Friedman *et al.* [124,126] suggested that root canal infection and associated apical periodontitis could occur subsequent to endodontic treatment, when microorganisms become established in the coronal part of the tooth, e.g., the pulp chamber. This suggestion supported earlier indications of microbial proliferation in the filled root canal *in vitro* [27,30,56–58,138,203,241–243,417,429]. Indeed, an impaired outcome has been reported when a permanent restoration had not been placed in the long term after retreatment [103]. The type of restoration (temporary, permanent, filling, cast) has not been significantly associated with the outcome of initial treatment [248,393] and retreatment [103]. However, in one study [391] teeth restored with crowns or serving as bridge abutments had a poorer outcome than teeth restored with fillings.

According to one cross-sectional study [218], presence or absence of posts was not associated with the outcome of treatment; however, the outcome was impaired when the remaining root canal filling under the post was reduced to less than 3 mm. In two other cross-sectional studies [41,372] posts have been associated with an increased prevalence of apical periodontitis, but the opposite was reported in a third cross-sectional study [439]. However, cross-sectional studies do not comply with the parameters of best evidence. The selected studies [103,248,391] have reported no significant association between the presence or absence of posts and the outcome of initial treatment and retreatment. *Thus, the type of restoration (intraradicular, intracoronal, or extracoronal) does not appear to influence the outcome of nonsurgical* endodontic treatment, as long as the tooth is permanently restored in a timely manner.

Nevertheless, it is clear that the restoration, and particularly its failure, plays an important role in the survival or loss of root-filled teeth [447]. For example, in the four Toronto study reports [*103,104,129,248*] of the total of 87 lost teeth, as many as 32 teeth (37%) were extracted because of restorative considerations. In a survival analysis, 53% of teeth lost after endodontic treatment were extracted because of fracture (root or crown not specified), with additional teeth extracted because of "prosthetic need" [60]. Posts have been implicated in longitudinal root fracture and tooth loss in approximately 9% of cases [447], and also in root perforations that impair the prognosis [217]. *Clearly, posts present a risk to root-filled teeth, and they should be used judiciously.*

14.7.4 Summary of prognostic factors: efficacy of bacterial elimination

When nonsurgical endodontic treatment is reviewed in general, there is a consensus among most studies that preoperative apical periodontitis is the most dominant factor that influences prognosis, but no such consensus exists with regard to other factors. Because apical periodontitis is caused and sustained primarily by root canal infection, it can be argued that "the bacteriological status of the root canal at the time of root canal filling is a critical factor in determining the outcome of endodontic treatment" [*393*]. Therefore, use of means that enhance bacterial elimination should be considered as enhancing prognosis. The efficacy of these means, measured by the proportion of root canal bacterial cultures below the level of detection (negative culture) and by the number (density) of bacteria in the cultures, is briefly reviewed.

Irrigation

The first critically important step in elimination of root canal bacteria is irrigation with effective bactericidal solutions. Several researchers [44,74,300] have observed that root canal instrumentation coupled with inactive irrigants does not predictably eliminate bacteria, regardless of whether it is carried out with stainless-steel hand instruments or with nickel–titanium engine-driven ones. The chance of eliminating bacteria to the extent of negative culture using filing and inactive irrigants is less than 50% [44,74,300]. In contrast, irrigation with sodium hypochlorite

(NaOCl), even if it is diluted to 0.5% or 1.25%, considerably improves the efficacy of bacterial elimination; the chance of obtaining negative cultures may increase to about 50–80%, and bacterial counts may be reduced over 99%, from approximately 10^5 to approximately 10^2 [45,47,220,251,261,309,325,383,392, 393,455]. Elimination of bacteria may be improved by subsequent irrigation with iodine–potassium iodide, with over 70% negative cultures reported [220]. A new immersion-irrigating agent, MTAD, has been introduced; however, no data are yet available from clinical trials to substantiate its potential benefit in enhancing bacterial elimination.

There are considerably fewer data about the efficacy of intracanal procedures in retreatment than in initial treatment. Two studies [312,477] reported a reduction of bacteria below the detection level (negative culture) in 70% and 77% of the teeth, respectively, after instrumentation and irrigation with NaOCl. This efficacy of bacterial elimination is comparable to that reported in studies on initial treatment. It may be further improved by additional irrigation with iodine–potassium iodide, with negative cultures reported at over 95% of teeth [312].

Dressing

The next step in elimination of root canal bacteria is dressing with an effective medication, which requires completion of treatment at a subsequent session. The importance of this step has met with considerable controversy. Byström *et al.* [46,48] have clearly demonstrated the superior efficacy of intracanal dressing with $Ca(OH)_2$ in bacterial elimination. According to these reports and more recent studies [251,383,392], the chance of obtaining a negative culture after such dressing may exceed 85%, and bacterial counts can be reduced to approximately 10^1. In other studies [263,300,472] the increase in negative cultures after dressing with $Ca(OH)_2$ was moderate, reaching 60–80%. However, three recent studies [220,325,455] have reported a decline in negative cultures to 70% or less, and an increase in bacterial counts to approximately 10^3–10^4. It is difficult to reconcile these contrary findings.

Other intracanal medicaments have also been investigated, although less often than $Ca(OH)_2$. Apparently, intracanal dressing with clindamycin yielded 76% negative cultures, a comparable result to that achieved with $Ca(OH)_2$ [261]. In a recent study [309], dressing with 2% chlorhexidine–gluconate liquid resulted in a decline of negative cultures from 68% to 45%, and an increase in bacterial counts from 10^2 to 10^3.

In spite of these results challenging the efficacy of intracanal medication, it is noteworthy that the proportion of negative cultures appears to have been higher, and the bacterial counts lower at the end of the second treatment session than at the end of the first one [300,309,325,455]. Thus, the two-session treatment with interim dressing may still enhance bacterial elimination, compared with treatment in one session.

The only retreatment study [477] that assessed the efficacy of intracanal dressing with $Ca(OH)_2$ added to the controversy from studies on initial treatment. The authors reported a reduction in negative cultures from 77% after canal preparation to 57% after dressing with $Ca(OH)_2$ alone or mixed with chlorhexidine. In the second treatment session, the proportion of negative cultures increased to 87%, but fell again to 70% after subsequent dressing.

Taking all the reports together, it becomes clear that more research is required to establish irrefutably whether dressing with $Ca(OH)_2$ or another effective medication, is critical in the elimination of root canal bacteria in nonsurgical endodontic treatment.

Apical enlargement

Early studies [300,472] have not established a significant improvement in bacterial elimination with progressive enlargement of the root canal. However, a recent study [74] suggested that bacterial counts were reduced when the canal was enlarged from ISO size 45 (size 25 in curved canals) to size 50 and 60 (size 30 and 35 in curved canals). The bacterial reduction is even more pronounced when NaOCl is used [383]. However, when the apical part of the canal was enlarged to even larger sizes with the use of nickel–titanium instruments a further reduction was demonstrated [53], supporting the premise that enlargement does promote microbial elimination.

Apical enlargement during retreatment has not been assessed in relation to bacterial elimination. However, many *in vitro* studies have shown consistently that, irrespective of the retreatment technique used, a considerable amount of root canal filling residue remains attached to the canal walls [24,106,121, 122,168,181,216,221,366,374,423,461–467]. Such residue is likely to shelter bacterial colonies. It appears that the amount of residue can be reduced by further enlargement of the canal beyond its dimensions before retreatment [168].

The data suggest that the combination of copious irrigation with NaOCl (with a small-gauge needle that can be inserted into the apical parts of the root canal) and substantial apical enlargement (possibly to sizes approximating those listed by Kerekes and Tronstad [199–201]), are the critical basic steps in elimination of root canal bacteria. Whether or not root canal dressing with a medication, $Ca(OH)_2$, chlorhexidine, or other, has the potential to improve the elimination of bacteria has been cast into doubt and requires clarification. Because bacteria are the primary cause of persistent apical periodontitis, the ability to maximize their elimination enhances the prognosis of nonsurgical endodontic treatment.

14.8 The expected outcome and prognosis after surgical endodontics

Apical surgery is a viable alternative to root canal retreatment for the management of persistent apical periodontitis. This section reviews the expected outcome of apical surgery (Table 14.6). The projected chance for healing is the benefit that should be weighed against that of root canal retreatment, as well as tooth extraction and replacement.

The selected seven studies on surgical endodontics [62,134,189,219,341,456,479] form the basis for this section. Although these studies were assessed as methodologically adequate, there are important variations in their cohort (population) and exposure (intervention) characteristics (Table 14.7). For example, all the teeth included in the study by Zuolo *et al.* [479] had received root canal retreatment at least once before surgery. Chong *et al.* [62] implied that many teeth included in their study were previously retreated, but the proportion of these teeth was not specified. Two other studies [341,456] included 37–39% of previously retreated teeth, while the remaining studies [134,189,219] did not mention the previous treatment history of their cohorts. The outcome of surgical endodontics after previous root canal retreatment is expected to be better. Similarly, in the studies of Rahbaran *et al.* [341], Gagliani *et al.* [134], and Wang *et al.* [456] teeth with previous history of surgical endodontics comprised 44%, 33%, and 10% of their cohorts, respectively. In contrast, Jensen *et al.* [189] included only teeth that required first-time surgery, while the other studies [62,219] did not characterize their cohorts in regards to previous surgery. As highlighted below, the outcome of repeat surgery is expected to

Table 14.6 Follow-up studies reporting on the outcome of surgical endodontics (apical surgery), appraised for inclusion/exclusion in this chapter review

Study	Follow-up (years)	Cases observed	Recall rate (%)	Cohort	Exposure	Assessment	Analysis	Orthograde and surgery	Surgery	Healed	Healing	Functional*
Mattila and Altonen 1968	0.8–5	164	81	y	n	y	n	39		63	11	≥74
									61	49	17	≥66
Harty et al. 1970	5	1016	74	y	n	y	n	83		90	–	–
									17	89	–	–
Nord 1970	0.5–6.5	354	80	n	y	n	n		100	60	13	≥73
Nordenram and Svärdström 1970	0.6–6	697	87	n	y	n	y	15		82	11	≥93
									85	60	16	≥76
Lehtinen and Aitasalo 1972	n/a	460 [p]	33	n	n	n	n	n/a		78	11	≥89
Rud et al. 1972	1–15	1000	72	n	n	y	y	100		90	6	≥96
Ericson et al. 1974	0.5–12	314	94	n	n	n	n		100	54	25	≥79
Persson et al. 1974	1	220	95	y	y	n	n		100	41	36	≥77
Altonen and Mattila 1976	1–6	46	80 [p]	n	n	n	n	69 [rt]		84	8	≥92
									31 [rt]	65	6	≥71
Finne et al. 1977 [a]	3	218	94	y	y	n	n		100	50	19	≥69
Tay et al. 1978 [b]	n/a	86	n/a	n	n	n	n	n/a		78	–	–
Hirsch et al. 1979	0.5–3	572	88	n	n	n	y	87	13	47	48	≥95
Malmström et al. 1982	2.4	154	25 [p]	n	y	n	n	57 [1]		74	24	≥98
									43	54	33	≥87
Persson 1982	1	26	96	y	y	n	n		100	73	15	≥88
Ioannides and Borstlap 1983	0.5–5	182 [rt]	81	n	y	n	n	75		72	18	≥90
									25	73	11	≥84
Mikkonen and Kullaa-Mikkonen 1983	1–2	174	100	y	y	n	n	93		56	28	≥84
									7	75	17	≥92
Skoglund and Persson 1985	0.5–7	27	100	n	y	n	n		100	37	33	≥70
Reit and Hirsch 1986	1–≥4	35	100	y	y	n	n		100 [r]	71	26	≥97
Forssell et al. 1988	1–4	358	n/a	n	n	y	n	71		68	21	≥89
									29	69	7	≥76
Allen et al. 1989	≥0.5	695	n/a	n	n	n	n		100	60	27	≥87
Amagasa et al. 1989	1–7.5	64	100	y	y	n	n		100 [r]	–	–	95
Crosher et al. 1989	2	85	91	n	y	n	n	100		92	–	–
Dorn and Gartner 1990	0.5	488	n/a	n	n	n	n	n/a		63	18	≥81
Grung et al. 1990	1–8	473	88	y	n	y	n	66		96	3	≥99
									34	72	12	≥84
Friedman et al. 1991	0.5–8	136 [rt]	n/a	n	n	y	y		100	44	23	≥67
Lasaridis et al. 1991	≥0.5	24	100	y	y	n	n	100		79	17	≥96
Lustmann et al. 1991 [c]	0.5–8	134 [rt]	n/a	n	n	y	y	7		70	30	≥100
									93	43	22	≥65
Molven et al. 1991 [d]	1–8	222	n/a	y	n	y	n	50		96	3	≥99
									50	73	14	≥87
Rapp et al. 1991 [e]	≤0.5–≥2	428	60	n	n	n	n		94	66	29	≥95
								6 [2]		56	33	≥89
Rud et al. 1991	0.5–1	388	97	n	y	y	n		100	78	15	≥93
Waikakul and Punwutikorn 1991	0.5–2	62	94	y	y	n	n		100	81	17	≥96
Zetterqvist et al. 1991	1	105	100	y	y	n	n		100	61	31	≥92
Frank et al. 1992	≥10	104	n/a	n	n	n	n	n/a		58	–	–

continued

Table 14.6 *Continued*

Study	Follow-up (years)	Cases observed	Recall rate (%)	Appraisal categories				Treatment approach (%)		Outcome (%)		
				Cohort	Exposure	Assessment	Analysis	Orthograde and surgery	Surgery	Healed	Healing	Functional*
Cheung and Lam 1993	≥2	32	n/a	n	n	n	n	n/a		62	22	≥84
Pantschev et al. 1994	3	79	79	n	y	y	n		100	54	21	≥75
Jesslén et al. 1995	5	93	94	y	y	n	n		100	59	28	≥87
August 1996	10–23	39	18	n	n	n	n			74	15	≥09
Danin et al. 1996	1	19	100	n	y	y	n		100	58	26	≥84
Rud et al. 1996	0.5–1.5	351 [rt]	62	n	y	y	n		100	82	12	≥94
Sumi et al. 1996	0.5–3	157	100	y	y	n	n		100	–	–	92
Jansson et al. 1997	0.9–1.3	62	100	y	y	n	n		100	31	55	≥86
Rud et al. 1997 [f]	0.5–1.5	551 [rt]	61	n	y	y	n		100	79	16	≥95
Bader and Lejeune 1998	1	254	79	n	y	n	n		100	–	–	81
Danin et al. 1999	1	10	100	n	y	y	n		100	50	50	≥100
Kvist and Reit 1999	*4*	*45*	*100*	*y*	*y*	*n*	*y*		*100*	*60*	*–*	*–*
Rubinstein and Kim 1999	1.2	94	73	n	y	n	n		100	97	–	–
Testori et al. 1999	1–6	134	76 [p]	n	y	n	n		100	78	9	≥87
von Arx and Kurt 1999	1	43	96	y	y	n	n		100	82	14	≥96
Zuolo et al. 2000	*1–4*	*102*	*96*	*y*	*y*	*y*	*n*		*100* [2]	*91*	*–*	*92*
Rahbaran et al. 2001	*≥4*	*129* [en]	*61* [p]	*y*	*y*	*y*	*y*		*100* [3]	*37*	*33*	*≥80*
Rud et al. 2001	0.5–12.5	834 [rt]	84	n	y	y	n		100	92	1	≥93
von Arx and Kurt 2001	1	25	96	y	y	n	n		100	88	8	≥96
Rubinstein and Kim 2002 [g]	5–7	59	86	y	y	n	n		100	92	–	–
Jensen et al. 2002	*1*	*60* [Rp]	*91*	*y*	*y*	*n*	*y*		*100*	*73*	*17*	*≥90*
Chong et al. 2003	2	108	59	n	y	y	y			90	6	≥96
Maddalone and Gagliani 2003	0.3–3	120	82	n	y	y	n		100	93	3	≥96
Schwartz-Arad et al. 2003	0.5–0.9	262	47	n	y	n	y		100	44	21	≥65
Wang et al. 2004	*4–8*	*94*	*85*	*y*	*y*	*y*	*y*		*100* [4]	*74*	*–*	*91*
Gagliani et al. 2005	*5*	*231* [rt]	*89*	*y*	*y*	*n*	*y*		*100*	*78*	*10*	*89*

Italicized font highlights studies conforming to at least three out of the four appraisal categories.

*	Asymptomatic, without or with residual radiolucency (≥ not reported; rate is sum of healed and healing).	[2] Treated for persistent disease after orthograde retreatment.
n/a	Not available.	[3] 39% of cases treated for persistent disease after orthograde retreatment.
y	Yes.	
n	No.	[4] 37% of cases treated for persistent disease after orthograde retreatment.
[p]	Patients (as opposed to teeth).	
[rt]	Roots (as opposed to teeth).	[a] Sample as in Persson et al. 1974.
[en]	Only teeth treated in the endodontic clinic included.	[b] Sample as in Harty et al. 1970.
[r]	Retrograde retreatment	[c] Sample as in Friedman et al. 1991.
[Rp]	Only teeth treated with Retroplast included.	[d] Sample as in Grung et al. 1990.
[1]	31% of cases treated for persistent disease after orthograde retreatment.	[e] Sample as in Allen et al. 1989.
		[f] Sample as in Rud et al. 1991 and Rud et al. 1996.
		[g] Sample as in Rubinstein et al. 1999.

Table 14.7 Methodological characteristics of selected follow-up studies on the outcome of surgical endodontics (apical surgery)

Methodological considerations		Kvist & Reit 1999	Zuolo et al. 2000	Rahbaran et al. 2001	Jensen et al. 2002	Chong et al. 2003	Wang et al. 2004	Gagliani et al. 2005
Type of study	Direction	Prospective	Prospective ?	Retrospective	Prospective	Prospective	Prospective	Prospective ?
	Design	RCT	Cohort	Cohort	RCT	RCT	Cohort	Cohort
Cohort	Tooth type	Anteriors	Anteriors 38% Premolars 24% Molars 38%	Anteriors 73% Premolars 19% Molars 8%	Anteriors 25% Premolars 33% Molars 42%	Single-rooted Molars (M roots)	Anteriors 39% Posterior 61%	Anteriors 17% Premolars 33% Molars 50%
	Inclusion criteria	AP present	AP present 1 tooth/subject At least 1 retreat Good restoration	20% w/o AP No probing Good root filling Good restoration	1 tooth/subject	AP present 1 tooth/subject No probing Good root filling Good restoration	All included	No probing Good root filling Lesion <10 mm
	Exclusion criteria	Recent retreatment Probing to apex	Fracture Perforation Resorption Trauma Probing >7 mm Loss of bone plate		Previous surgery		None	
	Previous retreatment		100%	39%		Yes; ?%	37%	
	Previous surgery		None	44%	None		10%	32%
Intervention	Operators	Endodontist	Endodontist	Endodontics residents	4 Oral surgery residents	Endodontist	Endodontics residents	Endodontist
	Resection level	1–2 mm	2–4 mm Bevel		2–3 mm	No bevel	3 mm	3 mm Little bevel
	Hemostasis				Epinephrin		Epinephrin Ferric sulfate	Ferric sulfate
	Cavity preparation	Bur 34% R-rtx	Ultrasonic	Bur or ultrasonic	Scooped	Ultrasonic	Ultrasonic 7% R-rtx	Ultrasonic
	Root-end filling material	GP softened with chloroform or heat	IRM	S-EBA, amalgam, IRM, GP, none	Retroplast GIC	IRM MTA	Amalgam, IRM, s-EBA, CR, MTA, none	ZOE with EBA
	Magnification					Microscope	Loops	Loops ×4.5
	Sutures		Monofilament 5×0 3–4 days	4–7 days	Vicryl 4×0	4–7 days		Silk
	Antibiotics		7 days Steroid	45% of teeth	Only when sinus invaded		44% of teeth	
	Antinflammatories							
	Antiseptic rinse		4 days	7 days		Used	7 days	

continued

Table 14.7 *Continued*

Assessment							
Radiographic aids	Stents	Stents		None used	Stents	Parallel device	Parallel device
Radiographic criteria	"Strict definition of healing/disease"	CH = success, IH = failure, >4 years, US = failure	CH = success, IH = uncertain, Failure	CH = success, IH = success, UH = doubtful, US = failure	CH = success, IH = success, UH = failure, US = failure	PAI 1, 2	CH = success, IH = improvement, Failure
Calibration		Yes	Yes	No	Yes	Yes	Yes
Blinding		Yes	Yes	No	Yes	Yes	Yes
Observers	2	2	3	3	2	1	2
Conflicts resolved	Joint assessment	Joint assessment	Joint assessment	Concensus or majority	Joint assessment	N/a	Worst accepted
Analysis							
Follow-up	6, 12, 24, 48 months	1–4 years Successful not followed further	1, 2, 4 years	1 year	1, 2 years	4–8 years	5 years
Evaluated unit	Tooth	Tooth	Tooth	Tooth	Root and tooth	Tooth	Root
Bivariate tests	Used	Used	Not used	Used	Used	Used	Used
Multivariate tests	N/a	Not used	Used	Used	N/a	Used	N/a

AP   Apical periodontitis.
R-rtx Retrograde retreatment.
GP   Gutta-percha.
GIC   Glass-ionomer cement.
CR   Composite resin.
ZOE   Zinc oxide/eugenol.
CH   Complete healing.
IH   Incomplete healing.
UH   Uncertain healing.
US   Unsatisfactory healing.
N/a   Not applicable.

be poorer than that of first-time surgery. Because of these differences among the selected studies, there is considerable inconsistency in their reported outcomes (Table 14.7).

Proportion of healed teeth

The greatest variation among the studies comprising the best evidence is in the healed rate, ranging from 37% [341] to 91% [479]. This range is almost as large as that observed across all studies (Table 14.6), in contrast to the expected uniformity of studies that satisfy the appraisal criteria. Still, the lowest healed rate of 37% [341] and the highest rates of 90% [62] and 91% [479] fall considerably outside the range of rates reported in the remaining studies [134,189,219,456]. These unusually low and high rates may be considered as outliers. *Thus, the chance for complete healing after surgical endodontics is 60–78%.*

Since the criteria for complete healing are well defined and fairly consistent in the selected studies, the variation in the reported outcomes must be related to other factors (see Section 14.3):

- Different outcomes may have resulted from assembly bias, particularly from inclusion of teeth with persistent disease after previous root canal retreatment, as opposed to previous initial treatment. These two scenarios may differ with regard to the site where persistent bacteria are located [128,456]. Persistence of apical periodontitis after retreatment suggests that "intracanal irritants and contamination" were reduced [479] and infection is sustained by bacteria situated beyond reach. The bacteria can be harbored in the apical ramifications of the canal [278,281,284], the outer surface of the root tip [228,286,387,435,437,438,440], or the periapical tissue [108,109,135,154,163,164,195,279,292,368,386, 390,409–413,440]. In all these sites, the infection would be eradicated by the surgical removal of the root tip and periapical tissue. Indeed, the reported healed rate in teeth that had been retreated at least once before the surgical treatment is 84% [456] to 91% [479]. In contrast, persistence of disease after initial treatment is more likely to be sustained by bacteria situated within the root canal [29,40,59,115,133,155,161,197,230,231,262,281,311, 312,335,336,349,388,414,415,477]. These bacteria are not eliminated during surgery, but an attempt is made to enclose them with a root-end filling. The proportion of teeth where surgical endodontics

was performed because of persisting disease after retreatment has been specified in only three of the studies [341,456,479].

- Different outcomes may have resulted from differences in treatment procedures. The techniques and materials used in one of the selected studies [219] differed from the current ones used in the more recent studies [62,134,189,341,456,479]. These current procedures included use of ultrasonic tips to prepare deeper, cleaner and better-aligned root-end cavities, with lesser risk of lingual perforation than with round burs used in the past [54,55,254,449,471]. Magnification and micro-instruments were used [62,134,456] that facilitate identification and treatment of accessory canals and isthmuses, as well as detection of root cracks [54,55,207,313]. These modern tools are amenable to work in smaller bony crypts and with lesser apical bevel, so that fewer dentinal tubules become exposed [55,204,254,449,471]. Instead of using amalgam for root-end filling, IRM, Super-EBA cement, MTA, or a dentin-bonded composite resin were used, with the expectation of improved clinical performance based on favorable outcomes in animal studies [14,338,339,358,430, 442]. Collectively, these current procedures may have improved the outcome of treatment in some of the more recent studies when compared with the study where these techniques were not used [219].

Proportion of healing teeth

When reported, the healing rates have varied between 6% [62] and 33% [341]. Similarly to nonsurgical treatment, a high proportion of teeth still demonstrating healing is typical of short-term studies that do not capture the completion of the healing process [127]. Therefore, it is atypical that the highest proportion of healing was reported after a follow-up of 4 years or longer [341]. Possibly, the cohort in this particular study included many large lesions that healed by formation of a scar and were included in the "uncertain" category (consistent with the definition of "healing"), whereas in the other selected studies scars were included in the "incomplete healing" category (consistent with the definition of "healed"). *Thus, the chance of teeth to demonstrate incomplete healing after surgical endodontics is approximately 5–30%, depending on the case selection and outcome classification used.*

Proportion of asymptomatic functional teeth

Four studies [134,341,456,479] suggested that 80–94% of the teeth were "asymptomatic and functional" at the follow-up examination. This rate of "asymptomatic function" is not synonymous with the lower "survival" rate reported in another study [457] because the former does not take into account all lost teeth. Thus, the reported rate of "asymptomatic function" overestimates the chances of teeth to be retained after surgical endodontics. Importantly, however, a survival analysis may underestimate the chance of teeth being retained, if the reported tooth loss includes functional teeth without disease that were extracted as part of a comprehensive treatment plan or to avoid costly restorative or periodontal treatment. *Thus, the chance of teeth to remain functional after surgical endodontics may approximate 80–90%.* This good potential for maintained asymptomatic function suggests that for root-filled teeth with apical periodontitis and with reasonable periodontal prognosis, *surgical endodontics is a conservative treatment option that should be attempted*, rather than having the tooth extracted and replaced.

Dynamics of healing

Healing progresses quickly after surgical endodontics, peaking within the first year after treatment [159,219]. Approximately 60% of the teeth that heal eventually, and almost all those that heal by scar, are already healed within a year [151,159,174,239,245, 267]. From those that appear as healing at 1 year, over one-half are healed by 3 years totaling approximately 85% of teeth that heal eventually, while about one-quarter revert to disease [151,159,289]. The majority of teeth that appear either healed or diseased at 1 year demonstrate the same outcome at 3–5 years [110,159,174,289,354]. Thus, apparently, the 1-year follow-up may be considered conclusive for the majority of cases, while longer follow-up is required only for those cases that appear as still healing [159,267]. However, recurrence of disease in the long-term has been reported in 5% to over 40% of healed cases [110, 117,159,190,219,289,354]. It is advisable, therefore, to follow-up the teeth periodically even if they appear healed at the 1-year examination.

Healing after surgical endodontics can be in the form of fibrous periapical tissue (scar) rather than deposition of bone at the surgery site [11,12,264,267,356]. This form of healing occurs particularly when a cavity is formed in the bone involving both the buccal and lingual plates [151,266]. Because the scar remains stable over time [267], the area is considered healed [264,267,356].

Persistence of disease

Persistent disease after surgical endodontics usually occurs when the attempt to seal bacteria within the root canal system is ineffective [118]. The root canal bacteria may interact with the periapical tissues by different pathways:

- Accessory canals or isthmuses between canals may not be sealed by the root-end filling [55,178].
- Exposed dentinal tubules cut open after root-end resection may communicate between the root canal space and periapical tissues [137,427,446]. The number of exposed tubules is related to the degree of beveling of the cut root surface [137].
- The root-end filling fails to seal the canal effectively, either because of poor placement and adaptation, or poor sealing ability [118].

14.9 Outcome predictors in surgical endodontics

In the first edition of this book [119] clinical factors were identified that appeared to influence the outcome of surgical endodontics, without an attempt to differentiate studies according to the level of evidence. Consequently, contradicting results were rather frequent. This review focuses primarily on the selected studies that comprise the best evidence for surgical endodontics [62,134,189,219,341,456,479] (Table 14.7). For easy identification in the following section, the reference numbers for these studies are highlighted in italicized type. The nonselected studies are cited only where selected studies are unavailable. As with nonsurgical treatment, the prognostic factors are divided into preoperative, intraoperative, and postoperative.

14.9.1 Preoperative factors

The preoperative factors form the basis for projecting the prognosis after surgical endodontics, and thus the expected benefit that the patient can weigh against those of alternative treatments. Therefore, it is important to recognize the preoperative factors and to take them into account when treatment decisions are formed.

Patient's age, gender, and systemic health

In the studies that examined the patients' age [341,456,479] and gender [341,456,479], these factors have not been significantly associated with the outcome of treatment. Systemic health has not been assessed as a prognostic factor in any of the studies. *Thus, age, gender, and health should not be considered to influence the outcome of surgical endodontics.*

Tooth location

In several studies [134,341,456,479] comparable outcomes have been reported for different tooth types, in both the maxilla and mandible. The only outcome feature related to tooth location is the frequent healing by scar tissue observed in maxillary lateral incisors [151,266]. *Apparently, the specific convenience of access and root anatomy influence the outcome of surgical endodontics to a greater extent than the location of the tooth.*

Clinical signs and symptoms

In one study [113], a poorer outcome was reported in teeth with a sinus tract present. Two selected studies [341,456], however, have reported a comparable treatment outcome for asymptomatic teeth and for teeth presenting with preoperative symptoms *Thus, presence or absence of symptoms should not be considered to influence the outcome of surgical endodontics.*

Lesion size

One study [341] suggested that the lesion size had no significant influence on the outcome of treatment. However, in another study [456] a better outcome was reported in teeth with small lesions, up to 5 mm in diameter, than in teeth with larger lesions. The authors hypothesized that when the lesion was small, surgical enlargement of the crypt was required to gain adequate access, resulting in eradication of the pathological lesion and creation of an excisional wound in the surrounding bone [165]. When the lesion was large the access was adequate and the crypt was not enlarged to avoid injury to adjacent anatomical structures; therefore, curettage of the pathological lesion might have been incomplete. When the lesion is very large, exceeding 10 mm in diameter, more healing by scar tissue occurs [151,266]. *Thus, a better outcome*

may be expected when the lesion diameter does not exceed 5 mm.

Supporting bone loss

The treatment of teeth where the entire buccal bone plate is missing has been assessed in several nonselected studies [110,113,174,355,394], suggesting a poor prognosis for teeth with considerable bone loss, either vertical or marginal. Such bone loss can compromise periodontal reattachment by apical migration of gingival epithelium. Consequently, bacteria present in the periodontal pocket may invade the periapical site and prevent healing. *Thus, considerable attachment loss of the treated tooth may have a negative influence on the outcome after surgical endodontics.*

Restoration of the tooth

Surgical endodontics is frequently performed on teeth that are already restored; in these teeth, the restorative status is a preoperative consideration. One study [341] reported a poorer treatment outcome in teeth with a faulty coronal seal or with a post; however, this finding has not been corroborated by another study [456]. Nevertheless, a defective restoration can impair the survival of root-filled teeth [447]. Indeed, Wang *et al.* [456] observed that of 10 teeth lost after surgical endodontics, seven teeth (70%) were extracted because of restorative considerations, while two teeth were extracted because of fracture and one tooth because of persistent apical periodontitis. *Thus, there is insufficient information available to assess the influence of the type of the restoration on the outcome of surgical endodontics, as long as the tooth is adequately restored.*

The existing root canal filling

The root canal filling with which the tooth presents for surgery can be characterized by its material, density, and length. The type of the filling material does not influence the outcome of surgical endodontics [341,456]. The filling density – absence or presence of voids – also does not appear to influence the outcome [341,456]. A significantly better outcome is reported when the filling is too short ($\geq$2 mm from the root end) or too long (extruded beyond the root end), than when its length is adequate [456]; however, this finding is not supported by another study [341]. *Thus, the type and density of the existing root canal filling should not be considered to influence the outcome of surgical endo-*

dontics; but there is insufficient information to assess the influence of the length of the filling on outcome.

Repeat (second-time) surgery

One study focusing on repeat surgery [*134*], a non-selected study [321], and a systematic review of several nonselected studies [328] have concluded that the prognosis after repeat surgery is poorer than after first-time surgery. This finding is not supported by two other studies [*341,456*]. Wang *et al.* [*456*] reported a nonsignificant difference in outcome between first-time (79% healed) and second-time (62% healed) surgery. As only eight teeth received repeat surgery, this analysis could be underpowered. Nevertheless, the authors speculated that in the other studies, surgery was frequently repeated using the same case selection criteria and techniques as in the first surgery, whereas in their study root canal retreatment was preferred over repeat surgery. In the few cases of repeat surgery, the technique differed from that of the first-time surgery. The authors suggested that the modified case selection and techniques might have resulted in a better outcome after repeat surgery in their study than in previous studies [*456*]. *Thus, the outcome of repeat surgery may be poorer than that of first-time surgery, unless the repeat procedure is performed with an improved approach.*

14.9.2 Intraoperative factors

The intraoperative prognostic factors can be instrumental in maximizing the patient's benefit by improving the outcome of the surgical procedure. Therefore, it is important to recognize the intraoperative factors and take them into account when treatment strategies and techniques are selected.

Level of apical resection and degree of beveling

In one study [7], a better outcome was reported after resection at the midroot level than at a more apical level. Resection close to the apex may expose many ramifications of the canal system that, if not sealed by the root-end filling, can comprise pathways for intracanal bacteria to sustain disease after surgery [55]. Therefore, the resection should be performed approximately 3 mm from the apex, where ramifications are fewer [206]. Furthermore, resection at a more coronal level facilitates preparation of the root-end cavity and filling. *Thus, a better outcome of surgical endodontics*

may be expected after a more radical resection of the root than after a very conservative resection.

The degree of beveling has not been assessed in relation to treatment outcome. Nevertheless, the bevel should be minimal to avoid the risk of missing canals emerging at the lingual aspect of the root [55]. A minimal bevel also reduces the number of exposed dentinal tubules on the cut root surface, which comprise a bacterial pathway for persistence of disease [137,427,450].

Presence/absence of a root-end filling

Placement of a root-end filling is consistent with the rationale of surgical endodontics to establish an effective barrier that will prevent interaction of intracanal bacteria with the periapical tissues [118]. This rationale applies in all teeth where it is assumed that apical periodontitis is sustained by persistent intracanal bacteria [118]. However, a root-end filling may be superfluous when the disease is assumed to be sustained by extraradicular bacteria [118,456]; indeed, in one study [*456*] seven out of eight teeth (88%) suspected for extraradicular infection healed without receiving a root-end filling.

It is noteworthy from the historical perspective that according to many studies [7,113,151,185,227,245,250, 266,289] presence of a root-end filling impairs the prognosis. For example, Grung *et al.* [151] concluded that "retrofills have a strong negative effect on the end results". In these studies, root-end fillings were placed in the teeth treated exclusively by surgical endodontics, but not in the teeth treated concurrently by surgery and root canal treatment. Therefore, comparison of teeth without and with root-end fillings was confounded by root canal treatment, performed in the former but not in the latter [118]. However, limiting the analysis in the same studies and others to teeth treated only surgically reveals better outcomes with than without root-end fillings [7,119,174,250,343]. *Thus, placement of a root-end filling may enhance the outcome of surgical endodontics, particularly when persistent root canal infection is assumed to be the cause of persistent disease.*

Root-end management

In the past two decades, the classical root-end cavity drilled with a small round bur has been modified in two ways. Rud *et al.* [16,357,358] developed the method of bonding a cap of Retroplast – a composite resin – over the cut root surface, to seal the main canal, accessory canals, isthmuses and exposed dentinal tubules. To avoid adverse effects of shrinkage Retroplast is not placed into a root-end cavity. Instead, it is placed as a thin layer into a concavity created in the resected surface with a large round bur. One of the selected studies [*189*] reports a healed rate of 73% and a healing rate of 17% 1 year after surgical endodontics with Retroplast. The outcomes in this study and others where Retroplast was used [357–361,363] appear to surpass the outcomes reported in studies where root-end cavities have been prepared and filled with a variety of materials (Table 14.6). Conceivably, Geristore [82,83] and OptiBond can be used as alternatives to Retroplast for establishing the apical cap [55]; however, their clinical effectiveness has not been reported.

To modify the root-end cavity, Carr [54,55] developed special angled tips for ultrasonic cavity preparation. Use of these tips requires less beveling of the cut root surface and a smaller crypt preparation than burs [55,254,449,450]. More importantly, the resulting cavities are deeper, allowing the root-end filling to seal exposed dentinal tubules from within the canal [254,449,471]. The cavities are also cleaner and better aligned with the long axis of the canal, so that the risk of perforation of the lingual wall of the root is reduced [143,229,449]. Two nonselected studies [22,424] have reported a better outcome in teeth where root-end cavities were prepared with ultrasonic tips than when cavities were prepared with burs; however, the analyses in both studies were confounded by extraneous factors, undermining their conclusions. Importantly, the healed rates (37–91%) reported in the selected studies in which root-end cavities were prepared with ultrasonic tips [*62,134,341,456,479*] are not different from those in other studies where root-end cavities were drilled with burs.

Thus, there is no strong evidence to suggest that the apical cap or the ultrasonic root-end cavity preparation offer a better prognosis after surgical endodontics; however, there is a sound clinical rationale for using both approaches. Both approaches also offer greater ease and consistency of application than drilling the root-end cavity with small round burs.

Root-end filling material

Many materials used in dentistry over the years have also been considered as root-end filling materials, including amalgam with or without varnish, plain or reinforced zinc oxide/eugenol cement, EBA and Super-EBA cement, polycarboxylate cement, glass-ionomer cement, burnished or injectable gutta-percha, composite resin, cyanoacrylate glue, Teflon, gold foil, titanium screws, and Cavit. These materials have been comprehensively reviewed by Friedman [118]. In the past decade, MTA, a material developed specifically for root-end filling, has also been used [430,431]. This plethora of materials has primarily been assessed by *in vitro* methods and characterized by inconsistent results [118,425]. To overcome the limitations of *in vitro* studies, an *in vivo* simulation model was developed by Friedman *et al.* [120]. Variations of this model have been used in several studies [14,338,339,430,442,469] with better consistency of results than in the *in vitro* studies. In these animal studies, IRM [14,338], Super-EBA [339,442], MTA [430], and Diaket [469] have performed better than other materials. However, these *in vivo* studies do not provide the evidence-base required for supporting the clinical effectiveness of these materials.

Several nonrandomized clinical trials have assessed different root-end filling materials, including Biobond [288], Cavit [110,322], glass-ionomer cement [73,190,478], Retroplast [358], IRM [81,343,375], EBA [81,308,343], gold leaf [453], and titanium inlay [408]. Amalgam has frequently been used as the control. The methodology in all these studies does not comply with an adequate level of evidence, negating their conclusions. For example, EBA cement was significantly superior to amalgam in one study (95% vs 51% success, respectively) [81], marginally superior in another study (57% vs 52%, respectively) [308], and marginally inferior in a third study (65% vs 71%, respectively) [343]. Better evidence can be derived from recent RCTs [*62,189*]. For use as an apical cap, Retroplast is significantly better than a glass-ionomer cement, that was observed to detach in several of the teeth [*189*]. For filling a root-end cavity, IRM and MTA were reported to be equally effective [*62*]; however, the validity of this finding could be disputed because the root canals sealed by these materials may not have been infected after a previous retreatment. A comparable outcome was also reported for root-end fillings with Super-EBA and other materials (IRM, MTA, composite resin, amalgam) in a recent cohort study [*456*]. *Thus, the outcome of surgical endodontics relying on a bonded cap critically depends on the bonding properties of the material used. When an intracanal root-end cavity is filled, a similar outcome may be expected if IRM, EBA, or MTA is used.*

Method of hemostasis

Different hemostatic agents, including epinephrine-saturated pellets, ferric sulfate, bone wax, thrombin, calcium sulfate, Gelfoam, Surgicel, and collagen wound dressing, have been routinely used for crypt control by many clinicians [55,188,205]. Good hemostasis is critically important for the quality of the root-end filling [55] and bonding of an apical cap [*189*]. However, in a recent study [*456*] there was no significant association between the outcome and the use of hemostatic agents. *Thus, use of hemostatic agents should not be considered to influence the outcome of surgical endodontics.*

Combination with root canal treatment

Surgical endodontics performed concurrently with initial root canal treatment or retreatment addresses all possible sites where bacteria colonize, including root canal ramifications, the apical root surface and the periapical tissue. Furthermore, according to Molven *et al.* [266] "infection is eliminated and reinfection is prevented". Consequently, studies in which both procedures were combined in the majority of the sample usually show a better outcome than those in which only surgical endodontics was performed [118,172]. The difference between the two approaches is also demonstrated in specific studies [7,151,227,245,250, 289,355]. Currently, however, surgical endodontics is not considered imminent when the root canal is accessible from the coronal pathway; rather, it is performed alone as an alternative to root canal retreatment. *Thus, the better outcome offered by combining surgical endodontics with root canal treatment is merely of academic interest.* It confirms that root canal bacteria are the predominant cause of posttreatment apical periodontitis [155,415], and that they may still sustain the disease process in spite of the root-end filling.

Retrograde root canal retreatment

A modified approach to surgical endodontics, focusing on instrumentation, irrigation and filling of the root canal as far coronally as can be reached from the apical end, can be used as an alternative to the typical root-end filling [8,111,139,291,346,381,404]. According to several clinical studies [8,140,346,456], the healed rate after such retrograde retreatment ranges from 71% to 100%, and the rate of persistent disease does not exceed 16%. Clearly, this procedure offers an advantage over the standard root-end filling, as it places a deeper barrier between intracanal bacteria and the periapical tissue. However, if bacterial ingress continues coronally under the restoration and along the post into the canal, with time bacteria may overcome this barrier resulting in recurrence of disease. *Thus, retrograde retreatment of the root canal can enhance the outcome of surgical endodontics, even though it cannot entirely prevent recurrence of disease.*

Quality and depth of root-end filling

Only one study [*341*] highlighted the significance of the quality of the root-end filling, particularly its correct placement. In another study [*456*] comparable outcomes were reported for root-end fillings extending up to 2 mm or deeper into the canal space. However, the depth of the root-end filling cannot be reliably assessed in radiographs because its apical surface is frequently beveled [341]. *Thus, there is insufficient information available to assess the influence of the root-end filling depth, ranging from 1 to 4 mm, on the outcome of surgical endodontics. The accurate placement of the root-end filling enhances the outcome.*

Magnification and illumination

In the past decade the use of aids to enhance visualization during surgical endodontics has become increasingly popular among clinicians. Magnification aids include loupes, operating microscopes [54,259,352], and endoscopes [451,452]. The latter two also greatly enhance illumination. Apart from convenience, these aids facilitate identification of intricate anatomical features and improve control of all aspects of the surgical procedure [54,55,204,207,313,445,451,452]. Reporting 97% success, one study [353] implied that the outcome of surgical endodontics was improved by use of the operating microscope and Super-EBA cement as the root-end filling. Among the selected studies loupes were used to enhance visualization [*134,456*], or the operating microscope was used to inspect the adaptation of the root-end filling [*62*]. However, the value of magnification and illumination in surgical endodontics has not been assessed at an adequate level of evidence. *Thus, there is no information available to assess the influence of magnification and illumination on the outcome of surgical endodontics. Nevertheless, there is a sound rationale for use of these aids to improve the quality of the surgical procedure.*

Laser irradiation

Laser irradiation of the resected root surface and crypt has been suggested as a means of sterilization and hemostasis [215,255,260], and to render the dentin on the cut root surface impermeable to bacteria [17,306,401,402,470]. Despite these theoretical benefits of laser irradiation, it has not been shown to influence the outcome of surgical endodontics when applied *in vivo* in animal studies [120,420] and in a clinical trial [22]. *Thus, use of laser irradiation should not be considered to influence the outcome of surgical endodontics.*

Barriers and bone grafting substances

The use of guided regeneration barriers in surgical endodontics has been advocated in case reports [314,316]. Similarly, the use of various bone grafting substances in the crypt has been described [274,315,317,385,473]. The handful of clinical studies and case reports published [147,314,342,364,428] do not provide evidence to support the routine use of these procedures in surgical endodontics. *Thus, use of barriers and bone grafting substances should not be considered to enhance the prognosis of surgical endodontics, while care must be taken to avoid infection of the foreign materials placed.*

Operator's skill

Two nonselected studies have suggested that the outcome of surgical endodontics may depend on the individual operator's skill [7,238]. In three of the selected studies [189,341,456] specialty trainees were the treatment providers, while in the remaining four studies treatment was performed by specialists, either oral surgeons or endodontists. Therefore, reference to operator skill is scarce. *Thus, the operator's skill may influence the outcome of surgical endodontics, but there is insufficient information to assess the extent of this influence.*

Complications

Occasionally during surgical endodontics, a perforation can occur in the opposing (lingual) aspect of the root or cortical bone plate, or the maxillary sinus may be exposed. Perforation of the opposing bone plate has not been significantly associated with the outcome beyond an increased rate of healing by scar tissue [151,266,456]. Similarly, perforation into the sinus has not been associated with the outcome [95,323,362]. *Thus, midtreatment complications should not be considered to influence the outcome of surgical endodontics.*

Antibiotics

Antibiotics may be prescribed to prevent infection of a postoperative hematoma. Two studies [*341,456*] have reported no significant association between a course of systemic antibiotics, starting before and continuing after treatment, and the outcome of surgical endodontics. *Thus, the use of systemic antibiotics should not be considered to influence the outcome of surgical endodontics.*

14.9.3 Postoperative factor

The only postoperative prognostic factor that may modify the prognosis is a biopsy report.

Results of biopsy

Periapical biopsies are frequently obtained during surgical endodontics. Theoretically, the biopsy results defining the pathological lesion – granuloma or cyst – might be used as indicators of the prognosis. Jensen *et al.* [*189*] reported a significant association between the biopsy results and the outcome of surgical endodontics; however, no such association has been reported in two other studies [*456,479*]. These conflicting reports may be the result of differences in processing of biopsy specimens. Routine biopsies are seldom subjected to serial sections, and therefore may not accurately reflect the nature of the pathological lesion. *Thus, a biopsy report on the nature of the lesion removed during surgical endodontics should not be considered in the estimation of prognosis.*

14.10 The expected outcome and prognosis after intentional replantation

Intentional replantation has been applied to address a variety of clinical conditions, including difficult endodontic treatment [208], surgical endodontics, and root canal retreatment [350] and even prevention of predictable failures [290]. Currently, it is applied considerably less than in the past, mainly as an alternative to extraction, when both retreatment and surgical endodontics are not feasible *in situ* [79,86,92,153].

In this context, survival of the replanted tooth is the expected goal, and may be considered as success [150], even if pathological processes persist. Therefore conceptually, intentional replantation cannot be simply compared with root canal retreatment and surgical endodontics on the basis of success and failure.

In contrast to the "conventional" treatment modalities, intentional replantation requires healing of the attachment apparatus without root resorption. Research reports have indicated that the treatment outcome of tooth replantation is determined by survival of the periodontal ligament and cementum along the root surface [13,15], as well as infection of the root canal [436] and the socket [441]. Resorption-free reattachment is governed by the trauma associated with exarticulation, extraoral manipulation and replantation, the extraoral time and environment, and the type and duration of splinting [160,295]. Accordingly, the following conditions are optimal for healing after intentional replantation: (i) gentle extraction and reinsertion; (ii) careful extraoral manipulation of the root, keeping it moist; (iii) retrograde cleaning and filling of the root canal as far coronally as possible; (iv) replantation within 15 minutes; (v) flexible splinting for 7–14 days and elimination of occlusal contacts; (vi) preoperative and postoperative antibiotic regimen; and (vii) preoperative and postoperative antiseptic mouth rinsing.

Current studies on the treatment outcome of intentional replantation are few, and the majority of the available studies (Table 14.8) were performed more than 20 years ago. According to these studies, the success rate of intentional replantation ranges from 34% [92] to 93% [208], whereas the survival rate appears to exceed 80%. However, the evaluation criteria are not clearly defined, and the treatment procedures differ considerably. Most importantly, in the majority of studies listed in Table 14.8 the clinical protocols did not meet the currently recognized requirements for successful replantation of teeth. For example, Grossman and Chacker [148] replanted 28 root-filled teeth with persistent apical periodontitis without placing root-end fillings; this was likely the cause of persistent infection observed in 27% of their material. Emmertsen and Andreasen [92] kept the teeth out of the socket for 30–60 minutes, then tapered some roots by grinding to facilitate replantation; both factors compromise the tissues on the root surface, increasing the risk of resorption. The root canal fillings, when performed, were done with the inefficient method of gutta-percha and Kloroperka N-Ø (see Section 14.7.2). Many roots

were only sealed apically by root-end filling, potentially allowing persisting intracanal bacteria to propagate through the dentinal tubules and infect the root surface [91]; these roots were frequently associated with inflammatory root resorption. A similar technique was used by Keller [198] and in a proportion of the teeth treated by Koenig *et al.* [214]. Deeb [79] performed root canal treatment and occasionally also the coronal restoration outside the mouth, probably extending the extraoral period over 20 minutes.

Because of procedural inadequacy, the realistic treatment outcome of correctly performed intentional replantation cannot be assessed on the basis of published studies. Projection from reported outcomes after replantation of traumatically avulsed teeth is inappropriate, because intentional replantation affords superior control over most of the factors influencing the treatment outcome. However, because animal studies on replantation and root resorption use intentional replantation as the actual experimental procedure, the results of these studies may be interpreted to suggest the outcome of intentional replantation in humans. From these studies it appears that, when the optimal conditions for replantation are provided, development of progressive root resorption is minimized, and it does not exceed 4% [160]. Indeed, in three of the clinical studies on intentional replantation root resorption occured only in 2–5% of the cases (Table 14.8). Replacement resorption should not occur at all [214] because of the optimal extraoral time and environment; indeed, in the study by Emmertsen and Andreasen [92] replacement resorption occurred in only 4% of the teeth, in spite of the compromised protocol. Apart from reattachment, healing of apical periodontitis appears to be rather predictable, because of the ability to seal off the infected root canal effectively when the root-end filling is carried out extraorally. The low incidence of both replacement resorption and persistent apical periodontitis after intentional replantation, is corroborated by a considerable number of case reports [84,105,153,196,232,235,236,240,257,290,350,351, 398,406], further supporting the premise that the treatment outcome of intentional replantation is predictable under well-controlled conditions, albeit at the lowest level of evidence.

Dynamics of resorption

In the majority of intentionally replanted teeth that succumb to inflammatory resorption, the resorptive

Table 14.8 Treatment outcome following intentional replantation

Study	Cases treated	Follow-up (years)	Treatment outcome (%)					
			Survival	Success	RR	IR	RES	AP
Schmidt 1954*	500	5	–	77			–	–
Tombeur 1953*	188	–	–	62			–	–
Bielas *et al.* 1959*	943	5	–	59			–	–
La Forgia 1955*	60	–	–	55			–	–
Emmertsen and Andreasen 1966	100	1–13	80	34	4	27	31	50
Grossman and Chacker 1968	61	3–11	100	57	–	–	18	27
Deeb 1968	117	0.5–2	93	67	–	–	33	–
Kingsbury and Wiesebaugh 1971	151	1–3	95	93	–	–	3	–
Will 1974	158	5–7	96	–	–	–	2	–
Koenig 1988	177	0.5–4	82	82	0	5	5	11
Kahnberg 1988	58	2–7	71	71	–	–	0	29
Keller 1990	34	3	91	91	–	–	0	9
Bender and Rossman 1993	31	0–22	81	81	–	–	6	10

*   Cited by Grossman and Chacker, 1968.
RR   Replacement resorption.
IR   Inflammatory resorption.
RES   Resorption of any kind.
AP   Apical periodontitis.

area is discernible within one year of treatment [92]. A recent report on replantation following traumatic avulsions indicated that replacement resorption might be first observed radiologically several years after replantation [15]. However, it may be indicated clinically much earlier than radiologically, by a specific pitch in response to percussion. In any event, occurrence of replacement resorption should be minimal.

endodontic treatment of apical periodontitis is good: the chances for the periapical tissues to heal are reasonably high, and the chances to retain a well-restored tooth in asymptomatic function over time are excellent. Therefore, whenever it is feasible, either nonsurgical or surgical endodontic treatment should be attempted before considering tooth extraction and replacement.

14.11 Case selection considerations

Selection of cases for endodontics takes into consideration the prognosis of dental interventions – endodontic, restorative, and periodontal – but also health and socioeconomic factors. Contraindications to treatment include nonrestorable and periodontally severely compromised teeth, patients with extensive dental problems and restricted resources (that should be selectively utilized to benefit as many teeth as possible), and medically compromised patients at high-risk of infection or, for surgical procedures, those with bleeding disorders.

From the endodontic perspective, none of the preoperative clinical factors truly contraindicates treatment. The prognosis and expected outcome of

14.12 References

1. Abbott P (1999) A retrospective analysis of the reasons for, and the outcome of, conservative endodontic retreatment and periradicular surgery. *Australian Dental Journal* **44**, 3–4.
2. Adenubi JO, Rule DC (1976) Success rate for root fillings in young patients. A retrospective analysis of treated cases. *British Dental Journal* **141**, 237–41.
3. Åkerblöm A, Hasselgren G (1988) The prognosis for endodontic treatment of obliterated root canals. *Journal of Endodontics* **14**, 565–7.
4. Allard U, Palmqvist S (1986) A radiographic survey of periapical conditions in elderly people in a Swedish county population. *Endodontics and Dental Traumatology* **2**, 103–8.
5. Allen RK, Newton CW, Brown CE (1989) A statistical analysis of surgical and nonsurgical endodontic retreatment cases. *Journal of Endodontics* **15**, 261–6.

6. Alley BS, Kitchens GG, Alley LW, Eleazer PD (2004) A comparison of survival of teeth following endodontic treatment performed by general dentists or by specialists. *Oral Surgery, Oral Medicine, Oral Pathology, Oral Radiology and Endodontics* **98**, 115–18.

7. Altonen M, Mattila K (1976) Follow-up study of apicoectomized molars. *International Journal of Oral Surgery* **5**, 33–40.

8. Amagasa T, Nagase M, Sato T, Shioda S (1989) Apicoectomy with retrograde gutta-percha root filling. *Oral Surgery, Oral Medicine, Oral Pathology* **68**, 339–42.

9. Ambrosio E, Walkerley S (1996) Broadening the ethical focus: a community perspective on patient autonomy. *Humane Health Care International* **12**, E10.

10. Anderson JD (2000) Need for evidence-based practice in prosthodontics. *Journal of Prosthetic Dentistry* **83**, 58–65.

11. Andreasen JO, Rud J (1972) Correlation between histology and radiography in the assessment of healing after endodontic surgery. *International Journal of Oral Surgery* **1**, 161–73.

12. Andreasen JO, Rud J (1972) Modes of healing histologically after endodontic surgery in 70 cases. *International Journal of Oral Surgery* **1**, 148–60.

13. Andreasen JO (1985) External root resorption: its implication in dental traumatology, paedodontics, periodontics, orthodontics and endodontics. *International Endodontic Journal* **18**, 109–18.

14. Andreasen JO, Pitt Ford TR (1994) A radiographic study of the effect of various retrograde fillings on periapical healing after replantation. *Endodontics and Dental Traumatology* **10**, 276–81.

15. Andreasen JO, Borum MK, Jacobsen HL, Andreasen FM (1995) Replantation of 400 avulsed permanent incisors. 4. Factors related to periodontal ligament healing. *Endodontics and Dental Traumatology* **11**, 76–89.

16. Andreasen JO, Munksgaard L, Rud J (1993) Periodontal tissue regeneration including cementogenesis adjacent to dentin-bonded retrograde composite fillings in humans. *Journal of Endodontics* **19**, 151–3.

17. Arens DL, Levy GC, Rizoiu IM (1993) A comparison of dentin permeability after bur and laser apicoectomies *Compendium* **14**, 1290–8.

18. Ashkenaz PJ (1979) One-visit endodontics – a preliminary report. *Dental Survey* **55**, 62–7.

19. Augsburger RA, Peters DD (1990) Radiographic evaluation of extruded obturation materials. *Journal of Endodontics* **16**, 492–7.

20. August DS (1996) Long-term, postsurgical results on teeth with periapical radiolucencies. *Journal of Endodontics* **22**, 380–3.

21. Avivi-Arber L, Zarb GA (1996) Clinical effectiveness of implant-supported single-tooth replacement: the Toronto study. *International Journal of Oral and Maxillofacial Implants* **11**, 311–21.

22. Bader G, Lejeune S (1998) Prospective study of two retrograde endodontic apical preparations with and without the use of CO_2 laser. *Endodontics and Dental Traumatology* **14**, 75–8.

23. Bader JD, Shugars DA (1995) Variation, treatment outcomes, and practice guidelines in dental practice. *Journal of Dental Education* **59**, 61–95.

24. Baldassari-Cruz LA, Wilcox LR (1999) Effectiveness of gutta-percha removal with and without the microscope. *Journal of Endodontics* **25**, 627–8.

25. Barbakow FH, Cleaton-Jones P, Friedman D (1980) An evaluation of 566 cases of root canal therapy in general dental practice. 2. Postoperative observations. *Journal of Endodontics* **6**, 485–9.

26. Barbakow FH, Cleaton-Jones PE, Friedman D (1981) Endodontic treatment of teeth with periapical radiolucent areas in a general dental practice. *Oral Surgery, Oral Medicine, Oral Pathology* **51**, 552–9.

27. Barrieshi KM, Walton RE, Johnson WT, Drake DR (1997) Coronal leakage of mixed anaerobic bacteria after obturation and post space preparation. *Oral Surgery, Oral Medicine, Oral Pathology, Oral Radiology and Endodontics* **84**, 310–14.

28. Barton S (2000) Editorial. Which clinical studies provide the best evidence? *British Medical Journal* **321**, 255–6.

29. Baumgartner JC, Falkler WA (1991) Bacteria in the apical 5 mm of infected root canals. *Journal of Endodontics* **17**, 380–3.

30. Beckham BM, Anderson RW, Morris CF (1993) An evaluation of three materials as barriers to coronal microleakage in endodontically treated teeth. *Journal of Endodontics* **19**, 388–91.

31. Bender IB, Seltzer S (1964) To culture or not to culture? *Oral Surgery, Oral Medicine, Oral Pathology* **18**, 527–40.

32. Bender IB, Rossman LE (1993) Intentional replantation of endodontically treated teeth *Oral Surgery, Oral Medicine, Oral Pathology* **76**, 623–30.

33. Benenati FW, Roane JB, Biggs JT, Simon JH (1986) Recall evaluation of iatrogenic root perforations repaired with amalgam and gutta-percha. *Journal of Endodontics* **12**, 161–6.

34. Benenati FW, Khajotia SS (2002) A radiographic recall evaluation of 894 endodontic cases treated in a dental school setting. *Journal of Endodontics* **28**, 391–5.

35. Benson K, Hartz AJ (2000) A comparison of observational studies and randomized, controlled trials *New England Journal of Medicine* **342**, 1878–86.

36. Bergenholtz G, Lekholm U, Milthon R, Heden G, Ödesjö B, Engström B (1979) Retreatment of endodontic fillings. *Scandinavian Journal of Dental Research* **87**, 217–24.

37. Bergström J, Eliasson S, Ahlberg KF (1987) Periapical status in subjects with regular dental care habits. *Community Dentistry and Oral Epidemiology* **15**, 236–9.

38. Bhaskar SN (1966) Oral surgery – oral pathology conference No. 17, Walter Reed Army Medical Center. Periapical lesions – types, incidence, and clinical features. *Oral Surgery, Oral Medicine, Oral Pathology* **21**, 657–71.

39. Boltacz-Rzepkowska E, Pawlicka H (2003) Radiographic features and outcome of root canal treatment carried out in the Lodz region of Poland. *International Endodontic Journal* **36**, 27–32.

40. Borssen E, Sundqvist G (1981) Actinomyces of infected dental root canals. *Oral Surgery, Oral Medicine, Oral Pathology* **51**, 643–8.

41. Boucher Y, Matossian L, Rilliard F, Machtou P (2002) Radiographic evaluation of the prevalence and technical quality of root canal treatment in a French subpopulation. *International Endodontic Journal* **35**, 229–38.

42. Brynolf L (1967) Histological and roentgenological study of periapical region of human upper incisors. *Odontoogiskl Revy* **18**, Suppl 11.

43. Buckley M, Spångberg LS (1995) The prevalence and technical quality of endodontic treatment in an American subpopulation. *Oral Surgery, Oral Medicine, Oral Pathology, Oral Radiology and Endodontics* **79**, 92–100.

44. Byström A, Sundqvist G (1981) Bacteriologic evaluation of the efficacy of mechanical root canal instrumentation in endodontic therapy. *Scandinavian Journal of Dental Research* **89**, 321–8.

45. Byström A, Sundqvist G (1983) Bacteriologic evaluation of the effect of 0.5 percent sodium hypochlorite in endodontic therapy. *Oral Surgery, Oral Medicine, Oral Pathology* **55**, 307–12.

46. Byström A, Claesson R, Sundqvist G (1985) The antibacterial effect of camphorated paramonochlorophenol, camphorated phenol and calcium hydroxide in the treatment of infected root canals. *Endodontics and Dental Traumatology* **1**, 170–5.

47. Byström A, Sundqvist G (1985) The antibacterial action of sodium hypochlorite and EDTA in 60 cases of endodontic therapy. *International Endodontic Journal* **18**, 35–40.

48. Byström A, Happonen RP, Sjögren U, Sundqvist G (1987) Healing of periapical lesions of pulpless teeth after endodontic treatment with controlled asepsis. *Endodontic and Dental Traumatology* **3**, 58–63.

49. Caliskan MK, Sen BH (1996) Endodontic treatment of teeth with apical periodontitis using calcium hydroxide: a long-term study. *Endodontics and Dental Traumatology* **12**, 215–21.

50. Caliskan MK (2004) Prognosis of large cyst-like periapical lesions following nonsurgical root canal treatment: a clinical review. *International Endodontic Journal* **37**, 408–16.

51. Caplan DJ, Weintraub JA (1997) Factors related to loss of root canal filled teeth. *Journal of Public Health Dentistry* **57**, 31–9.

52. Caplan DJ, Kolker J, Rivera EM, Walton RE (2002) Relationship between number of proximal contacts and survival of root canal treated teeth. *International Endodontic Journal* **35**, 193–99.

53. Card SJ, Sigurdsson A, Ørstavik D, Trope M (2002) The effectiveness of increased apical enlargement in reducing intracanal bacteria. *Journal of Endodontics* **28**, 779–83.

54. Carr GB (1992) Microscopes in endodontics. *Journal of the California Dental Association* **20**, 55–61.

55. Carr GB, Bentkover SK (1998) Surgical endodontics. In Cohen S, Burns RC, editors. *Pathways of the Pulp*, pp. 608–56, 7th edn. St. Louis, MO: Mosby.

56. Chailertvanitkul P, Saunders WP, MacKenzie D (1996) The effect of smear layer on microbial coronal leakage of gutta-percha root fillings. *International Endodontic Journal* **29**, 242–8.

57. Chailertvanitkul P, Saunders WP, Mackenzie D (1996) An assessment of microbial coronal leakage in teeth root filled with gutta-percha and three different sealers. *International Endodontic Journal* **29**, 387–92.

58. Chailertvanitkul P, Saunders WP, MacKenzie D, Weetman DA (1996) An in vitro study of the coronal leakage of two root canal sealers using an obligate anaerobe microbial marker. *International Endodontic Journal* **29**, 249–55.

59. Cheung GS, Ho MW (2001) Microbial flora of root canal-treated teeth associated with asymptomatic periapical radiolucent lesions. *Oral Microbiology and Immunology* **16**, 332–7.

60. Cheung GS (2002) Survival of first-time nonsurgical root canal treatment performed in a dental teaching hospital. *Oral Surgery, Oral Medicine, Oral Pathology, Oral Radiology and Endodontics* **93**, 596–604.

61. Cheung LK, Lam J (1993) Apicectomy of posterior teeth – a clinical study. *Australian Dental Journal* **38**, 17–21.

62. Chong BS, Pitt Ford TR, Hudson MB (2003) A prospective clinical study of mineral trioxide aggregate and IRM when used as root-end filling materials in endodontic surgery. *International Endodontic Journal* **36**, 520–6.

63. Chu C, Lo ECM, Cheung GS (2005) Outcome of root canal treatment using Thermafil and cold lateral condensation filling techniques. *International Endodontic Journal* **38**, 179–85.

64. Chugal NM, Clive JM, Spångberg LS (2001) A prognostic model for assessment of the outcome of endodontic treatment: Effect of biologic and diagnostic variables. *Oral Surgery, Oral Medicine, Oral Pathology, Oral Radiology and Endodontics* **91**, 342–52.

65. Chugal NM, Clive JM, Spångberg LS (2003) Endodontic infection: some biologic and treatment factors associated with outcome. *Oral Surgery, Oral Medicine, Oral Pathology, Oral Radiology and Endodontics* **96**, 81–90.

66. Concato J, Shah N, Horwitz RI (2000) Randomized, controlled trials, observational studies, and the hierarchy of research designs. *New England Journal of Medicine* **342**, 1887–92.

67. Creugers NH, Kreulen CM, Snoek PA, de Kanter RJ (2000) A systematic review of single-tooth restorations supported by implants. *Journal of Dentistry* **28**, 209–17.

68. Crosher RF, Dinsdale RC, Holmes A (1989) One visit apicectomy technique using calcium hydroxide cement as the canal filling material combined with retrograde amalgam. *International Endodontic Journal* **22**, 283–9.

69. Cvek M (1972) Treatment of non-vital permanent incisors with calcium hydroxide. I. Follow-up of periapical repair and apical closure of immature roots. *Odontologisk Revy* **23**, 27–44.

70. Cvek M, Hollender L, Nord CE (1976) Treatment of non-vital permanent incisors with calcium hydroxide. VI. A clinical, microbiological and radiological evaluation of treatment in one sitting of teeth with mature or immature root. *Odontologisk Revy* **27**, 93–108.

71. Cvek M, Granath L, Lundberg M (1982) Failures and healing in endodontically treated non-vital anterior teeth with posttraumatically reduced pulpal lumen. *Acta Odontologica Scandinavica* **40**, 223–8.

72. Cvek M (1992) Prognosis of luxated non-vital maxillary incisors treated with calcium hydroxide and filled with gutta-percha. A retrospective clinical study. *Endodontics and Dental Traumatology* **8**, 45–55.

73. Dalal MB, Gohil KS (1983) Comparison of silver amalgam, glass ionomer cement and gutta percha as retrofilling materials, an in vivo and an in vitro study. *Journal of the Indian Dental Association* **55**, 153–8.

74. Dalton BC, Ørstavik D, Phillips C, Pettiette M, Trope M (1998) Bacterial reduction with nickel-titanium rotary instrumentation. *Journal of Endodontics* **24**, 763–7.

75. Danin J, Strömberg T, Forsgren H, Linder LE, Ramsköld LO (1996) Clinical management of nonhealing periradicular pathosis. Surgery versus endodontic retreatment. *Oral Surgery, Oral Medicine, Oral Pathology, Oral Radiology and Endodontics* **82**, 213–17.

76. Danin J, Linder LE, Lundqvist G, Ohlsson L, Ramsköld LO, Strömberg T (1999) Outcomes of periradicular surgery in cases with apical pathosis and untreated canals. *Oral Surgery, Oral Medicine, Oral Pathology, Oral Radiology and Endodontics* **87**, 227–32.

77. De Cleen MJ, Schuurs AH, Wesselink PR, Wu MK (1993) Periapical status and prevalence of endodontic treatment in an adult Dutch population. *International Endodontic Journal* **26**, 112–19.

78. De Moor RJ, Hommez GM, De Boever JG, Delme KI, Martens GE (2000) Periapical health related to the quality of root canal treatment in a Belgian population. *International Endodontic Journal* **33**, 113–20.

79. Deeb E (1968) Intentional replantation of endodontically treated teeth. *Transactions of Fourth International Conference on Endodontics*, Philadelphia, PA: University of Pennsylvania. pp. 147–57.

80. Department of Clinical Epidemiology and Biostatistics MUHSC (1981) How to read clinical journals: III. To learn the clinical course and prognosis of disease. *Canadian Medical Association Journal* **124**, 869–72.

81. Dorn SO, Gartner AH (1990) Retrograde filling materials: a retrospective success-failure study of amalgam, EBA, and IRM. *Journal of Endodontics* **16**, 391–3.

82. Dragoo MR (1996) Resin-ionomer and hybrid-ionomer cements: Part I. Comparison of three materials for the treatment of subgingival root lesions. *International Journal of Periodontics and Restorative Dentistry* **16**, 594–601.

83. Dragoo MR, Wheeler BG (1996) Clinical evaluation of subgingival debridement with ultrasonic instruments used by trained and untrained operators. *General Dentistry* **44**, 234–7.

84. Dryden JA (1986) Ten-year follow-up of intentionally replanted mandibular second molar. *Journal of Endodontics* **12**, 265–7.

85. Dugas NN, Lawrence HP, Teplitsky PE, Pharoah MJ, Friedman S (2003) Periapical health and treatment quality assessment of root-filled teeth in two Canadian populations. *International Endodontic Journal* **36**, 181–92.

86. Dumsha TC, Gutmann JL (1985) Clinical guidelines for intentional replantation. *Compendium of Continuing Education in Dentistry* **6**, 604.

87. Eckerbom M, Andersson JE, Magnusson T (1986) Interobserver variation in radiographic examination of endodontic variables. *Endodontics and Dental Traumatology* **2**, 243–6.

88. Eckerbom M, Andersson JE, Magnusson T (1987) Frequency and technical standard of endodontic treatment in a Swedish population. *Endodontics and Dental Traumatology* **3**, 245–8.

89. Eckerbom M, Andersson JE, Magnusson T (1989) A longitudinal study of changes in frequency and technical standard of endodontic treatment in a Swedish population. *Endodontics and Dental Traumatology* **5**, 27–31.

90. Eckerbom M, Magnusson T, Martinsson T (1991) Prevalence of apical periodontitis, crowned teeth and teeth with posts in a Swedish population. *Endodontics and Dental Traumatology* **7**, 214–20.

91. Ehnevid H, Jansson L, Lindskog S, Weintraub A, Blomlof L (1995) Endodontic pathogens: propagation of infection through patent dentinal tubules in traumatized monkey teeth. *Endodontics and Dental Traumatology* **11**, 229–34.

92. Emmertsen E, Andreasen JO (1966) Replantation of extracted molars. A radiographic and histological study. *Acta Odontologica Scandinavica* **24**, 327–46.

93. Engström B, Hård af Segerstad L, Ramström G, Frostell G (1964) Correlation of positive cultures with the prognosis for root canal treatment. *Odontologisk Revy* **15**, 257–70.

94. Engström B, Lundberg M (1965) The correlation between positive culture and the prognosis of root canal therapy after pulpectomy. *Odontologisk Revy* **16**, 193–203.

95. Ericson S, Finne K, Persson G (1974) Results of apicoectomy of maxillary canines, premolars and molars with special reference to oroantral communication as a prognostic factor. *International Journal of Oral Surgery* **3**, 386–93.

96. Eriksen HM, Bjertness E, Ørstavik D (1988) Prevalence and quality of endodontic treatment in an urban adult population in Norway. *Endodontics and Dental Traumatology* **4**, 122–6.

97. Eriksen HM, Ørstavik D, Kerekes K (1988) Healing of apical periodontitis after endodontic treatment using three different root canal sealers. *Endodontics and Dental Traumatology* **4**, 114–17.

98. Eriksen HM (1991) Endodontology – epidemiologic considerations. *Endodontics and Dental Traumatology* **7**, 189–95.

99. Eriksen HM, Bjertness E (1991) Prevalence of apical periodontitis and results of endodontic treatment in middle-aged adults in Norway. *Endodontics and Dental Traumatology* **7**, 1–4.

100. Eriksen HM, Berset GP, Hansen BF, Bjertness E (1995) Changes in endodontic status 1973–1993 among 35-year-olds in Oslo, Norway. *International Endodontic Journal* **28**, 129–32.

101. Eriksen HM (1998) Epidemiology of apical periodontitis. In Ørstavik D, Pitt Ford TR, editors. *Essential endodontology: prevention and treatment of apical periodontitis*, pp. 179–91. Oxford: Blackwell.

102. Fager FK, Messer HH (1986) Systemic distribution of camphorated monochlorophenol from cotton pellets

sealed in pulp chambers. *Journal of Endodontics* **12**, 225–30.

103. Farzaneh M, Abitbol S, Friedman S (2004) Treatment outcome in endodontics: the Toronto study. Phases I and II: Orthograde retreatment. *Journal of Endodontics* **30**, 627–33.

104. Farzaneh M, Abitbol S, Lawrence HP, Friedman S (2004) Treatment outcome in endodontics – the Toronto study. Phase II: initial treatment *Journal of Endodontics* **30**, 302–9.

105. Feldman G, Solomon C, Notaro P, Moskowitz E (1971) Intentional replantation of a molar tooth. *New York Journal of Dentistry* **41**, 352–3.

106. Ferreira JJ, Rhodes JS, Pitt Ford TR (2001) The efficacy of gutta-percha removal using ProFiles. *International Endodontic Journal* **34**, 267–74.

107. Field JW, Gutmann JL, Solomon ES, Rakusin H (2004) A clinical radiographic retrospective assessment of the success rate of single-visit root canal treatment. *International Endodontic Journal* **37**, 70–82.

108. Figdor D (2004) Microbial aetiology of endodontic treatment failure and pathogenic properties of selected species. *Australian Endodontic Journal* **30**, 11–14.

109. Figures KH, Douglas CW (1991) Actinomycosis associated with a root-treated tooth: report of a case. *International Endodontic Journal* **24**, 326–9.

110. Finne K, Nord PG, Persson G, Lennartsson B (1977) Retrograde root filling with amalgam and Cavit. *Oral Surgery, Oral Medicine, Oral Pathology* **43**, 621–6.

111. Flath RK, Hicks ML (1987) Retrograde instrumentation and obturation with new devices. *Journal of Endodontics* **13**, 546–9.

112. Fletcher RH, Fletcher SW, Wagner EH (1996) *Clinical epidemiology: the essentials*, 3rd edn. Baltimore, MD: Williams & Wilkins.

113. Forssell H, Tammisalo T, Forssell K (1988) A follow-up study of apicectomized teeth. *Proceedings of the Finnish Dental Society* **84**, 85–93.

114. Fouad A, Burleson J (2003) The effect of diabetes mellitus on endodontic treatment outcome: data from an electronic patient record. *Journal of the American Dental Association* **134**, 43–51.

115. Fouad AF, Zerella J, Barry J, Spångberg LS (2005) Molecular detection of Enterococcus species in root canals of therapy-resistant endodontic infections. *Oral Surgery, Oral Medicine, Oral Pathology, Oral Radiology and Endodontics* **99**, 112–18.

116. Fournier V (2005) The balance between beneficence and respect for patient autonomy in clinical medical ethics in France. *Cambridge Quarterly of Healthcare Ethics* **14**, 281–6.

117. Frank AL, Glick DH, Patterson SS, Weine FS (1992) Long-term evaluation of surgically placed amalgam fillings. *Journal of Endodontics* **18**, 391–8.

118. Friedman S (1991) Retrograde approaches in endodontic therapy. *Endodontics and Dental Traumatology* **7**, 97–107.

119. Friedman S, Lustmann J, Shaharabany V (1991) Treatment results of apical surgery in premolar and molar teeth. *Journal of Endodontics* **17**, 30–3.

120. Friedman S, Rotstein I, Mahamid A (1991) In vivo efficacy of various retrofills and of CO_2 laser in apical surgery. *Endodontics and Dental Traumatology* **7**, 19–25.

121. Friedman S, Moshonov J, Trope M (1992) Efficacy of removing glass ionomer cement, zinc oxide eugenol, and epoxy resin sealers from retreated root canals. *Oral Surgery, Oral Medicine, Oral Pathology* **73**, 609–12.

122. Friedman S, Moshonov J, Trope M (1993) Residue of gutta-percha and a glass ionomer cement sealer following root canal retreatment. *International Endodontic Journal* **26**, 169–72.

123. Friedman S, Löst C, Zarrabian M, Trope M (1995) Evaluation of success and failure after endodontic therapy using a glass ionomer cement sealer. *Journal of Endodontics* **21**, 384–90.

124. Friedman S, Torneck CD, Komorowski R, Ouzounian Z, Syrtash P, Kaufman A (1997) In vivo model for assessing the functional efficacy of endodontic filling materials and techniques. *Journal of Endodontics* **23**, 557–61.

125. Friedman S (1998) Treatment outcome and prognosis of endodontic therapy. In Ørstavik D, Pitt Ford TR, editors. *Essential Endodontology: Prevention and treatment of apical periodontitis*, pp. 367–401. Oxford: Blackwell.

126. Friedman S, Komorowski R, Maillet W, Klimaite R, Nguyen HQ, Torneck CD (2000) In vivo resistance of coronally induced bacterial ingress by an experimental glass ionomer cement root canal sealer. *Journal of Endodontics* **26**, 1–5.

127. Friedman S (2002) Prognosis of initial endodontic therapy. *Endodontic Topics* **2**, 59–88.

128. Friedman S (2002) Considerations and concepts of case selection in the management of post-treatment endodontic disease (treatment failure). *Endodontic Topics* **1**, 54–78.

129. Friedman S, Abitbol S, Lawrence HP (2003) Treatment outcome in endodontics: the Toronto study. Phase 1: initial treatment. *Journal of Endodontics* **29**, 787–93.

130. Friedman S (2006) The prognosis and expected outcome of apical surgery. *Endodontic Topics* **11**, 219–62.

131. Friedman S, Mor C (2004) The success of endodontic therapy – healing and functionality. *California Dental Association Journal* **32**, 493–503.

132. Fristad I, Molven O, Halse A (2004) Nonsurgically retreated root-filled teeth – radiographic findings after 20–27 years. *International Endodontic Journal* **37**, 12–18.

133. Fukushima H, Yamamoto K, Hirohata K, Sagawa H, Leung KP, Walker CB (1990) Localization and identification of root canal bacteria in clinically asymptomatic periapical pathosis. *Journal of Endodontics* **16**, 534–8.

134. Gagliani MM, Gorni FG, Strohmenger L (2005) Periapcial resurgery versus periapical surgery: a 5-year longitudinal comparison. *International Endodontic Journal* **38**, 320–7.

135. Gatti JJ, Dobeck JM, Smith C, White RR, Socransky SS, Skobe Z (2000) Bacteria of asymptomatic periradicular endodontic lesions identified by DNA–DNA hybridization. *Endodontics and Dental Traumatology* **16**, 197–204.

136. Georgopoulou MK, Spanaki-Voreadi AP, Pantazis N, Kontakiotis EG (2005) Frequency and distribution of

root filled teeth and apical periodontitis in a Greek population. *International Endodontic Journal* **38**, 105–11.

137. Gilheany PA, Figdor D, Tyas MJ (1994) Apical dentin permeability and microleakage associated with root end resection and retrograde filling. *Journal of Endodontics* **20**, 22–6.

138. Gish SP, Drake DR, Walton RE, Wilcox L (1994) Coronal leakage: bacterial penetration through obturated canals following post preparation. *Journal of the American Dental Association* **125**, 1369–72.

139. Goldberg F, Torres MD, Bottero C (1990) Thermoplasticized gutta-percha in endodontic surgical procedures. *Endodontics and Dental Traumatology* **6**, 109–13.

140. Goldberg F, Torres MD, Bottero C, Alvarez AF (1991) Use of thermoplasticized gutta-percha in retrograde obturation. *Revista de la Asociacion Odontologica Argentina* **79**, 142–6.

141. Goldman M, Pearson AH, Darzenta N (1972) Endodontic success – who's reading the radiograph? *Oral Surgery, Oral Medicine, Oral Pathology* **33**, 432–7.

142. Goldman M, Pearson AH, Darzenta N (1974) Reliability of radiographic interpretations. *Oral Surgery, Oral Medicine, Oral Pathology* **38**, 287–93.

143. Gorman MC, Steiman HR, Gartner AH (1995) Scanning electron microscopic evaluation of root-end preparations. *Journal of Endodontics* **21**, 113–17.

144. Gorni F, Gagliani MM (2004) The outcome of endodontic retreatment: a 2-yr follow-up. *Journal of Endodontics* **30**, 1–4.

145. Grahnén H, Hansson L (1961) The prognosis of pulp and root canal therapy. *Odontologisk Revy* **12**, 146–65.

146. Green SB, Byar DP (1984) Using observational data from registries to compare treatments: the fallacy of omnimetrics. *Statistics in Medicine* **3**, 361–73.

147. Grimes EW (1994) A use of freeze-dried bone in endodontics. *Journal of Endodontics* **20**, 355–6.

148. Grossman L, Chacker F (1968) Clinical evaluation and histologic study of intentionally replanted teeth. *Transactions of Fourth International Conference on Endodontics*, pp. 127–44 Philadelphia, PA: University of Pennsylvania.

149. Grossman LI, Shepard LI, Pearson LA (1964) Roentgenologic and clinical evaluation of endodontically treated teeth. *Oral Surgery, Oral Medicine, Oral Pathology* **17**, 368–74.

150. Grossman LI (1982) Intentional replantation of teeth: a clinical evaluation. *Journal of the American Dental Association* **104**, 633–9.

151. Grung B, Molven O, Halse A (1990) Periapical surgery in a Norwegian county hospital: follow-up findings of 477 teeth. *Journal of Endodontics* **16**, 411–17.

152. Gutierrez JH, Jofre A, Villena F (1990) Scanning electron microscope study on the action of endodontic irrigants on bacteria invading the dentinal tubules. *Oral Surgery, Oral Medicine, Oral Pathology* **69**, 491–501.

153. Guy SC, Goerig AC (1984) Intentional replantation: technique and rationale. *Quintessence International* **15**, 595–603.

154. Haapasalo M, Ranta K, Ranta H (1987) Mixed anaerobic periapical infection with sinus tract. *Endodontics and Dental Traumatology* **3**, 83–5.

155. Haapasalo M, Udnaes T, Endal U (2003) Persistent, recurrent, and acquired infection of the root canal system post-treatment. *Endodontic Topics* **6**, 29–56.

156. Haas R, Polak C, Furhauser R, Mailath-Pokorny G, Dortbudak O, Watzek G (2002) A long-term follow-up of 76 Branemark single-tooth implants. *Clinical Oral Implants Research* **13**, 38–43.

157. Halse A, Molven O (1986) A strategy for the diagnosis of periapical pathosis. *Journal of Endodontics* **12**, 534–8.

158. Halse A, Molven O (1987) Overextended gutta-percha and Kloroperka N-O root canal fillings. Radiographic findings after 10–17 years. *Acta Odontologica Scandinavica* **45**, 171–7.

159. Halse A, Molven O, Grung B (1991) Follow-up after periapical surgery: the value of the one-year control. *Endodontics and Dental Traumatology* **7**, 246–50.

160. Hammarström L, Pierce A, Blömlof L, Feiglin B, Lindskog S (1986) Tooth avulsion and replantation – a review. *Endodontics and Dental Traumatology* **2**, 1–8.

161. Hancock HH, Sigurdsson A, Trope M, Moiseiwitsch J (2001) Bacteria isolated after unsuccessful endodontic treatment in a North American population. *Oral Surgery, Oral Medicine, Oral Pathology, Oral Radiology and Endodontics* **91**, 579–86.

162. Hansen BF, Johansen JR (1976) Oral roentgenologic findings in a Norwegian urban population. *Oral Surgery, Oral Medicine, Oral Pathology* **41**, 261–6.

163. Happonen RP, Soderling E, Viander M, Linko-Kettunen L, Pelliniemi LJ (1985) Immunocytochemical demonstration of Actinomyces species and Arachnia propionica in periapical infections. *Journal of Oral Pathology* **14**, 405–13.

164. Happonen RP (1986) Periapical actinomycosis: a follow-up study of 16 surgically treated cases. *Endodontics and Dental Traumatology* **2**, 205–9.

165. Harrison J, Jurosky K (1992) Wound healing in the tissues of the periodontium following periradicular surgery. 3. The excisional wound. *Journal of Endodontics* **18**, 76–81.

166. Harty FJ, Parkins BJ, Wengraf AM (1970) The success rate of apicectomy. A retrospective study of 1,016 cases. *British Dental Journal* **129**, 407–13.

167. Harty FJ, Parkins BJ, Wengraf AM (1970) Success rate in root canal therapy. A retrospective study of conventional cases. *British Dental Journal* **128**, 65–70.

168. Hassanloo A, Watson P, Finer Y, Friedman S (2007) Retreatment efficacy of the Epiphany soft resin obturation system. *International Endodontic Journal* **40**, 633–43.

169. Heling B, Tamshe A (1970) Evaluation of the success of endodontically treated teeth. *Oral Surgery, Oral Medicine, Oral Pathology* **30**, 533–6.

170. Heling B, Shapira J (1978) Roentgenologic and clinical evaluation of endodontically treated teeth, with or without negative culture. *Quintessence International* **9**, 79–84.

171. Heling I, Bialla-Shenkman S, Turetzky A, Horwitz J, Sela J (2001) The outcome of teeth with periapical periodontitis treated with nonsurgical endodontic treatment: a computerized morphometric study. *Quintessence International* **32**, 397–400.

172. Hepworth MJ, Friedman S (1997) Treatment outcome of surgical and non-surgical management of endodontic failures. *Journal of the Canadian Dental Association* **63**, 364–71.

173. Hession RW (1981) Long-term evaluation of endodontic treatment: anatomy, instrumentation, obturation – the endodontic practice triad. *International Endodontic Journal* **14**, 179–84.

174. Hirsch JM, Ahlström U, Henrikson PA, Heyden G, Peterson LE (1979) Periapical surgery. *International Journal of Oral Surgery* **8**, 173–85.

175. Hoen MM, Pink FE (2002) Contemporary endodontic retreatments: an analysis based on clinical treatment findings. *Journal of Endodontics* **28**, 834–6.

176. Hommez G, Coppens CRM, DeMoor RJG (2002) Periapical health related to the quality of coronal restorations and root fillings. *International Endodontic Journal* **35**, 680–9.

177. Hoskinson SE, Ng YL, Hoskinson AE, Moles DR, Gulabivala K (2002) A retrospective comparison of outcome of root canal treatment using two different protocols. *Oral Surgery, Oral Medicine, Oral Pathology, Oral Radiology and Endodontics* **93**, 705–15.

178. Hsu YY, Kim S (1997) The resected root surface. The issue of canal isthmuses. *Dental Clinics of North America* **41**, 529–40.

179. Hugoson A, Koch G (1979) Oral health in 1000 individuals aged 3–70 years in the community of Jonkoping, Sweden. A review. *Swedish Dental Journal* **3**, 69–87.

180. Hugoson A, Koch G, Bergendal T *et al.* (1986) Oral health of individuals aged 3–80 years in Jonkoping, Sweden, in 1973 and 1983. II. A review of clinical and radiographic findings. *Swedish Dental Journal* **10**, 175–94.

181. Hulsmann M, Bluhm V (2004) Efficacy, cleaning ability and safety of different rotary NiTi instruments in root canal retreatment. *International Endodontic Journal* **37**, 468–76.

182. Huumonen S, Lenander-Lumikari M, Sigurdsson A, Ørstavik D (2003) Healing of apical periodontitis after endodontic treatment: a comparison between a silicone-based and a zinc oxide–eugenol-based sealer. *International Endodontic Journal* **36**, 296–301.

183. Imfeld TN (1991) Prevalence and quality of endodontic treatment in an elderly urban population of Switzerland. *Journal of Endodontics* **17**, 604–7.

184. Ingle JI, Beveridge EE, Glick DH, Weichman JA (1994) Modern endodontic therapy. In Ingle BLK editor. *Endodontics*, pp. 27–53, 4th edn. Baltimore, MD: Williams & Wilkins.

185. Ioannides C, Borstlap WA (1983) Apicoectomy on molars: a clinical and radiographical study. *International Journal of Oral Surgery* **12**, 73–9.

186. Jansson L, Sandstedt P, Laftmån AC, Skoglund A (1997) Relationship between apical and marginal healing in periradicular surgery. *Oral Surgery, Oral Medicine, Oral Pathology, Oral Radiology and Endodontics* **83**, 596–601.

187. Jaoui L, Machtou P, Ouhayoun JP (1995) Long-term evaluation of endodontic and periodontal treatment. *International Endodontic Journal* **28**, 249–54.

188. Jeansonne BG, Boggs WS, Lemon RR (1993) Ferric sulfate hemostasis: effect on osseous wound healing. II. With curettage and irrigation. *Journal of Endodontics* **19**, 174–6.

189. Jensen SS, Nattestad A, Egdø P, Sewerin I, Munksgaard EC, Schou S (2002) A prospective, randomized, comparative clinical study of resin composite and glass ionomer cement for retrograde root filling. *Clinical Oral Investigations* **6**, 236–43.

190. Jesslen P, Zetterqvist L, Heimdahl A (1995) Long-term results of amalgam versus glass ionomer cement as apical sealant after apicectomy. *Oral Surgery, Oral Medicine, Oral Pathology, Oral Radiology and Endodontics* **79**, 101–3.

191. Jimenez-Pinzon A, Segura-Egea JJ, Poyato-Ferrera M, Velasco-Ortega E, Rios-Santos JV (2004) Prevalence of apical periodontitis and frequency of root-filled teeth in an adult Spanish population. *International Endodontic Journal* **37**, 167–73.

192. Jokinen MA, Kotilainen R, Poikkeus P, Poikkeus R, Sarkki L (1978) Clinical and radiographic study of pulpectomy and root canal therapy. *Scandinavian Journal of Dental Research* **86**, 366–73.

193. Kabak Y, Abbott PV (2005) Prevalence of apical periodontitis and the quality of endodontic treatment in an adult Belarusian population. *International Endodontic Journal* **38**, 238–45.

194. Kahnberg KE (1988) Surgical extrusion of root-fractured teeth – a follow-up study of two surgical methods. *Endodontics and Dental Traumatology* **4**, 85–9.

195. Kalfas S, Figdor D, Sundqvist G (2001) A new bacterial species associated with failed endodontic treatment: identification and description of Actinomyces radicidentis. *Oral Surgery, Oral Medicine, Oral Pathology, Oral Radiology and Endodontics* **92**, 208–14.

196. Kaufman AY (1982) Intentional replantation of a maxillary molar. A 4-year follow-up. *Oral Surgery, Oral Medicine, Oral Pathology* **54**, 686–8.

197. Kaufman B, Spångberg L, Barry J, Fouad AF (2005) *Enterococcus* spp. in endodontically treated teeth with and without periradicular lesions. *Journal of Endodontics* **31**, 851–6.

198. Keller U (1990) A new method of tooth replantation and autotransplantation: aluminum oxide ceramic for extraoral retrograde root filling. *Oral Surgery, Oral Medicine, Oral Pathology* **70**, 341–4.

199. Kerekes K, Tronstad L (1977) Morphometric observations on the root canals of human molars. *Journal of Endodontics* **3**, 114–18.

200. Kerekes K, Tronstad L (1977) Morphometric observations on root canals of human anterior teeth. *Journal of Endodontics* **3**, 24–9.

201. Kerekes K, Tronstad L (1977) Morphometric observations on root canals of human premolars. *Journal of Endodontics* **3**, 74–9.

202. Kerekes K, Tronstad L (1979) Long-term results of endodontic treatment performed with a standardized technique. *Journal of Endodontics* **5**, 83–90.

203. Khayat A, Lee SJ, Torabinejad M (1993) Human saliva penetration of coronally unsealed obturated root canals. *Journal of Endodontics* **19**, 458–61.

204. Kim S (1997) Principles of endodontic microsurgery. *Dental Clinics of North America* **41**, 481–97.

205. Kim S, Rethnam S (1997) Hemostasis in endodontic microsurgery. *Dental Clinics of North America* **41**, 499–511.

206. Kim S (2002) Endodontic microsurgery. In Cohen S, Burns RC, editors. *Pathways of the pulp*, pp. 683–725, 8th edn. St. Louis, MO: Mosby.

207. Kim S, Baek S (2004) The microscope and endodontics. *Dental Clinics of North America* **48**, 11–18.

208. Kingsbury BC, Wiesenbaugh JM (1971) Intentional replantation of mandibular premolars and molars. *Journal of the American Dental Association* **83**, 1053–7.

209. Kirkevang LL, Hørsted-Bindslev P, Ørstavik D, Wenzel A (2001) A comparison of the quality of root canal treatment in two Danish subpopulations examined 1974–75 and 1997–98. *International Endodontic Journal* **34**, 607–12.

210. Kirkevang LL, Vaeth M, Hørsted-Bindslev P, Wenzel A (2006) Longitudinal study of periapical and endodontic status in a Danish population. *International Endodontic Journal* **39**, 100–7.

211. Kirkevang LL, Ørstavik D, Hørsted-Bindslev P, Wenzel A (2000) Periapical status and quality of root fillings and coronal restorations in a Danish population. *International Endodontic Journal* **33**, 509–15.

212. Kirkevang LL, Hørsted-Bindslev P, Ørstavik D, Wenzel A (2001) Frequency and distribution of endodontically treated teeth and apical periodontitis in an urban Danish population. *International Endodontic Journal* **34**, 198–205.

213. Klevant FJ, Eggink CO (1983) The effect of canal preparation on periapical disease. *International Endodontic Journal* **16**, 68–75.

214. Koenig KH, Nguyen NT, Barkhordar RA (1988) Intentional replantation: a report of 192 cases. *General Dentistry* **36**, 327–31.

215. Komori T, Yokoyama K, Takato T, Matsumoto K (1997) Clinical application of the erbium:YAG laser for apicoectomy. *Journal of Endodontics* **23**, 748–50.

216. Kosti E, Lambrianidis T, Economides N, Neofitou C (2006) Ex vivo study of the efficacy of H-files and rotary Ni-Ti instruments to remove gutta-percha and four types of sealer. *International Endodontic Journal* **39**, 48–54.

217. Kvinnsland I, Oswald RJ, Halse A, Gronningsaeter AG (1989) A clinical and roentgenological study of 55 cases of root perforation. *International Endodontic Journal* **22**, 75–84.

218. Kvist T, Rydin E, Reit C (1989) The relative frequency of periapical lesions in teeth with root canal-retained posts. *Journal of Endodontics* **15**, 578–80.

219. Kvist T, Reit C (1999) Results of endodontic retreatment: a randomized clinical study comparing surgical and nonsurgical procedures. *Journal of Endodontics* **25**, 814–17.

220. Kvist T, Molander A, Dahlén G, Reit C (2004) Microbiological evaluation of one- and two-visit endodontic treatment of teeth with apical periodontitis: a randomized, clinical trial. *Journal of Endodontics* **30**, 572–6.

221. Ladley RW, Campbell AD, Hicks ML, Li SH (1991) Effectiveness of halothane used with ultrasonic or hand instrumentation to remove gutta-percha from the root canal. *Journal of Endodontics* **17**, 221–4.

222. Lambjerg-Hansen H (1974) Vital and mortal pulpectomy on permanent human teeth. An experimental comparative histologic investigation. *Scandinavian Journal of Dental Research* **82**, 243–332.

223. Lambrianidis T (1985) Observer variations in radiographic evaluation of endodontic therapy. *Endodontics and Dental Traumatology* **1**, 235–41.

224. Lasaridis N, Zouloumis L, Antoniadis K (1991) Bony lid approach for apicoectomy of mandibular molars. *Australian Dental Journal* **36**, 366–8.

225. Laupacis A, Wells G, Richardson WS, Tugwell P (1994) Users' guides to the medical literature. V. How to use an article about prognosis. Evidence-Based Medicine Working Group. *Journal of the American Medical Association* **272**, 234–7.

226. Lazarski MP, Walker WA, Flores CM, Schindler WG, Hargreaves KM (2001) Epidemiological evaluation of the outcomes of nonsurgical root canal treatment in a large cohort of insured dental patients. *Journal of Endodontics* **27**, 791–6.

227. Lehtinen R, Aitasalo K (1972) Comparison of the clinical and roentgenological state at the re-examination of root resections. *Proceedings of the Finnish Dental Society* **68**, 209–11.

228. Leonardo MR, Rossi MA, Silva LA, Ito IY, Bonifacio KC (2002) EM evaluation of bacterial biofilm and microorganisms on the apical external root surface of human teeth. *Journal of Endodontics* **28**, 815–18.

229. Lin CP, Chou HG, Kuo JC, Lan WH (1998) The quality of ultrasonic root-end preparation: a quantitative study. *Journal of Endodontics* **24**, 666–70.

230. Lin LM, Pascon EA, Skribner J, Gangler P, Langeland K (1991) Clinical, radiographic, and histologic study of endodontic treatment failures. *Oral Surgery, Oral Medicine, Oral Pathology* **71**, 603–11.

231. Lin LM, Skribner JE, Gaengler P (1992) Factors associated with endodontic treatment failures. *Journal of Endodontics* **18**, 625–7.

232. Lindeberg RW, Girardi AF, Troxell JB (1986) Intentional replantation: management in contraindicated situations. *Compendium of Continuing Education in Dentistry* **7**, 248.

233. Loftus JJ, Keating AP, McCartan BE (2005) Periapical status and quality of endodontic treatment in an adult Irish population. *International Endodontic Journal* **38**, 81–6.

234. Love RM (1996) Regional variation in root dentinal tubule infection by *Streptococcus gordonii*. *Journal of Endodontics* **22**, 290–3.

235. Lu DP (1986) Intentional replantation of periodontally involved and endodontically mistreated tooth. *Oral Surgery, Oral Medicine, Oral Pathology* **61**, 508–13.

236. Lubin H (1982) Intentional reimplantation: report of case *Journal of the American Dental Association* **104**, 858–9.

237. Lupi-Pegurier L, Bertrand, MF, Muller-Bolla M, Rocca, JP, Bolla M (2002) Periapical status, prevalence and quality of endodontic treatment in an adult

French population. *International Endodontic Journal* **35**, 690–7.

238. Lustmann J, Friedman S, Shaharabany V (1991) Relation of pre- and intraoperative factors to prognosis of posterior apical surgery. *Journal of Endodontics* **17**, 239–41.

239. Maddalone M, Gagliani M (2003) Periapical endodontic surgery: a 3-year follow-up study. *International Endodontic Journal* **36**, 193–8.

240. Madison S (1986) Intentional replantation. *Oral Surgery, Oral Medicine, Oral Pathology* **62**, 707–9.

241. Madison S, Swanson K, Chiles SA (1987) An evaluation of coronal microleakage in endodontically treated teeth. Part II. Sealer types. *Journal of Endodontics* **13**, 109–12.

242. Madison S, Wilcox LR (1988) An evaluation of coronal microleakage in endodontically treated teeth. Part III. In vivo study. *Journal of Endodontics* **14**, 455–8.

243. Magura ME, Kafrawy AH, Brown CE, Newton CW (1991) Human saliva coronal microleakage in obturated root canals: an in vitro study. *Journal of Endodontics* **17**, 324–31.

244. Main C, Mirzayan N, Shabahang S, Torabinejad M (2004) Repair of root perforations using mineral trioxide aggregate: a long-term study. *Journal of Endodontics* **30**, 80–3.

245. Malmström M, Perkki K, Lindquist K (1982) Apicectomy. A retrospective study. *Proceedings of the Finnish Dental Society* **78**, 26–31.

246. Marending M, Peters OA, Zehnder M (2005) Factors affecting the outcome of orthograde root canal therapy in a general dentistry hospital practice. *Oral Surgery, Oral Medicine, Oral Pathology, Oral Radiology and Endodontics* **99**, 119–24.

247. Marques MD, Moreira B, Eriksen HM (1998) Prevalence of apical periodontitis and results of endodontic treatment in an adult, Portuguese population. *International Endodontic Journal* **31**, 161–5.

248. Marquis V, Dao T, Farzaneh M, Abitbol S, Friedman S (2006) Treatment outcome in endodontics: The Toronto study. Phase III: Initial treatment. *Journal of Endodontics* **32**, 299–306.

249. Matsumoto T, Nagai T, Ida K *et al.* (1987) Factors affecting successful prognosis of root canal treatment. *Journal of Endodontics* **13**, 239–42.

250. Mattila K, Altonen M (1968) A clinical and roentgenological study of apicoectomized teeth. *Odontologisk Tidskrift* **76**, 389–408.

251. McGurkin-Smith R, Trope M, Caplan D, Sigurdsson A (2005) Reduction of intracanal bacteria using GT rotary instrumentation, 5.25% NaOCl, EDTA, and $Ca(OH)_2$. *Journal of Endodontics* **31**, 359–63.

252. Mead C, Javidan-Nejad S, Mego ME, Nash B, Torabinejad M (2005) Levels of evidence for the outcome of endodontic surgery. *Journal of Endodontics* **31**, 19–24.

253. Meeuwissen R, Eschen S (1983) Twenty years of endodontic treatment. *Journal of Endodontics* **9**, 390–3.

254. Mehlhaff DS, Marshall JG, Baumgartner JC (1997) Comparison of ultrasonic and high-speed-bur root-end preparations using bilaterally matched teeth. *Journal of Endodontics* **23**, 448–52.

255. Melcer J (1986) Latest treatment in dentistry by means of the CO_2 laser beam. *Lasers in Surgery and Medicine* **6**, 396–8.

256. Messer HH, Chen RS (1984) The duration of effectiveness of root canal medicaments. *Journal of Endodontics* **10**, 240–5.

257. Messkoub M (1991) Intentional replantation: a successful alternative for hopeless teeth. *Oral Surgery, Oral Medicine, Oral Pathology* **71**, 743–7.

258. Mikkonen M, Kullaa-Mikkonen A, Kotilainen R (1983) Clinical and radiologic re-examination of apicoectomized teeth. *Oral Surgery, Oral Medicine, Oral Pathology* **55**, 302–6.

259. Mines P, Loushine RJ, West LA, Liewehr FR, Zadinsky JR (1999) Use of the microscope in endodontics: a report based on a questionnaire. *Journal of Endodontics* **25**, 755–8.

260. Miserendino LJ (1988) The laser apicoectomy: endodontic application of the CO_2 laser for periapical surgery. *Oral Surgery, Oral Medicine, Oral Pathology* **66**, 615–19.

261. Molander A, Reit C, Dahlén G (1990) Microbiological evaluation of clindamycin as a root canal dressing in teeth with apical periodontitis. *International Endodontic Journal* **23**, 113–18.

262. Molander A, Reit C, Dahlén G, Kvist T (1998) Microbiological status of root-filled teeth with apical periodontitis. *International Endodontic Journal* **31**, 1–7.

263. Molander A, Reit C, Dahlén G (1999) The antimicrobial effect of calcium hydroxide in root canals pretreated with 5% iodine potassium iodide. *Endodontics and Dental Traumatology* **15**, 205–9.

264. Molven O, Halse A, Grung B (1987) Observer strategy and the radiographic classification of healing after endodontic surgery. *International Journal of Oral and Maxillofacial Surgery* **16**, 432–9.

265. Molven O, Halse A (1988) Success rates for gutta-percha and Kloroperka N-Ø root fillings made by undergraduate students: radiographic findings after 10–17 years. *International Endodontic Journal* **21**, 243–50.

266. Molven O, Halse A, Grung B (1991) Surgical management of endodontic failures: indications and treatment results. *International Dental Journal* **41**, 33–42.

267. Molven O, Halse A, Grung B (1996) Incomplete healing (scar tissue) after periapical surgery – radiographic findings 8 to 12 years after treatment. *Journal of Endodontics* **22**, 264–8.

268. Molven O, Halse A, Fristad I (2002) Long-term reliability and observer comparisons in the radiographic diagnosis of periapical disease. *International Endodontic Journal* **35**, 142–7.

269. Molven O, Halse A, Fristad I, MacDonald-Jankowksi D (2002) Periapical changes following root-canal treatment observed 20–27 years postoperatively. *International Endodontic Journal* **35**, 784–90.

270. Morse DR, Esposito JV, Pike C, Furst ML (1983) A radiographic evaluation of the periapical status of teeth treated by the gutta-percha – eucapercha endodontic method: a one-year follow-up study of 458 root canals. Part III. *Oral Surgery, Oral Medicine, Oral Pathology* **56**, 190–7.

271. Morse DR, Esposito JV, Pike C, Furst ML (1983) A radiographic evaluation of the periapical status of teeth treated by the gutta-percha – eucapercha endodontic method: a one-year follow-up study of 458 root canals. Part I. *Oral Surgery, Oral Medicine, Oral Pathology* **55**, 607–10.

272. Morse DR, Esposito JV, Pike C, Furst ML (1983) A radiographic evaluation of the periapical status of teeth treated by the gutta-percha – eucapercha endodontic method: a one-year follow-up study of 458 root canals. Part II. *Oral Surgery, Oral Medicine, Oral Pathology* **56**, 89–96.

273. Moshonov J, Slutzky-Goldberg I, Gottlieb A, Peretz B (2005) The effect of the distance between post and residual gutta-percha on the clinical outcome of endodontic treatment. *Journal of Endodontics* **31**, 177–9.

274. Murashima Y, Yoshikawa G, Wadachi R, Sawada N, Suda H (2002) Calcium sulfate as a bone substitute for various osseous defects in conjunction with apicectomy. *International Endodontic Journal* **35**, 768–74.

275. Murphy WK, Kaugars GE, Collett WK, Dodds RN (1991) Healing of periapical radiolucencics after nonsurgical endodontic therapy. *Oral Surgery, Oral Medicine, Oral Pathology* **71**, 620–4.

276. Nair P (2003) Non-microbial etiology: foreign body reaction maintaining post-treatment apical periodontitis. *Endodontic Topics* **6**, 114–34.

277. Nair P (2003) Non-microbial etiology: periapical cysts sustain post-treatment apical periododontitis. *Endodontic Topics* **6**, 96–113.

278. Nair P (2004) Pathogenesis of apical periodontitis and the causes of endodontic failures. *Critical Reviews in Oral Biology and Medicine* **15**, 348–81.

279. Nair PN, Shroeder JH (1984) Periapical actinomycosis. *Journal of Endodontics* **10**, 567–70.

280. Nair PN (1987) Light and electron microscopic studies of root canal flora and periapical lesions. *Journal of Endodontics* **13**, 29–39.

281. Nair PN, Sjögren U, Krey G, Kahnberg KE, Sundqvist G (1990) Intraradicular bacteria and fungi in root-filled, asymptomatic human teeth with therapy-resistant periapical lesions: a long-term light and electron microscopic follow-up study. *Journal of Endodontics* **16**, 580–8.

282. Nair PN, Sjögren U, Krey G, Sundqvist G (1990) Therapy-resistant foreign body giant cell granuloma at the periapex of a root-filled human tooth. *Journal of Endodontics* **16**, 589–95.

283. Nair PN, Sjögren U, Schumacher E, Sundqvist G (1993) Radicular cyst affecting a root-filled human tooth: a long-term post-treatment follow-up. *International Endodontic Journal* **26**, 225–33.

284. Nair PN, Sjögren U, Figdor D, Sundqvist G (1999) Persistent periapical radiolucencies of root-filled human teeth, failed endodontic treatments, and periapical scars. *Oral Surgery, Oral Medicine, Oral Pathology, Oral Radiology and Endodontics* **87**, 617–27.

285. Nelson IA (1982) Endodontics in general practice – a retrospective survey. *International Endodontic Journal* **15**, 168–72.

286. Noiri Y, Ehara A, Kawahara T, Takemura N, Ebisu S (2002) Participation of bacterial biofilms in refractory and chronic periapical periodontitis. *Journal of Endodontics* **28**, 679–83.

287. Nord PG (1970) Retrograde rootfilling with Cavit: a clinical and roentgenological study. *Svensk Tandlakare Tidskrift* **63**, 261–73.

288. Nordenram A (1970) Biobond for retrograde root filling in apicoectomy. *Scandinavian Journal of Dental Research* **78**, 251–5.

289. Nordenram A, Svardström G (1970) Results of apicectomy. *Svensk Tandlakare Tidskrift* **63**, 593–604.

290. Nosonowitz DM, Stanley HR (1984) Intentional replantation to prevent predictable endodontic failures. *Oral Surgery, Oral Medicine, Oral Pathology* **57**, 423–32.

291. Nygaard-Østby B (1971) *Introduction to endodontics*, pp. 73–5. Oslo: Universitetsforlaget.

292. O'Grady JF, Reade PC (1988) Periapical actinomycosis involving *Actinomyces israelii*. *Journal of Endodontics* **14**, 147–9.

293. Ödesjo B, Hellden L, Salonen L, Langeland K (1990) Prevalence of previous endodontic treatment, technical standard and occurrence of periapical lesions in a randomly selected adult, general population. *Endodontics and Dental Traumatology* **6**, 265–72.

294. Oguntebi BR (1994) Dentine tubule infection and endodontic therapy implications. *International Endodontic Journal* **27**, 218–22.

295. Oikarinen K (1993) Dental tissues involved in exarticulation, root resorption and factors influencing prognosis in relation to replanted teeth. A review. *Proceedings of the Finnish Dental Society* **89**, 29–44.

296. Oliet S, Sorin SM (1969) Evaluation of clinical results based upon culturing root canals. *Journal of the British Endodontic Society* **3**, 3–6.

297. Oliet S (1983) Single-visit endodontics: a clinical study. *Journal of Endodontics* **9**, 147–52.

298. Ørstavik D, Kerekes K, Eriksen HM (1986) The periapical index: a scoring system for radiographic assessment of apical periodontitis. *Endodontics and Dental Traumatology* **2**, 20–34.

299. Ørstavik D, Kerekes K, Eriksen HM (1987) Clinical performance of three endodontic sealers. *Endodontics and Dental Traumatology* **3**, 178–86.

300. Ørstavik D, Kerekes K, Molven O (1991) Effects of extensive apical reaming and calcium hydroxide dressing on bacterial infection during treatment of apical periodontitis: a pilot study. *International Endodontic Journal* **24**, 1–7.

301. Ørstavik D, Horsted-Bindslev P (1993) A comparison of endodontic treatment results at two dental schools. *International Endodontic Journal* **26**, 348–54.

302. Ørstavik D (1996) Time-course and risk analyses of the development and healing of chronic apical periodontitis in man. *International Endodontic Journal* **29**, 150–5.

303. Ørstavik D, Pitt Ford TR (1998) Apical periodontitis: microbial infection and host responses. In Ørstavik D, Pitt Ford TR, editors. *Essential endodontology: prevention and treatment of apical periodontitis*, pp. 1–8. Oxford: Blackwell.

304. Ørstavik D, Qvist V, Stoltze K (2004) A mutlivariate analysis of the outcome of endodontic treatment. *European Journal of Oral Sciences* **112**, 224–30.

305. Oxman AD (1994) Checklists for review articles. *British Medical Journal* **309**, 648–51.

306. Paghdiwala AF (1993) Root resection of endodontically treated teeth by erbium: YAG laser radiation. *Journal of Endodontics* **19**, 91–4.

307. Paik S, Sechrist C, Torabinejad M (2004) Levels of evidence for the outcome of endodontic retreatment. *Journal of Endodontics* **30**, 745–50.

308. Pantschev A, Carlsson AP, Andersson L (1994) Retrograde root filling with EBA cement or amalgam. A comparative clinical study. *Oral Surgery, Oral Medicine, Oral Pathology* **78**, 101–4.

309. Paquette L, Legner M, Fillery ED, Friedman S (2006) Antibacterial efficacy of chlorhexidine gluconate intracanal medication in vivo. *Journal of Endodontics* **33**, 788–95.

310. Peak JD, Hayes SJ, Bryant ST, Dummer PM (2001) The outcome of root canal treatment. A retrospective study within the armed forces (Royal Air Force). *British Dental Journal* **190**, 140–4.

311. Peciuliene V, Balciuniene I, Eriksen HM, Haapasalo M (2000) Isolation of Enterococcus faecalis in previously root-filled canals in a Lithuanian population. *Journal of Endodontics* **26**, 593–5.

312. Peciuliene V, Reynaud AH, Balciuniene I, Haapasalo M (2001) Isolation of yeasts and enteric bacteria in root-filled teeth with chronic apical periodontitis. *International Endodontic Journal* **34**, 429–34.

313. Pecora G, Andreana S (1993) Use of dental operating microscope in endodontic surgery. *Oral Surgery, Oral Medicine, Oral Pathology* **75**, 751–8.

314. Pecora G, Kim S, Celletti R, Davarpanah M (1995) The guided tissue regeneration principle in endodontic surgery: one-year postoperative results of large periapical lesions. *International Endodontic Journal* **28**, 41–6.

315. Pecora G, Andreana S, Margarone JE, Covani U, Sottosanti JS (1997) Bone regeneration with a calcium sulfate barrier. *Oral Surgery, Oral Medicine, Oral Pathology, Oral Radiology and Endodontics* **84**, 424–9.

316. Pecora G, Baek SH, Rethnam S, Kim S (1997) Barrier membrane techniques in endodontic microsurgery. *Dental Clinics of North America* **41**, 585–602.

317. Pecora G, De Leonardis D, Ibrahim N, Bovi M, Cornelini R (2001) The use of calcium sulphate in the surgical treatment of a 'through and through' periradicular lesion. *International Endodontic Journal* **34**, 189–97.

318. Pekruhn RB (1986) The incidence of failure following single-visit endodontic therapy. *Journal of Endodontics* **12**, 68–72.

319. Pellegrino ED (1994) Patient autonomy and the physician's ethics. *Annals of the Royal College of Physicians and Surgeons of Canada* **27**, 171–3.

320. Penick EC (1961) Periapical repair by dense fibrous connective tissue following conservative endodontic therapy. *Oral Surgery, Oral Medicine, Oral Pathology* **14**, 239–42.

321. Persson G (1973) Prognosis of reoperation after apicectomy. A clinical-radiological investigation. *Svensk Tandlakare Tidskrift* **66**, 49–68.

322. Persson G, Lennartson B, Lundstrom I (1974) Results of retrograde root-filling with special reference to amalgam and Cavit as root-filling materials. *Svensk Tandlakare Tidskrift* **67**, 123–43.

323. Persson G (1982) Periapical surgery of molars. *International Journal of Oral Surgery* **11**, 96–100.

324. Peters LB, Wesselink PR, Buijs JF, van Winkelhoff AJ (2001) Viable bacteria in root dentinal tubules of teeth with apical periodontitis. *Journal of Endodontics* **27**, 76–81.

325. Peters LB, van Winkelhoff AJ, Buijs JF, Wesselink PR (2002) Effects of instrumentation, irrigation and dressing with calcium hydroxide on infection in pulpless teeth with periapical bone lesions. *International Endodontic Journal* **35**, 13–21.

326. Peters LB, Wesselink PR (2002) Periapical healing of endodontically treated teeth in one and two visits obturated in the presence or absence of detectable microorganisms. *International Endodontic Journal* **35**, 660–7.

327. Peters O, Barbakow F, Peters, CI (2004) An analysis of endodontic treatment with three nickel-titanium rotary root canal preparation techniques. *International Endodontic Journal* **37**, 849–59.

328. Peterson J, Gutmann JL (2001) The outcome of endodontic resurgery: a systematic review. *International Endodontic Journal* **34**, 169–75.

329. Petersson K, Petersson A, Olsson B, Hakansson J, Wennberg A (1986) Technical quality of root fillings in an adult Swedish population. *Endodontics and Dental Traumatology* **2**, 99–102.

330. Petersson K, Lewin B, Hakansson J, Olsson B, Wennberg A (1989) Endodontic status and suggested treatment in a population requiring substantial dental care. *Endodontics and Dental Traumatology* **5**, 153–8.

331. Petersson K, Hakansson R, Hakansson J, Olsson B, Wennberg A (1991) Follow-up study of endodontic status in an adult Swedish population. *Endodontics and Dental Traumatology* **7**, 221–5.

332. Petersson K (1993) Endodontic status of mandibular premolars and molars in an adult Swedish population. A longitudinal study 1974–1985. *Endodontics and Dental Traumatology* **9**, 13–18.

333. Pettiette MT, Delano EO, Trope M (2001) Evaluation of success rate of endodontic treatment performed by students with stainless-steel K-files and nickel-titanium hand files. *Journal of Endodontics* **27**, 124–7.

334. Piatowska D, Pawlicka H, Laskiewicz J, Boltacz-Rzepkowska E, Brauman-Furmanek S (1997) Evaluation of endodontic re-treatment. *Czasopismo Stomatologiczne* **L**, 451–8.

335. Pinheiro ET, Gomes BP, Ferraz CC, Sousa EL, Teixeira FB, Souza-Filho FJ (2003) Microorganisms from canals of root-filled teeth with periapical lesions. *International Endodontic Journal* **36**, 1–11.

336. Pinheiro ET, Gomes BP, Ferraz CC, Teixeira FB, Zaia AA, Souza Filho FJ (2003) Evaluation of root canal microorganisms isolated from teeth with endodontic failure and their antimicrobial susceptibility. *Oral Microbiology and Immunology* **18**, 100–3.

337. Pitt Ford TR (1982) The effects on the periapical tissues of bacterial contamination of the filled root canal. *International Endodontic Journal* **15**, 16–22.

338. Pitt Ford TR, Andreasen JO, Dorn SO, Kariyawasam SP (1994) Effect of IRM root end fillings on healing after replantation. *Journal of Endodontics* **20**, 381–5.

339. Pitt Ford TR, Andreasen JO, Dorn SO, Kariyawasam SP (1995) Effect of super-EBA as a root end filling on healing after replantation. *Journal of Endodontics* **21**, 13–15.

340. Priest G (1999) Single-tooth implants and their role in preserving remaining teeth: a 10-year survival study. *International Journal of Oral and Maxillofacial Implants* **14**, 181–8.

341. Rahbaran S, Gilthorpe MS, Harrison SD, Gulabivala K (2001) Comparison of clinical outcome of periapical surgery in endodontic and oral surgery units of a teaching dental hospital: a retrospective study. *Oral Surgery, Oral Medicine, Oral Pathology, Oral Radiology and Endodontics* **91**, 700–9.

342. Rankow HJ, Krasner PR (1996) Endodontic applications of guided tissue regeneration in endodontic surgery. *Oral Health* **86**, 33–43.

343. Rapp EL, Brown CE, Newton CW (1991) An analysis of success and failure of apicoectomies. *Journal of Endodontics* **17**, 508–12.

344. Ray HA, Trope M (1995) Periapical status of endodontically treated teeth in relation to the technical quality of the root filling and the coronal restoration. *International Endodontic Journal* **28**, 12–18.

345. Reit C, Hollender L (1983) Radiographic evaluation of endodontic therapy and the influence of observer variation. *Scandinavian Journal of Dental Research* **91**, 205–12.

346. Reit C, Hirsch J (1986) Surgical endodontic retreatment. *International Endodontic Journal* **19**, 107–12.

347. Reit C (1987) Decision strategies in endodontics: on the design of a recall program. *Endodontics and Dental Traumatology* **3**, 233–9.

348. Reit C (1987) The influence of observer calibration on radiographic periapical diagnosis. *International Endodontic Journal* **20**, 75–81.

349. Rolph HJ, Lennon A, Riggio MP *et al.* (2001) Molecular identification of microorganisms from endodontic infections. *Journal of Clinical Microbiology* **39**, 3282–9.

350. Rosenberg ES, Rossman LE, Sandler AB (1980) Intentional replantation: a case report. *Journal of Endodontics* **6**, 610–13.

351. Ross WJ (1985) Intentional replantation: an alternative. *Compendium of Continuing Education in Dentistry* **6**, 734.

352. Rubinstein R (1997) The anatomy of the surgical operating microscope and operating positions. *Dental Clinics of North America* **41**, 391–413.

353. Rubinstein RA, Kim S (1999) Short-term observation of the results of endodontic surgery with the use of a surgical operation microscope and Super-EBA as root-end filling material. *Journal of Endodontics* **25**, 43–8.

354. Rubinstein RA, Kim S (2002) Long-term follow-up of cases considered healed one year after apical microsurgery. *Journal of Endodontics* **28**, 378–83.

355. Rud J, Andreasen JO, Jensen JE (1972) A follow-up study of 1,000 cases treated by endodontic surgery. *International Journal of Oral Surgery* **1**, 215–28.

356. Rud J, Andreasen JO, Jensen JE (1972) Radiographic criteria for the assessment of healing after endodontic surgery. *International Journal of Oral Surgery* **1**, 195–214.

357. Rud J, Munksgaard EC, Andreasen JO, Rud V (1991) Retrograde root filling with composite and a dentin-bonding agent. 2. *Endodontics and Dental Traumatology* **7**, 126–31.

358. Rud J, Munksgaard EC, Andreasen JO, Rud V, Asmussen E (1991) Retrograde root filling with composite and a dentin-bonding agent. 1. *Endodontics and Dental Traumatology* **7**, 118–24.

359. Rud J, Rud V, Munksgaard EC (1996) Retrograde root filling with dentin-bonded modified resin composite. *Journal of Endodontics* **22**, 477–80.

360. Rud J, Rud V, Munksgaard EC (1996) Long-term evaluation of retrograde root filling with dentin-bonded resin composite. *Journal of Endodontics* **22**, 90–3.

361. Rud J, Rud V, Munksgaard EC (1997) Effect of root canal contents on healing of teeth with dentin-bonded resin composite retrograde seal. *Journal of Endodontics* **23**, 535–41.

362. Rud J, Rud V (1998) Surgical endodontics of upper molars: relation to the maxillary sinus and operation in acute state of infection. *Journal of Endodontics* **24**, 260–1.

363. Rud J, Rud V, Munksgaard EC (2001) Periapical healing of mandibular molars after root-end sealing with dentine-bonded composite. *International Endodontic Journal* **34**, 285–92.

364. Saad AY, Abdellatief ESM (1991) Healing assessment of osseous defects of periapical lesions associated with failed endodontically treated teeth with use of freeze-dried bone allograft. *Oral Surgery, Oral Medicine, Oral Pathology* **71**, 612–17.

365. Sackett DL, Haynes RB, Guyatt GH, Tugwell P (1991) *Clinical epidemiology: a basic science of clinical medicine*, 2nd edn. Boston, MA: Little, Brown.

366. Sae-Lim V, Rajamanickam I, Lim BK, Lee HL (2000) Effectiveness of ProFile .04 taper rotary instruments in endodontic retreatment. *Journal of Endodontics* **26**, 100–4.

367. Safavi KE, Dowden WE, Langeland K (1987) Influence of delayed coronal permanent restoration on endodontic prognosis. *Endodontics and Dental Traumatology* **3**, 187–91.

368. Sakellariou PL (1996) Periapical actinomycosis: report of a case and review of the literature. *Endodontics and Dental Traumatology* **12**, 151–4.

369. Salehrabi R, Rotstein I (2004) Endodontic treatment outcomes in a large patient population in the USA: an epidemiological study. *Journal of Endodontics* **30**, 846–50.

370. Sathorn C, Parashos P, Messer HH (2005) Effectiveness of single- versus multiple-visit endodontic treatment of teeth with apical periodontitis: a systematic review and meta-analysis. *International Endodontic Journal* **38**, 347–55.

371. Saunders WP, Saunders EM (1997) The root filling and restoration continuum – prevention of long-term endodontic failures. *Alpha Omegan* **90**, 40–6.

372. Saunders WP, Saunders EM, Sadiq J, Cruickshank E (1997) Technical standard of root canal treatment in an adult Scottish sub-population. *British Dental Journal* **182**, 382–6.

373. Schattner A, Tal M (2002) Truth telling and patient autonomy: the patient's point of view. *American Journal of Medicine* **113**, 66–9.

374. Schirrmeister JF, Meyer KM, Hermanns P, Altenburger MJ, Wrbas KT (2006) Effectiveness of hand and rotary instrumentation for removing a new synthetic polymer-based root canal obturation material (Epiphany) during retreatment. *International Endodontic Journal* **39**, 150–6.

375. Schwartz-Arad D, Yaorm N, Lustig JP, Kaffe I (2003) A retrospective radiographic study of root-end surgery with amalgam and intermediate restorative material. *Oral Surgery, Oral Medicine, Oral Pathology, Oral Radiology and Endodontics* **96**, 472–7.

376. Segura-Egea JJ, Jimenez-Pinzon A, Poyato-Ferrera M, Velasco-Ortega E, Rios-Santos JV (2004) Periapical status and quality of root fillings and coronal restorations in an adult Spanish population. *International Endodontic Journal* **37**, 525–30.

377. Selden HS (1974) Pulpoperiapical disease: diagnosis and healing. A clinical endodontic study. *Oral Surgery, Oral Medicine, Oral Pathology* **37**, 271–83.

378. Selden HS (1999) Periradicular scars: a sometime diagnostic conundrum. *Journal of Endodontics* **25**, 829–30.

379. Seltzer S, Bender IB, Turkenkopf S (1963) Factors affecting successful repair after root canal therapy. *Journal of the American Dental Association* **52**, 651–62.

380. Sen BH, Piskin B, Demirci T (1995) Observation of bacteria and fungi in infected root canals and dentinal tubules by SEM. *Endodontics and Dental Traumatology* **11**, 6–9.

381. Serota KS, Krakow AA (1983) Retrograde instrumentation and obturation of the root canal space. *Journal of Endodontics* **9**, 448–51.

382. Shah N (1988) Nonsurgical management of periapical lesions: a prospective study. *Oral Surgery, Oral Medicine, Oral Pathology* **66**, 365–71.

383. Shuping GB, Ørstavik D, Sigurdsson A, Trope M (2000) Reduction of intracanal bacteria using nickel-titanium rotary instrumentation and various medications. *Journal of Endodontics* **26**, 751–5.

384. Sidaravicius B, Aleksejuniene J, Eriksen HM (1999) Endodontic treatment and prevalence of apical periodontitis in an adult population of Vilnius, Lithuania. *Endodontics and Dental Traumatology* **15**, 210–15.

385. Sikri K, Dua SS, Kapur R (1986) Use of tricalcium phosphate ceramic in apicoectomized teeth and in their peri-apical areas – clinical and radiological evaluation. *Journal of the Indian Dental Association* **58**, 441–7.

386. Siqueira J (2003) Periapical actinomycosis and infection with *Propionibacterium Propionicum*. *Endodontic Topics* **6**, 78–95.

387. Siqueira JF, Lopes HP (2001) Bacteria on the apical root surfaces of untreated teeth with periradicular lesions: a scanning electron microscopy study. *International Endodontic Journal* **34**, 216–20.

388. Siqueira JF (2001) Aetiology of root canal treatment failure: why well-treated teeth can fail. *International Endodontic Journal* **34**, 1–10.

389. Sirén EK, Haapasalo MP, Ranta K, Salmi P, Kerosuo EN (1997) Microbiological findings and clinical treatment procedures in endodontic cases selected for microbiological investigation. *International Endodontic Journal* **30**, 91–5.

390. Sjögren U, Happonen RP, Kahnberg KE, Sundqvist G (1988) Survival of *Arachnia propionica* in periapical tissue. *International Endodontic Journal* **21**, 277–82.

391. Sjögren U, Hagglund B, Sundqvist G, Wing K (1990) Factors affecting the long-term results of endodontic treatment. *Journal of Endodontics* **16**, 498–504.

392. Sjögren U, Figdor D, Spångberg L, Sundqvist G (1991) The antimicrobial effect of calcium hydroxide as a short-term intracanal dressing. *International Endodontic Journal* **24**, 119–25.

393. Sjögren U, Figdor D, Persson S, Sundqvist G (1997) Influence of infection at the time of root filling on the outcome of endodontic treatment of teeth with apical periodontitis. *International Endodontic Journal* **30**, 297–306.

394. Skoglund A, Persson G (1985) A follow-up study of apicoectomized teeth with total loss of the buccal bone plate. *Oral Surgery, Oral Medicine, Oral Pathology* **59**, 78–81.

395. Smith CS, Setchell DJ, Harty FJ (1993) Factors influencing the success of conventional root canal therapy – a five-year retrospective study. *International Endodontic Journal* **26**, 321–33.

396. Smith DE, Zarb GA (1989) Criteria for success of osseointegrated endosseous implants. *Journal of Prosthetic Dentistry* **62**, 567–72.

397. Soikkonen K (1995) Endodontically treated teeth and periapical findings in the elderly. *International Endodontic Journal* **28**, 200–3.

398. Solomon CS, Abelson J (1981) Intentional replantation: report of case. *Journal of Endodontics* **7**, 317–19.

399. Soltanoff W (1978) A comparative study of the single-visit and the multiple-visit edodontic procedure. *Journal of Endodontics* **4**, 278–81.

400. Spili P, Parashos P, Messer HH (2005) The impact of instrument fracture on outcome of endodontic treatment. *Journal of Endodontics* **31**, 845–50.

401. Stabholz A, Khayat A, Ravanshad SH, McCarthy DW, Neev J, Torabinejad M (1992) Effects of Nd:YAG laser on apical seal of teeth after apicoectomy and retrofill. *Journal of Endodontics* **18**, 371–5.

402. Stabholz A, Khayat A, Weeks DA, Neev J, Torabinejad M (1992) Scanning electron microscopic study of the apical dentine surfaces lased with ND:YAG laser following apicectomy and retrofill. *International Endodontic Journal* **25**, 288–91.

403. Storms JL (1969) Factors that influence the success of endodontic treatment. *Journal of the Canadian Dental Association* **35**, 83–97.

404. Storms JL (1978) Root canal therapy via the apical foramen – radical or conservative? *Oral Health* **68**, 60–5.

405. Strindberg LZ (1956) The dependence of the results of pulp therapy on certain factors. An analytic study based

on radiographic and clinical follow-up examination. *Acta Odontologica Scandinavica* **14**, suppl 21.

406. Stroner WF, Laskin DM (1981) Replantation of a mandibular molar: report of case. *Journal of the American Dental Association* **103**, 730–1.

407. Sumi Y, Hattori H, Hayashi K, Ueda M (1996) Ultrasonic root-end preparation: clinical and radiographic evaluation of results. *Journal of Oral and Maxillofacial Surgery* **54**, 590–3.

408. Sumi Y, Hattori H, Hayashi K, Ueda M (1997) Titanium-inlay – a new root-end filling material. *Journal of Endodontics* **23**, 121–3.

409. Sunde PT, Olsen I, Lind PO, Tronstad L (2000) Extraradicular infection: a methodological study. *Endodontics and Dental Traumatology* **16**, 84–90.

410. Sunde PT, Tronstad L, Eribe ER, Lind PO, Olsen I (2000) Assessment of periradicular microbiota by DNA-DNA hybridization. *Endodontics and Dental Traumatology* **16**, 191–6.

411. Sunde PT, Olsen I, Debelian GJ, Tronstad L (2002) Microbiota of periapical lesions refractory to endodontic therapy. *Journal of Endodontics* **28**, 304–10.

412. Sunde PT, Olsen I, Gobel UB *et al.* (2003) Fluorescence in situ hybridization (FISH) for direct visualization of bacteria in periapical lesions of asymptomatic root-filled teeth. *Microbiology* **149**, 1095–102.

413. Sundqvist G, Reuterving CO (1980) Isolation of *Actinomyces israelii* from periapical lesion. *Journal of Endodontics* **6**, 602–6.

414. Sundqvist G, Figdor D, Persson S, Sjögren U (1998) Microbiologic analysis of teeth with failed endodontic treatment and the outcome of conservative re-treatment. *Oral Surgery, Oral Medicine, Oral Pathology, Oral Radiology and Endodontics* **85**, 86–93.

415. Sundqvist G, Figdor D (2003) Life as an endodontic pathogen. Ecological differences between the untreated and the root-filled root canals. *Endodontic Topics* **6**, 3–28.

416. Sutherland SE (2001) Evidence-based dentistry: Part VI. Critical appraisal of the dental literature: papers about diagnosis, etiology and prognosis. *Journal of the Canadian Dental Association* **67**, 582–5.

417. Swanson K, Madison S (1987) An evaluation of coronal microleakage in endodontically treated teeth. Part I. Time periods. *Journal of Endodontics* **13**, 56–9.

418. Swartz DB, Skidmore AE, Griffin JA (1983) Twenty years of endodontic success and failure. *Journal of Endodontics* **9**, 198–202.

419. Taintor JF, Ingle JI, Fahid A (1983) Retreatment versus further treatment. *Clin Preventive Dentistry* **5**, 8–14.

420. Takeda A (1989) An experimental study upon the application of Nd:YAG laser to surgical endodontics. *Japanese Journal of Conservative Dentistry* **32**, 541–53.

421. Tamse A, Heling B (1973) Success of endodontically treated anterior teeth in young and adult patients. *Annals of Dentistry* **32**, 20–6.

422. Tay WM, Gale KM, Harty FJ (1978) The influence of periapical radiolucencies on the success or failure of apicectomies. *Journal of the British Endodontic Society* **11**, 3–6.

423. Teplitsky PE, Rayner D, Chin I, Markowsky R (1992) Gutta percha removal utilizing GPX instrumentation. *Journal of the Canadian Dental Association* **58**, 53–8.

424. Testori T, Capelli M, Milani S, Weinstein RL (1999) Success and failure in periradicular surgery: a longitudinal retrospective analysis. *Oral Surgery, Oral Medicine, Oral Pathology, Oral Radiology and Endodontics* **87**, 493–8.

425. Theodosopoulou JN, Niederman R (2005) A systematic review of in vitro retrograde obturation materials. *Journal of Endodontics* **31**, 341–9.

426. Thilander B, Odman J, Jemt T (1999) Single implants in the upper incisor region and their relationship to the adjacent teeth. An 8-year follow-up study. *Clinical Oral Implants Research* **10**, 346–55.

427. Tidmarsh BG, Arrowsmith MG (1989) Dentinal tubules at the root ends of apicected teeth: a scanning electron microscopic study. *International Endodontic Journal* **22**, 184–9.

428. Tobon SI, Arismendi JA, Marin ML, Mesa AL, Valencia JA (2002) Comparison between a conventional technique and two bone regeneration techniques in periradicular surgery. *International Endodontic Journal* **35**, 635–41.

429. Torabinejad M, Ung B, Kettering JD (1990) In vitro bacterial penetration of coronally unsealed endodontically treated teeth. *Journal of Endodontics* **16**, 566–9.

430. Torabinejad M, Hong CU, Lee SJ, Monsef M, Pitt Ford TR (1995) Investigation of mineral trioxide aggregate for root-end filling in dogs. *Journal of Endodontics* **21**, 603–8.

431. Torabinejad M, Chivian N (1999) Clinical applications of mineral trioxide aggregate. *Journal of Endodontics* **25**, 197–205.

432. Torabinejad M, Bahjri K (2005) Essential elements of evidence-based endodontics: steps involved in conducting clinical research. *Journal of Endodontics* **31**, 563–9.

433. Torabinejad M, Kutsenko D, Machnick TK, Ismail A, Newton CW (2005) Levels of evidence for the outcome of nonsurgical endodontic treatment. *Journal of Endodontics* **31**, 637–46.

434. Tronstad L, Yang ZP, Trope M, Barnett F, Hammond B (1985) Controlled release of medicaments in endodontic therapy. *Endodontics and Dental Traumatology* **1**, 130–4.

435. Tronstad L, Barnett F, Riso K, Slots J (1987) Extraradicular endodontic infections. *Endodontics and Dental Traumatology* **3**, 86–90.

436. Tronstad L (1988) Root resorption – etiology, terminology and clinical manifestations. *Endodontics and Dental Traumatology* **4**, 241–52.

437. Tronstad L, Barnett F, Cervone F (1990) Periapical bacterial plaque in teeth refractory to endodontic treatment. *Endodontics and Dental Traumatology* **6**, 73–7.

438. Tronstad L, Kreshtool D, Barnett F (1990) Microbiological monitoring and results of treatment of extraradicular endodontic infection. *Endodontics and Dental Traumatology* **6**, 129–36.

439. Tronstad L, Asbjornsen K, Doving L, Pedersen I, Eriksen HM (2000) Influence of coronal restorations on the

periapical health of endodontically treated teeth. *Endodontics and Dental Traumatology* **16**, 218–21.

440. Tronstad L, Sunde PT (2003) The evolving new understanding of endodontic infections. *Endodontic Topics* **6**, 57–77.

441. Trope M, Friedman S (1992) Periodontal healing of replanted dog teeth stored in Viaspan, milk and Hank's balanced salt solution. *Endodontics and Dental Traumatology* **8**, 183–8.

442. Trope M, Löst C, Schmitz HJ, Friedman S (1996) Healing of apical periodontitis in dogs after apicoectomy and retrofilling with various filling materials. *Oral Surgery, Oral Medicine, Oral Pathology, Oral Radiology and Endodontics* **81**, 221–8.

443. Trope M, Delano EO, Ørstavik D (1999) Endodontic treatment of teeth with apical periodontitis: single vs. multivisit treatment. *Journal of Endodontics* **25**, 345–50.

444. Van Nieuwenhuysen JP, Aouar M, D'Hoore W (1994) Retreatment or radiographic monitoring in endodontics. *International Endodontic Journal* **27**, 75–81.

445. Velvart P, Peters CI (2005) Soft tissue management in endodontic surgery. *Journal of Endodontics* **31**, 4–16.

446. Vertucci FJ, Beatty RG (1986) Apical leakage associated with retrofilling techniques: a dye study. *Journal of Endodontics* **12**, 331–6.

447. Vire DE (1991) Failure of endodontically treated teeth: classification and evaluation. *Journal of Endodontics* **17**, 338–42.

448. von Arx T, Kurt B (1999) Root-end cavity preparation after apicoectomy using a new type of sonic and diamond-surfaced retrotip: a 1-year follow-up study. *Journal of Oral and Maxillofacial Surgery* **57**, 656–61.

449. von Arx T, Walker WA, (2000) Microsurgical instruments for root-end cavity preparation following apicoectomy: a literature review. *Endodontics and Dental Traumatology* **16**, 47–62.

450. von Arx T, Gerber C, Hardt N (2001) Periradicular surgery of molars: a prospective clinical study with a one-year follow-up. *International Endodontic Journal* **34**, 520–5.

451. von Arx T, Montagne D, Zwinggi C, Lussi A (2003) Diagnostic accuracy of endoscopy in periradicular surgery – a comparison with scanning electron microscopy. *International Endodontic Journal* **36**, 691–9.

452. von Arx T (2005) Frequency and type of canal isthmuses in first molars detected by endoscopic inspection during periradicular surgery. *International Endodontic Journal* **38**, 160–8.

453. Waikakul A, Punwutikorn J (1991) Clinical study of retrograde filling with gold leaf: comparison with amalgam. *Oral Surgery, Oral Medicine, Oral Pathology* **71**, 228–31.

454. Waltimo T, Boiesen, J, Eriksen, HM, Ørstavik, D (2001) Clinical performance of 3 endodontic sealers. *Oral Surgery, Oral Medicine, Oral Pathology, Oral Radiology and Endodontics* **92**, 89–92.

455. Waltimo T, Trope M, Haapasalo M, Ørstavik D (2005) Clinical efficacy of treatment procedures in endodontic infection control and one year follow-up of periapical healing. *Journal of Endodontics* **31**, 863–6.

456. Wang N, Knight K, Dao T, Friedman S (2004) Treatment outcome in endodontics – The Toronto study. Phases I and II: apical surgery. *Journal of Endodontics* **30**, 751–61.

457. Wang Q, Cheung GS, Ng RP (2004) Survival of surgical endodontic treatment performed in a dental teaching hospital: a cohort study. *International Endodontic Journal* **37**, 764–75.

458. Weiger R, Hitzler S, Hermle G, Löst C (1997) Periapical status, quality of root canal fillings and estimated endodontic treatment needs in an urban German population. *Endodontics and Dental Traumatology* **13**, 69–74.

459. Weiger R, Rosendahl R, Löst C (2000) Influence of calcium hydroxide intracanal dressings on the prognosis of teeth with endodontically induced periapical lesions. *International Endodontic Journal* **33**, 219–26.

460. Wertz DC (1998) Patient and professional views on autonomy: a survey in the United States and Canada. *Health Law Review* **7**, 9–10.

461. Wilcox LR, Krell KV, Madison S, Rittman B (1987) Endodontic retreatment: evaluation of gutta-percha and sealer removal and canal reinstrumentation. *Journal of Endodontics* **13**, 453–7.

462. Wilcox LR (1989) Endodontic retreatment: ultrasonics and chloroform as the final step in reinstrumentation. *Journal of Endodontics* **15**, 125–8.

463. Wilcox LR, Swift ML (1991) Endodontic retreatment in small and large curved canals. *Journal of Endodontics* **17**, 313–15.

464. Wilcox LR, Van Surksum R (1991) Endodontic retreatment in large and small straight canals. *Journal of Endodontics* **17**, 119–21.

465. Wilcox LR (1993) Thermafil retreatment with and without chloroform solvent. *Journal of Endodontics* **19**, 563–6.

466. Wilcox LR, Juhlin JJ (1994) Endodontic retreatment of Thermafil versus laterally condensed gutta-percha. *Journal of Endodontics* **20**, 115–17.

467. Wilcox LR (1995) Endodontic retreatment with halothane versus chloroform solvent. *Journal of Endodontics* **21**, 305–7.

468. Will R (1974) Reimplantation – a form of therapy. *Quintessence International* **5**, 13–17.

469. Witherspoon DE, Gutmann JL (2000) Analysis of the healing response to gutta-percha and Diaket when used as root-end filling materials in periradicular surgery. *International Endodontic Journal* **33**, 37–45.

470. Wong SW, Rosenberg PA, Boylan RJ, Schulman A (1994) A comparison of the apical seal achieved using retrograde amalgam fillings and the Nd:YAG laser. *Journal of Endodontics* **20**, 595–7.

471. Wuchenich G, Meadows D, Torabinejad M (1994) A comparison between two root end preparation techniques in human cadavers. *Journal of Endodontics* **20**, 279–82.

472. Yared GM, Dagher FE (1994) Influence of apical enlargement on bacterial infection during treatment of apical periodontitis. *Journal of Endodontics* **20**, 535–7.

473. Yoshikawa G, Murashima Y, Wadachi R, Sawada N, Suda H (2002) Guided bone regeneration (GBR) using membranes and calcium sulphate after apicectomy: a comparative histomorphometrical study. *International Endodontic Journal* **35**, 255–64.

474. Yusuf H (1982) The significance of the presence of foreign material periapically as a cause of failure of root treatment. *Oral Surgery, Oral Medicine, Oral Pathology* **54**, 566–74.

475. Zakariasen KL, Scott DA, Jensen JR (1984) Endodontic recall radiographs: how reliable is our interpretation of endodontic success or failure and what factors affect our reliability? *Oral Surgery, Oral Medicine, Oral Pathology* **57**, 343–7.

476. Zeldow B, Ingle JI (1963) Correlation of the positive culture to the prognosis of endodontically treated teeth: a clinical study. *Journal of the American Dental Association* **66**, 23–7.

477. Zerella JA, Fouad AF, Spångberg LS (2005) Effectiveness of a calcium hydroxide and chlorhexidine digluconate mixture as disinfectant during retreatment of failed endodontic cases. *Oral Surgery, Oral Medicine, Oral Pathology, Oral Radiology and Endodontics* **100**, 756–61.

478. Zetterqvist L, Hall G, Holmlund A (1991) Apicectomy: a comparative clinical study of amalgam and glass ionomer cement as apical sealants. *Oral Surgery, Oral Medicine, Oral Pathology* **71**, 489–91.

479. Zuolo ML, Ferreira MO, Gutmann JL (2000) Prognosis in periradicular surgery: a clinical prospective study. *International Endodontic Journal* **33**, 91–8.

Index